Advanced Researches in Diabetes

Advanced Researches in Diabetes

Edited by **Rex Slavin**

hayle medical

New York

Published by Hayle Medical,
30 West, 37th Street, Suite 612,
New York, NY 10018, USA
www.haylemedical.com

Advanced Researches in Diabetes
Edited by Rex Slavin

International Standard Book Number: 978-1-63241-398-7 (Hardback)

Printed in the United States of America.

Contents

Preface

Diabetes is a common disease as it has affected a large number of people around the globe. It is a pancreatic disease in which the secretion of insulin gets lowered due to improper functioning of the organ. Type1 and type2 diabetes are more prevalent forms of diabetes although there is a third form present called gestational diabetes, primarily affecting pregnant women. There are many medicines present to regulate the blood sugar levels but the cure is yet to be found. The ever growing need for advanced medicines and treatments that could provide a complete cure for this disease is the reason that has fueled the research in this field. From theories to research to practical applications, case studies related to all contemporary topics of relevance to this area have been included in this book. It is a vital tool for all researching and studying this field.

The researches compiled throughout the book are authentic and of high quality, combining several disciplines and from very diverse regions from around the world. Drawing on the contributions of many researchers from diverse countries, the book's objective is to provide the readers with the latest achievements in the area of research. This book will surely be a source of knowledge to all interested and researching the field.

In the end, I would like to express my deep sense of gratitude to all the authors for meeting the set deadlines in completing and submitting their research chapters. I would also like to thank the publisher for the support offered to us throughout the course of the book. Finally, I extend my sincere thanks to my family for being a constant source of inspiration and encouragement.

Editor

1

Transgenerational Glucose Intolerance of Tumor Necrosis Factor with Epigenetic Alteration in Rat Perirenal Adipose Tissue Induced by Intrauterine Hyperglycemia

Rina Su, Jie Yan, and Huixia Yang

Department of Obstetrics and Gynecology, Peking University First Hospital, No. 8, Xishiku Street, Xicheng District, Beijing 100034, China

Correspondence should be addressed to Huixia Yang; yanghuixia@bjmu.edu.cn

Academic Editor: Kimber Stanhope

Changes in DNA methylation may play a role in the genetic mechanism underlying glucose intolerance in the offspring of mothers with diabetes. Here, we established a rat model of moderate intrauterine hyperglycemia induced by streptozotocin to detect glucose and lipid metabolism of first-generation (F1) and second-generation (F2) offspring. Moderate intrauterine hyperglycemia induced high body weight in F1 and F2 offspring of diabetic mothers. F1 offspring had impaired glucose tolerance and abnormal insulin level. Additionally, F1 and F2 offspring that were exposed to intrauterine hyperglycemia had impaired insulin secretion from the islets. The tumor necrosis factor (*Tnf*) gene was upregulated in perirenal adipose tissue from F1 offspring and relatively increased in F2 offspring. Both F1 and F2 offspring showed similar hypomethylation level at the −1952 site of *Tnf*. We confirmed that DNA methylation occurs in offspring exposed to intrauterine hyperglycemia and that the DNA methylation is intergenerational and inherited.

1. Introduction

Gestational diabetes mellitus (GDM) is characterized by intrauterine hyperglycemia and has been reported to affect 17.5% of pregnant women in China [1]. GDM is associated with health issues in offspring. The offspring of mothers with GDM have been shown to have higher birth weights and are reportedly prone to obesity, hypertension, and dyslipidemia compared to offspring of mothers without diabetes [2, 3]. It has been suggested that, apart from genetic influences, the intrauterine environment may also influence the phenotype of the offspring.

"Programming" refers to the process by which a stimulus at a critical window of development has long-term effects. Numerous studies have investigated the effects of adverse intrauterine environment and found that it is correlated with poor fetal growth and increased risk of type 2 diabetes and obesity in adulthood [4]. Some studies have shown that obesity and type 2 diabetes are a global metabolic disorder and systemic inflammation, and the intersection of these phenomena is especially evident in visceral adipose tissue [5, 6]. Nevertheless, the potential mechanism of glucose intolerance induced by intrauterine hyperglycemia remains to be fully understood, and it is yet unknown whether inflammation is related to metabolic disturbances in offspring exposed to intrauterine hyperglycemia.

It has been suggested that epigenetic mechanisms may be the link between environmental and nutritional factors and regulation of gene expression. DNA methylation is one of the major epigenetic modifications. We hypothesized that changes in DNA methylation could participate in the expression of genes related to glucose intolerance in offspring. Furthermore, DNA methylation might also determine the transgenerational disease transmission.

In this study, we established a rat model of streptozotocin-(STZ-) induced moderate intrauterine hyperglycemia. F1 female rats were fed either normal diet or high-fat diets after weaning. The F1 adult female rats obtained from the control and diabetic rats were mated with control male rats, and the phenotypes of F2 female offspring were characterized to study transgenerational influences. Furthermore, we analyzed the methylation status in perirenal adipose tissue to investigate whether intrauterine hyperglycemia affected gene expression of inflammatory cytokines by regulating epigenetic modification.

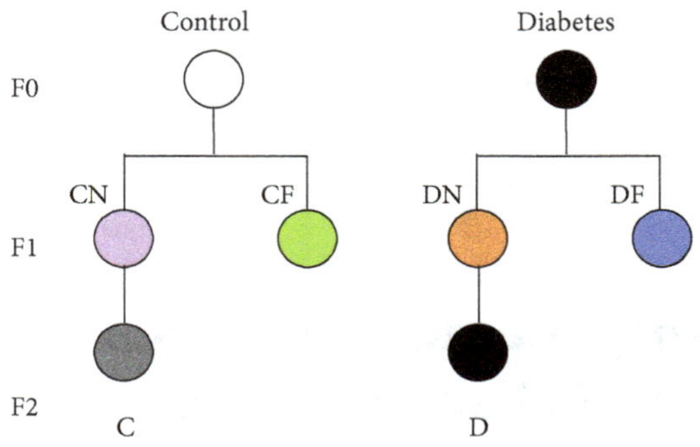

FIGURE 1: GDM rat model with moderate hyperglycemia induced by streptozotocin. Study design: female offspring were fed either normal or high-fat diets after weaning: control groups were fed normal diet (F1-CN) or high-fat diet (F1-CF) and rats in the diabetic group were fed normal diet (F1-DN) or high-fat diet (F1-DF). Adult females of the F1-CN and F1-DN groups were mated with control males to obtain F2 female offspring (F2-C and F2-D). Purple denotes the F1-CN group; green, F1-DN; orange, F1-CF; blue, F1-DF; and grey, F2-C group; and the plain circle denotes the F2-D group.

2. Materials and Methods

2.1. Animals and Tissue Isolation. Twenty-one Wistar rats were used in this study. All the rats were fed in the specific-pathogen-free (SPF) grade animal test room with stable room temperature and humidity. The rats were housed in a 12 : 12 light : dark cycle. All animal protocols were reviewed and approved by the Institutional Animal Care and Use Committee of Peking University First Hospital (J201010). At 12 weeks, female Wistar rats (Vital River Laboratory Animal Technology Co., Ltd., Beijing, China) were mated with male rats. Onset of pregnancy was determined by the presence of a vaginal plug after overnight mating (designated as day 0 [D0] of pregnancy). After the rats were made to fast for a 12 h period, the female rats were randomly divided into two groups: intrauterine hyperglycemia group (F0-D), in which fourteen rats were injected with a single intraperitoneal injection of 25 mg/kg STZ (Sigma) in citrate buffer (pH 4.4) on D0.5, and control group (F0-C), in which the seven pregnant rats received an equal volume of citrate buffer on D0.5. On D4 of pregnancy and every three days thereafter, the blood glucose concentration was measured via the tail vein to check for diabetes. The pregnant rats were allowed to deliver spontaneously. Female offspring were studied and fed either a normal diet (12% kcal fat, 24% kcal protein, and 64% kcal carbohydrates; Beijing KeAoXieLi Feeds Co., Ltd., Beijing, China) or a high-fat diet (45% kcal fat, 20% kcal protein, and 45% kcal carbohydrates; Beijing KeAoXieLi Feeds Co., Ltd., Beijing, China) after weaning: the control group rats were fed a normal diet (F1-CN, $n = 9$) or high-fat diet (F1-CF, $n = 9$), and the diabetic group rats were fed a normal diet (F1-DN, $n = 9$) or high-fat diet (F1-DF, $n = 9$). The F1-CN and F1-DN female adult rats were then mated with control male rats. The phenotypes of F2 female offspring were characterized. F2 female offspring were divided into F2-C and F2-D groups (Figure 1). The F1 and F2 offspring were sacrificed at 28 weeks. Blood from the abdominal aorta was obtained and centrifuged at 3,000 ×g for 10 min to separate the serum and stored at −80°C until analysis. The heart, liver, pancreas, kidney, and fat pads (including mesenteric, perirenal, and ovarian fat) were carefully dissected and weighed. Perirenal adipose tissues were dissected from visible blood vessels and immediately frozen in liquid nitrogen, and the perirenal adipose tissue samples were stored at −80°C before further processing.

2.2. Oral Glucose Tolerance Test. F1 rats from all the four F1 groups (F1-CN, F1-DN, F1-CF, and F1-DF) were fasted overnight and given 2 g/kg glucose by gavage for the oral glucose tolerance test (OGTT) conducted at 16, 20, and 24 weeks. Blood samples were collected from the tail vein before ($t = 0$) and at 30, 60, and 120 min of glucose administration.

2.3. Biochemical Test and Analysis. The fasting insulin (FINS) levels were measured in the F1-CN, F1-DN, F2-C, and F2-D groups by enzyme-linked immunosorbent assay (ELISA) at 28 weeks (rat insulin ELISA kit, Cayman Chemical, 589501, USA), according to the manufacturer's instructions. The total triglyceride (TG) and high-density lipoprotein (HDL) levels in the F1-CN, F1-DN, F2-C, and F2-D groups were detected in a fully automatic biochemical analyzer at 28 weeks. The reagents used in the assays were provided by Beijing BHKT Clinical Reagent Co., Ltd., China.

2.4. Histology and Morphometric Analysis. Morphological evaluation was carried out as follows: briefly, pancreases were dissected rapidly, cleaned of connective tissue, weighed, and fixed in 4% paraformaldehyde solution for 48 h. The pancreases were then embedded in wax and serially sliced to obtain 5 μm wide histological sections. The sections were stained with hematoxylin and eosin and then the morphological features were analyzed under a microscope. The areas and diameters of pancreatic islets were measured using Image-Pro Plus 6.0 (Media Cybernetics). Ten different fields were analyzed per rat, and six rats in each of the F1-CN, F1-DN, F2-C, and F2-D groups were analyzed.

2.5. Immunohistochemistry of Pancreatic Islets. Immunolocalization was performed for anti-insulin reaction on 5 μm thick sections, and the sections were subsequently stained with streptavidin biotin peroxidase. Paraffin sections were deparaffinized in xylene and rehydrated in descending grades of alcohol followed by heat-induced epitope retrieval. Endogenous peroxidase and nonspecific antibody binding sites were suppressed by treating the sections with 0.3% hydrogen peroxide for 10 min at room temperature.

The sections were then washed in phosphate-buffered saline and incubated for 1 h with primary antibodies for rat insulin (ZSGB-BIO, Beijing, China). The sections were washed again with phosphate-buffered saline and incubated with biotinylated secondary antibody (PV6000, ZSGB-BIO, Beijing, China) for 40 min. Finally, the nuclei were stained using hematoxylin and eosin and mounted in 3,3′-diaminobenzidine (DAB). Antibody binding was evaluated by high-power light microscopy (cellSens, Olympus DP72, Japan). The pancreatic islet area and fluorescence intensity were measured using Image-Pro Plus 6.0 (Media Cybernetics). Ten different fields were analyzed per rat, and six rats per group were analyzed.

2.6. MeDIP Array. A purified genomic DNA pool was prepared from three perirenal adipose tissue samples from the F1-CN and F1-DN groups and digested overnight with *Mse*I restriction enzyme (NEB, R0525S). Denatured DNA was immunoprecipitated using monoclonal antibodies against 5-methyl cytidine (Abcam, Ab10805). Immunoprecipitated DNA was recovered with proteinase K digestion followed by column-based purification, amplified, and hybridized on a Rat DNA Methylation 3 × 720 K CpG Island Plus RefSeq Promoter Array according to the protocol of Roche NimbleGen. Immunoprecipitated (IP) and input DNA samples were labeled with Cy5 and Cy3, respectively. Hybridization was performed using a NimbleGen Hybridization Kit and NimbleGen Hybridization System 12. Scanning was done using high-resolution NimbleGen MS 200 Microarray Scanner. MeDIP array data were analyzed using NimbleScan software, and the array results could be visualized using SignalMap software. Microarray data reported in the paper were deposited to the Gene Expression Omnibus (GEO) at the National Center for Biotechnology Information (NCBI) under the series accession number GSE65779.

2.7. DNA Methylation ChIP Analysis. MeDIP samples from the F1-CN and F1-DN groups were hybridized to Rat DNA Methylation 3 × 720 K CpG Island Plus RefSeq Promoter Array representing 15,287 putative promoters (−3.88 kb to +0.97 kb to the transcription start site (TSS)) and 15,790 CpG islands. Chromatin immunoprecipitation (ChIP) analysis was carried out by CapitalBio Corporation (Beijing, China). We identified 923 and 2150 promoters as significantly hypermethylated and significantly hypomethylated, respectively. The biological significance of the microarray data was analyzed by the Molecular Annotation System (CB-MAS, CapitalBio Corporation, Beijing, China, http://bioinfo.capitalbio.com/mas3/).

2.8. DNA Methylation Analysis Using Bisulfite Sequencing. Genomic DNA of three perirenal adipose tissue samples from the F1-CN, F1-DN, F2-C, and F2-D groups was treated and purified with the EpiTect bisulfite kit (Qiagen), according to the manufacturer's instructions. The methylation status was evaluated by cloning and sequencing the bisulfite-treated DNA. The following primers were used to amplify region −2012 to −1829 of the *Tnf* promoter: sense 5′-GGT TTT TTT TGG AGA AAG TTG TTT-3′, antisense 5′-AAA AAC ACA ACC CCC TAA TAC ATT A-3′. The following primers were used to amplify region −220 to +26 of the *Tnf* promoter: sense 5′-TTT TGA TGT TTG GGT GTT TTT AAT T-3′, antisense 5′-TTC TCC CTC CTA ACT AAT CCC TTA A-3′. The purified PCR products were cloned using a pEASY-T1 Simple Cloning Vector system (TransGen Biotech, Beijing, China), and ten individual clones in each sample were sequenced. A total of three samples were evaluated in each group. The sequence obtained by cloning was analyzed at Beijing General GeneTest Co., Ltd. (Beijing, China).

2.9. Nucleic Acid Purification and Real-Time PCR. For RNA extraction, perirenal adipose tissues from the F1-CN, F1-DN, F2-C, and F2-D groups were homogenized in 1 mL of TRIzol reagent and RNA was purified according to the manufacturer's recommendations. The RNA was used as a template for synthesis of the same amount of cDNA (2 μg) using First Strand Synthesis Kit (Applied Biosystems, USA). cDNA quantity was measured using real-time PCR with the ABI PRISM 7500 sequence detection system and fluorescence-based SYBR Green technology. The PCR reaction mixture consisted of 2 μg of diluted cDNA sample, 2x SYBR Green PCR Master Mix (Molecular Probes, USA), primers optimized for each target gene, and nuclease-free water to achieve a final volume of 20 μL. All the samples were analyzed in duplicate. Primers were designed using Primer Express 3.0 software. The following primers were used: *Rplp0*, sense 5′-GGC GAC CTG GAA GTC CAA-3′ and antisense 5′-TCT GCT CCC ACA ATG AAG CA-3′; *Tnf*, sense 5′-TGA TCG GTC CCA ACA AGG A-3′ and antisense 5′-GGG CCA TGG AAC TGA TGA GA-3′; *IL-1β*, sense 5′-CCCAAGCACCTTCTTTTCCTT-3′ and antisense 5′-CGTCATCATCCCACGAGTCA-3′; *IL-6*, sense 5′-ACAGAGGATACCACCCACAACAG-3′ and antisense 5′-TCAGAATTGCCATTGCACAAC-3′; *IL-10*, sense 5′-CAGTCAGCCAGACCCACATG-3′ and antisense 5′-TGTTGTCCAGCTGGTCCTTCT-3′; *IFN-γ*, sense 5′-ATCGAATCGCACCTGATCACT-3′ and antisense 5′-GTGCTGGATCTGTGGGTTGTT-3′.

2.10. Western Blot Analysis. Perirenal adipose biopsies from the F1-CN, F1-DN, F2-C, and F2-D groups were homogenized in RIPA lysis buffer (KeyGen Biotech, KGP702, Nanjing, China) and 1 mM phenylmethylsulfonyl fluoride (PMSF; Amresco, M221, USA). The protein content was determined using a bicinchoninic acid (BCA) protein assay kit from KeyGen Biotech (Nanjing, China). Protein samples were placed at equal concentrations on polyacrylamide gel and separated using 12% sodium dodecyl sulfate-polyacrylamide gel electrophoresis (SDS-PAGE). Proteins were transferred to polyvinylidene difluoride (PVDF) membranes (Applygen, P2110, Beijing, China) and subjected to Western blot analysis. After incubation with primary antibodies (Cell Signaling Technology, 11948S, USA) overnight, the PVDF membranes were washed and incubated with horseradish peroxidase-conjugated secondary antibodies (ZSGB-BIO, Beijing, China) for 1 h at room temperature. The results were

Table 1: Body weight (grams) of F1 and F2 females.

	N	Birth	3 weeks	7 weeks	11 weeks	15 weeks	19 weeks	23 weeks	28 weeks
F1-CN	8	6.26 ± 0.13	37.51 ± 1.25	171.88 ± 4.73	242.00 ± 7.70	259.38 ± 7.52	284.25 ± 10.70	301.13 ± 11.02	309.50 ± 12.84
F1-DN	9	6.90 ± 0.14^a	41.93 ± 4.08	179.11 ± 7.86	255.56 ± 9.29	284.33 ± 8.57^a	305.44 ± 8.92	318.22 ± 10.11	325.44 ± 10.91
F1-CF	8	6.37 ± 0.08	38.01 ± 1.68	169.38 ± 4.38	248.63 ± 6.70	281.50 ± 8.20^a	311.50 ± 11.34	328.38 ± 14.23	332.57 ± 15.16
F1-DF	8	7.04 ± 0.09^b	42.56 ± 1.91	179.50 ± 4.32	259.50 ± 7.08	292.50 ± 9.43	306.86 ± 10.07	317.43 ± 14.78	318.86 ± 14.85
F2-C	6	7.2 ± 0.4	57.62 ± 1.49	187 ± 3.96	248.66 ± 6.11	274.17 ± 3.7	286.5 ± 7.53	288.66 ± 9.61	300.17 ± 6.63
F2-D	6	7.1 ± 0.8	56.80 ± 1.94	198.83 ± 6.69	256.66 ± 9.59	284 ± 9.08	299.17 ± 6.62	310.83 ± 5.64*	322.33 ± 6.65*

Data are means ± SEM. Significance was determined by ANOVA. $^a p < 0.05$ versus F1-CN, $^b p < 0.05$ versus F1-CF, and $^* p < 0.05$ versus F2-C.

Table 2: Body composition (grams) of F1 and F2 females at 28 weeks.

	N	Mesenteric adipose tissue weight (g)	Perirenal adipose tissue weight (g)	Ovarian adipose tissue weight (g)	Visceral adipose tissue weight (g)	Pancreas weight (g)	Liver weight (g)	Heart weight (g)	Kidney weight (g)
F1-CN	8	4.34 ± 0.79	3.79 ± 0.89	7.69 ± 1.42	15.82 ± 3.03	1.97 ± 0.06	7.68 ± 0.21	0.92 ± 0.04	1.98 ± 0.06
F1-DN	7	3.78 ± 0.44	4.21 ± 0.42	9.57 ± 0.96	17.56 ± 1.72	1.96 ± 0.08	7.67 ± 0.46	0.89 ± 0.04	1.96 ± 0.08
F1-CF	7	5.34 ± 1.18	6.93 ± 1.96	11.88 ± 2.10	24.16 ± 4.99	1.90 ± 0.10	7.13 ± 0.47	0.90 ± 0.05	1.90 ± 0.10
F1-DF	4	3.9 ± 1.01	4.28 ± 0.92	8.87 ± 1.92	17.05 ± 3.81	1.98 ± 0.06	8.49 ± 0.64	0.77 ± 0.03	1.98 ± 0.06
F2-C	8	3.87 ± 0.43	3.56 ± 0.30	9.95 ± 0.44	17.37 ± 0.75	0.91 ± 0.09	9.31 ± 0.33	0.91 ± 0.03	2.38 ± 0.05
F2-D	8	4.18 ± 0.63	4.49 ± 0.27*	8.88 ± 0.69	17.89 ± 1.46	0.89 ± 0.07	8.68 ± 0.44	0.89 ± 0.02	2.11 ± 0.34

Data are means ± SEM. Significance was determined by ANOVA. $^* p < 0.05$ versus F2-C.

quantified by densitometry using AlphaEaseFC FluorChem SA software for Windows (Alpha Innotech Corporation, California, USA).

2.11. Statistics. One-way ANOVA was used to determine the comparisons among the four groups. Post hoc comparisons using Tukey's test were performed when a significant F-score was detected. Comparisons between two groups were performed using two-tailed unpaired Student's t-test. All the values are presented as mean ± SEM. Statistically significant differences were defined at $p < 0.05$.

3. Results

3.1. Moderate Intrauterine Hyperglycemia Induced High Body Weight in F1 Females. As previously described [7], we established a moderate intrauterine hyperglycemia rat model by injecting Wistar rats with a single intraperitoneal injection of streptozotocin (STZ). The average glucose level of diabetic mothers during pregnancy was 11.2–15.0 mmol/L. Further morphological studies of the pancreas samples confirmed that rats with GDM had smaller pancreatic islets than rats without GDM.

The birth weight was significantly higher in the F1-DN group than in the F1-CN group (Table 1). The body weight was also significantly higher in the F1-DN group than in the F1-CN group at 15 weeks (Table 1). Furthermore, intrauterine hyperglycemia was found to induce adipopexis in F1 offspring, and the perirenal adipose tissue, ovarian adipose tissue, and whole visceral adipose tissue weighed more in the F1-DN group than in the F1-CN group; however, the tissue weights did not significantly differ between the two groups (Table 2). The pancreas, liver, heart, and kidney weights also showed no significant differences between the F1-DN and F1-CN groups (Table 2).

The body weight was higher in the F1-CF group than in the F1-CN group at 15 weeks (Table 1). The high-fat diet did not further exacerbate the effect of intrauterine hyperglycemia exposure on body weight (F1-DF versus F1-DN, Table 1).

The weights of perirenal adipose tissue and whole visceral adipose tissue were higher in the F1-CF group than in the F1-CN group with borderline significance ($p = 0.065$ and $p = 0.094$, resp.). There were no significant differences in the weights of the pancreas, liver, heart, and kidney in each group (Table 2).

3.2. Moderate Intrauterine Hyperglycemia Induced Glucose Intolerance and Abnormal Insulin and Lipid Levels in F1 Females. At birth, there was no significant difference in the blood glucose level between the F1-CN and F1-DN groups (Figure 2(a)). The fasting glucose levels were monitored in the F1 rats at 16, 20, 24, and 28 weeks. The fasting glucose level was higher in the F1-DN group than in the F1-CN group at 20 weeks (Figure 2(b)). The fasting glucose level was also elevated in the F1-DF group compared to that in the F1-CF group at 24 and 28 weeks (Figure 2(b)). Results of the GTT revealed impaired glucose tolerance (IGT) in the F1-DN group at 20 weeks. In this group, the blood glucose level had significantly increased at 0, 30, 60, and 120 min after glucose load, and the AUC was significantly higher in the F1-DN group than in the F1-CN group (Figures 3(b) and 3(e)). The GTT revealed IGT at 30 and 120 min in the F1-DN group at

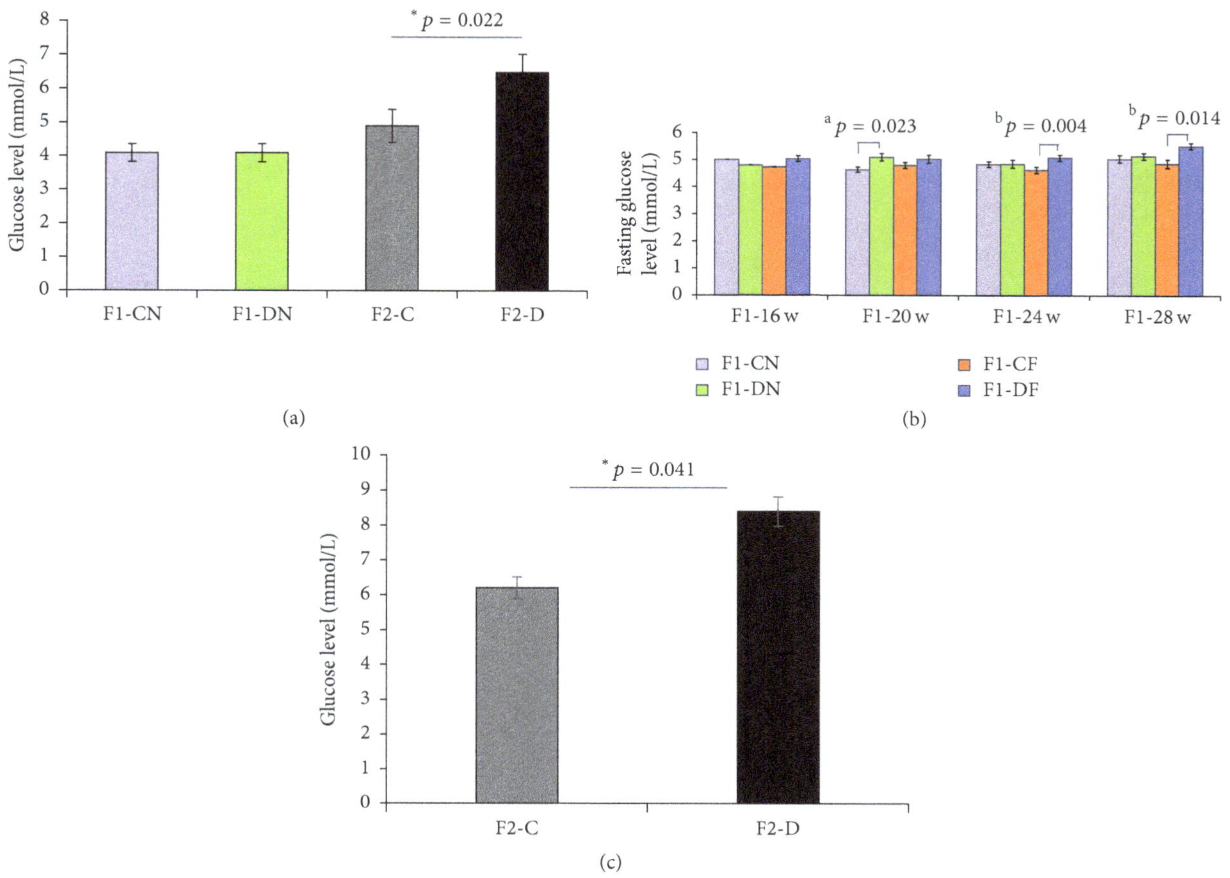

FIGURE 2: Glucose levels in F1 and F2 offspring. (a) The F2 offspring in the F2-D group have a higher glucose level at birth. (b) Rats in the F1-DN group have a higher fasting glucose level at 20 weeks, and rats in the F1-DF group have a higher fasting glucose level at 24 and 28 weeks than rats in the F1-CF group. (c) Rats in the F2-D group have a higher glucose level at 28 weeks. The results are means ± SEM, $N = 8\text{-}9$; $^{a}p < 0.05$ versus F1-CN; $^{b}p < 0.05$ versus F1-CF; $^{*}p < 0.05$ versus F2-C.

24 weeks, and there were no differences in the AUC between the F1-DN and F1-CN groups at 24 weeks (Figures 3(c) and 3(f)). The GTT revealed no difference in the glucose tolerance at 16 weeks (Figures 3(a) and 3(d)).

The high-fat diet also induced glucose intolerance. The blood glucose level significantly increased at 60 min after glucose load at 16 weeks, at 60 and 120 min at 20 weeks, and at 30 min at 24 weeks in the F1-CF group compared to the F1-CN group (Figures 3(a)–3(c)). The high-fat diet could exacerbate glucose intolerance of offspring exposed to intrauterine hyperglycemia, as evidenced by the blood glucose level, which was significantly increased at 30 min after glucose load at both 16 and 24 weeks in the F1-DF group compared to the F1-DN group, and the AUC was significantly increased at 24 weeks (Figures 3(a), 3(c), and 3(f)). Moreover, IGT was found in the F1-DF group compared to the F1-CF group, and the blood glucose level of the former group significantly increased at 30 min at 16 weeks; 30 min at 20 weeks; and 0, 30, and 60 min at 24 weeks. Furthermore, the AUC was significantly higher at 20 and 24 weeks (Figures 3(a), 3(b), 3(c), 3(e), and 3(f)).

The FINS, triglyceride, and HDL levels in the F1 rats were monitored at 28 weeks (Figures 4(a)–4(c)). The FINS and HDL levels were significantly decreased in the F1-DN group compared to the F1-CN group (Figures 4(a) and 4(c)).

3.3. Moderate Intrauterine Hyperglycemia Induced High Body Weight and Hyperglycemia in F2 Females. The birth weights of F2 females were similar between the diabetes and control groups, and body weight increased in the F2-D group compared to the controls at 23 and 28 weeks (Table 1). In addition, the blood glucose levels at birth and at 28 weeks were significantly increased in the F2-D group compared to those in the F2-C group (Figures 2(a) and 2(c)). Moreover, the weight of perirenal adipose tissue was significantly higher in the F2-D than that in the F2-C group, whereas the weights of the pancreas, liver, heart, and kidney did not significantly differ between the two groups (Table 2). In addition, the FINS, TG, and HDL levels were similar between the two F2 groups (Figures 4(a)–4(c)).

3.4. Moderate Intrauterine Hyperglycemia Induced Transgenerational Effects on Islet Structure and Impaired Insulin

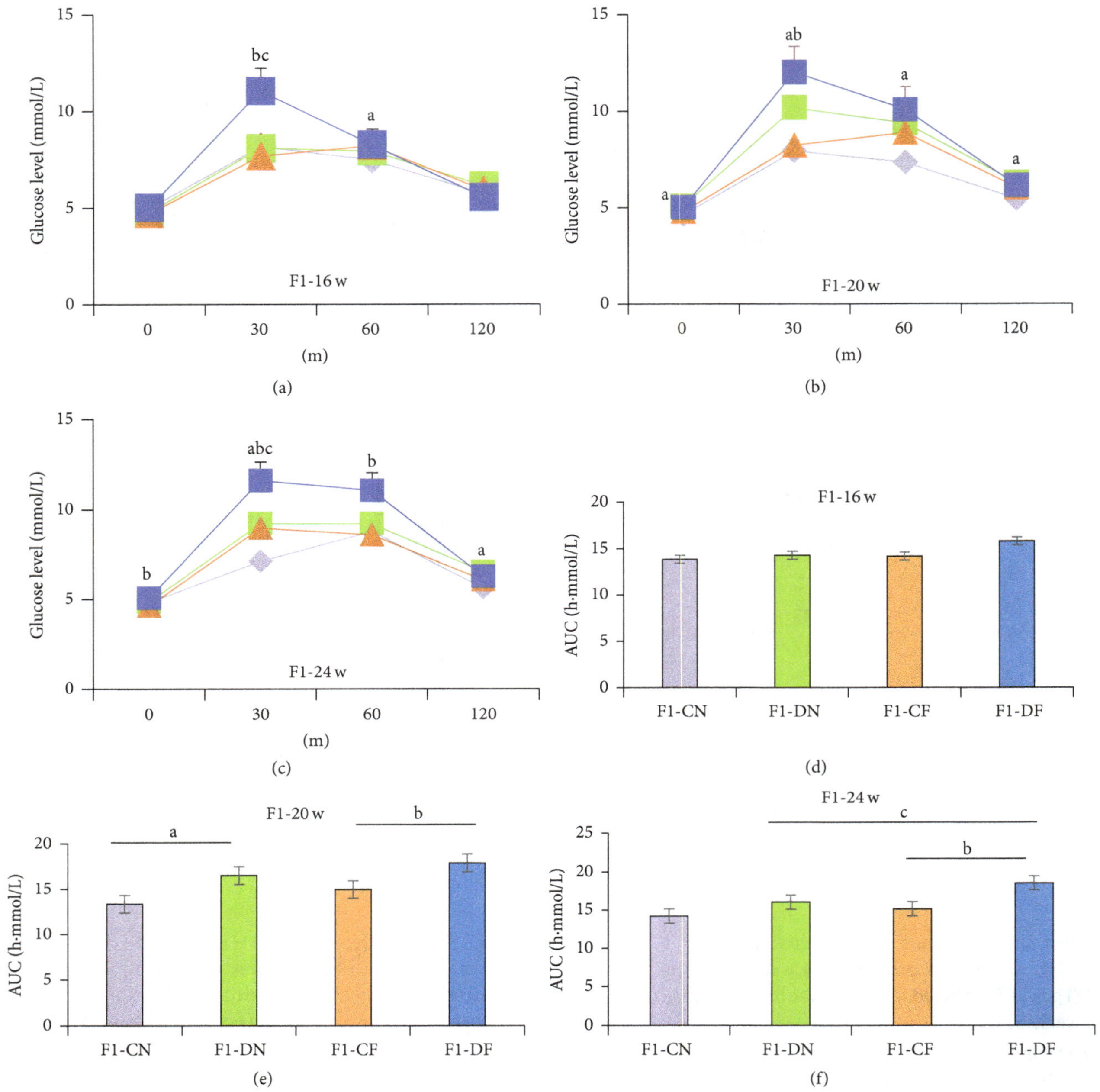

FIGURE 3: Glucose tolerance test. (a–c) Glucose tolerance test (GTT) was performed at 16, 20, and 24 weeks using 2 g glucose/kg body weight given by gavage. (d–f) AUC was performed at 16, 20, and 24 weeks. The results are presented as means ± SEM, $N = 8\text{-}9$; $^{a}p < 0.05$ versus F1-CN; $^{b}p < 0.05$ versus F1-CF; $^{c}p < 0.05$ versus F1-DN.

Secretion. A morphological study of the pancreas samples confirmed that the F1-DN group had obviously smaller pancreatic islets and atrophied β-cell mass compared to the F1-CN group (Figures 5(a) and 5(b)). Pancreatic islets in the F2-D group were similar to those in the control group (Figures 5(a) and 5(b)). To further define the potential secretory defects that may be related to the abnormal structure of islets in offspring exposed to intrauterine hyperglycemia, pancreatic islets were immunohistochemically analyzed. The level of insulin-positive cells in the islets was borderline significantly reduced in F1-DN group compared to F1-CN group (Figures 5(c) and 5(d)); interestingly, the level of insulin-positive cell area of islets was borderline significantly increased in F2-D group compared to that in F2-C group (Figures 5(c) and 5(d)).

3.5. Altered Genome-Wide Methylation Levels in F1 Female Offspring Exposed to Intrauterine Hyperglycemia. We used methylated DNA immunoprecipitation (MeDIP) combined with microarray technology to discover whether changes in DNA methylation are specific to intrauterine hyperglycemia

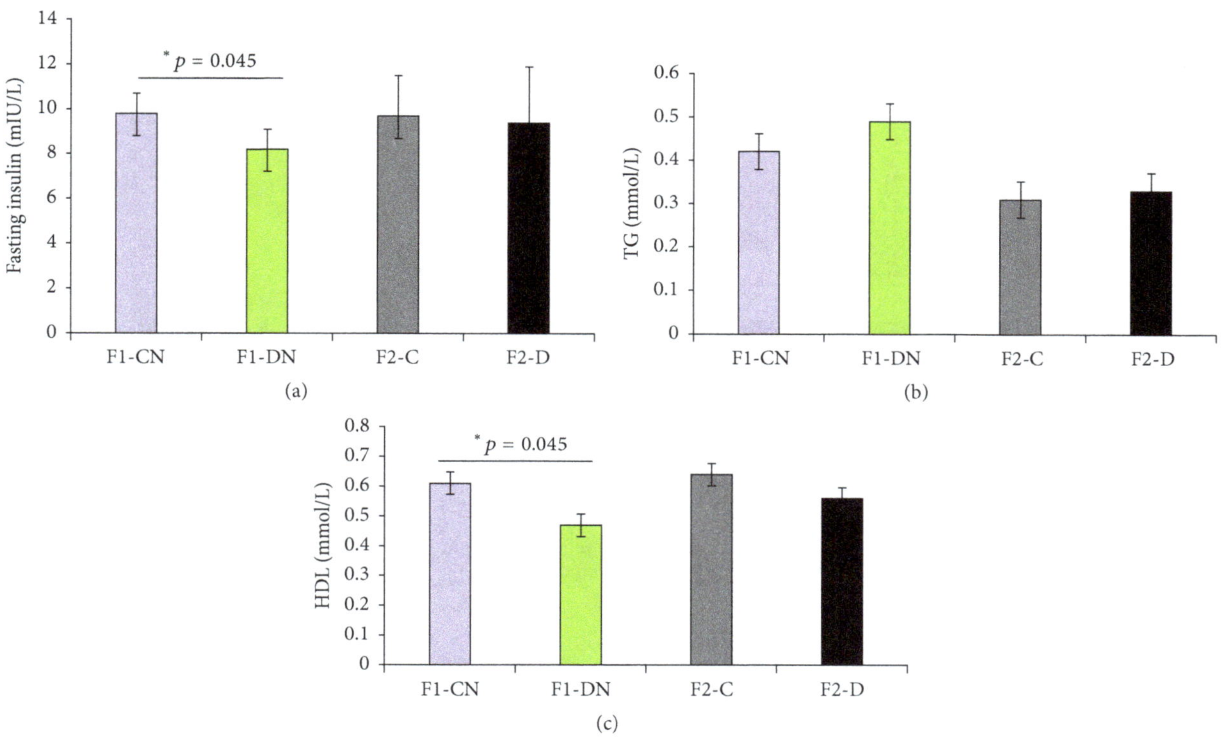

FIGURE 4: Biochemical analysis of F1 and F2 offspring at 28 weeks. (a) Level of fasting insulin in F1 and F2 offspring. (b) TG level in F1 and F2 offspring. (c) HDL level in F1 and F2 offspring. Results are presented as means ± SEM, $N = 6$ per group; $^*p < 0.05$ versus F1-CN.

exposure. We identified differentially methylated genes in the F1-DN group using Rat DNA Methylation 3 × 720 K CpG Island Plus RefSeq Promoter Array representing 15,287 putative promoters (−3.88 kb to +0.97 kb respective to the TSS) and 15,790 CpG islands. A total of 923 and 2150 promoters were significantly hypermethylated and hypomethylated, respectively, compared to the controls in perirenal adipose tissue.

In order to identify groups of genes with similar changes in methylation in perirenal adipose tissue from offspring in the F1-DN and F1-CN groups, we defined the biological processes of the identified genes using a molecular annotation system. Genes were ranked by the level of significance (p values) according to the difference in methylation (Figure 6, Tables S1 and S2 in Supplementary Material available online at http://dx.doi.org/10.1155/2016/4952801). It is noteworthy that some genes associated with adipocytokine signaling pathway were significantly hypomethylated, including *Camkk2*, *Pck1*, *Rxrb*, *Adipoq*, *Tnf*, *Prkag3*, *Nfkbib*, and *Mapk10*. Moreover, the methylation level of genes related to type II diabetes mellitus was also prominently decreased, including *Prkce*, *Prkcz*, *Adipoq*, *Tnf*, *Slc2a2*, *Prkcd*, and *Mapk10* (Figure S1). As a key gene associated with adipocytokine signaling pathway and diabetes, the *Tnf* promoter was hypomethylated in perirenal adipose tissue from F1-DN group compared to controls ($p < 0.05$).

3.6. Methylation Levels of Tnf Promoter Region in F1 and F2 Offspring. MeDIP data showed that the portion of the *Tnf* promoter region from −2914 to −1717 was hypomethylated. Bisulfite sequencing was used to validate results of MeDIP for *Tnf*. Genomic DNA was extracted from perirenal adipose tissue obtained from F1 and F2 female offspring. Bisulfite sequencing was performed on a portion of the promoter region encompassing −2012 to −1829 relative to the +1 TSS of the *Tnf* gene, including 5 CpG sites (−1952, −1901, −1881, −1866, and −1858). We found a significant decrease in methylation in the −1952 site in the F1-DN group compared to the F1-CN group (Figure 7(a)). Interestingly, the hypomethylation level at the −1952 site was similar in the F2-D and the F1-DN groups (Figure 7(a)).

We further carried out bisulfite sequencing on another portion of the *Tnf* promoter region encompassing −220 to +26 relative to the +1 TSS, which included 8 CpG sites (−178, −138, −91, −89, −66, −35, −20, and −7). The methylation level did not significantly differ between the F1-DN and F1-CN groups, and similar results were obtained for the F2 generation (Figure 7(a)).

3.7. Tnf Methylation May Control the Expression of Tnf. In order to investigate the physiological importance of methylation in gene and protein expression, we measured the *Tnf* gene and protein expression levels using real-time PCR and Western blot analysis, respectively. The *Tnf* gene expression was significantly higher in the F1-DN group than in the F1-CN group ($p < 0.05$), and the *Tnf* gene expression showed an increasing trend in the F2-D group compared to the F2-C

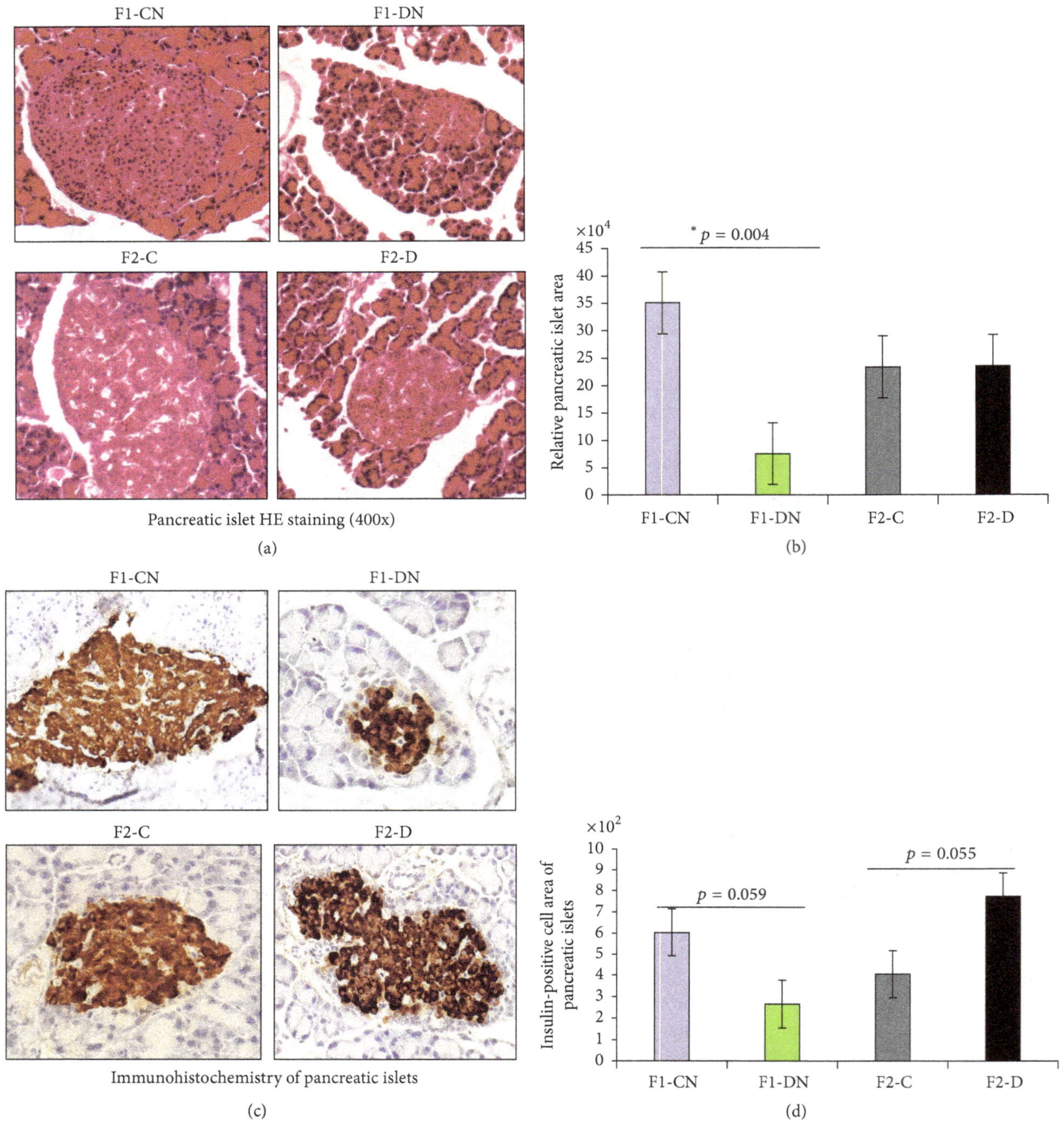

Figure 5: Histology and immunohistochemistry of pancreatic islets. (a) HE staining images (400x) of pancreatic islets obtained from F1 and F2 offspring. (b) The area and diameters of pancreatic islets were measured using Image-Pro Plus 6.0, Media Cybernetics. Ten different fields were analyzed for each rat, with a total of six rats per group. (c) Immunohistochemistry of pancreatic islets. (d) Insulin-positive cell area of pancreatic islets was measured using Image-Pro Plus 6.0. Ten different fields were analyzed for each rat; totally six rats in each group were analyzed. Results are presented as means ± SEM, $N = 6$ per group; $^*p < 0.05$ versus F1-CN.

group, but this difference was not statistically significant ($p = 0.09$; Figure 7(b)). The protein expression did not significantly differ in the F1-DN and F2-D groups compared to the corresponding control groups (Figure 7(c)).

Hypomethylation of the *Tnf* promoter region at −1952 site was negatively correlated with the increased gene expression in diabetic offspring ($r = -0.36$). The transcription factors *Tfap2a*, *Tfap2c*, *Ebf1*, *Egr1*, *Rxra*, *c-Rel*, *RelA*, and *Nfic*

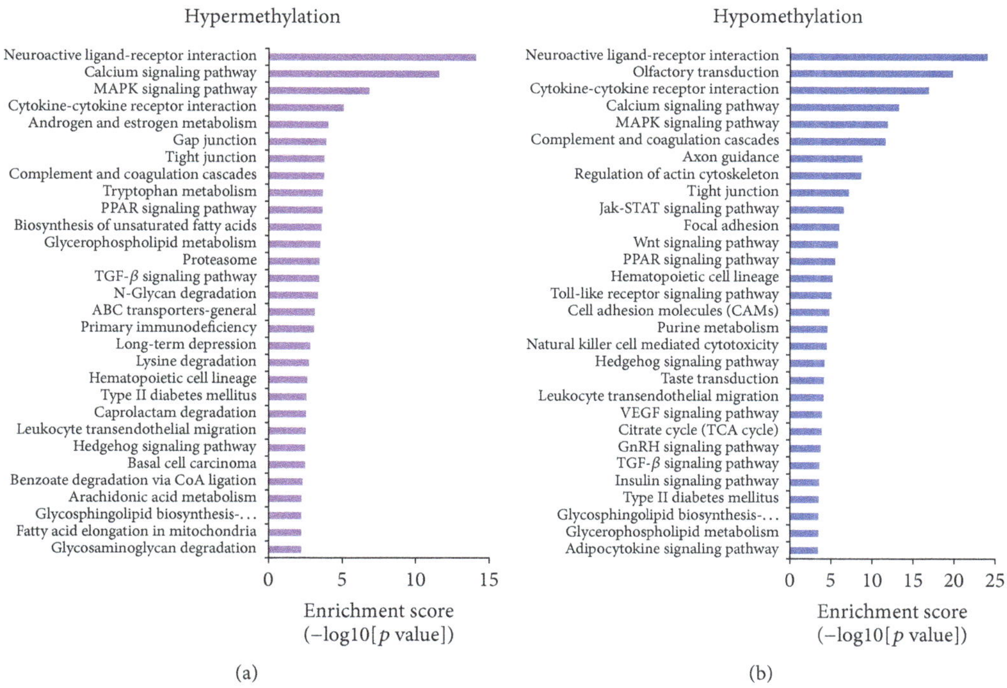

FIGURE 6: The pathways of DNA methylation changes in F1 offspring exposed to intrauterine hyperglycemia. Immunoprecipitated DNA was amplified and hybridized on Rat DNA Methylation 3 × 720 K CpG Island Plus RefSeq Promoter Array according to the Roche NimbleGen protocol. Microarray data was extracted and analyzed by the Molecular Annotation System (CB-MAS, CapitalBio Corporation, Beijing, China, http://bioinfo.capitalbio.com/mas3/).

predicted by the JASPAR database may be involved in the regulation of *Tnf* expression by binding to the specific CpG site in a methylation-sensitive manner.

3.8. Expression of Inflammatory Cytokines in Perirenal Adipose Tissue. Expression of inflammatory cytokines in perirenal adipose tissue was detected, and the expression levels of *IL-1β*, *IL-6*, *IL-10*, and *IFN-γ* did not significantly differ between the F1-DN and F2-D groups compared to controls (Figure 8).

4. Discussion

A GDM rodent model can be established using streptozotocin, which is directly toxic to maternal pancreatic β-cells. A previous study found that small fetuses were delivered following severe intrauterine hyperglycemia induced by a high dose of streptozotocin [8]. Nevertheless, GDM women with moderate hyperglycemia and large babies are more common in the clinical setting. Previous studies have found that administering a low dose of streptozotocin for five consecutive days can also induce moderate intrauterine hyperglycemia [8]. We established a GDM rat model with a single intraperitoneal injection of 25 mg/kg streptozotocin. The resultant moderate glucose level and the large fetus were used to mimic human macrosomia in offspring from mothers with GDM.

The birth weight of F1 offspring was significantly higher in offspring of the GDM group than in the control group; furthermore, the body weight and fat mass were increased in the offspring during adulthood. Although the F1 offspring of mothers in the GDM group had normal blood glucose levels at birth, impaired glucose tolerance and abnormal insulin and HDL levels were displayed in adulthood. The pancreatic islets were smaller in size and disordered and the insulin secretion was affected in F1 offspring of mothers with GDM, indicating that intrauterine hyperglycemia may lead to abnormal structure of fetal islets. The impaired β-cells may be related to the development of IGT.

The birth weights did not significantly differ between F2 offspring of mothers with GDM and controls. Nevertheless, the F2 offspring showed higher body weight and fat mass in adulthood. Furthermore, F2 offspring displayed hyperglycemia at birth and increased insulin secretion from the pancreatic islets in adulthood.

Together, these data contribute to the idea that early-life exposure to hyperglycemia in utero can influence glucose metabolism and induce insulin resistance in offspring up to the F2 generation. In addition, transgenerational offspring will be prone to obesity and hyperlipidemia in adulthood. It is indicated that a certain developmental pattern is programmed in utero. Ding et al. [9] demonstrated that intrauterine hyperglycemia induced IGT and abnormal insulin levels in both F1 and F2 offspring, which are partly due to the deficient islet ultrastructure. Future studies should aim to

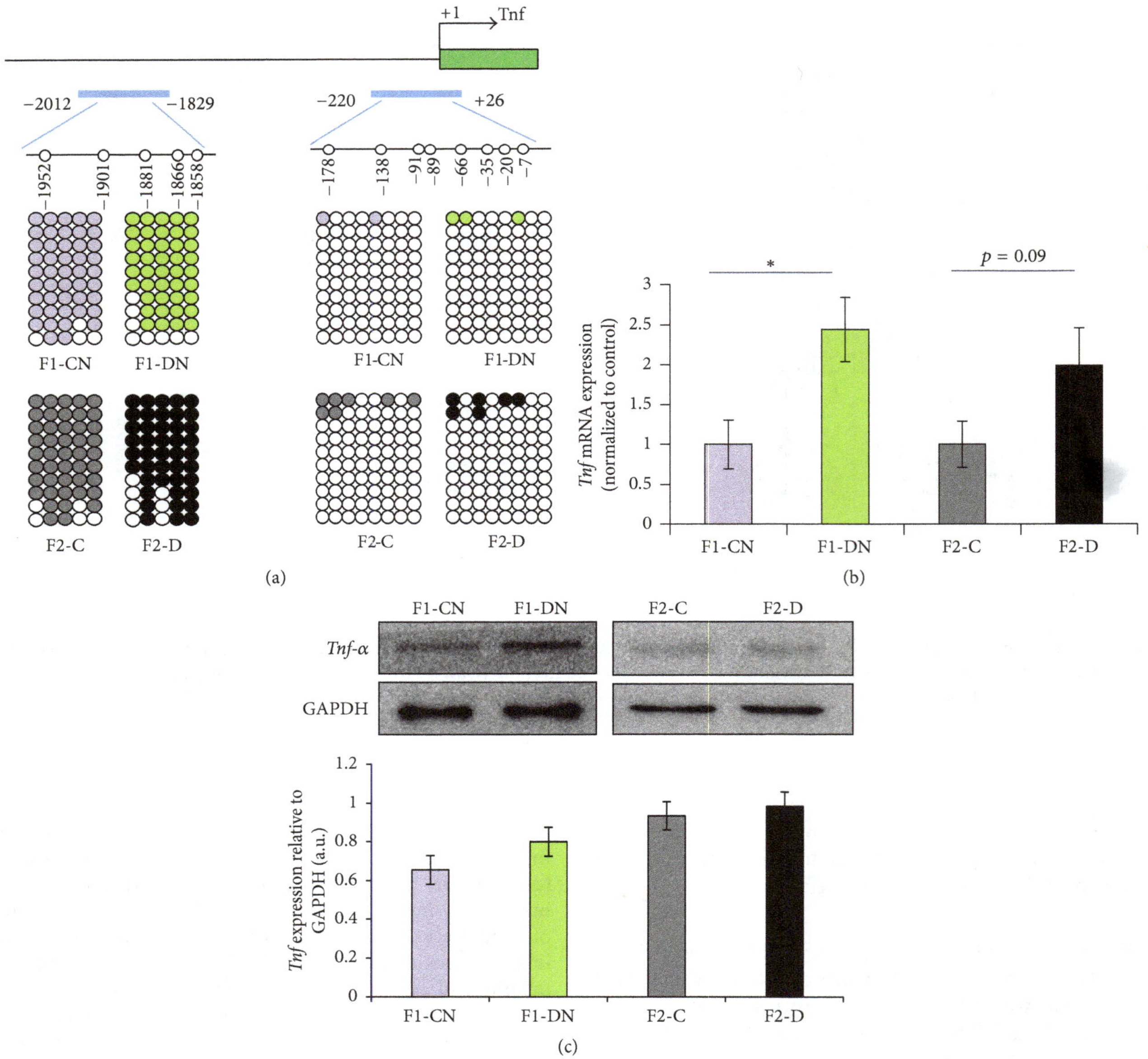

FIGURE 7: Methylation analysis and gene expression of *Tnf*. (a) Bisulfite sequencing was performed on the portion of the promoter regions encompassing −2012 to −1829 relative to the +1 transcription start site of the *Tnf* gene including 5 CpG sites and −220 to +26 including 8 CpG sites. Each line represents the average methylation level of the sequence of all the clones. CpG sites are shown as blank (unmethylated) or filled (methylated) circles ($N = 3$ per group). (b) The expression of *Tnf* was identified using real-time PCR ($N = 8$-9). (c) The protein expression of *Tnf* was identified using Western blotting ($N = 5$ per group). Results are presented as the means ± SEM. $^*p < 0.05$ versus F1-CN. $N = 4$–9.

investigate the potential mechanisms by which environmental factors can influence the expression of genes involved in insulin resistance.

Previous studies have showed that a low-grade inflammation characterized by increased circulating levels of proinflammatory cytokines in adipose tissue, such as *IL-6* and *Tnf*, and chemokines is a common feature of obesity and diabetes [10]. The overexpression of *Tnf* is closely related to insulin resistance, reduced lipoprotein lipase activity, and increased lipase activity. Moreover, *Tnf* is an adipokine involved in systemic inflammation, and inflammatory factors secreted from adipocytes may interfere with the insulin signaling pathway and impair the action of insulin and glucose transport [11–14]. In our study, *Tnf* expression was increased in the F1 generation born from mothers with GDM and relatively increased in F2 offspring. Additionally, chronic inflammation was found in adipose tissue, and the levels of *IL-1β* and *IL-10* tended to increase in both F1 and F2 offspring obtained from F0 mothers with GDM. Transgenerational transmission of inflammatory state may be presented between F1 and

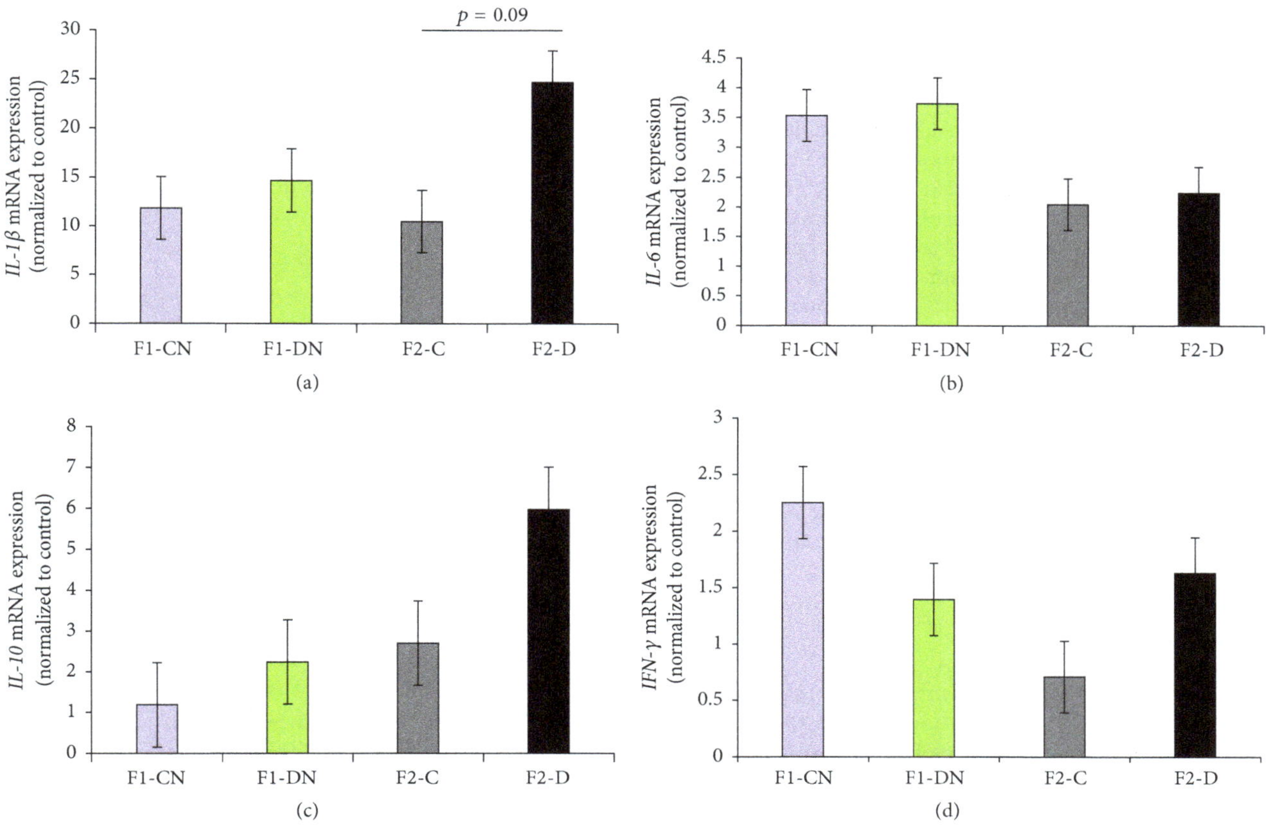

FIGURE 8: Inflammatory cytokines in perirenal adipose tissue. (a) *IL-1β* expression was identified using real-time PCR. (b) *IL-6* expression was identified using real-time PCR. (c) *IL-10* expression was identified using real-time PCR. (d) *IFN-γ* expression was identified using real-time PCR. Results are presented as the means ± SEM. $N = 4$-5.

F2 offspring. Consistent with our study, Ding et al. [15] showed that a feed-forward cycle exists in female mice after continuous high-fat diet stress, as demonstrated by increased adiposity and progressive inflammation in adipose tissue across generations.

Epigenetic mechanisms have been cited as a possible link between environmental and nutritional factors and the regulation of gene expression. DNA methylation is a major epigenetic modification. Evidence suggests that gene expression can be regulated by DNA methylation in diabetic patients, and the differential methylation may be responsible for the progression of type 2 diabetes [16]. Environmental events and nutritional conditions during early pregnancy may induce permanent DNA methylation changes in the fetus in utero. These studies emphasized the effect of early intrauterine exposure on epigenetic changes, which may be "memorized" and last throughout the lifetime of the offspring. Additionally, these epigenetic changes could also be transmitted to the F2 generation and show transgenerational effects [17, 18]. Nevertheless, most studies in this area have only focused on restricted intrauterine nutrition and reported the epigenetic modifications in intrauterine growth restriction (IUGR) models [19–21]. Our study is the first to provide further evidence of intrauterine exposure to excess nutrition.

We identified specific changes in DNA methylation induced by intrauterine hyperglycemia using MeDIP array. We identified a total of 923 and 2150 promoters in the visceral adipose tissue of F1 offspring that had been significantly hypermethylated and hypomethylated, respectively. It is noteworthy that the *Tnf* promoter was hypomethylated in diabetic offspring compared to the controls. Further bisulfite sequencing of the *Tnf* promoter encompassing −220 to +26 revealed that, overall, hypomethylation did not broadly alter the chromatin in diabetic offspring; rather, it was confined to the specific cytosine.

The *Tnf* promoter sequence contains CpG dinucleotides within or next to transcription factor-binding sites. The CpG site at site −1952 of the *Tnf* promoter was distinctly hypomethylated both in F1 and F2 offspring of diabetic mothers and the 1952-bp 5′-flanking region of the promoter may be a *c-Rel*-, *EBF1*-, *NFIC*-, *RelA*-, and *NF-κB*-binding site. Therefore, DNA methylation is proposed to participate in regulating the expression of the *Tnf* gene by interfering with transcription binding sites, playing a role in the progression of insulin resistance. Consistent with our findings, a study by Lou et al. [22] showed that the activation and upregulation of proinflammatory cytokines such as *IL-1β*, *IL-6*, *TNF-α*, and *IFN-γ* mainly occurred in the arterial intima of diabetic rats, and reduced levels of DNA methylation at the specific cytosine-phosphate-guanosine sites of *IL-1β*, *IL-6*, *TNF-α*, and *IFN-γ* may be one of the mechanisms to regulate the expression of these genes. Our results emphasized the effect of early intrauterine exposure on insulin sensitivity via epigenetic changes, which may persist throughout the lifetime as well as get transmitted to the next generation.

Another factor related to insulin resistance is lifestyle, and previous studies have reported that accumulation of intracellular lipid metabolites from incomplete lipid oxidation could inhibit signal transduction to glucose transport [23–25], suggesting the involvement of a high-fat diet in the development of insulin resistance. In the current study, offspring were given high-fat diets, and we found that fat overload could exaggerate the programmed glucose intolerance in offspring exposed to intrauterine hyperglycemia. The underlying mechanism for this phenomenon is not yet fully understood. Barrès et al. reported that elevated free fatty acids might induce insulin resistance through epigenetic mechanisms [16].

5. Conclusions

Overall, our results revealed that intrauterine hyperglycemia can influence the DNA methylation level in the promoter regions of inflammatory factors involved in insulin resistance, such as *TNF-α*, and the DNA methylation is intergenerational and inherited.

Abbreviations

GDM: Gestational diabetes mellitus
MeDIP: Methylated DNA immunoprecipitation
STZ: Streptozotocin
GTT: Glucose tolerance test
IGT: Impaired glucose tolerance
IUGR: Intrauterine growth restriction
OGTT: Oral glucose tolerance test
IP: Immunoprecipitated
TNF: Tumor necrosis factor
IL-1β: Interleukin-1β
IL-6: Interleukin-6
IL-10: Interleukin-10
IFN-γ: Interferon-γ.

Conflict of Interests

No potential conflict of interests relevant to this paper was reported.

Authors' Contribution

Rina Su and Jie Yan contributed equally to this work.

Acknowledgments

This study was supported by the National Natural Science Foundation of China (81370722, 30973212) and the Scientific Research Foundation for the Returned Overseas Chinese Scholars, State Education Ministry ([2014]1685).

References

[1] W. W. Zhu, H. X. Yang, Y. M. Wei et al., "Evaluation of the value of fasting plasma glucose in the first prenatal visit to diagnose gestational diabetes mellitus in China," *Diabetes Care*, vol. 36, no. 3, pp. 586–590, 2013.

[2] P. W. Franks, H. C. Looker, S. Kobes et al., "Gestational glucose tolerance and risk of type 2 diabetes in young Pima Indian offspring," *Diabetes*, vol. 55, no. 2, pp. 460–465, 2006.

[3] J. G. Manderson, B. Mullan, C. C. Patterson, D. R. Hadden, A. I. Traub, and D. McCance, "Cardiovascular and metabolic abnormalities in the offspring of diabetic pregnancy," *Diabetologia*, vol. 45, no. 7, pp. 991–996, 2002.

[4] D. J. P. Barker, "The fetal origins of type 2 diabetes mellitus," *Annals of Internal Medicine*, vol. 130, no. 4, pp. 322–324, 1999.

[5] O. Izaola, D. De Luis, I. Sajoux, J. C. Domingo, and M. Vidal, "Inflammation and obesity (lipoinflammation)," *Nutrición Hospitalaria*, vol. 31, no. 6, pp. 2352–2358, 2015.

[6] E. D. Buras, L. Yang, P. Saha et al., "Proinsulin-producing, hyperglycemia-induced adipose tissue macrophages underlie insulin resistance in high fat-fed diabetic mice," *The FASEB Journal*, vol. 29, no. 8, pp. 3537–3548, 2015.

[7] J. Yan, X. Li, R. Su, K. Zhang, and H. Yang, "Long-term effects of maternal diabetes on blood pressure and renal function in rat male offspring," *PLoS ONE*, vol. 9, no. 2, Article ID e88269, 2014.

[8] F. A. Van Assche, K. Holemans, and L. Aerts, "Long-term consequences for offspring of diabetes during pregnancy," *British Medical Bulletin*, vol. 60, pp. 173–182, 2001.

[9] G.-L. Ding, F.-F. Wang, J. Shu et al., "Transgenerational glucose intolerance with Igf2/H19 epigenetic alterations in mouse islet induced by intrauterine hyperglycemia," *Diabetes*, vol. 61, no. 5, pp. 1133–1142, 2012.

[10] B. D. Kayser, C. M. Toledo-Corral, T. L. Alderete, M. J. Weigensberg, and M. I. Goran, "Temporal relationships between adipocytokines and diabetes risk in Hispanic adolescents with obesity," *Obesity*, vol. 23, no. 7, pp. 1479–1485, 2015.

[11] G. S. Hotamisligil, P. Peraldi, A. Budavari, R. Ellis, M. F. White, and B. M. Spiegelman, "IRS-1-mediated inhibition of insulin receptor tyrosine kinase activity in TNF-α- and obesity-induced insulin resistance," *Science*, vol. 271, no. 5249, pp. 665–668, 1996.

[12] K. T. Uysal, S. M. Wiesbrock, M. W. Marino, and G. S. Hotamisligil, "Protection from obesity-induced insulin resistance in mice lacking TNF-alpha function," *Nature*, vol. 389, no. 6651, pp. 610–614, 1997.

[13] M. Yuan, N. Konstantopoulos, J. Lee et al., "Reversal of obesity- and diet-induced insulin resistance with salicylates or targeted disruption of *Ikkβ*," *Science*, vol. 293, no. 5535, pp. 1673–1677, 2001.

[14] S. N. Vallerie, M. Furuhashi, R. Fucho, and G. S. Hotamisligil, "A predominant role for parenchymal c-Jun amino terminal kinase (JNK) in the regulation of systemic insulin sensitivity," *PLoS ONE*, vol. 3, no. 9, Article ID e3151, 2008.

[15] Y. Ding, J. Li, S. Liu et al., "DNA hypomethylation of inflammation-associated genes in adipose tissue of female mice after multigenerational high fat diet feeding," *International Journal of Obesity*, vol. 38, no. 2, pp. 198–204, 2014.

[16] R. Barrès, M. E. Osler, J. Yan et al., "Non-CpG methylation of the PGC-1α promoter through DNMT3B controls mitochondrial density," *Cell Metabolism*, vol. 10, no. 3, pp. 189–198, 2009.

[17] R. C. Painter, C. Osmond, P. Gluckman, M. Hanson, D. I. W. Phillips, and T. J. Roseboom, "Transgenerational effects of prenatal exposure to the Dutch famine on neonatal adiposity and health in later life," *BJOG: An International Journal of Obstetrics & Gynaecology*, vol. 115, no. 10, pp. 1243–1249, 2008.

[18] G. C. Burdge, J. Slater-Jefferies, C. Torrens, E. S. Phillips, M. A. Hanson, and K. A. Lillycrop, "Dietary protein restriction of pregnant rats in the F0 generation induces altered methylation of hepatic gene promoters in the adult male offspring in the F1 and F2 generations," *British Journal of Nutrition*, vol. 97, no. 3, pp. 435–439, 2007.

[19] J. H. Park, D. A. Stoffers, R. D. Nicholls, and R. A. Simmons, "Development of type 2 diabetes following intrauterine growth retardation in rats is associated with progressive epigenetic silencing of Pdx1," *The Journal of Clinical Investigation*, vol. 118, no. 6, pp. 2316–2324, 2008.

[20] Q. Fu, R. A. McKnight, C. W. Callaway, X. Yu, R. H. Lane, and A. V. Majnik, "Intrauterine growth restriction disrupts developmental epigenetics around distal growth hormone response elements on the rat hepatic IGF-1 gene," *The FASEB Journal*, vol. 29, no. 4, pp. 1176–1184, 2015.

[21] D. Goodspeed, M. D. Seferovic, W. Holland et al., "Essential nutrient supplementation prevents heritable metabolic disease in multigenerational intrauterine growth-restricted rats," *The FASEB Journal*, vol. 29, no. 3, pp. 807–819, 2015.

[22] X. D. Lou, H. D. Wang, S. J. Xia, S. Skog, and J. Sun, "Effects of resveratrol on the expression and DNA methylation of cytokine genes in diabetic rat aortas," *Archivum Immunologiae et Therapia Experimentalis*, vol. 62, pp. 329–340, 2014.

[23] K. F. Petersen, S. Dufour, D. Befroy, R. Garcia, and G. I. Shulman, "Impaired mitochondrial activity in the insulin-resistant offspring of patients with type 2 diabetes," *The New England Journal of Medicine*, vol. 350, no. 7, pp. 664–671, 2004.

[24] V. B. Ritov, E. V. Menshikova, J. He, R. E. Ferrell, B. H. Goodpaster, and D. E. Kelley, "Deficiency of subsarcolemmal mitochondria in obesity and type 2 diabetes," *Diabetes*, vol. 54, no. 1, pp. 8–14, 2005.

[25] J.-Y. Kim, R. C. Hickner, R. L. Cortright, G. L. Dohm, and J. A. Houmard, "Lipid oxidation is reduced in obese human skeletal muscle," *American Journal of Physiology—Endocrinology and Metabolism*, vol. 279, no. 5, pp. E1039–E1044, 2000.

2

Comparison of Clinical Trajectories before Initiation of Renal Replacement Therapy between Diabetic Nephropathy and Nephrosclerosis on the KDIGO Guidelines Heat Map

Masanori Abe,[1] Kazuyoshi Okada,[1] Noriaki Maruyama,[1] Hiroyuki Takashima,[1] Osamu Oikawa,[1] and Masayoshi Soma[1,2]

[1]*Division of Nephrology, Hypertension and Endocrinology, Department of Internal Medicine, Nihon University School of Medicine, Tokyo 173-8610, Japan*
[2]*Division of General Medicine, Department of Internal Medicine, Nihon University School of Medicine, Tokyo 173-8610, Japan*

Correspondence should be addressed to Masanori Abe; abe.masanori@nihon-u.ac.jp

Academic Editor: Monika A. Niewczas

This study investigated differences between the clinical trajectories of diabetic nephropathy and nephrosclerosis using the Kidney Disease: Improving Global Outcomes (KDIGO) heat map and the clinical characteristics between the two diseases at RRT initiation. This single-center, retrospective study enrolled 100 patients whose estimated glomerular filtration rate (eGFR) was $\geq$45 mL/min/1.73 m^2 at their first visit and who were initiated on RRT. Fifty consecutive patients were assigned to each of the diabetic nephropathy and nephrosclerosis groups. All data for simultaneously measured eGFR and urinary albumin to creatinine ratio (UACR) were collected from first visit to RRT initiation and were plotted on the KDIGO heat map. Diabetic nephropathy was characterized by higher blood pressure and UACR and lower age, eGFR, and serum albumin levels compared with nephrosclerosis at RRT initiation. The vast majority of patients with diabetic nephropathy and eGFR < 60 mL/min/1.73 m^2 had concomitant macroalbuminuria, whereas for patients with nephrosclerosis, even when eGFR was <45 mL/min/1.73 m^2, many still had normoalbuminuria or microalbuminuria. The rate of decline of eGFR was significantly faster in the diabetic nephropathy group than that in the nephrosclerosis group. The clinical trajectories of diabetic nephropathy and nephrosclerosis differed markedly on the KDIGO heat map.

1. Background

Chronic kidney disease (CKD) progressively increases the risk of end-stage kidney disease (ESKD) and cardiovascular disease in line with its severity [1]. The prevalence of ESKD is expected to rise steeply over the next few decades, driven by population ageing and the increasing prevalence of diabetes and hypertension [2–4]. Although renal replacement therapy (RRT), via dialysis or renal transplantation, is a potentially lifesaving treatment for patients with ESKD, it is costly.

Type 2 diabetes mellitus is among the leading causes of CKD, including ESKD, in both developed and developing countries; in various countries including the USA and Japan, type 2 diabetes mellitus accounts for nearly 50% of patients on incident dialysis [2, 3]. In the USA in 2012, nephrosclerosis was the second most common primary disease after diabetic nephropathy [2], and in Japan in 2011, nephrosclerosis was the third most common primary disease (12.3%) after diabetic nephropathy and chronic glomerulonephritis [5]. In relation to the aging of new dialysis patients, the percentage of patients who had nephrosclerosis and were newly started on dialysis continuously increased. Since about 2000, the rate of increase in the annual number of new dialysis patients with chronic glomerulonephritis has been negative [5]. Therefore, in the future, nephrosclerosis will likely be the second most common primary disease in Japan as well as the USA. The management of diabetic nephropathy and nephrosclerosis is thus very important for helping prevent these patients from newly requiring RRT.

The Kidney Disease: Improving Global Outcomes (KDIGO) Clinical Practice Guideline for the Evaluation and Management of CKD was released in January 2013 [6]. KDIGO recommends CKD classifications based on cause, glomerular filtration rate (GFR) category, and albuminuria category. The cause of CKD is considered because it provides important prognostic information and influences treatment decisions. Albuminuria and estimated GFR (eGFR) provide independent information regarding the risk of CKD progression, cardiovascular disease, and mortality. In addition, clinicians and researchers are advised to categorize patients using a heat map generated by composite rankings of relative risk. However, differences between the clinical trajectories for diabetic nephropathy and nephrosclerosis, the two major primary causes of CKD, have not been revealed clearly on the KDIGO heat map.

Against this background, this retrospective study investigated differences between the clinical courses of diabetic nephropathy and nephrosclerosis using the KDIGO heat map and sought to determine how the clinical characteristics differed between the two diseases at the time of the RRT initiation.

2. Methods

This single-center, retrospective study, conducted between January 2011 and December 2013, was designed to compare the clinical courses of diabetic nephropathy and nephrosclerosis with respect to eGFR and the urinary albumin to creatinine ratio (UACR) in patients with CKD who were already receiving treatment from a nephrologist. Specifically, the study compared the clinical progression of the two diseases as represented by the heat map based on the prognosis of CKD by GFR and albuminuria category stated in the KDIGO 2012 Clinical Practice Guideline for the Evaluation and Management of Chronic Kidney Disease [6]. All data used in the analysis were collected from medical records. All study participants provided written informed consent, and the study protocol was approved by the Research Review Board of our University and conducted in accordance with the Declaration of Helsinki (Clinical Trial Registration Number: UMIN000017502).

Inclusion criteria were (1) patients who underwent RRT initiation at our hospital during January 2011 and December 2013 and (2) eGFR $\geq$ 45 mL/min/1.73 m^2 at the first visit to our hospital. Exclusion criteria were (1) age $<$ 20 years at RRT initiation, (2) RRT initiated due to acute kidney injury (AKI), and (3) primary cause of CKD other than diabetic nephropathy and nephrosclerosis (i.e., glomerulonephritis, cystic disease, or vasculitis). Diabetic nephropathy and nephrosclerosis were diagnosed by renal biopsy or medical history. Specifically, diabetic nephropathy was defined as diagnosis based on kidney biopsy (n = 15), on the presence of type 1 diabetes (n = 2), or on fulfillment of all the following criteria (n = 33): (1) diabetes duration $\geq$ 10 years; (2) clear presence of diabetic retinopathy; (3) no history of proteinuria or hematuria prior to the first visit; (4) other primary kidney disease, such as secondary, hereditary, cystic, or drug-induced kidney disease or vasculitis completely ruled out by blood work or imaging diagnostics. Nephrosclerosis was diagnosed by kidney biopsy (n = 10) or fulfillment of all of the following criteria (n = 40): (1) no history of comorbid diabetes prior to the first visit or during the observational period; (2) duration of hypertension $\geq$ 10 years; (3) no history of proteinuria or hematuria prior to the first visit; (4) presence of hypertensive retinopathy by fundus examination; and (5) other primary kidney disease, such as secondary, hereditary, cystic, drug-induced kidney disease, or vasculitis completely ruled out by blood work or imaging diagnostics. Subjects were assigned to either the diabetic nephropathy group or nephrosclerosis group at RRT initiation, with 50 consecutive subjects enrolled per group for a total of 100 subjects.

All data for simultaneously measured eGFR and UACR were used to monitor the clinical course from the first visit to RRT initiation and were collected from the medical records. These data were plotted on the heat map according to the KDIGO guidelines. Serum samples were assayed for creatinine (sCr) at a central laboratory (Central Laboratory; SRL Co., Tokyo, Japan) with the enzymatic Cr assay method using a Japan electron Cr auto-analyzer (JCA-BM8060; JEOL Ltd., Tokyo, Japan) and enzyme solution (Preauto-S CRE-L; Sekisui Medical Co., Ltd., Tokyo, Japan). To assess urinary albumin excretion, we measured urinary concentrations of albumin and Cr (albumin/Cr ratio) in spot urine samples. Urinary albumin was measured using the immunoturbidimetric assay. Glomerular filtration rate was estimated using the modified, final recommended equation for Japanese patients issued by the Japanese Society of Nephrology-CKD Initiatives, as eGFR values obtained by this method are more accurate for Japanese patients with CKD [7]. The formula was as follows:

$$\begin{aligned} \text{eGFR } &\left(\text{mL/min per } 1.73\,\text{m}^2\right) \\ &= 194 \times \text{sCr}^{-1.094} \\ &\quad \times \text{age}^{-0.287} \quad (\times\, 0.739 \text{ for women}). \end{aligned} \tag{1}$$

The composite ranking of relative risk by GFR and albuminuria levels was calculated according to the 2012 KDIGO guidelines using the following definitions: no CKD (green zone), G1A1 and G2A1; moderate risk (yellow zone), G1A2, G2A2, and G3aA1; high risk (orange zone), G1A3, G2A3, G3aA2, and G3bA1; and very high risk (red zone), G3aA3, G3bA2-3, all G4, and all G5 [6]. Blood pressure (BP) was measured at the outpatient clinic according to the Japanese Society of Hypertension 2009 guidelines [8]. Measurements were performed in duplicate every month using a sphygmomanometer (Nippon Colin, Tokyo, Japan) with the patient in a sitting position after a 5 min period of rest. Patients, particularly those with dietary restrictions, were given guidance on how to maintain their diet. Doses of antihypertensive agents, including angiotensin receptor blockers (ARBs), angiotensin-converting enzyme (ACE) inhibitors, calcium channel blockers, and diuretics, were adjusted during the study period to maintain the target BP level of <130/80 mmHg.

2.1. Statistical Analysis. Data were analyzed on the basis of assigned groups and are expressed as the mean ± SD

Table 1: Clinical characteristics at the first visit in the two groups.

	Diabetic nephropathy	Nephrosclerosis	P value
n (male/female)	50 (34/16)	50 (35/15)	0.833
Age (years)	57.1 ± 9.2	65.6 ± 8.4	<0.0001
Body mass index (kg/m^2)	24.7 ± 2.5	22.5 ± 1.7	<0.0001
Systolic blood pressure (mmHg)	149 ± 8	146 ± 10	0.038
Diastolic blood pressure (mmHg)	86 ± 7	82 ± 10	0.012
Heart rate (bpm)	76 ± 8	76 ± 7	0.989
Serum creatinine (mg/dL)	0.9 ± 0.2	1.1 ± 0.2	<0.0001
eGFR (mL/min/1.73 m^2)	65.6 ± 10.5	50.0 ± 6.3	<0.0001
UACR (mg/gCr)	131 [57, 189]	25 [15, 31]	<0.0001
Hemoglobin (g/dL)	13.7 ± 0.9	13.5 ± 0.7	0.129
Serum albumin (g/dL)	4.0 ± 0.3	4.0 ± 0.2	0.580
Type of diabetes (type 1/2)	2/48	—	—
Glycated hemoglobin (%)	7.6 ± 0.6	5.4 ± 0.3	<0.00001

Data are expressed as mean ± SD, median [interquartile range], or n.
GFR, glomerular filtration rate; UACR, urinary albumin to creatinine ratio.

or median [interquartile range], as appropriate. Continuous variables were compared using Student's t-test or the Mann-Whitney U test, and categorical variables were compared by the chi-square or Fisher's exact test as appropriate to the data distribution. To analyze the time course changes in eGFR, we fitted scatterplot smoothing curves to all the eGFR measures for all the patients in each group. Then, we used the Mann-Whitney U test to compare the eGFR decline (mL/min/1.73 m^2 per year) between the groups. The eGFR time course data within groups were analyzed by repeated-measures analysis of variance (ANOVA), while changes between the two groups were analyzed by two-way ANOVA followed by Dunnett's test. To analyze the time course changes in albuminuria, we fitted scatterplot smoothing curves to all UACR measures for all the patients in each group. Then, we used the Mann-Whitney U test to compare the regression coefficients between the groups. Statistical significance was set at $P < 0.05$. All analyses were performed using JMP ver. 11 software (SAS Institute Ltd., Cary, NC, USA).

3. Results

3.1. Study Population and Characteristics at the First Visit and RRT Initiation. The clinical characteristics of the patients at the first visit are shown in Table 1. At the first visit, mean age was significantly higher in the nephrosclerosis group than in the diabetic nephropathy group. Body mass index (BMI) was significantly higher in the diabetic nephropathy group. Although there was no significant difference in heart rate, both systolic and diastolic BP was significantly higher in the diabetic nephropathy group. Serum Cr level was significantly lower and eGFR was significantly higher in the diabetic nephropathy group. There was no significant difference in hemoglobin or serum albumin level between the groups. Mean glycated hemoglobin level was 7.6 ± 0.6% in the diabetic nephropathy group.

The patients' clinical characteristics and medications being taken at RRT initiation are shown for each group in Table 2. Mean retrospective observational period and mean time of simultaneous measurement of eGFR and albuminuria did not significantly differ between the groups. At RRT initiation, mean age was significantly higher in the nephrosclerosis group than in the diabetic nephropathy group. BMI was significantly higher in the diabetic nephropathy group. Although there was no significant difference in heart rate, both systolic and diastolic BP was significantly higher in the diabetic nephropathy group. There was a significantly higher occurrence of cardiovascular comorbidity, in particular ischemic heart disease, in the diabetic nephropathy group. All patients had hypertension and were taking antihypertensive medication, with renin-angiotensin system (RAS) inhibitors including ARBs, ACE inhibitors, and direct renin inhibitors being the most common, followed by calcium channel blockers. Although 49 patients in the diabetic nephropathy group and 46 patients in the nephrosclerosis group had used diuretics, thiazide diuretics were used by only 3 patients in the diabetic nephropathy group and none in the nephrosclerosis group; other patients used loop diuretics. Although there was no significant difference in the type of antihypertensive agents used in the two groups, the number of such agents used per person was significantly greater in the diabetic nephropathy group.

3.2. Laboratory Data at RRT Initiation. The final data set collected before RRT initiation is shown in Table 3. The nephrosclerosis group had significantly higher serum Cr levels and lower eGFR values than the diabetic nephropathy group. The diabetic nephropathy group had a significantly higher UACR and a significantly lower serum albumin level. The diabetic nephropathy group had significantly higher triglyceride, N-terminal pro-brain natriuretic peptide (NT-proBNP), and C-reactive protein (CRP) levels and significantly lower high-density lipoprotein (HDL)-cholesterol levels. Hemoglobin level did not differ significantly between the groups. The glycated hemoglobin level was significantly

TABLE 2: Clinical characteristics and medications at the initiation of RRT in the two groups.

	Diabetic nephropathy	Nephrosclerosis	P value
n (male/female)	50 (34/16)	50 (35/15)	0.833
Age (years)	67.2 ± 9.6	78.8 ± 6.4	<0.0001
Observational periods (months)	115 ± 57	122 ± 35	0.447
Measurement times (/year)	4.4 ± 2.5	4.4 ± 2.6	0.955
Measurement times (/person)	34 ± 11	37 ± 10	0.109
Body mass index (kg/m^2)	24.8 ± 2.5	22.1 ± 1.7	<0.0001
Systolic blood pressure (mmHg)	147 ± 15	137 ± 9	<0.0001
Diastolic blood pressure (mmHg)	80 ± 12	73 ± 10	0.0003
Heart rate (bpm)	77 ± 7	76 ± 8	0.541
Mode of renal replacement therapy % (n)			
Hemodialysis	92 (46)	92 (46)	—
Peritoneal dialysis	8 (4)	8 (4)	—
Kidney transplantation	0 (0)	0 (0)	—
Cardiovascular comorbidities % (n)	34 (17)	18 (9)	0.069
Ischemic heart disease	28 (14)	12 (6)	0.046
Cerebrovascular disease	6 (3)	4 (2)	0.650
Peripheral artery disease	4 (2)	2 (1)	0.562
Diabetic retinopathy % (n)	100 (50)	—	—
Medication % (n)			
Antihypertensive agents			
Angiotensin receptor blockers	98 (49)	90 (45)	0.093
Angiotensin-converting enzyme inhibitors	14 (7)	4 (2)	0.082
Direct renin inhibitors	8 (4)	2 (1)	0.173
Calcium channel blockers	98 (49)	94 (47)	0.312
Diuretics	98 (49)	92 (46)	0.172
β-blockers	30 (15)	14 (7)	0.054
α-blockers	30 (15)	14 (7)	0.054
Number of antihypertensive agents (per person)	3.76 ± 0.2	3.10 ± 0.1	0.0006
Antidiabetic agents			
Insulin	38 (19)	—	—
Oral hypoglycemic agents	58 (29)	—	—
Diet therapy alone	4 (2)	—	—
Erythropoiesis stimulating agents	100 (50)	98 (49)	0.319
Statins	80 (40)	78 (39)	0.808
Active vitamin D	94 (47)	92 (46)	0.698

Data are expressed as mean ± SD, %, or n.

decreased at RRT initiation compared with that at the first visit in the diabetic nephropathy group ($P < 0.0001$).

3.3. Time Course of eGFR Decline and Urinary Albumin Excretion Rate. Figure 1 shows the eGFR trajectories of individuals in the diabetic nephropathy (a) and nephrosclerosis (b) groups. The mean eGFR slopes from first visit to RRT initiation for the diabetic nephropathy group and nephrosclerosis group were −6.6 ± 2.4 and −3.6 ± 1.2 mL/min/1.73 m^2 per year, respectively ($P < 0.0001$). The duration between the observation of eGFR < 45 mL/min/1.73 m^2 and RRT initiation was 59 ± 26 months in the diabetic nephropathy group and 94 ± 28 months in the nephrosclerosis group, showing a significant difference between the groups ($P < 0.0001$). Furthermore, the rates of decline in eGFR in the diabetic nephropathy group and nephrosclerosis group were −9.9 ± 5.3 and −4.8 ± 2.2 mL/min/1.73 m^2 per year, respectively ($P < 0.0001$). Figure 2 shows the UACR trajectories of individuals in the diabetic nephropathy (a) and nephrosclerosis (b) groups. The regression coefficient was −23.3 [−34 to −13] in the diabetic nephropathy group and −4.7 [−9.7 to −2.2] in the nephrosclerosis group, again showing a significant difference between the groups ($P < 0.0001$).

3.4. Clinical Course on the KDIGO Heat Map. Figure 3 shows all plotted data for simultaneously measured eGFR and UACR from the first visit to our hospital to final data collection before RRT initiation in the two groups. In

Table 3: Laboratory data before the initiation of RRT in the two groups.

Variables	Diabetic nephropathy	Nephrosclerosis	P value
Serum creatinine (mg/dL)	8.8 ± 1.4	9.9 ± 1.6	0.004
eGFR (mL/min/1.73 m^2)	5.5 ± 1.1	4.2 ± 0.8	<0.0001
UACR (mg/gCr)	3000 [2084, 4184]	972 [490, 1830]	<0.0001
Hemoglobin (g/dL)	10.1 ± 0.9	10.7 ± 0.9	0.290
Serum albumin (g/dL)	3.3 ± 0.6	3.7 ± 0.4	0.0012
Total cholesterol (mg/dL)	173 ± 38	167 ± 35	0.341
HDL-cholesterol (mg/dL)	45 ± 13	52 ± 13	0.013
Triglyceride (mg/dL)	141 [96, 178]	94 [76, 127]	<0.0001
Glycated hemoglobin (%)	6.5 ± 0.7	5.6 ± 0.4	<0.0001
NT-proBNP (pg/mL)	2670 [1531, 7209]	1298 [594, 3226]	0.021
C-reactive protein (mg/dL)	0.17 [0.10, 0.29]	0.09 [0.03, 0.14]	<0.0001

Data are expressed as mean ± SD or median [interquartile range]. eGFR, estimated glomerular filtration rate; HDL, high-density lipoprotein; NT-proBNP, N-terminal pro-brain natriuretic peptide; UACR, urinary albumin to creatinine ratio.

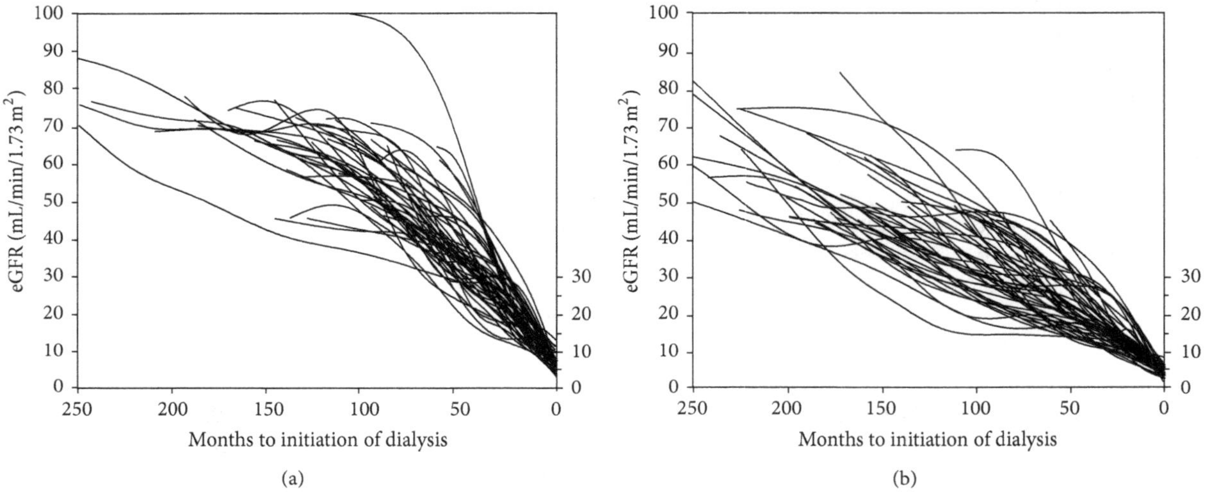

Figure 1: Estimated glomerular filtration rate (eGFR) trajectories with individual slopes during the observation period in the two groups. (a) Smoothing curve for the diabetic nephropathy group; (b) smoothing curve for the nephrosclerosis group.

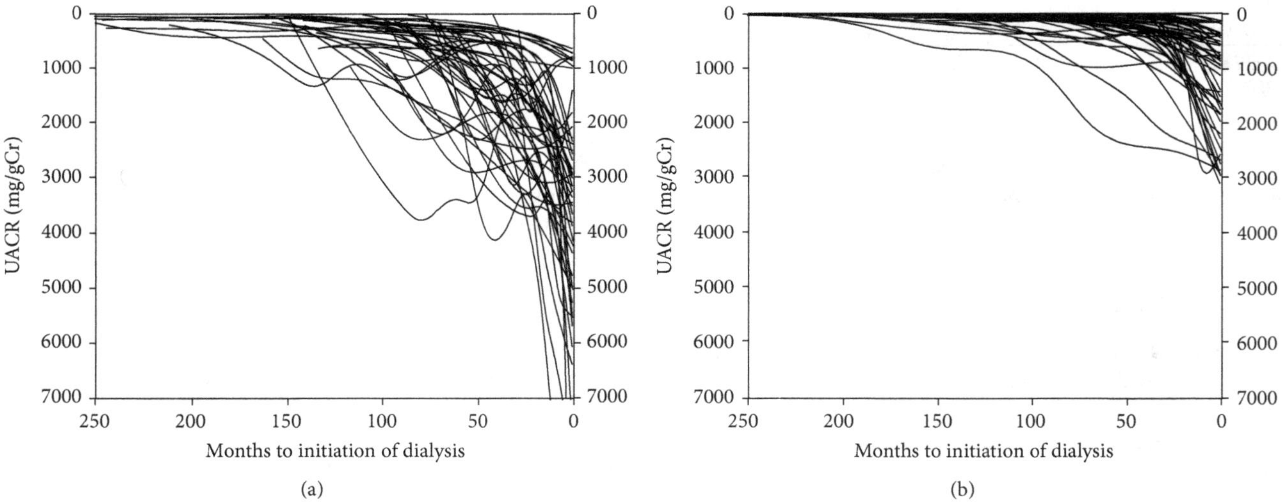

Figure 2: Urinary albumin to creatinine ratio (UACR) trajectories with individual slopes during the observation period in the two groups. (a) Smoothing curve for the diabetic nephropathy group; (b) smoothing curve for the nephrosclerosis group.

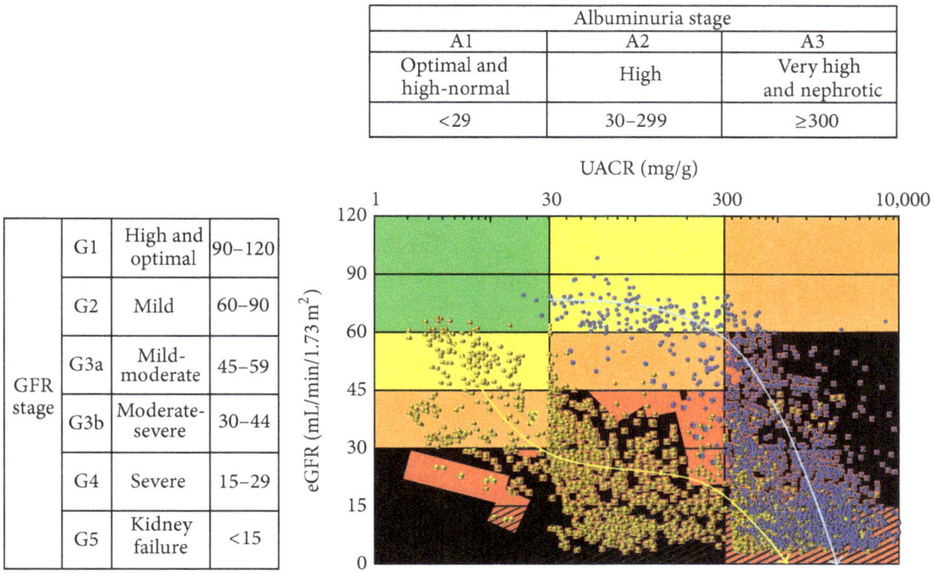

FIGURE 3: Data of simultaneously measured eGFR and UACR from the first visit to RRT initiation in the diabetic nephropathy group and nephrosclerosis group as represented on the KDIGO heat map. Blue and yellow bold arrows indicate clinical trajectories of the diabetic nephropathy and nephrosclerosis groups, respectively. eGFR, estimated glomerular filtration rate; GFR, glomerular filtration rate; KDIGO, Kidney Disease: Improving Global Outcomes; UACR, urinary albumin to creatinine ratio.

the diabetic nephropathy group, only 3 patients (6%) were plotted into the no CKD (G2A1) category at the first visit. Five patients (10%) and 2 patients (4%) were plotted into the high risk G3aA2 and G2A3 categories, respectively; the remaining 40 patients (80%) were plotted into the moderate risk category. In the nephrosclerosis group, 3 patients (6%) were plotted into the no CKD (G2A1) category at the first visit. However, 6 patients (12%) were plotted into the high risk category (G3aA2), and the remaining 41 patients (82%) were plotted into the moderate risk category (G3aA1). None of the patients in the nephrosclerosis group were plotted into G2A2 or G2A3, unlike many patients in the diabetic nephropathy group. In the diabetic nephropathy group, risk categories progressed from moderate or high risk to very high risk when GFR was reduced to <60 mL/min/1.73 m^2. In other words, when eGFR was reduced to <60 mL/min/1.73 m^2, albuminuria showed progression from the A2 to A3 stage. Moreover, the eGFR decline resulted in further elevation of albuminuria up to 3000 (interquartile range, 2084 to 4184) mg/gCr at RRT initiation. All cases underwent RRT initiation at the G5A3 stage. On the other hand, in the nephrosclerosis group, when eGFR was reduced to <45 mL/min/1.73 m^2 and albuminuria had progressed from the A1 to A2 stage, the risk category changed from moderate or high risk to very high risk. Thereafter, eGFR gradually decreased and albuminuria gradually increased. Eight patients (16%) were started on RRT while remaining at the A2 stage, whereas the other 42 patients (84%) had progressed to A3 at RRT initiation.

4. Discussion

These results reveal that the clinical courses of the two primary causative diseases of CKD—diabetic nephropathy and nephrosclerosis—differ considerably when represented on the KDIGO heat map. As shown in Figure 3, diabetic nephropathy and nephrosclerosis showed contrasting characteristic courses. Furthermore, there was a significant difference in the rate of decline of eGFR between patients with diabetic nephropathy and those with nephrosclerosis. This indicates that even when eGFR levels are comparable, the subsequent progression in diabetic nephropathy would be more rapid compared with that for nephrosclerosis. It is recommended that patients be referred to nephrology at stage 4 CKD to prepare for RRT. Nephrologists and general physicians should be aware of the different clinical courses of these two CKDs and should aim to differentiate the causes of CKD upon physician examination.

Declines in eGFR, such as a 30% reduction over 2 years, were reported to be strongly and consistently associated with the risks for ESKD and mortality and have been considered an alternative endpoint for CKD progression [9]. Although the traditional view of kidney function decline in CKD is a steady linear decline (or slope), albeit at different rates among individuals, recent studies have evaluated the trajectories of decline and have shown they are often not linear [10–12]. The average overall rate of decline reported in 1441 adult individuals with stage 3–5 CKD was 1.47 mL/min/1.73 m^2; however, the rate was faster in individuals with eGFR < 30 mL/min/1.73 m^2 and accelerated in the year before the development of ESKD [10]. Individuals with steeper trajectories were more likely to have been hospitalized and to receive a diagnosis of AKI during hospitalization [12]. Although the patients who began RRT due to AKI were not included in the present study, diabetic nephropathy might be predisposed to rapid decline compared with nephrosclerosis. These findings highlight the heterogeneity of the rates of decline of eGFR and should lead to more individualized approaches to preparation for ESKD and transplant referral. Further studies should focus on identifying risk factors for the rapid decline of eGFR to allow for more timely intervention, as trajectories according to the primary disease of CKD have not been considered in previous studies.

Recently, the prognostic significance of identifying individuals with diabetes and an early decline (starting at <60 mL/min/1.73 m^2) in GFR (>3.5 mL/min/1.73 m^2 per year) that is over and above what would be expected with aging alone has been highlighted, with this early decline being linked to the development of ESKD in type 1 diabetes [13, 14]. Krolewski reported that 25% of patients with diabetes can be considered to have rapid progressive renal decline (eGFR slope < −7 mL/min/year) and these patients progressed to ESKD within 2–10 years. Another 25% showed moderate progressive renal decline (eGFR slope −7 to −3 mL/min/year), and most of them progressed or will progress to ESKD within 10–30 years. The remaining patients (50%) will have slow or no progressive renal decline and few may progress to ESKD during 30 years of follow-up [15]. Furthermore, the prevalence rate of patients showing such renal decline is 10%, 32%, and 50% among patients with normoalbuminuria, microalbuminuria, and proteinuria, respectively [16]. In the present study, the GFR decline rate in the diabetic nephropathy group was −6.6 mL/min/1.73 m^2 per year during 115 months overall. However, when the eGFR declined to less than 45 mL/min/1.73 m^2, the decline rate accelerated to −9.9 mL/min/1.73 m^2 per year.

However, some studies have shown microalbuminuria remission rates of 21–64% in patients with diabetes [17–22]. These high rates of microalbuminuria remission have been linked to the use of RAS inhibitors in some studies. Currently, there is known to be a four- to fivefold magnitude increase in the risk for ESKD in patients with type 1 diabetes or type 2 diabetes and microalbuminuria [23]. However, many of our patients with ESKD due to diabetic nephropathy had resistant hypertension and higher blood pressures compared with those with ESKD due to nephrosclerosis, despite taking significantly larger numbers of antihypertensive agents. In the absence of antihypertensive therapy, GFR may decrease by 10–15 mL/min per year during stage 4, which is characterized by clinically detectable proteinuria, hypertension, and declining GFR [24]. Therefore, our data demonstrate that, in patients with diabetic nephropathy, the inhibition of progression from microalbuminuria to macroalbuminuria is important for preventing progression to ESKD. Although RAS inhibitors remain the cornerstone of therapy, the management of patients who do not respond to them remains an issue.

Recent studies demonstrated that normoalbuminuric renal insufficiency is not uncommon for diabetic patients, especially those with type 2 diabetes [25]. There are several possible pathogenic mechanisms that may account for the development of normoalbuminuric renal insufficiency. Renal ischemia due to intrarenal arteriosclerosis and disproportionately advanced tubulointerstitial lesions, despite minor diabetic glomerular lesions, which denote the presence of diabetic kidney lesions as well as nephrosclerosis, are likely to be related to the development of normoalbuminuric renal insufficiency [26, 27]. The clinical characteristics of such patients include older age, female predilection, shorter duration of diabetes, lower prevalence of hypertension, smoking, previous cardiovascular disease, and antihypertensive agents including RAS inhibitors, lower levels of glycated hemoglobin, and higher levels of HDL-cholesterol [28–30]. The diabetic nephropathy group in the present study included patients in whom diabetic nephropathy showed a typical clinical course, since none had normoalbuminuric renal insufficiency.

We recognize that our study is limited by the diagnostic methods used for diabetic nephropathy and nephrosclerosis. Moreover, there were only 17 and 10 biopsy-proven patients in the diabetic nephropathy and nephrosclerosis groups, respectively. Therefore, patients with chronic glomerulonephritis might have been included in the diabetic nephropathy group. However, all patients in the diabetic nephropathy group had diabetic retinopathy and a prolonged duration of diabetes. Therefore, we believe that the diagnosis of diabetic nephropathy was fairly certain in our patients. A second limitation is that the frequency of simultaneous measurement of eGFR and UACR was lower for the duration from the first visit to an eGFR of 45 mL/min/1.73 m^2, because in Japan, many patients are commonly followed by a general physician. Patients were thereafter treated by a nephrologist only when eGFR decreased to <45–30 mL/min/1.73 m^2. Therefore, there was less data for the duration in the moderate and high risk categories than for the very high risk category, and the precise duration from the no CKD to moderate risk categories (G2A2 and G3aA1) could not be determined. Although some patients with diabetic nephropathy rapidly progress to ESKD, these patients were excluded from the present analysis because they had less data available for simultaneous measurements and most of them already had eGFR < 30 mL/min/1.73 m^2 at the first visit. Moreover, we could not clarify the eGFR and UACR trajectories of patients who had no or minimal decline in eGFR over the study period, since our study design allowed for only the investigation of subjects that ultimately progressed to ESKD. Lastly, the sample size was relatively small, and our study was retrospective. However, if this study were to be performed as a prospective study, we would need a relatively long period to complete it, as the endpoint of the study is RRT initiation. Nevertheless, additional studies are necessary to more firmly establish whether the risk categories of the KDIGO classification precisely reflect prognosis; not only the requirements for RRT but also cardiovascular events should be considered as endpoints since the risk categories of the KDIGO classification have three distinct indications, namely, risks for ESKD, cardiovascular events, and all-cause mortality.

5. Conclusions

This retrospective analysis showed that the clinical trajectories to RRT initiation on the KDIGO heat map differed between diabetic nephropathy and nephrosclerosis. The rate of decline of eGFR in the diabetic nephropathy group was significantly faster than that in the nephrosclerosis group. Therefore, identification of the primary disease of CKD by kidney biopsy might be important for determining the likelihood of progression to ESKD. Furthermore, compared with nephrosclerosis, diabetic nephropathy was characterized at RRT initiation by higher BMI, higher systolic and diastolic BPs, and higher CRP, NT-proBNP, and albuminuria levels as well as lower age and serum albumin levels. Further studies are needed to clarify the factors that influence the progression to ESKD.

Conflict of Interests

The authors declare no conflict of interests.

Authors' Contribution

Masanori Abe conceived of the study and participated in its design, advised throughout the study and at final approval, and helped draft the paper. Kazuyoshi Okada, Noriaki Maruyama, Osamu Oikawa, and Hiroyuki Takashima participated in its design and coordination, drafted the paper, and performed statistical analysis. Masayoshi Soma reviewed the study design and revised the paper. All authors read and approved the final paper.

References

[1] A. S. Levey, P. E. de Jong, J. Coresh et al., "The definition, classification, and prognosis of chronic kidney disease: a KDIGO Controversies Conference report," *Kidney International*, vol. 80, no. 1, pp. 17–28, 2011.

[2] A. J. Collins, R. N. Foley, C. Herzog et al., "US renal data system 2012 annual data report," *American Journal of Kidney Diseases*, vol. 61, no. 1, supplement 1, article A7, pp. e1–e476, 2013.

[3] M. Abe and K. Kalantar-Zadeh, "Haemodialysis-induced hypoglycaemia and glycaemic disarrays," *Nature Reviews Nephrology*, vol. 11, no. 5, pp. 302–313, 2015.

[4] S. L. White, S. J. Chadban, S. Jan, J. R. Chapman, and A. Cass, "How can we achieve global equity in provision of renal replacement therapy?" *Bulletin of the World Health Organization*, vol. 86, no. 3, pp. 229–237, 2008.

[5] S. Nakai, Y. Watanabe, I. Masakane et al., "Overview of regular dialysis treatment in Japan (as of 31 December 2011)," *Therapeutic Apheresis and Dialysis*, vol. 17, no. 6, pp. 567–611, 2013.

[6] Kidney Disease Improving Global Outcomes (KDIGO) CKD Work Group, "KDIGO 2012 clinical practice guideline for the evaluation and management of chronic kidney disease," *Kidney International Supplements*, vol. 3, no. 5, pp. 1–150, 2013.

[7] S. Matsuo, E. Imai, M. Horio et al., "Revised equations for estimated GFR from serum creatinine in Japan," *American Journal of Kidney Diseases*, vol. 53, no. 6, pp. 982–992, 2009.

[8] Japanese Society of Hypertension, "Japanese Society of Hypertension guidelines for the management of hypertension (JSH 2009)," *Hypertension Research*, vol. 32, no. 4, pp. 4–107, 2009.

[9] J. Coresh, T. C. Turin, K. Matsushita et al., "Decline in estimated glomerular filtration rate and subsequent risk of end-stage renal disease and mortality," *The Journal of the American Medical Association*, vol. 311, no. 24, pp. 2518–2531, 2014.

[10] J. G. Heaf and L. S. Mortensen, "Uraemia progression in chronic kidney disease stages 3–5 is not constant," *Nephron: Clinical Practice*, vol. 118, no. 4, pp. c367–c374, 2011.

[11] L. Li, B. C. Astor, J. Lewis et al., "Longitudinal progression trajectory of GFR among patients with CKD," *American Journal of Kidney Diseases*, vol. 59, no. 4, pp. 504–512, 2012.

[12] A. M. O'Hare, A. Batten, N. R. Burrows et al., "Trajectories of kidney function decline in the 2 years before initiation of long-term dialysis," *American Journal of Kidney Diseases*, vol. 59, no. 4, pp. 513–522, 2012.

[13] R. J. Macisaac, E. I. Ekinci, and G. Jerums, "Markers of and risk factors for the development and progression of diabetic kidney disease," *American Journal of Kidney Diseases*, vol. 63, no. 2, pp. S39–S62, 2014.

[14] J. Skupien, J. H. Warram, A. M. Smiles et al., "The early decline in renal function in patients with type 1 diabetes and proteinuria predicts the risk of end-stage renal disease," *Kidney International*, vol. 82, no. 5, pp. 589–597, 2012.

[15] A. S. Krolewski, "Progressive renal decline: the new paradigm of diabetic nephropathy in type 1 diabetes," *Diabetes Care*, vol. 38, no. 6, pp. 954–962, 2015.

[16] A. S. Krolewski, M. A. Niewczas, J. Skupien et al., "Early progressive renal decline precedes the onset of microalbuminuria and its progression to macroalbuminuria," *Diabetes Care*, vol. 37, no. 1, pp. 226–234, 2014.

[17] B. A. Perkins, L. H. Ficociello, K. H. Silva, D. M. Finkelstein, J. H. Warram, and A. S. Krolewski, "Regression of microalbuminuria in type 1 diabetes," *The New England Journal of Medicine*, vol. 348, no. 23, pp. 2285–2293, 2003.

[18] P. Hovind, L. Tarnow, P. Rossing et al., "Predictors for the development of microalbuminuria and macroalbuminuria in patients with type 1 diabetes: inception cohort study," *British Medical Journal*, vol. 328, no. 7448, pp. 1105–1108, 2004.

[19] P. Gæde, L. Tarnow, P. Vedel, H.-H. Parving, and O. Pedersen, "Remission to normoalbuminuria during multifactorial treatment preserves kidney function in patients with type 2 diabetes and microalbuminuria," *Nephrology Dialysis Transplantation*, vol. 19, no. 11, pp. 2784–2788, 2004.

[20] S. Araki, M. Haneda, T. Sugimoto et al., "Factors associated with frequent remission of microalbuminuria in patients with type 2 diabetes," *Diabetes*, vol. 54, no. 10, pp. 2983–2987, 2005.

[21] J. M. Steinke, A. R. Sinaiko, M. S. Kramer, S. Suissa, B. M. Chavers, and M. Mauer, "The early natural history of nephropathy in type 1 diabetes: III. Predictors of 5-year urinary albumin excretion rate patterns in initially normoalbuminuric patients," *Diabetes*, vol. 54, no. 7, pp. 2164–2171, 2005.

[22] T. Yamada, M. Komatsu, I. Komiya et al., "Development, progression, and regression of microalbuminuria in Japanese patients with type 2 diabetes under tight glycemic and blood pressure control: the Kashiwa study," *Diabetes Care*, vol. 28, no. 11, pp. 2733–2738, 2005.

[23] M. E. Molitch, A. I. Adler, A. Flyvbjerg et al., "Diabetic kidney disease: a clinical update from Kidney Disease: improving Global Outcomes," *Kidney International*, vol. 87, no. 1, pp. 20–30, 2015.

[24] H.-H. Parving, U. Smidt, A. Andersen, and P. Svendsen, "Early aggressive antihypertensive treatment reduces rate of decline in kidney function in diabetic nephropathy," *The Lancet*, vol. 321, no. 8335, pp. 1175–1179, 1983.

[25] M. Shimizu, K. Furuichi, H. Yokoyama et al., "Kidney lesions in diabetic patients with normoalbuminuric renal insufficiency,"

Clinical and Experimental Nephrology, vol. 18, no. 2, pp. 305–312, 2014.

[26] H. Taniwaki, Y. Nishizawa, T. Kawagishi et al., "Decrease in glomerular filtration rate in Japanese patients with type 2 diabetes is linked to atherosclerosis," *Diabetes Care*, vol. 21, no. 11, pp. 1848–1855, 1998.

[27] R. J. MacIsaac, S. Panagiotopoulos, K. J. McNeil et al., "Is nonalbuminuric renal insufficiency in type 2 diabetes related to an increase in intrarenal vascular disease?" *Diabetes Care*, vol. 29, no. 7, pp. 1560–1566, 2006.

[28] H. Yokoyama, H. Sone, M. Oishi, K. Kawai, Y. Fukumoto, and M. Kobayashi, "Prevalence of albuminuria and renal insufficiency and associated clinical factors in type 2 diabetes: the Japan Diabetes Clinical Data Management study (JDDM15)," *Nephrology Dialysis Transplantation*, vol. 24, no. 4, pp. 1212–1219, 2009.

[29] G. Penno, A. Solini, E. Bonora et al., "Clinical significance of nonalbuminuric renal impairment in type 2 diabetes," *Journal of Hypertension*, vol. 29, no. 9, pp. 1802–1809, 2011.

[30] V. Rigalleau, C. Lasseur, C. Raffaitin et al., "Normoalbuminuric renal-insufficient diabetic patients: a lower-risk group," *Diabetes Care*, vol. 30, no. 8, pp. 2034–2039, 2007.

3

CCL2 Serum Levels and Adiposity Are Associated with the Polymorphic Phenotypes -2518A on CCL2 and 64ILE on CCR2 in a Mexican Population with Insulin Resistance

Milton-Omar Guzmán-Ornelas,[1,2] Marcelo Heron Petri,[1,3] Mónica Vázquez-Del Mercado,[1,4,5] Efraín Chavarría-Ávila,[1,2,6] Fernanda-Isadora Corona-Meraz,[1,2] Sandra-Luz Ruíz-Quezada,[2,7] Perla-Monserrat Madrigal-Ruíz,[1,2,4] Jorge Castro-Albarrán,[2] Flavio Sandoval-García,[1] and Rosa-Elena Navarro-Hernández[1,2,4,7]

[1] *Instituto de Investigación en Reumatología y del Sistema Musculo Esquelético, Centro Universitario de Ciencias de la Salud, Universidad de Guadalajara, Sierra Mojada No. 950, Colonia Independencia, 44340 Guadalajara, JAL, Mexico*
[2] *UDG-CA-701, Grupo de Investigación Inmunometabolismo en Enfermedades Emergentes (GIIEE), Centro Universitario de Ciencias de la Salud, Universidad de Guadalajara, Sierra Mojada No. 950, Colonia Independencia, 44340 Guadalajara, JAL, Mexico*
[3] *Translational Cardiology, Center for Molecular Medicine, Department of Medicine, Karolinska Institutet, L8:03, 17176 Stockholm, Sweden*
[4] *Departamento de Biología Molecular y Genómica, Centro Universitario de Ciencias de la Salud, Universidad de Guadalajara, Sierra Mojada No. 950, Colonia Independencia, 44340 Guadalajara, JAL, Mexico*
[5] *Servicio de Reumatología, División de Medicina Interna, Hospital Civil "Dr. Juan I. Menchaca", Universidad de Guadalajara, Salvador de Quevedo y Zubieta No. 750, 44340 Guadalajara, JAL, Mexico*
[6] *Departamento de Disciplinas Filosófico, Metodológico e Instrumentales, Centro Universitario de Ciencias de la Salud, Universidad de Guadalajara, Sierra Mojada No. 950, Colonia Independencia, 44340 Guadalajara, JAL, Mexico*
[7] *Departamento de Farmacobiología, Centro Universitario de Ciencias Exactas e Ingenierías, Universidad de Guadalajara, Boulevard Marcelino García Barragán No. 1421, 44430 Guadalajara, JAL, Mexico*

Correspondence should be addressed to Rosa-Elena Navarro-Hernández; rosa_elena_n@hotmail.com

Academic Editor: Michal Ciborowski

Genetic susceptibility has been described in insulin resistance (IR). Chemokine (C-C motif) ligand-2 (CCL2) is overexpressed in white adipose tissue and is the ligand of C-C motif receptor-2 (CCR2). The *CCL2* G-2518A polymorphism is known to regulate gene expression, whereas the physiological effects of the *CCR2*Val64Ile polymorphism are unknown. The aim of the study is to investigate the relationship between these polymorphisms with soluble CCL2 levels (sCCL2), metabolic markers, and adiposity. In a cross-sectional study we included 380 Mexican-Mestizo individuals, classified with IR according to Stern criteria. Polymorphism was identified using PCR-RFLP/sequence-specific primers. Anthropometrics and metabolic markers were measured by routine methods and adipokines and sCCL2 by ELISA. The CCL2 polymorphism was associated with IR (polymorphic *A*+ phenotype frequencies were 70.9%, 82.6%, in individuals with and without IR, resp.). Phenotype carriers CCL2 (*A*+) displayed lower body mass and fat indexes, insulin and HOMA-IR, and higher adiponectin levels. Individuals with IR presented higher sCCL2 compared to individuals without IR and was associated with CCR2 (*Ile*+) phenotype. The double-polymorphic phenotype carriers (*A*+/*Ile*+) exhibited higher sCCL2 than double-wild-type phenotype carriers (*A*−/*Ile*−). The present findings suggest that sCCL2 production possibly will be associated with the adiposity and polymorphic phenotypes of *CCL2* and *CCR2*, in Mexican-Mestizos with IR.

1. Introduction

The insulin resistance (IR) presents many subclinical manifestations, characterized by alterations in lipids and carbohydrates metabolism at different levels. Most of these changes is due to a low-grade systemic chronic inflammation [1, 2]. Adipose tissue is the primary anatomical site where the disease takes place. In early stage, this tissue became inflamed with the following pathological mechanism: first, monocytes migrate to adipose tissue, these cells express high levels of C-C motif receptor 2 (CCR2) and release monocyte chemoattractant protein-1 (MCP-1), also known as chemokine (C-C motif) ligand 2 (CCL2). This chemokine can promote further local inflammation and/or acts in paracrine way. The signaling through CCR2 may polarize the monocytes to M1 macrophages; these cells present a proinflammatory profile. Nevertheless, CCL2-CCR2 interaction is known to regulate continuous migration of monocytes to adipose tissue [3–5].

CCL2 is produced in soluble form by monocytes and macrophages and binds with high affinity to the CCR2 receptor. The later one is constitutively expressed in monocytes and its levels decrease as it differentiate into macrophages [4].

The human *CCL2* gene is located on chromosome 17q11.2 [6, 7]. It has two remote kappa B binding sites known as A1 (-2640/-2632) and A2 (−2612/−2603) that regulates the transcription of *CCL2* gene. Whereas the *CCR2* belongs to the family of seven transmembrane-spanning receptors that are coupled to heterotrimeric G proteins, the gene is located on the chromosome 3p21 within a cluster of chemokine receptor genes [7, 8].

The IR is considered a multifactor and polygenic disease; nevertheless, it has not determine the environmental and genetic factors contribution. In this context the study of candidate genes to make a contribution in clarifying this point is important. It has been reported that single nucleotide polymorphisms (SNP) in *CCL2* and *CCR2* are related with IR, G-2518A (rs 1024611), and Val64Ile (rs 17998649), respectively. The SNP of *CCL2* is located at 85 base pairs (bp) of remote kappa B binding site A2, while in *CCR2* gene, the SNP is conservative and the amino acid change (Val>Ile) takes place in the first transmembrane domain. This change decreases the affinity CCL2 binding, since the join of CCL2 with CCR2 receptor is through the second transmembrane domain [9–11].

Clinical phenotype has been described with these polymorphisms; type 2 diabetes mellitus (T2DM), cardiometabolic risk factors, obesity indexes, and insulin secretion association were found [12]. Interestingly, another study failed to show effect of this polymorphism in adipokines levels in patients with essential hypertension and T2DM [13]. Studies in animal models were performed to demonstrate the functional effect of these polymorphisms, but the results were not conclusive [14].

With this in mind, the aim of this study is to describe the presence of polymorphism of *CCL2* and *CCR2* in a population with IR, compared to healthy subjects, and to elucidate the clinical/metabolic features that these polymorphisms may present.

2. Material and Methods

2.1. Subjects' Assessment. In this cross-sectional study, a total of 380 nonrelated Mexican-Mestizos (i.e., an individual that were born in Mexico, with a Spanish last name and a family history of Mexican ancestors for at least three generations), and aged 20–69 years, were recruited from population of Western Mexico and classified according to Stern criteria in two groups: group 1 individuals with IR, if any of the following conditions were met: HOMA-IR > 4.65 or BMI > 27.5 kg/m^2 and HOMA-IR > 3.6, and group 2 individuals without IR, therefore negative for those who did not meet the above conditions (i.e., HOMA-IR ≤ 4.65 or BMI ≤ 27.5 kg/m^2 and HOMA-IR ≤ 3.60) [15]. Inclusion criteria for the study were considered as follows: individuals who at the time of the study did not present glucose intolerance, infectious diseases, hypertension, history of cardiovascular disease, malignancy, and renal and metabolic diseases such as T2DM. The subjects were questioned and denied any medication or weight change at least 3 weeks.

2.2. Ethics Conduct. Before enrolment, participants were informed about the study and signed a consent form following the Helsinki declaration guidelines, and the institutional (Guadalajara University) review boards' committees ensured appropriate ethical and biosecurity conduct [16].

2.3. Medical History and Physical Examination. All individuals who fulfil inclusion criteria were clinically evaluated by a physician who performed a complete medical history and assessment of general health status and vital signs were included: blood pressure (executed 3 times with the subject in the sitting position and relaxing for 15 minutes before the measurement), heart and respiratory rate, and body temperature.

2.4. Body Fat Storage Measurements. We evaluated the following body measurements: height, measured to the nearest 1 mm by using a stadiometer (Seca GmbH & Co. KG. Hamburg, Germany), weight, body mass index (BMI), and total body fat, determined by using bioelectrical impedance analysis (TANITA TBF304.Tokio, JPN) to the nearest 0.1 kg. Waist and hip circumferences where measured to the nearest 0.1 cm by using an anthropometric fiberglass tape (GULICK length 0–180 cm precision ±1 mm; USA) following the procedures recommended by the anthropometric indicators measurement guide [17, 18]. We calculated the waist-hip ratio [19] [WHR = waist (cm)/hip (cm)], body fat ratio [BFR = body fat mass (kg)/height^2 (m^2)], and waist to height ratio [WHtR = waist (cm)/height (cm)], as indicators of adiposity [20, 21].

2.5. Laboratory Techniques and Procedures. Individuals included in the study were fasting 12 hours before the blood samples were taken, after allowing them to clot at room temperature; then the blood was centrifuged at 1509 RCF (Rotanta 460R, Andreas Hettich GmbH & Co. KG) for 10 minutes at 20°C. Serum was collected and stored at −86°C until further analysis. We quantified the serum concentration of C reactive protein (CRP, with a limit of detection of 0.15 mg/L), basal glucose, lipid profile that included triglycerides, total cholesterol, HDLc, LDLc, and VLDLc (high, low, and very low density lipoprotein cholesterol, resp.), and apolipoproteins A1 and B (Apo-A1 and Apo-B, Randox Laboratories 55 Diamond Road, Crumlin Co. Antrim, Northern Ireland UK). By using commercial enzyme-linked immunoabsorbent assays (ELISA) were determined soluble levels of insulin (sensitivity of 0.399 μUI/mL), sCCL2 (limit of detection of 2.3 pg/mL), sAdiponectin (limit of detection 0.019 ng/mL) (ALPCO Diagnostics 26-G Keewaydin Drive, Salem, NH), and sResistin (sensitivity 0.026 ng/mL, R&D Systems Inc., Minneapolis, MN, USA).

2.6. SNPs Analysis. Genomic DNA was obtained from total blood using a standard protocol for extraction with the modified Miller method as described previously [22] and was stored at −20°C until being used for genotyping. For each gene studied, polymorphic regions were amplified by polymerase chain reaction (PCR) method as described previously [23, 24].

To analyze the *CCR2* Val64Ile SNP was determined using sequence-specific primers (SSP): forward, Val 5′-TGGGCA-ACATGCTGGTCG-3′, Ile 5′-TGGGCAACATGCTGG-TCA-3′, and reverse: 5′-TGGAAAATAAGGGCCACA-GAC-3′ annealing 62°C, PCR product 413 bp [11], and *CCL2* G-2518A SNP, forward primer 5′-TCACGCCAGCACTGA-CCTCC-3′, and reverse: 5′-ACTTCCCAGCTTTGCTGG-CTGAG-3′ with annealing temperature 56°C, PCR product 250 bp.

The PCR were performed in a 25 μL total volume (mixture with 100 ng of DNA, 2 nM of each primer, 0.20 mM of each dNTP, 0.25 U *Taq* polymerase, and 1x PCR buffer) and 1.5 or 3.0 mM of $MgCl_2$ for *CCL2* or *CCR2*, respectively.

To determine *CCL2* genotypes a PCR was performed and then a digestion of obtained products with *PVU II* restriction enzyme. The lengths of fragments observed were as follows: 175 and 75 bp (allele A) and 250 bp (allele G). Electrophoresis was done at a constant voltage of 180 V on 6% polyacrylamide gels stained with silver nitrate. For quality control, a blank and samples previously confirmed as positive for each genotype were used as controls. To ensure the accuracy of genotype data, we used internal controls and repetitive experiments. In addition, both polymorphisms were identified in duplicate by two different analysts. The genotyping success rate was 100%.

2.7. Statistical Analysis. Data were analyzed with the Statistics program SPSS v21 (IBM Inc., Chicago, IL, USA) and GraphPad Prism v6.01 (2014 Inc. 2236 Beach Avenue Jolla, CA 92037). Results are given as mean ± SD or median with 25, 75 percentiles or percentages based on normal distribution. The data distribution of clinical and laboratory variables of the study group was evaluated with *Z* Kolmogorov-Smirnov test, and we performed parametric and nonparametric test, as appropriate. The most important variables were adjusted by gender and age with an ANCOVA analysis. About these results we performed multifactorial analysis for the most important variables. The clinical and laboratory characteristics of the study group were performed with the unpaired Student's t-test or Mann-Whitney U test, and to compare quantitative data in four groups, a one-way ANOVA and post hoc Tukey test were used.

Data from serum concentrations of adipokines, the laboratorial assessment, and disease variables were subjected to Pearson or Spearman correlation tests. The Hardy-Weinberg equilibrium text for individual *loci* was performed with http://ihg.gsf.de/cgi-bin/hw/hwa1.pl. Contingency tables (2 × 2 and 2 × 3) with χ^2 trend test or Fisher exact test, as appropriate, were used for testing the differences of genotype distribution and allele frequencies between study groups. Two genetic models were used for these analyses: (1) the dominant model where each SNP was modeled categorically and separated into three categories, one for each genotype, and (2) the phenotype model, where each SNP was modeled into two categories, with two genotypes combined into one category (polymorphic homozygotes plus heterozygotes), choosing one genotype (homozygotes wild type) as the reference group. A two-tailed P value less than 0.05 was considered statistically significant.

3. Results

3.1. Adiposity Is Associated with Metabolic Markers. Anthropometrics characteristics and metabolic markers of the subjects included in this study split by IR Stern classification are shown in Table 1. The study group included 380 Mexican-Mestizo individuals of which 237 (62%) were women, they were classified without IR or with IR, ANCOVA was performed, adjusted for sex and age, and no differences were observed (data not showed). Twenty-one percent has been classified with obesity and 32% with IR. Sixty-five percent of individuals, included in the study, were determined with excess body fat according to the Deurenberg criteria [21], and 31% had dyslipidemic profile (data no shown). A positive correlation of soluble levels of sCCL2, adipokines, metabolic markers, and lipid profile (except HDLc, LDLc, and Apo-A1) was observed along body fat storage (Table 2).

3.2. Individuals with IR Presented Inflammatory State. According to IR classification, individuals with IR displayed higher soluble levels of CCL2, resistin, and CRP and lower levels of adiponectin than individuals without IR (Figure 1). Soluble levels of CCL2, CRP, sResistin, and metabolic markers correlated positively with body adiposity, whereas levels of soluble adiponectin correlated negatively (Table 2).

3.3. CCL2 Polymorphism Is Associated with IR. All genotype frequencies were in Hardy-Weinberg equilibrium.

TABLE 1: Anthropometric characteristics and metabolic markers in individuals included in the study.

Measurement	Study group: Individuals without IR	Study group: Individuals with IR	P
n (%)	270 (68)	110 (32)	
Age (years)	35 ± 14	34 ± 14	NS
Height (cm)	163.8 ± 5.7	165.7 ± 1.1	NS
Weight (kg)	**68.7 ± 13.2**	**79.4 ± 16.3**	**<0.001***
BMI (kg/m^2)	**24.9 (22.6–28.9)**	**28.6 (24.4–31.7)**	**<0.001⁺**
Body fat mass (kg)	**20.1 ± 9.2**	**25.9 ± 11.3**	**<0.001***
Total body fat mass (%)	**28.8 ± 9.4**	**32.80 ± 9.2**	**<0.001***
BFR (kg/m^2)	**7.03 (5.24–9.40)**	**9.40 (6.37–12.20)**	**0.001⁺**
Waist circumference (cm)	**86.5 (77.1–93.1)**	**95.0 (83–103)**	**<0.001⁺**
Hip circumference (cm)	**99.5 (95–105.9)**	**104 (99–110)**	**0.002⁺**
WHR	0.854 (0.68–1.17)	0.866 (0.70–1.28)	NS⁺
WHtR	**0.533 ± 0.076**	**0.568 ± 0.085**	**<0.001***
Glucose (mg/dL)	**89 ± 10**	**98 ± 18**	**<0.001***
Insulin (μUI/mL)	**8.6 ± 3.5**	**35.2 ± 32.5**	**<0.001***
HOMA-IR	**1.86 (1.34–2.58)**	**6.05 (4.40–9.03)**	**<0.001⁺**
Triglycerides (mg/dL)	**134 ± 83**	**162 ± 95**	**0.005***
Total cholesterol (mg/dL)	184 ± 40	185 ± 34	NS
HDLc (mg/dL)	39.5 ± 15.1	37.6 ± 14.9	NS
LDLc (mg/dL)	111 ± 36	110 ± 31	NS
VLDLc (mg/dL)	**26 ± 16**	**32 ± 19**	**0.005***
Apo-A1 (mg/dL)	114 ± 25	117 ± 27	NS
Apo-B (mg/dL)	111 ± 32	117 ± 32	NS

$n = 380$. Data are presented as mean ± standard deviation and median (25–75 percentiles). *Student's t-test and ⁺Mann-Whitney U test with P significantly, comparing the groups: individuals with IR versus individuals without IR. IR: insulin resistance; BMI: body mass index; WHR: waist to hip ratio; WHtR: waist to height ratio; BFR: body fat ratio; HOMA-IR: homeostasis model assessment-insulin resistance; HDLc, LDLc, and VLDLc: high, low, and very low density lipoprotein cholesterol, respectively; Apo: apolipoprotein.

TABLE 2: Correlations soluble levels of adipokines and metabolic markers with body adiposity.

Measurements	*Weight (kg)	⁺BMI (kg/m^2)	⁺Body fat mass (%)	⁺BFR (kg/m^2)	⁺WC (cm)	⁺WHtR
	% Correlation					
sCCL2 (pg/mL)	20.1	29.4	21.8	29.3	25.0	24.8
CRP (mg/L)	30.6	52.7	52.8	53.0	44.8	52.8
sAdiponectin (ng/mL)	−34.7	−25.0	−17.5	−25.1	−23.7	−17.2
sResistin (ng/mL)	43.3	27.1	30.1	27.3	32.5	24.9
Glucose (mg/dL)	22.7	38.1	24.0	35.4	32.5	35.6
Insulin (μUI/mL)	23.1	39.8	29.9	40.1	27.1	26.4
HOMA-IR	25.0	43.6	32.4	43.5	30.5	30.6
Triglycerides (mg/dL)	22.5	34.9	16.9	33.7	40.1	36.0
Total cholesterol (mg/dL)	19.5	32.2	27.3	30.8	37.5	39.6
VLDLc (mg/dL)	22.4	34.2	16.4	33.0	39.6	35.4
Apo-B (mg/dL)	21.0	34.5	17.5	34.3	46.7	44.3

$n = 380$. BMI: body mass index; BFR: body fat ratio; WC: waist circumference; WHtR: waist to height ratio; CCL2: chemokine (C-C motif) ligand 2; HOMA-IR: homeostasis model assessment-insulin resistance; CRP: C reactive protein; VLDLc: very low density lipoprotein cholesterol; Apo: apolipoprotein. Significant differences: $P < 0.05$, *Pearson or ⁺Spearman correlations test.

The individuals without IR presented a higher frequency of the phenotype $A+$ of the *CCL2* polymorphism, while phenotype $A-$ is more common in the individuals with IR. These differences were also observed in genotype and allele frequencies (Table 3). Higher levels of total adiponectin as well as a parallel decrease in insulin levels and HOMA-IR index were associated with $A+$ phenotype carriers (Figure 2), as long as phenotype $A+$ was associated with low measures of BMI and BFR (Table 4).

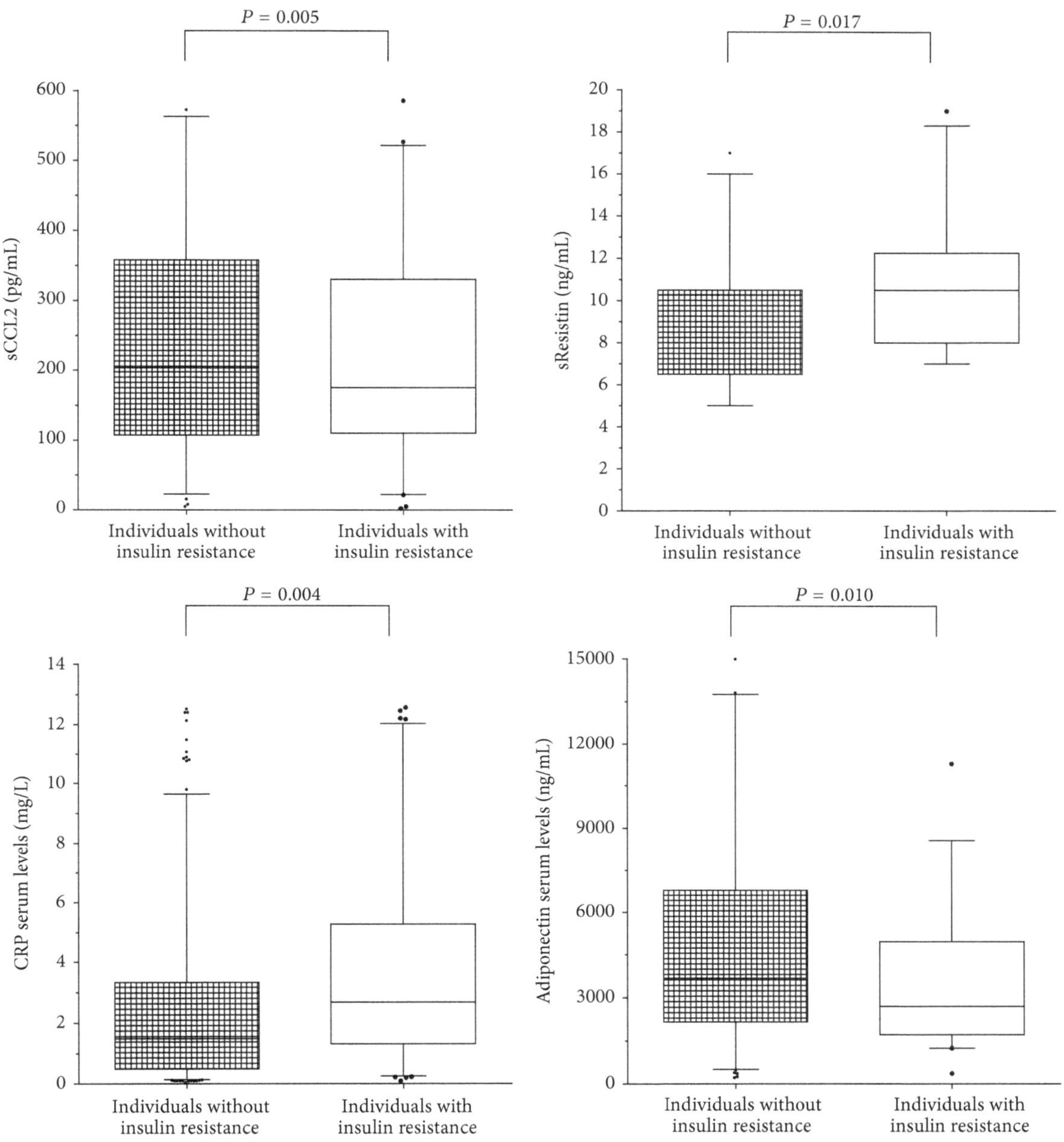

FIGURE 1: Soluble levels of adipokines and CRP by study group. $n = 380$. Student's t-test with P significantly, comparing the groups: individuals with IR versus individuals without IR.

3.4. CCR2 Polymorphism Was Not Associated with IR but Promoted Clinical Features of IR. None of the *CCR2* variants had an association with IR (Table 3). The detailed analysis showed association of phenotype *Ile+* with high BMI, levels of glucose and lipids (Table 4). The same as *CCL2 A+* phenotype, in *CCR2 Ile+* carriers presented higher levels of CCL2 compared to *Ile−* phenotypes (Figure 2).

3.5. A+ Phenotype of CCL2 and Ile+ of CCR2 Are Associated with High Levels of Circulating CCL2. No metabolic profile explored in this study was associated with A+ phenotype (Table 4). However, significant phenotype-by-phenotype association was observed between the *CCL2*-2518A allele and the *CCR2* 64Ile allele; carriers of the *CCR2* phenotype 64Ile+ who at the same time also were phenotype A+ of *CCL2* (polymorphic genotypes for the both polymorphisms) presented higher levels of soluble CCL2, than any other phenotype combinations (Figure 3).

4. Discussion

The IR is a disease of multifactorial etiology product of the interaction between the genetic component and the environment, epidemiological data describes IR as an emerging disease with epidemic proportions [19, 25, 26]. In prior information it has been postulated that there may exist

TABLE 3: Distribution of *CCL2* (G-2518A) and *CCR2* (Val64Ile) gene polymorphism in Mexican-Mestizo population.

Study group	Genotype, n (%)			Phenotype, n (%)		Allele, n (%)	
				CCL2 G-2518A			
	G/G	G/A	A/A	A+	A−	G	A
Individuals without IR	47 (17.4)	135 (50.0)	88 (32.6)	223 (82.6)	47 (17.4)	229 (42.4)	311 (57.6)
Individuals with IR	32 (29.0)	51 (46.4)	27 (24.6)	78 (70.9)	32 (29.1)	115 (52.3)	105 (47.7)
*P		**0.01378**		**0.01131**		**0.01321**	
Study group	Genotype, n (%)			Phenotype, n (%)		Allele, n (%)	
				CCR2 Val64Ile			
	Val/Val	Val/Ile	Ile/Ile	Ile+	Ile−	Val	Ile
Individuals without IR	173 (64.1)	82 (30.4)	15 (5.5)	97 (35.9)	173 (64.1)	428 (79.3)	112 (20.7)
Individuals with IR	67 (60.9)	37 (33.6)	6 (5.5)	43 (39.1)	67 (60.9)	171 (77.7)	49 (22.3)
*P		0.64924		0.94889		0.63925	

n = 380. IR: insulin resistance. *Significant differences: Pearson's goodness-of-fit test χ^2 or Fishers' exact test; G or Val: wild-type alleles; A+ phenotype: A/A plus G/A genotypes; Ile+ phenotype: Ile/Ile plus Ile/Val genotypes.

TABLE 4: Comparisons of body fat measurements and lipid profile between *CCL2* G-2518A and *CCR2* Val64Ile phenotype carriers.

Measurements	*CCL2* G-2518A			*CCR2* Val64Ile		
	Phenotype A+	Phenotype A−	P	Phenotype Ile+	Phenotype Ile−	P
n (%)	301 (79)	79 (21)		140 (37)	240 (63)	
Weight (kg)	72.0 ± 15.55	72.8 ± 13.56	NS	73.2 ± 14.82	71.5 ± 15.32	NS
BMI (kg/m^2)	**25.9 (22.9–29.1)**	**27.5 (24.3–29.65)**	**$^+$0.028**	**27.3 (23.8–29.7)**	**25.4 (23.0–28.9)**	**0.018$^+$**
Total body fat (%)	29.6 ± 9.81	31.7 ± 8.57	NS	31.2 ± 9.05	29.4 ± 9.85	NS
BFR (kg/m^2)	**7.31 (5.24–9.92)**	**8.25 (6.24–11.40)**	**$^+$0.039**	7.63 (5.57–10.90)	7.37 (5.31–9.93)	NS
Waist circumference (cm)	88.0 (78.4–98.0)	89.4 (79.3–96.5)	NS	89.1 (79.5–99.0)	88.1 (78.3–97.6)	NS
Glucose (mg/dL)	92 ± 12	93 ± 14	NS	**95 ± 13**	**91 ± 12**	**0.004***
Triglycerides (mg/dL)	142 ± 85.6	146 ± 94.2	NS	**156 ± 8.5**	**135 ± 5.0**	**0.039***
Total cholesterol (mg/dL)	181 ± 40.1	185 ± 34.3	NS	**190 ± 43.7**	**180 ± 35.5**	**0.031***
HDLc (mg/dL)	39 ± 14.8	37 ± 15.8	NS	38 ± 13.6	38 ± 15.8	NS
LDLc (mg/dL)	111 ± 35.6	109 ± 30.4	NS	114 ± 39.1	108 ± 31.2	NS
VLDLc (mg/dL)	28 ± 16.9	29 ± 18.8	NS	**31 ± 20.1**	**26 ± 15.3**	**0.032***
Apo-A1 (mg/dL)	114 ± 25.1	121 ± 29.1	NS	117 ± 24.4	114 ± 27.1	NS
Apo-B (mg/dL)	112 ± 30.0	121 ± 41.5	NS	**119 ± 36.8**	**109 ± 27.8**	**0.045***

n = 380. BMI: body mass index; BFR: body fat ratio; HDLc, LDLc, and VLDLc: high, low, and very low density lipoprotein cholesterol, respectively; Apo: apolipoprotein. A− or Ile−: wild-type phenotypes; polymorphic A+ phenotype (A/A plus G/A genotypes); polymorphic Ile+ phenotype (Ile/Ile plus Val/Ile genotypes). Data are presented as mean ± standard deviation and median (25–75 percentiles). *Student's t-test and $^+$Mann-Whitney U test with P significantly, comparing the polymorphic phenotype carriers versus wild-type phenotypes carriers.

susceptibility genes involved in adipogenesis and energy metabolism [27, 28]; in the current study we explored the distribution of polymorphisms G-2518A and Val64Ile of *CCL2* and *CCR2*, respectively, in individuals with IR.

In addition, the individuals' carriers of different genotypes according to gene dosage were evaluated on the possible association with CCL2 levels, metabolic markers, and adiposity within the population with IR.

In the present work 380 individuals, were classified with or without IR by Stern criteria and obesity by BMI WHO criteria. The frequencies found in IR and obesity, clinical data, and anthropometric measurements are consistent with previous reports in the Mexican population [26, 29].

There are several reasons why a certain obese phenotype possibly will not be equally expressed (e.g., different physical activity levels among participants); however, the aim of the study was to investigate the relationship between the polymorphisms of *CCL2* and *CCR2* with CCL2 soluble levels, metabolic markers, and adiposity (like indicator of body fat status, absolute and/or relative) measured by BIA. Most studies report that the impedance method is reliable and valid. Baumgartner's contribution reviews the assumptions, applicability, equipment, measurement procedure, precision, and accuracy of the BIA method and determined that they were highly recommended [30–32]. Unfortunately we did not evaluate the fat distribution in study subjects; hence, we were not able to include a body fat distribution analysis.

In this set, clinic profile and the ratio of prevalence of IR, presented in the present study, suggest that IR is a complex disease, meaning that different phenotypes are observed with various clinical stages during the development of the pathogenic process. It has been postulated that in

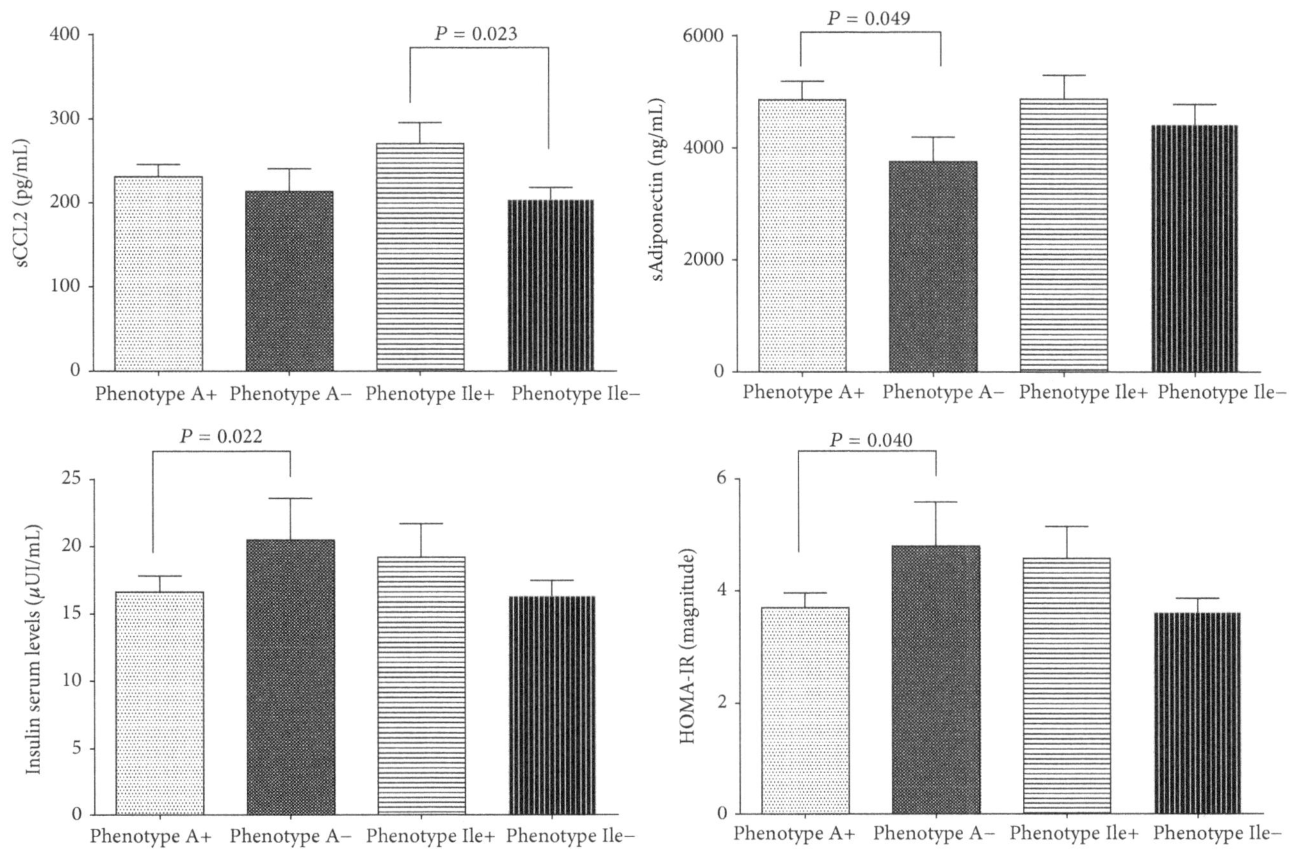

FIGURE 2: Soluble levels of adipokines, insulin, and HOMA-IR by *CCL2* G-2518A and *CCR2* Val64Ile phenotype carriers. $n = 380$. A+ phenotype: A/A plus G/A genotypes; Ile+ phenotype: Ile/Ile plus Val/Ile genotypes. Student's t-test with P significantly, comparing the polymorphic phenotype carriers versus wild-type phenotypes carriers.

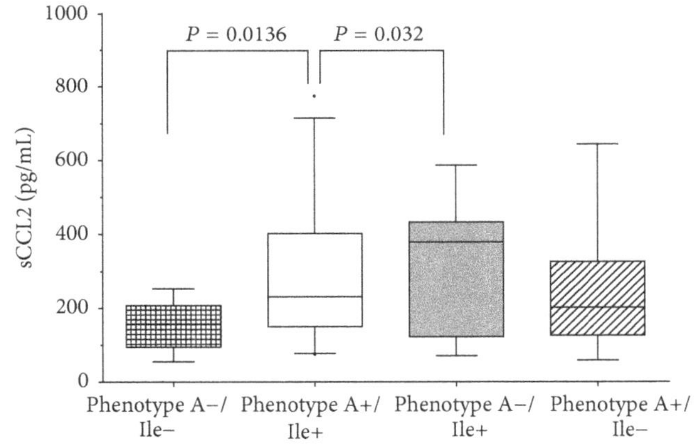

FIGURE 3: Soluble levels of CCL2 by phenotypes. Phenotype A−/Ile− (genotypes GG/ValVal) $n = 48$; phenotype A+/Ile+ (genotypes AA plus GA/ValIle plus IleIle) $n = 108$; phenotype A−/Ile+ (genotypes GG/ValIle plus IleIle) $n = 32$; phenotype A+/Ile− (genotypes AA plus GA/ValVal) $n = 192$. One way ANOVA and Tukey's post hoc test with P significantly, comparing the double-polymorphic phenotype carriers, (A+/Ile+) versus double-wild-type phenotype carriers (A−/Ile−).

course of the natural history of the IR, the hallmark is a low-grade subclinical inflammatory process, in which circulating monocytes infiltrate to adipose tissue, in a redundant manner, and polarize to M1 macrophages, becoming the main producers of chemokines and their receptors [33].

Two important observations lead this study to supporting that adiposity is associated with metabolic markers, in IR development. First, increased adiposity indicators and triglyceride levels were observed, and secondly no differences were found in other components of lipid profile. The first results are in agreement with previous studies [21, 33–35] that was attributed to the presence of obesity; in this case the expansion and accumulation of fat promotes the progress to IR. The second point given by the present study can be explained by the fact that IR is just component during the development of a mayor disease, since dyslipidemia is a later event, that could generate metabolic syndrome [36].

We observe that IR individuals presented higher inflammatory state, due to increased CCL2 levels in contrast to individuals without IR. These results can be explained by the increased levels of expression of adipokines, chemokines, and proinflammatory cytokines associated with a parallel increase in the number, macrophages in the adipose tissue. The later ones, mainly macrophages with M1 phenotype, are crucial in IR, based on the fact that these cells are the important source of proinflammatory markers: TNF-α, IL-6, and CRP [2, 33, 37].

Alongside, in the individuals with IR was confirmed the presence of a low-grade inflammatory process represented by the increased levels of sResistin, CRP, and the decreased levels of total adiponectin and the correlation of them with adiposity status, parallel to the increase in BMI, BFR, and metabolic markers.

The importance of the present results lies in the biological relationship that exists between IR and obesity for the development of other diseases, for instance, metabolic syndrome. Insulin has the following functions: on one side, it promotes synthesis of insulin-like growth factor 1, which correlates with fat accumulation, and increase of white adipose tissue; on other side, it is the leader in the deregulations in the secretion of adipokines and metabolic markers that has been associated with certain types of cancer and other chronic diseases such as T2DM [1, 4, 6, 38].

The main pathological mechanism that connect the increase of adipose tissue with IR is the disfunction of the immune system and the establishment of a low-grade subclinical systemic chronic inflammation state, as a result of increased adiposity. This dysregulation of the immune system can be explained on two mechanisms: first, the adipose tissue in obese subjects has an increased amount of infiltrated macrophages who present an M1 phenotype and have an increase in the expression of 4 retinol binding protein (RPB4); and second, it has been found that high concentrations of fatty acids and RPB4 induce the expression of TNF-α and the signaling mediated by the toll-like receptor 4 [1, 27].

In this context, the inflammatory process in IR is an underlying clinical sign in the course of the disease and is identified by an increase in levels of inflammatory markers, as well as deregulation in the production of adipokines; in this respect there is evidence based on animal model studies and in humans, in which the important role of white adipose tissue is demonstrated in the maintenance of an inflammatory response associated with the development of IR [6].

There are numerous studies that have found interactions between polymorphisms and development of diseases such as metabolic syndrome. Due to the link of inflammation with development of IR, numerous genes have been studied [2, 28]. The chemokine CCL2 and their CCR2 receptor have been studied in recent years because of their involvement in the recruitment of macrophages to adipose tissue and subsequent differentiation into proinflammatory M1 phenotype [27, 33, 39].

The polymorphism G-2518A, in *CCL2* gene, was identified as a G to A transition; this change is near to a response site of NF-kB and has been speculated that increases affinity to its ligand; this results in increased levels of CCL2 in the bloodstream and further recruitment of macrophages to adipose tissue compared to those individuals exhibiting wild-type allele. Concerning polymorphism in *CCR2*, Val64Ile, is a transition G to A at position 190 of *CCR2*, changing valine codon (GTC) to isoleucine (ATC) at position 64, a conservative change of neutral nonpolar amino acids. This change makes the CCR2A isoform more stable and increases its half-life but does not affect the stability of the isoform CCR2B [1, 40].

On the stage of genetic diversity between populations, the reported frequencies for polymorphic alleles -2518A and 64Ile ranging from 39.1% to 83.2% and 9.5% to 25.6%, respectively, with differences with the frequencies reported in this study (Tables 5(a) and 5(b)), show that wild-type allele changes in some populations, such as Asiatic. In the present study the allele polymorphic frequencies are similar to those reported in Mexican-Mestizos by González-Enríquez et al. and different from Vázquez-Lavista et al. [41, 42].

We found differences when comparing frequencies of alleles of our Mexican population with other populations of different nations, for example, the Asiatic, Caucasian European, or American populations, with a different genetic background, which is explained by the distribution of alleles as result of their anthropological relationships. Since the conquest by the Spanish, European genetics was introduced on the natures, over the centuries. Hence, individuals included in the present study were not pure endogenous Mexican population. Therefore the differences in genotype distribution with other Mexican populations may be because of the fact that in our study group participants were characterized as Mexican-Mestizos of Western Mexico (Tables 5(a) and 5(b)).

In this study group, *CCL2* polymorphism was associated with IR, according to the results showing differences in the distribution of frequencies of genotypes, phenotypes, and alleles, with a higher contribution of the A+ phenotype than A− phenotype for the presence of IR. A+ phenotype was associated with higher levels of total sAdiponectin and lower levels of insulin and HOMA-IR magnitude, while a decrease was shown in BMI and BFR. The opposite was observed for individuals carrying of polymorphic phenotype Ile+; they had an increase in lipid profile; these results show influence of both polymorphisms in the accumulation of body fat and its relation to the metabolic status of individuals.

This can be explained because this is the main tissue involved in the production of adipokines and increases its volume in the presence of a proinflammatory environment [5, 33]. Previous studies have demonstrated the interference of proinflammatory cytokine in the signaling pathway of insulin receptor [27]. Parallel to this stage, we observed increased levels of glucose in individuals with phenotype Ile+ which indicates involvement of this polymorphism in the establishment of IR.

The adiposity status shown in the individuals of this study regarding the polymorphisms in *CCL2* and *CCR2* and its association with metabolic and inflammatory markers, and levels of adipokines have not been previously described for Mexican-Mestizo population.

Among the most important results of this study are that A+ phenotype of *CCL2* and Ile+ of *CCR2* carriers are associated with higher levels of circulating CCL2; this difference is attributed to the fact that this variant generates a more stable form of the receptor CCR2 membrane which has a longer half-life, allowing for longer signaling that in people with wild-type polymorphism variant [40].

TABLE 5: (a) Distribution of G-2518A polymorphism in *CCL2* gene in other populations. (b) Distribution of Val64Ile polymorphism in *CCR2* gene in other populations.

(a)

Author	Population	*n*	G	A	G/G	A/G	A/A	*P*
The present study	**Mexican-Mestizo**	**380**	**45.2**	**54.6**	**20.7**	**48.9**	**30.3**	—
Vázquez-Lavista et al. [41]	Mexican-Mestizo	126	57.5	42.5	29.4	56.3	14.3	**<0.001**
González-Enríquez et al. [42]	Mexican-Mestizo	21	52.4	47.6	27.0	50.0	23.0	0.370
Bektas-Kayhan et al. [24]	Caucasian	140	16.8	83.2	0.8	32.1	67.1	**<0.001**
Kruszyna et al. [43]	Caucasian	323	29.9	70.1	7.4	44.9	47.7	**<0.001**
Kucukgergin et al. [44]	Caucasian	197	30.2	69.8	9.1	42.1	48.7	**<0.001**
Kouyama et al. [13]	Asian	361	34.6	65.4	—	—	—	—
Singh et al. [7]	Asian	200	35.3	64.7	11.0	48.5	40.5	**<0.001**
Mandal et al. [45]	Asian	390	37.2	62.8	13.2	48.0	38.8	**0.001**
Chen et al. [23]	Asian	344	51.7	48.3	26.7	50.0	23.3	**0.015**
Wu et al. [46]	Asian	253	60.1	39.1	34.8	52.2	13.0	**<0.001**

Pearson's goodness-of-fit test χ^2 or Fishers' exact test with *P* significantly, comparing alleles and/or genotypes polymorphism distribution in Mexican-Mestizos population in this study versus distribution in other populations. G wild-type allele, A polymorphic allele.

(b)

Author	Population	*n*	Val	Ile	Val/Val	Val/Ile	Ile/Ile	*P*
The present study	**Mexican-Mestizo**	**380**	**78.8**	**21.2**	**63.2**	**31.3**	**5.5**	—
Vázquez-Lavista et al. [41]	Mexican-Mestizo	126	75.8	24.2	58.7	34.1	7.2	0.330
González-Enríquez et al. [42]	Mexican-Mestizo	21	90.5	9.5	82.6	17.3	0	**0.006**
Bektas-Kayhan et al. [24]	Caucasians	140	88.5	11.42	80.0	17.1	2.9	**<0.001**
Kucukgergin et al. [44]	Caucasians	197	89.6	10.4	80.7	17.8	1.5	**<0.001**
González et al. [47]	Caucasians	280	90.0	10.0	80.0	19.0	1.0	**<0.001**
Mandal et al. [45]	Asian	390	74.4	25.6	54.8	39.2	6.0	**0.046**
Wu et al. [46]	Asian	253	80.6	19.4	64.4	32.4	3.2	0.438
Singh et al. [7]	Asian	200	80.5	19.5	63.0	35.0	2.0	0.501
Zandifar et al. [48]	Asian	100	87.5	12.5	75.0	25.0	0	**0.007**
Chen et al. [23]	Asian	344	89.1	10.9	80.2	17.7	2.1	**<0.001**

Pearson's goodness-of-fit test χ^2 or Fishers' exact test with *P* significantly, comparing alleles and/or genotypes polymorphism distribution in Mexican-Mestizos population in this study versus distribution in other populations. Val: wild-type allele; Ile: polymorphic allele.

Taking all results together, the present work shows new evidence that suggests that genetic factors contribute to the development of IR and this triggers pathobiological processes. These changes could influence the clinical course and severity of obesity-related diseases, such as IR. Therefore, the genetic load on individuals could play an important role in the genesis of diseases observed in obese subjects.

5. Conclusions

The most important results in the individuals of the present study are summarized as follows: association of adiposity with metabolic markers alongside with inflammatory state, *CCL2* polymorphism is associated with IR, while *CCR2* was associated with clinical features of IR besides it was seen that the individuals that had both polymorphic phenotypes had increased levels of CCL2.

These data suggests that the *CCL2*A+ phenotype could impact the reduced body fat storage, metabolic and healthy adipokine profile in Mexican-Mestizo individuals. The opposite, *CCR2*64Ile+ phenotype is associated with altered profile of metabolic markers and BMI. All this data suggests that the *CCL2* and *CCR2* polymorphisms and the signaling through this interactions could play a role in the metabolic changes associated with IR in Mexican-Mestizo population.

As a final remark we can conclude that an increase of CCL2 serum levels is associated with the polymorphic phenotypes (A+/Ile+) of the polymorphisms G-2518A in *CCL2* and Val64Ile in *CCR2* in individuals with insulin resistance of Mexican population.

Conflict of Interests

The authors declare that there is no conflict of interests regarding the publication of this paper.

Authors' Contribution

Milton-Omar Guzmán-Ornelas and Marcelo Heron Petri equally contributed to this work.

Acknowledgment

This work was supported by Grant no. PS-2009-552 to Rosa-Elena Navarro-Hernández of the State Council of Science and Technology (COECyTJal-University of Guadalajara).

References

[1] T. Ota, "Chemokine systems link obesity to insulin resistance," *Diabetes & Metabolism Journal*, vol. 37, no. 3, pp. 165–172, 2013.

[2] C. de Luca and J. M. Olefsky, "Inflammation and insulin resistance," *FEBS Letters*, vol. 582, no. 1, pp. 97–105, 2008.

[3] R. A. Bastarrachea, J. C. López-Alvarenga, V. E. Bolado-García, J. Téllez-Mendoza, H. Laviada-Molina, and A. G. Comuzzie, "Macrophages, inflammation, adipose tissue, obesity and insulin resistance," *Gaceta Médica de México*, vol. 143, no. 6, pp. 505–512, 2007.

[4] T. O'Connor, L. Borsig, and M. Heikenwalder, "CCL2-CCR2 signaling in disease pathogenesis," *Endocrine, Metabolic & Immune Disorders-Drug Targets*, vol. 15, no. 2, pp. 105–118, 2015.

[5] B. Gustafson, "Adipose tissue, inflammation and atherosclerosis," *Journal of Atherosclerosis and Thrombosis*, vol. 17, no. 4, pp. 332–341, 2010.

[6] A. Ueda, Y. Ishigatsubo, T. Okubo, and T. Yoshimura, "Transcriptional regulation of the human monocyte chemoattractant protein-1 gene: cooperation of two NF-κB sites and NF-κB/Rel subunit specificity," *Journal of Biological Chemistry*, vol. 272, no. 49, pp. 31092–31099, 1997.

[7] V. Singh, P. Srivastava, N. Srivastava, R. Kapoor, and R. D. Mittal, "Association of inflammatory chemokine gene CCL2I/D with bladder cancer risk in North Indian population," *Molecular Biology Reports*, vol. 39, no. 10, pp. 9827–9834, 2012.

[8] T. Yoshimura and J. J. Oppenheim, "Chemokine-like receptor 1 (CMKLRl) and chemokine (C-C motif) receptor-like 2 (CCRL2); two multifunctional receptors with unusual properties," *Experimental Cell Research*, vol. 317, no. 5, pp. 674–684, 2011.

[9] A. M. Valdes, M. L. Wolfe, E. J. O'Brien et al., "Val64Ile polymorphism in the C-C chemokine receptor 2 is associated with reduced coronary artery calcification," *Arteriosclerosis, Thrombosis, and Vascular Biology*, vol. 22, no. 11, pp. 1924–1928, 2002.

[10] J. Petrkova, Z. Cermakova, J. Drabek, J. Lukl, and M. Petrek, "CC chemokine receptor (CCR)2 polymorphism in Czech patients with myocardial infarction," *Immunology Letters*, vol. 88, no. 1, pp. 53–55, 2003.

[11] K. Chatterjee, C. Dandara, M. Hoffman, and A.-L. Williamson, "CCR2-V64I polymorphism is associated with increased risk of cervical cancer but not with HPV infection or pre-cancerous lesions in African women," *BMC Cancer*, vol. 10, article 278, 2010.

[12] E. Simeoni, M. M. Hoffmann, B. R. Winkelmann et al., "Association between the A-2518G polymorphism in the monocyte chemoattractant protein-1 gene and insulin resistance and Type 2 diabetes mellitus," *Diabetologia*, vol. 47, no. 9, pp. 1574–1580, 2004.

[13] K. Kouyama, K. Miyake, M. Zenibayashi et al., "Association of serum MCP-1 concentration and MCP-1 polymorphism with insulin resistance in Japanese individuals with obese type 2 diabetes," *Kobe Journal of Medical Sciences*, vol. 53, no. 6, pp. 345–354, 2007.

[14] W. R. Bolus, D. A. Gutierrez, A. J. Kennedy, E. K. Anderson-Baucum, and A. H. Hasty, "CCR2 deficiency leads to increased eosinophils, alternative macrophage activation, and type 2 cytokine expression in adipose tissue," *Journal of Leukocyte Biology*, vol. 98, no. 4, pp. 467–477, 2015.

[15] S. E. Stern, K. Williams, E. Ferrannini, R. A. DeFronzo, C. Bogardus, and M. P. Stern, "Identification of individuals with insulin resistance using routine clinical measurements," *Diabetes*, vol. 54, no. 2, pp. 333–339, 2005.

[16] DOF 07-02-1984, ú.r.D., Reglamento de la Ley General de Salud en Materia de Investigación para la Salud.

[17] R. Ness-Abramof and C. M. Apovian, "Waist circumference measurement in clinical practice," *Nutrition in Clinical Practice*, vol. 23, no. 4, pp. 397–404, 2008.

[18] WHO, "Physical status: the use and interpretation of anthropometry. Report of a WHO Expert Committee," World Health Organization Technical Report Series 854, WHO, 1995.

[19] World Health Organization, *Obesity: Preventing and Managing the Global Epidemic*, World Health Organization, Geneva, Switzerland, 1st edition, 2012.

[20] R. Fernandez-Vazquez, Á. Millán Romero, M. Á. Barbancho, and J. R. Alvero-Cruz, "Abdominal bioelectrical impedance analysis and anthropometry for predicting metabolic syndrome in middle aged men," *Nutrición Hospitalaria*, vol. 32, no. 3, pp. 1122–1130, 2015.

[21] P. Deurenberg, M. Yap, and W. A. van Staveren, "Body mass index and percent body fat: a meta analysis among different ethnic groups," *International Journal of Obesity*, vol. 22, no. 12, pp. 1164–1171, 1998.

[22] S. A. Miller, D. D. Dykes, and H. F. Polesky, "A simple salting out procedure for extracting DNA from human nucleated cells," *Nucleic Acids Research*, vol. 16, no. 3, p. 1215, 1988.

[23] M.-K. K. Chen, K.-T. Yeh, H.-L. Chiou, C.-W. Lin, T.-T. Chung, and S.-F. Yang, "CCR2-64I gene polymorphism increase susceptibility to oral cancer," *Oral Oncology*, vol. 47, no. 7, pp. 577–582, 2011.

[24] K. Bektas-Kayhan, M. Unur, Z. Boy-Metin, and B. Cakmakoglu, "MCP-1 and CCR2 gene variants in oral squamous cell carcinoma," *Oral Diseases*, vol. 18, no. 1, pp. 55–59, 2012.

[25] OMS, *Obesity: Preventing and Managing the Global Epidemic*, OMS, 1st edition, 2012.

[26] G. Olaiz-Fernández, J. Rivera, T. Shamah et al., *Encuesta Nacional de Salud y Nutrición 2006*, Instituto Nacional de Salud Pública, 2006.

[27] A. Rull, J. Camps, C. Alonso-Villaverde, and J. Joven, "Insulin resistance, inflammation, and obesity: role of monocyte chemoattractant protein-1 (orCCL2) in the regulation of metabolism," *Mediators of Inflammation*, vol. 2010, Article ID 326580, 11 pages, 2010.

[28] M. L. R. Curti, P. Jacob, M. C. Borges, M. M. Rogero, and S. R. G. Ferreira, "Studies of gene variants related to inflammation, oxidative stress, dyslipidemia, and obesity: implications for a nutrigenetic approach," *Journal of Obesity*, vol. 2011, Article ID 497401, 31 pages, 2011.

[29] J. P. Gutiérrez, J. Rivera, T. Shamah, C. Oropez, and M. H. Ávila, *Encuesta Nacional de Salud y Nutrición 2012. Resultados Nacionales*, Instituto Nacional de Salud Pública, Cuernavaca, México, 2012.

[30] D. Brodie, V. Moscrip, and R. Hutcheon, "Body composition measurement: a review of hydrodensitometry, anthropometry, and impedance methods," *Nutrition*, vol. 14, no. 3, pp. 296–310, 1998.

[31] U. G. Kyle, I. Bosaeus, A. D. de Lorenzo et al., "Bioelectrical impedance analysis—part II: utilization in clinical practice," *Clinical Nutrition*, vol. 23, no. 6, pp. 1430–1453, 2004.

[32] M. Y. Jaffrin and H. Morel, "Body fluid volumes measurements by impedance: a review of bioimpedance spectroscopy (BIS) and bioimpedance analysis (BIA) methods," *Medical Engineering and Physics*, vol. 30, no. 10, pp. 1257–1269, 2008.

[33] B. Feng, T. Zhang, and H. Xu, "Human adipose dynamics and metabolic health," *Annals of the New York Academy of Sciences*, vol. 1281, no. 1, pp. 160–177, 2013.

[34] C. T. Lichtash, J. Cui, X. Guo et al., "Body adiposity index versus body mass index and other anthropometric traits as correlates of cardiometabolic risk factors," *PLoS ONE*, vol. 8, no. 6, Article ID e65954, 2013.

[35] F. Taverne, C. Richard, P. Couture, and B. Lamarche, "Abdominal obesity, insulin resistance, metabolic syndrome and cholesterol homeostasis," *PharmaNutrition*, vol. 1, no. 4, pp. 130–136, 2013.

[36] A. V. Castro, C. M. Kolka, S. P. Kim, and R. N. Bergman, "Obesity, insulin resistance and comorbidities? Mechanisms of association," *Arquivos Brasileiros de Endocrinologia e Metabologia*, vol. 58, no. 6, pp. 600–609, 2014.

[37] M. C. Morrison and R. Kleemann, "Role of macrophage migration inhibitory factor in obesity, insulin resistance, type 2 diabetes, and associated hepatic co-morbidities: a comprehensive review of human and rodent studies," *Frontiers in Immunology*, vol. 6, article 308, 2015.

[38] L. Yao, O. Herlea-Pana, J. Heuser-Baker, Y. Chen, and J. Barlic-Dicen, "Roles of the chemokine system in development of obesity, insulin resistance, and cardiovascular disease," *Journal of Immunology Research*, vol. 2014, Article ID 181450, 11 pages, 2014.

[39] S. L. Deshmane, S. Kremlev, S. Amini, and B. E. Sawaya, "Monocyte chemoattractant protein-1 (MCP-1): an overview," *Journal of Interferon and Cytokine Research*, vol. 29, no. 6, pp. 313–325, 2009.

[40] Y. Huang, H. Chen, J. Wang et al., "Relationship between CCR2-V64I polymorphism and cancer risk: a meta-analysis," *Gene*, vol. 524, no. 1, pp. 54–58, 2013.

[41] L. G. Vázquez-Lavista, G. Lima, F. Gabilondo, and L. Llorente, "Genetic association of monocyte chemoattractant protein 1 (MCP-1)-2518 polymorphism in Mexican patients with transitional cell carcinoma of the bladder," *Urology*, vol. 74, no. 2, pp. 414–418, 2009.

[42] G. V. González-Enríquez, M. I. Rubio-Benítez, V. García-Gallegos, E. Portilla-de Buen, R. Troyo-Sanromán, and C. Á. Leal-Cortés, "Contribution of TNF-308A and CCL2-2518A to carotid intima-media thickness in obese mexican children and adolescents," *Archives of Medical Research*, vol. 39, no. 8, pp. 753–759, 2008.

[43] Ł. Kruszyna, M. Lianeri, B. Rubis et al., "CCL2-2518 A/G single nucleotide polymorphism as a risk factor for breast cancer," *Molecular Biology Reports*, vol. 38, no. 2, pp. 1263–1267, 2011.

[44] C. Kucukgergin, F. K. Isman, S. Dasdemir et al., "The role of chemokine and chemokine receptor gene variants on the susceptibility and clinicopathological characteristics of bladder cancer," *Gene*, vol. 511, no. 1, pp. 7–11, 2012.

[45] R. K. Mandal, T. Agrawal, and R. D. Mittal, "Genetic variants of chemokine CCL2 and chemokine receptor CCR2 genes and risk of prostate cancer," *Tumor Biology*, vol. 36, no. 1, pp. 375–381, 2015.

[46] H.-H. H. Wu, T.-H. Lee, Y.-T. Tee et al., "Relationships of single nucleotide polymorphisms of monocyte chemoattractant protein 1 and chemokine receptor 2 with susceptibility and clinicopathologic characteristics of neoplasia of uterine cervix in Taiwan women," *Reproductive Sciences*, vol. 20, no. 10, pp. 1175–1183, 2013.

[47] P. González, R. Alvarez, A. Batalla et al., "Genetic variation at the chemokine receptors CCR5/CCR2 in myocardial infarction," *Genes and Immunity*, vol. 2, no. 4, pp. 191–195, 2001.

[48] A. Zandifar, M. Taheriun, S. Soleimani, F. Haghdoost, M. Tajaddini, and S. H. Javanmard, "Investigation of chemokine receptor CCR2V64Il gene polymorphism and migraine without aura in the iranian population," *The Scientific World Journal*, vol. 2013, Article ID 836309, 5 pages, 2013.

4

Renal Protection by Genetic Deletion of the Atypical Chemokine Receptor ACKR2 in Diabetic OVE Mice

Shirong Zheng,[1] Susan Coventry,[2] Lu Cai,[1] David W. Powell,[3] Venkatakrishna R. Jala,[4] Bodduluri Haribabu,[4] and Paul N. Epstein[1]

[1] *Department of Pediatrics, University of Louisville, Louisville, KY 40202, USA*
[2] *Department of Pathology, University of Louisville, Louisville, KY 40202, USA*
[3] *Department of Medicine, University of Louisville, Louisville, KY 40202, USA*
[4] *Department of Microbiology and Immunology, University of Louisville, Louisville, KY 40202, USA*

Correspondence should be addressed to Shirong Zheng; shirong.zheng@louisville.edu

Academic Editor: Carlos Martinez Salgado

In diabetic nephropathy (DN) proinflammatory chemokines and leukocyte infiltration correlate with tubulointerstitial injury and declining renal function. The atypical chemokine receptor ACKR2 is a chemokine scavenger receptor which binds and sequesters many inflammatory CC chemokines but does not transduce typical G-protein mediated signaling events. ACKR2 is known to regulate diverse inflammatory diseases but its role in DN has not been tested. In this study, we utilized ACKR2$^{-/-}$ mice to test whether ACKR2 elimination alters progression of diabetic kidney disease. Elimination of ACKR2 greatly reduced DN in OVE26 mice, an established DN model. Albuminuria was significantly lower at 2, 4, and 6 months of age. ACKR2 deletion did not affect diabetic blood glucose levels but significantly decreased parameters of renal inflammation including leukocyte infiltration and fibrosis. Activation of pathways that increase inflammatory gene expression was attenuated. Human biopsies stained with ACKR2 antibody revealed increased staining in diabetic kidney, especially in some tubule and interstitial cells. The results demonstrate a significant interaction between diabetes and ACKR2 protein in the kidney. Unexpectedly, ACKR2 deletion reduced renal inflammation in diabetes and the ultimate response was a high degree of protection from diabetic nephropathy.

1. Introduction

Although hyperglycemia is the initiating and essential cause for all diabetic complications there is accumulating evidence that inflammatory processes activated by chronic elevated glucose are integral to the development of diabetic complications [1]. Diabetic nephropathy (DN) is one of the most severe and common complications of diabetes and it is the leading cause of end stage renal failure in the world. Immune modulation and inflammatory process contribute to the development and progression of DN [2, 3]. In diabetic kidneys expression of proinflammatory chemokines rises and infiltration of inflammatory cells increases [4–7]. These changes are correlated with progression of tubulointerstitial injury and deterioration of kidney function [8–10]. Inhibition of renal inflammation by small molecule inhibitors or by antibodies directed against chemokines or chemokine receptors has been shown to reduce renal damage in DN [11–14]. More complete understanding of how the kidney modulates immune and inflammatory processes in diabetes may lead to the discovery of improved biomarkers and new therapeutic targets for treatment of DN.

ACKR2 is a chemokine decoy receptor [15] which can bind and internalize chemokines without activating an intracellular response [16]. ACKR2 binds most inflammatory CC-chemokines (CCL2, CCL5, CCL3, CCL4, CCL7, CCL8, CCL11, CCL13, CCL17, CCL22, CCL23, and CCL24) leading to their degradation, thereby reducing local levels of inflammatory chemokines. This makes ACKR2 a likely modulator of local inflammation. The function of ACKR2 has been tested in knockout animals in which deletion of ACKR2 coding sequences increased the inflammatory response in cutaneous tissue [17], placenta [18], lung [19], liver [20], and colon [21]. The role of ACKR2 has not been examined for a complication of diabetes. In this study, we examined the effect of crossing an established ACKR2 knockout mouse (designated herein as ACKR2 mice) with the diabetic mouse model, OVE26 (OVE). This diabetic model exhibits several features of human DN [22] and extensive renal inflammation [23, 24].

2. Methods

2.1. Animals. All animal procedures followed the NIH Guide for the Care and Use of Laboratory Animals and were approved by the University of Louisville Institutional Animal Care and Use Committee. ACKR2 mice on the C57BL/6 background originally from Charles River Italia (Calco, Italy) [17] were bred to FVB mice for at least 10 generations to transfer the ACKR2 deletion to the FVB background (henceforth designated as ACKR2). These ACKR2 mice were bred for two generations to diabetic OVE mice on the background FVB to produce OVE mice homozygous for the ACKR2 deletion (OVE-ACKR2). Mice were maintained up to 6 months of age. Animals had free access to standard rodent chow and water throughout the study.

2.2. Glucose and Albumin Assays. Glucose was assayed in serum samples obtained from nonfasted mice at 6 months of age by the Glucose (HK) Assay Kit (Sigma-Aldrich). At 2 months urine glucose was evaluated with Clinistix (Bayer). Albumin was measured from spot urine samples with a mouse albumin ELISA kit (Bethyl Laboratories, Montgomery, TX) within the linear range of the assay. Urine creatinine was measured with a creatinine assay kit (DICT-500, BioAssay Systems). Urine albumin was expressed as the ratio of albumin to creatinine (μg/mg).

2.3. Assessment of Renal Fibrosis and Inflammatory Cell Infiltration. Kidneys were fixed overnight in 10% neutral buffered formalin and embedded in paraffin. Sagittal tissue sections from the center of the kidney were stained with Masson's trichrome using standard protocols. Stained slides were imaged with a 20x objective. Fibrosis was semiquantitatively scored by a blinded observer for the number of blue stained fibrotic areas per section. Renal inflammatory cell infiltration was evaluated by staining sections with rat anti-mouse CD45 antibody (Angio-Proteomie, Boston, MA). Positive staining was detected with HRP conjugated second antibody and diaminobenzidine (DAB). CD45 positive cell infiltration was evaluated by quantitating the DAB stained pixel area in 8 random, nonoverlapping 200x image fields from the cortical region per mouse with 3 mice per group. Digital images were taken by an observer blind to the identity of the section and the number of positive pixels was quantified by another observer blind to section identity. Pixel number was determined using the ability of Adobe Photoshop to select areas of matching color intensity.

2.4. Microarray Hybridization and Gene Expression Analysis. RNA extraction was done with the RNeasy Mini Kit (Qiagen, Santa Clarita, CA, USA) from frozen kidneys. Extracted RNA was checked for quality on Agilent 2100 Bioanalyzer (Agilent Technologies, Palo Alto, USA). The RNA samples having RNA integrity number (RIN) above 8.8 (average 9.1) were used for probe preparation. A 100 ng aliquot of RNA from each mouse was used for probe preparation with an Ambion WT Expression kit. The kit generates sense-strand cDNA from total RNA for fragmentation and labeling was done with an Affymetrix GeneChip WT Terminal Labeling Kit (PN90067). Probes from 3 six-month-old female mice in each group were hybridized to Affymetrix mouse gene 1.0 ST exon arrays and scanned with a GCS 3000 7G scanner and signals were analyzed with Command Console software (Affymetrix, Santa Clara, CA). Gene expression profiles were uploaded to Ingenuity software (Ingenuity Systems, http://www.ingenuity.com/, Ingenuity Pathway Analysis, Redwood City, CA) for data analysis. Gene array data was uploaded to GEO and the access number is GSE51205.

2.5. Quantitative Reverse Transcription-PCR. Total RNA was extracted from whole kidney using TRIzol reagent (Invitrogen, Carlsbad, CA). The cDNA was synthesized with high-capacity cDNA archive kit (p/n 4322171, Applied Biosystems, Foster City, CA) and PCR was performed on an Applied Biosystems 7300 thermocycler with commercially available Taqman reagents (Assay on Demand, Applied Biosystems) for ccbp2 (ACKR2) (Mm00445551_m1), ccl2 (Mm00441242_m1), ccl5 (Mm01302428_m1), ccr2 (Mm04207877_m1), and ccr5 (Mm01216171_m1). Amplification was performed in duplicate using 40 cycles of denaturation at 95°C for 15 sec and primer annealing/extension at 60°C for 1 min. Expression data were normalized to 18s ribosomal RNA (Hs99999901-sl) or GAPDH RNA measured on the same samples. Relative expression ratio was calculated according to the $2^{-\Delta\Delta CT}$ method.

2.6. ACKR2 Immunohistochemistry Staining in Human Kidney. Immunohistochemistry with anti-human ACKR2 antibody was used for detection of ACKR2 expression in human kidneys: renal tissue biopsies ($n = 9$) from diabetic patients with confirmed diabetic nephropathy and 6 nondiabetic control renal tissue samples (2 donor kidneys, 1 normal portion from renal cancer patient, and 3 renal biopsy specimens with proteinuria, lacking visible tubulointerstitial alterations). The research protocol was approved by our Medical Ethics Committee. Tissue was embedded in paraffin, stained with rat anti-human ACKR2 antibody (R&D SYSTEMS, Inc., Minneapolis, MN), and detected with DAB. ACKR2 staining in each section was scored semiquantitatively in tubular and interstitial regions with the criteria of 0 for none, 1 for rare, 2 for some, 3 for common, and 4 for common plus intense. The scorer had no knowledge of group identification of the slides. ACKR2 expression was presented as the average score of each group. In some samples tissues were double labeled with FITC conjugated *Lotus tetragonolobus* lectin (Vector labs), a marker for tubule epithelial cell brush border [25], and the ACKR2 antibody binding was visualized with Cy3 conjugated anti-rat second antibody.

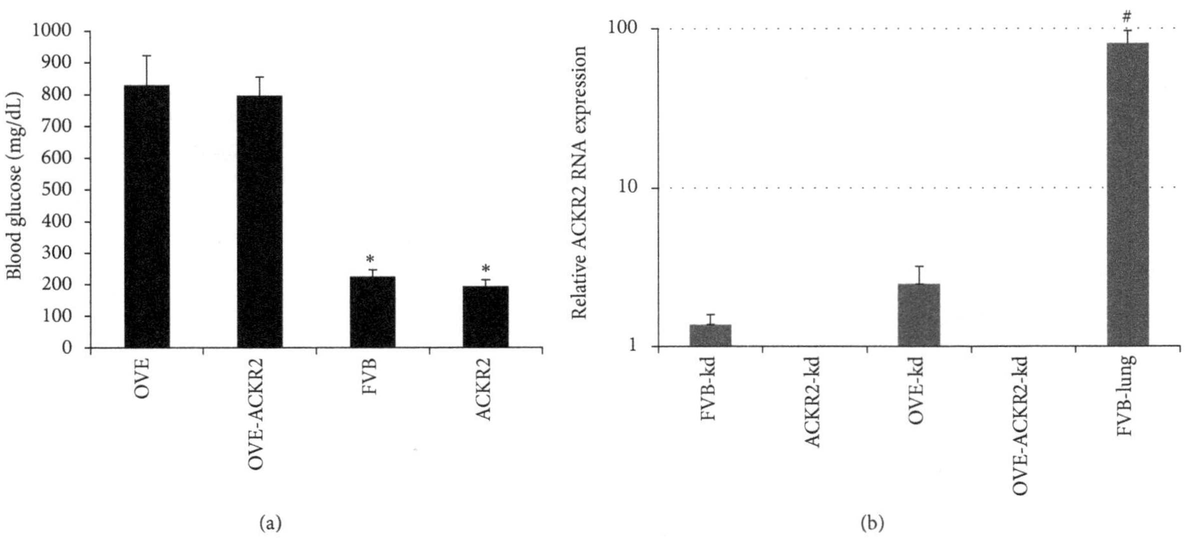

FIGURE 1: Blood glucose and ACKR2 RNA in diabetic and normal mice, with and without deletion of the ACKR2 gene. (a) ACKR2 knockout did not affect blood glucose levels in free fed normal or diabetic mice. $^*p < 0.02$ for both nondiabetic groups versus both diabetic groups. $N = 4, 6, 6$, and 11 in FVB, ACKR2, OVE, and OVE-ACKR2 groups, respectively. (b) Low level ACKR2 RNA expression in kidney is eliminated in ACKR2 KO mice. No ACKR2 RNA was detected in any ACKR2 kidney sample. $N = 4$ for nondiabetic kidney groups, 3 for diabetic kidney groups, and 2 for normal lung. Data are presented on a log 10 graph to include expression values for lung. # indicates that ACKR2 RNA expression in FVB lung was significantly higher than in normal FVB kidney. ACKR2 expression in diabetic kidney tended to be higher than in FVB kidney.

2.7. Statistical Analyses. Data are expressed as means ± SE. Comparisons between two groups were performed by t-test. Comparisons between more than 2 groups were performed by one-way ANOVA. Statistical analyses were performed with SigmaStat software.

3. Results

3.1. ACKR2 Deletion Did Not Alter Diabetes Development in OVE26 Mice. Enzymatic assays, necessary for accurate measurement of blood glucose in OVE diabetic mice [22, 26], indicated that deletion of the ACKR2 gene did not significantly reduce blood glucose levels in 6-month-old OVE-ACKR2$^{-/-}$ mice (Figure 1(a)). Urine glucose, undetectable in normal mice, exceeded 2000 mg/dL at 2 months of age in all OVE and OVE-ACKR2 spot urine samples tested ($n = 4$ per group, data not shown). Expression of ACKR2 RNA was 80% higher in diabetic kidneys compared to normal kidneys (Figure 1(b)), though this difference was not significant ($p = 0.11$). Interestingly high levels of ACKR2 in lungs were observed. Knockout mice served as negative controls for expression analysis.

3.1.1. Knockout of the ACKR2 Gene Reduced Diabetic Albuminuria. Albuminuria was assessed by measuring albumin/creatinine ratio (ACR expressed as μg/mg) in all groups at 2, 4, and 6 months of age (Figure 2). By 2 months ACR was already significantly elevated in OVE mice compared to FVB controls. ACR increased in OVE mice with age, from 600 at 2 months to over 10,000 at 4 months and over 35,000 at 6 months. These values were significantly higher than FVB mice at all ages and significantly higher than ACKR2 mice at 4 and 6 months. Interestingly, ACR values of OVE-ACKR2 mice were significantly lower than OVE values at all ages. The difference between ACR levels of OVE and OVE-ACKR2 groups increased from about 2-fold at 2 months to about 15-fold at 4 months and 7-fold at 6 months.

3.1.2. Reduced Renal Fibrosis and Inflammation in ACKR2 Mice. We evaluated the glomerular and tubular damage in OVE and OVE-ACKR2 mice at the age of 6 months as previously described [22–24]. Trichrome staining (Figure 3(a)) showed that fibrosis in OVE kidneys was much greater than in nondiabetic or OVE-ACKR2$^{-/-}$ kidneys. Semiquantitative scoring of trichrome staining (Figure 3(b)) by an observer blind to genotype confirmed that deletion of the ACKR2 gene significantly reduced fibrosis in diabetic OVE-ACKR2 mice compared to OVE mice.

Infiltration of leukocytes in kidney was determined by staining with anti-CD45 antibody (Figure 4). In nondiabetic FVB and ACKR2 mice, CD45 positive cells were sparsely distributed in the interstitial vessels and in the glomerular tuft. In OVE kidneys many more CD45 positive cells were observed, located mostly in the peritubular, interstitial space in a clustered distribution. Positive staining of CD45 cells was much less evident in kidneys of OVE-ACKR2 mice and appeared similar to staining in nondiabetic mice. Quantitation of CD45 positive pixel area confirmed significantly less leukocyte accumulation in the OVE-ACKR2 mice compared to the OVE mice (Figure 4(b)). Staining for CD3 to identify T cells demonstrated that CD3 positive cells were also more abundant in OVE kidneys than in any other genotype (data not shown).

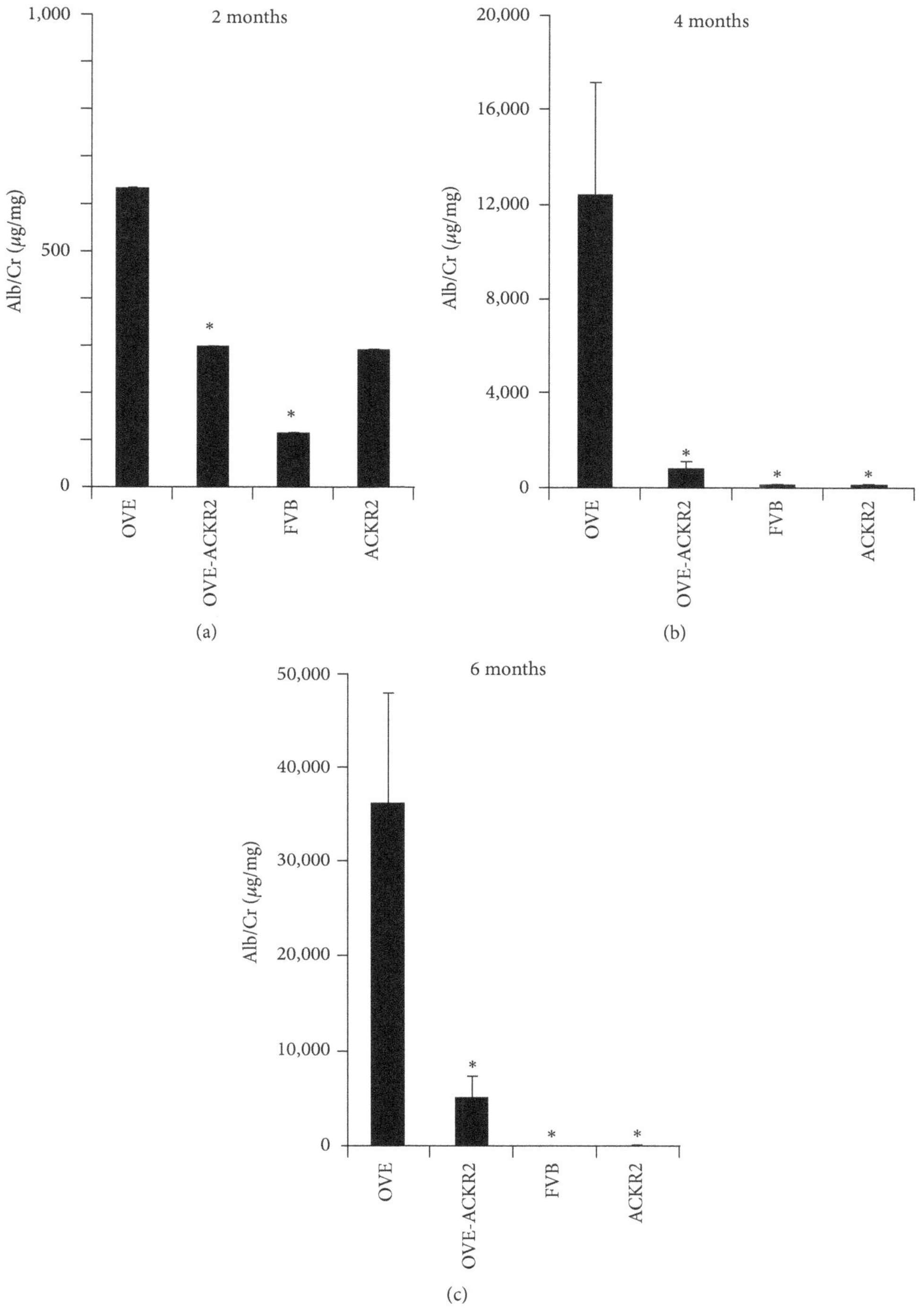

FIGURE 2: Diabetic albuminuria was reduced by knockout of the ACKR2 gene at 2, 4, and 6 months of age. Urine albumin and creatinine were determined as described in Methods. $*$ indicates $p < 0.05$ versus OVE. Comparisons were performed by one-way ANOVA. $n \geq 12$ in each OVE and OVE-ACKR2 group. For FVB $n = 14, 9$, and 6 at 2, 4, and 6 months, respectively. For ACKR2 $n = 3, 7$, and 7 at 2, 4, and 6 months, respectively.

Inflammatory chemokines CCL2 and CCL5 (ligands for ACKR2) are elevated in DN [6, 27, 28]. Quantitative RT-PCR for CCL2, CCL5, and their receptors was performed on RNA samples extracted from kidneys of all groups at 6 months of age (Figure 5). Levels of CCL2 and CCL5 mRNA significantly increased in OVE mice compared to FVB mice and OVE-ACKR2$^{-/-}$ mice (Figure 5).

3.2. Microarray Analysis of Kidneys from OVE and OVE-ACKR2 Mice. The global changes in gene expression profiles

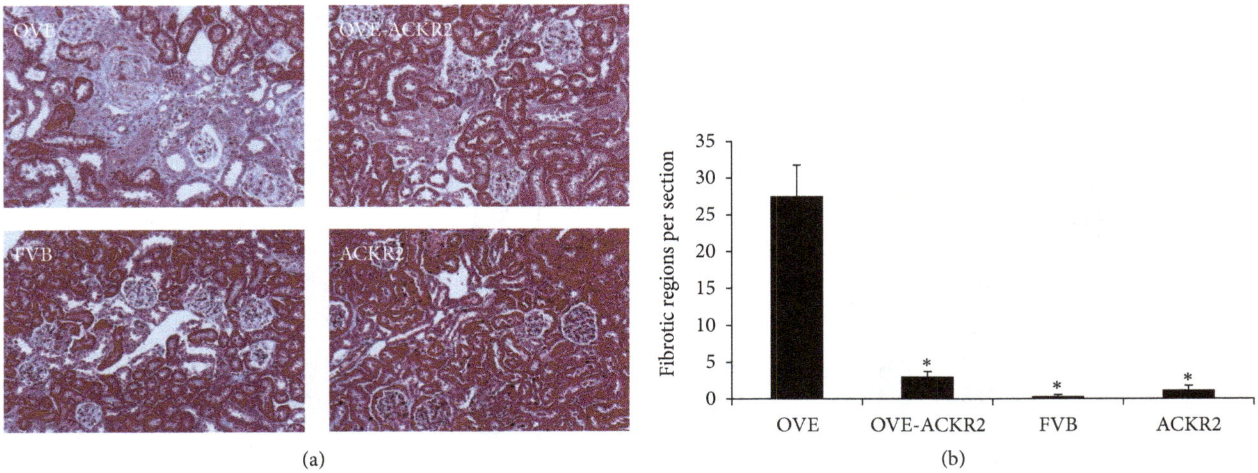

FIGURE 3: Renal fibrosis is reduced by knockout of the ACKR2 gene in diabetic OVE-ACKR2 mice. (a) Representative images of renal fibrosis illustrated by trichrome staining in a kidney section for each genotype. Original magnification 200x. (b) Scoring of renal fibrosis by blind counting of blue stained fibrotic regions in trichrome stained kidney sections. $^*p < 0.02$ versus OVE by one-way ANOVA. 6 sections from 3 mice per group were counted.

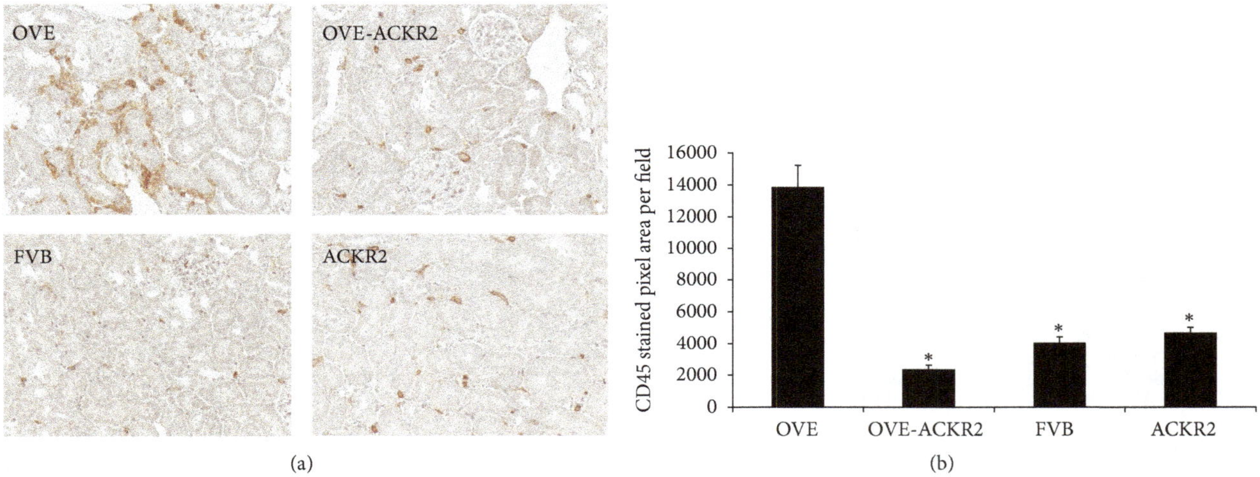

FIGURE 4: Knockout of the ACKR2 gene reduces leukocyte infiltration in diabetic mice. (a) Representative images of CD45 staining, original magnification 200x. (b) Quantitative analysis of leukocyte infiltration scored as CD45 positive pixel area per visual field. Twenty-four random fields from 3 mice per group were measured. $*$ indicates $p < 0.05$ versus OVE. Statistical comparisons were performed by one-way ANOVA.

were evaluated by microarray. To confirm the reliability of the microarray results correlation coefficients were calculated between RT-PCR and microarray results for CCL2, CCL5, CCR2, and CCR5 based on the 12 samples used in both assays. For all but CCR5 the correlation was at least 0.96 ($p \leq 0.000001$) and for CCR5 the correlation coefficient was 0.6 ($p \leq 0.05$).

Only 18 of 30,000 genes differed at the 0.05 level between the nondiabetic groups, FVB and ACKR2. Therefore, RNA expression of the OVE and OVE-ACKR2$^{-/-}$ diabetic groups was compared to one nondiabetic group, FVB. Using a minimal criterion of 1.5-fold change in expression and a p value of 0.05 versus FVB, there were 715 genes in OVE, 181 in OVE-ACKR2, and 18 in ACKR2 samples that reached this criterion. Expression data was analyzed with Ingenuity Pathway Analysis (IPA) software. Table 1 shows 40 IPA canonical pathways significantly affected by OVE diabetes arranged in 8 biological categories. Signaling pathways for hepatic fibrosis and leukocyte extravasation contained a large number of genes (26 and 27 genes, resp.) altered in expression in OVE samples. This is consistent with the extensive fibrosis and CD45 positive cell infiltration of OVE kidneys (Figures 3 and 4). OVE-ACKR2 kidneys, which showed minimal histological changes, had only 6 induced genes in the fibrosis pathway and 2 in the leukocyte extravasation pathway.

In OVE kidney, many protective pathways such as immune response and cytokine signaling were activated, as indicated by the high number of RNAs with significantly

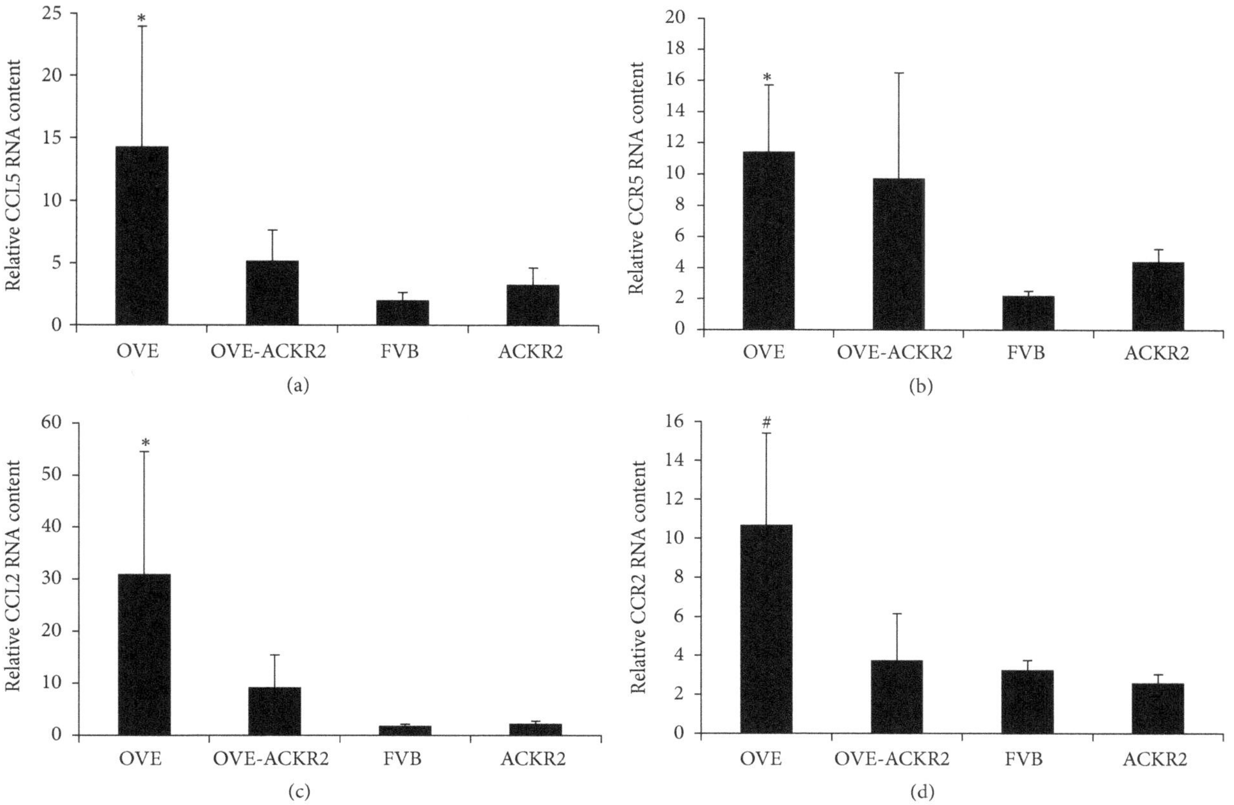

FIGURE 5: Kidney RNA levels of ACKR2 ligands CCL2 and CCL5 and their receptors. Values were determined by RT-PCR with Taqman probes using 18S as standard. Columns are mean + SE. $n = 3$ OVE, 4 OVE-ACKR2, 5 ACKR2, and 6 FVB. $*$ indicates $p \leq 0.05$ versus FVB and # indicates a trend of $p \leq 0.08$ versus FVB. All determined by one-way ANOVA.

altered expression. The same pathways in OVE-ACKR2 contained only a few RNAs with altered expression. With few exceptions, most of the biological pathways in Table 1 contained at least 4 times as many significantly modified RNAs for OVE as they did for OVE-ACKR2. Also, only 5 of the 40 pathways significantly affected by OVE diabetes were significantly affected by OVE-ACKR2 diabetes. The conclusion that inflammation was reduced by deletion of ACKR2 was also evident at the individual RNA level: transcripts reduced in OVE-ACKR2 kidneys relative to OVE kidneys included RNAs indicative of complement activation (C7 and C1qc) and macrophage and T cell infiltration (Mpegl, Cd68, and Itgam) and other cytokines (CCL8, CCL9, and CCL28) (Supplementary Tables 1 and 2, in Supplementary Material available online at http://dx.doi.org/10.1155/2016/5362506, show the 50 transcripts most reduced and increased in OVE-ACKR2 relative to OVE, resp.).

3.3. ACKR2 Protein Expression in Kidneys of Diabetic Patients. The effect of diabetes on kidney ACKR2 protein expression was evaluated in human DN and nondiabetic samples using a rat anti-human ACKR2 monoclonal antibody, previously evaluated on human samples [18, 29, 30]. A reliable antibody to mouse ACKR2 is not available. Positive but sporadic ACKR2 staining was visible in diabetic kidneys (Figures 6(a) and 6(d)–6(f)) in tubule epithelial cells and in the interstitium. Stained tubule epithelial cells were positively identified by the presence of a brush border by staining with *Lotus tetragonolobus* lectin [25]. ACKR2 staining was never seen in glomeruli. Positive cells in the interstitium appeared to be either mononuclear cells (lymphocytes or monocytes) or endothelial cells belonging to capillaries or lymphatics. Staining was more frequent and more intense in diabetic samples, which was confirmed by semiquantitative scoring of epithelial cells and interstitial cells (Figure 6(g)).

4. Discussion

This study demonstrates that the ACKR2 chemokine scavenger receptor has an unexpected important role in the development of diabetic kidney disease. Deletion of the ACKR2 gene in OVE diabetic mice produced a great reduction in albuminuria, accompanied by reduced severity of renal fibrosis, leucocyte infiltration, and inflammatory chemokine gene expression. In addition, ACKR2 protein content was elevated in several cell types in kidneys of DN patients.

Chemokines and cytokines regulate the inflammatory processes and contribute to progressive kidney damage in diabetes [31]. Chemokine scavenging has been proposed as a significant mechanism for controlling ongoing inflammation. This suggests that scavenger receptors like ACKR2 could limit DN progression by reducing kidney chemokine levels.

Table 1: Ingenuity pathways in kidney affected by OVE diabetes and/or OVE-ACKR2 diabetes.

Ingenuity canonical pathway	OVE versus FVB		OVE-ACKR2 versus FVB	
	p value	Ratio*	p value	Ratio*
Diseases-specific pathways				
Hepatic fibrosis	$4.27E-10$	26/147	0.003	6/147
Atherosclerosis signaling	$7.76E-10$	23/129	NS	2/129
Altered T cell and B cell signaling in rheumatoid arthritis	$3.38E-08$	17/92	NS	1/92
Graft-versus-host disease signaling	$3.71E-06$	10/50	NS	1/50
Glioma invasiveness signaling	$6.31E-06$	12/60	NS	1/60
Cellular immune response				
Communication between innate and adaptive immune cells	$3.89E-10$	18/109	NS	1/109
Dendritic cell maturation	$2.39E-08$	23/185	NS	0
Altered T cell and B cell signaling in rheumatoid arthritis	$3.38E-08$	17/92	NS	1/92
Pattern recognition receptors of bacteria and viruses	$3.38E-08$	19/106	NS	2/106
Leukocyte extravasation signaling	$6.61E-08$	27/199	NS	2/199
Humoral immune response				
Complement system	$7.94E-11$	13/35	NS	1/35
B cell development	$5.49E-06$	8/36	NS	0
NF-κB signaling	$7.94E-05$	19/175	NS	0
p38 MAPK signaling	0.00017	14/106	NS	0
Antigen presentation pathway	0.0002	7/40	NS	0
Intracellular and second messenger signaling				
p38 MAPK signaling	0.0002	14/106	NS	0
Role of NFAT in regulation of the immune response	0.002	16/198	NS	0
Nitrogen metabolism	0.0037	6/120	NS	1/120
Histidine metabolism	0.0044	7/112	0.00012	5/112
Arginine and proline metabolism	0.0141	8/176	0.00676	4/176
Cellular stress and injury				
Intrinsic prothrombin activation pathway	$1.55E-05$	8/32	NS	1/32
Coagulation system	$1.73E-05$	9/38	NS	0
Extrinsic prothrombin activation pathway	$5.25E-05$	6/20	NS	0
p38 MAPK signaling	0.00017	14/106	NS	0
HMGB1 signaling	0.00245	11/100	NS	0
Cytokine signaling				
Dendritic cell maturation	$2.39E-08$	23/185	NS	0
Acute phase response signaling	$8.91E-08$	25/177	0.00813	6/177
TREM1 signaling	$6.92E-05$	10/66	NS	0
IL-8 signaling	$7.41E-05$	20/193	NS	2/193
NF-κB signaling	$7.94E-05$	19/175	NS	0
Pathogen-influenced signaling				
Dendritic cell maturation	$2.39E-08$	23/185	NS	0
Pattern recognition receptors of bacteria and viruses	$3.38E-08$	19/106	NS	2/106
Virus entry via endocytic pathways	0.00014	13/100	NS	2/100
Clathrin-mediated endocytosis signaling	0.00019	20/195	NS	2/195
Caveolar-mediated endocytosis signaling	0.0015	10/85	NS	1/85
Nuclear receptor signaling				
LXR/RXR activation	$1.63E-13$	28/136	0.0002	7/136
TR/RXR activation	0.0017	11/96	NS	2/96
Aryl hydrocarbon receptor signaling	0.0028	14/159	NS	6/159
Nitrogen metabolism	0.0037	6/120	NS	1/120
LPS/IL-1 mediated inhibition of RXR function	0.0039	18/235	NS	9/235

*Ratio: RNAs altered versus FVB divided by the number of genes in the pathway. NS, not significant.

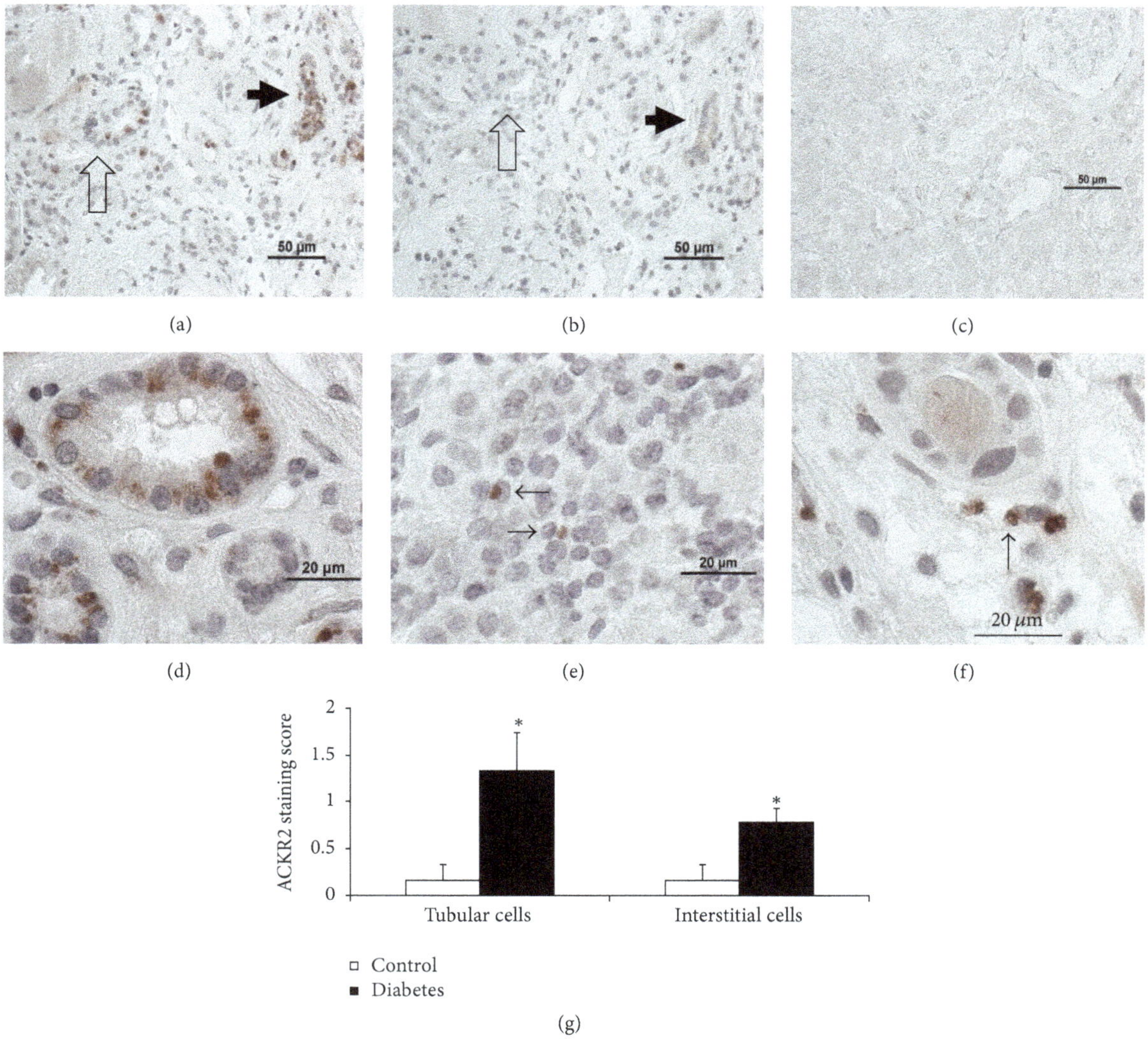

FIGURE 6: Increased ACKR2 protein in diabetic human kidney sections stained with rat monoclonal antibody to human ACKR2. (a) Positive ACKR2 staining in diabetic kidney. Strongest staining in tubules (arrows) especially in a collapsed (arrow) tubule. (b) Minimal staining is seen on a serial section without primary antibody. The arrows indicate the same 2 tubules in images (a) and (b). (c) Sparse ACKR2 staining in a nondiabetic section. (d) At higher magnification granule-like deposits of ACKR2 can be seen in cytoplasm of proximal tubular epithelial cells in diabetic kidney. In the interstitial space ACKR2 staining is also visible in diabetic kidney monocytes (e) and endothelial cells (f). (g) Semiquantitative scoring of ACKR2 staining by a scorer blind to sample identity. Scores for proximal tubule and interstitial cells are higher in diabetic than nondiabetic samples. $^*p < 0.05$ by t-test, $n = 9$ diabetic and 6 nondiabetic samples.

Surprisingly little information is available for the ACKR2 chemokine scavenger receptor in the kidney, and only previous study indicated that the level of ACKR2 RNA in mouse kidney is low [15]. The current study also found low expression of ACKR2 RNA in normal kidney, approximately fiftyfold lower than in lung. We further observed a tendency for diabetes to increase ACKR2 RNA expression in OVE mouse kidney.

To determine if the ACKR2 RNA results indicate that diabetes alters ACKR2 protein immunohistochemistry studies were performed on human tissue since only an anti-human ACKR2 antibody has been validated [18, 29, 30]. Diabetic kidneys had significantly stronger ACKR2 staining in tubule and interstitial cells. Staining increased primarily in proximal tubule cells and in tubule cells that were too abnormal to distinguish as proximal or distal (Figure 6(a)). ACKR2 positive interstitial cells seen in diabetic samples appeared to be a mix of infiltrating monocytes and endothelial cells which could belong to blood or lymphatic vessels. The ACKR2 positive cell profile in kidney was not unusual. Positive stromal cells were expected, since ACKR2 staining in other organs has been reported for monocytes, lymphocytes, dendritic cells, and endothelial cells. Increased infiltration of inflammatory cells is common in diabetic kidneys [7, 8, 32]. Tubule cell staining for ACKR2 is unsurprising considering ACKR2 has been shown in parenchymal cells of several organs: ACKR2 antibodies stain epidermis in psoriatic skin [33], syncytiotrophoblast cells of placenta [18], and breast cancer cells [34]. The absence of ACKR2 staining in diabetic glomeruli indicates that direct actions of ACKR2 are limited to the tubular and interstitial portions of the diabetic kidney.

The primary finding of this study was that ACKR2 deletion dramatically reduced DN. The reduction of albuminuria in OVE-ACKR2 mice was significant at the earliest age tested, two months. As OVE mice aged DN progressed and the protection by ACKR2 KO became more striking. At 6 months ACKR2 deletion produced a greater reduction in diabetic albuminuria. In addition several markers demonstrated reduced inflammation in OVE-ACKR2 kidneys compared to OVE kidneys. Histologically this was indicated by decreased leukocyte infiltration and less fibrosis. Gene expression data demonstrated that absence of ACKR2 prevented activation of multiple molecular pathways involved in immune or inflammatory processes in kidneys of diabetic mice. The finding of such potent renal protection from diabetes by deletion of ACKR2 was contradictory to our expectation, which was that deletion of ACKR2 would exacerbate DN by increasing renal inflammation. This expectation was based on the damage inflammation produces in DN and the anti-inflammatory potency of ACKR2 as a scavenger of proinflammatory chemokines. In several studies manipulation of ACKR2 levels modified tissue inflammation in a manner that would be predicted based on anti-inflammatory potency of ACKR2 as a chemokine scavenger: this was shown in experimental models of colitis and psoriasis, where deletion of ACKR2 increased colon [21] or skin [17] inflammation, and in inflamed NOD mouse islets where transgenic overexpression of ACKR2 reduced local islet inflammation [35].

Mechanisms to explain protection from DN by deletion of ACKR2 are not obvious. Protection was not due to reduced OVE diabetes since hyperglycemia was equivalent in OVE and OVE-ACKR2 mice (Figure 1). In considering potential mechanisms of protection by ACKR2 KO it needs to be considered that this is not the first such report. Unexpected protection by deletion of ACKR2 has been reported to reduce pathology of several inflammatory diseases: ACKR2 deletion inhibits spinal cord inflammation and autoimmune encephalomyelitis [36], reduces susceptibility and symptoms of dextran sulfate-induced colitis [37], and reduces airway reactivity in allergen-induced airway disease [19]. In addition to these inflammatory disease models, KO of host ACKR2 can suppress transplant graft rejection [38, 39]. The unexpected but repeated finding of beneficial effects of ACKR2 deletion in multiple disease models indicates that our anti-inflammatory concept of ACKR2 was overly simplistic and the chemokine scavenging properties of ACKR2 may produce complex and not purely anti-inflammatory results. For example, deletion of ACKR2 releases chemokines that promote increased production of immunosuppressive monocytes [39] that reduce graft-versus-host disease. During chronic DN progression complex and changing interactions occur between the immune system and the kidney. At this time, the underlying molecular mechanisms involved in diabetic kidney disease are not clear. It is possible that kidney damage initiated by hyperglycemia is more efficiently cleared in ACKR2 mice. More rapid damage removal decreases the chances of developing chronic inflammation. Despite uncertainty about the mechanism, the strength of protection produced by elimination of ACKR2 indicates that it has a key role in the pathology which needs to be dissected at a finer level.

In *summary*, we found that deletion of the ACKR2 gene produced a dramatic reduction in albuminuria and renal inflammation in the OVE diabetic mouse without decreasing diabetes. In human samples diabetes increased the expression of ACKR2 protein in tubule cells, leukocytes, and endothelial cells.

Conflict of Interests

The authors declare that there is no conflict of interests regarding the publication of this paper.

Acknowledgments

The authors thank Yun Huang for mice mating and genotyping, Patricia Kralik for albuminuria assay, and Sabina J Waigel for gene array data discussion. This work was supported by Juvenile Diabetes Research Foundation Grants 1-INO-2014-116-A-N and 1-2011-588.

References

[1] C. Mora and J. F. Navarro, "Inflammation and diabetic nephropathy," *Current Diabetes Reports*, vol. 6, no. 6, pp. 463–468, 2006.

[2] A. K. H. Lim and G. H. Tesch, "Inflammation in diabetic nephropathy," *Mediators of Inflammation*, vol. 2012, Article ID 146154, 12 pages, 2012.

[3] F. B. Hickey and F. Martin, "Diabetic kidney disease and immune modulation," *Current Opinion in Pharmacology*, vol. 13, no. 4, pp. 602–612, 2013.

[4] Y. Wang, J. Chen, L. Chen, Y.-C. Tay, G. K. Rangan, and D. C. H. Harris, "Induction of monocyte chemoattractant protein-1 in proximal tubule cells by urinary protein," *Journal of the American Society of Nephrology*, vol. 8, no. 10, pp. 1537–1545, 1997.

[5] C. Sassy-Prigent, D. Heudes, C. Mandet et al., "Early glomerular macrophage recruitment in streptozotocin-induced diabetic rats," *Diabetes*, vol. 49, no. 3, pp. 466–475, 2000.

[6] A. A. Eddy and C. M. Giachelli, "Renal expression of genes that promote interstitial inflammation and fibrosis in rats with protein-overload proteinuria," *Kidney International*, vol. 47, no. 6, pp. 1546–1557, 1995.

[7] D. Nguyen, F. Ping, W. Mu, P. Hill, R. C. Atkins, and S. J. Chadban, "Macrophage accumulation in human progressive diabetic nephropathy," *Nephrology*, vol. 11, no. 3, pp. 226–231, 2006.

[8] F. Y. Chow, D. J. Nikolic-Paterson, R. C. Atkins, and G. H. Tesch, "Macrophages in streptozotocin-induced diabetic nephropathy: potential role in renal fibrosis," *Nephrology Dialysis Transplantation*, vol. 19, no. 12, pp. 2987–2996, 2004.

[9] J. F. Navarro, F. J. Milena, C. Mora, C. León, and J. García, "Renal pro-inflammatory cytokine gene expression in diabetic

nephropathy: effect of angiotensin-converting enzyme inhibition and pentoxifylline administration," *American Journal of Nephrology*, vol. 26, no. 6, pp. 562–570, 2007.

[10] P. P. Wolkow, M. A. Niewczas, B. Perkins et al., "Association of urinary inflammatory markers and renal decline in microalbuminuric type 1 diabetics," *Journal of the American Society of Nephrology*, vol. 19, no. 4, pp. 789–797, 2008.

[11] B. Rodríguez-Iturbe, Y. Quiroz, A. Shahkarami, Z. Li, and N. D. Vaziri, "Mycophenolate mofetil ameliorates nephropathy in the obese Zucker rat," *Kidney International*, vol. 68, no. 3, pp. 1041–1047, 2005.

[12] Y.-G. Wu, H. Lin, X.-M. Qi et al., "Prevention of early renal injury by mycophenolate mofetil and its mechanism in experimental diabetes," *International Immunopharmacology*, vol. 6, no. 3, pp. 445–453, 2006.

[13] S. G. Sayyed, M. Ryu, O. P. Kulkarni et al., "An orally active chemokine receptor CCR2 antagonist prevents glomerulosclerosis and renal failure in type 2 diabetes," *Kidney International*, vol. 80, no. 1, pp. 68–78, 2011.

[14] B. Y. Nam, J. Paeng, S. H. Kim et al., "The MCP-1/CCR2 axis in podocytes is involved in apoptosis induced by diabetic conditions," *Apoptosis*, vol. 17, no. 1, pp. 1–13, 2012.

[15] R. J. B. Nibbs, S. M. Wylie, I. B. Pragnell, and G. J. Graham, "Cloning and characterization of a novel murine beta chemokine receptor, D6. Comparison to three other related macrophage inflammatory protein-1alpha receptors, CCR-1, CCR-3, and CCR-5," *The Journal of Biological Chemistry*, vol. 272, no. 19, pp. 12495–12504, 1997.

[16] M. Locati, Y. M. De La Torre, E. Galliera et al., "Silent chemoattractant receptors: D6 as a decoy and scavenger receptor for inflammatory CC chemokines," *Cytokine and Growth Factor Reviews*, vol. 16, no. 6, pp. 679–686, 2005.

[17] T. Jamieson, D. N. Cook, R. J. B. Nibbs et al., "The chemokine receptor D6 limits the inflammatory response in vivo," *Nature Immunology*, vol. 6, no. 4, pp. 403–411, 2005.

[18] Y. M. de la Torre, C. Buracchi, E. M. Borroni et al., "Protection against inflammation- and autoantibody-caused fetal loss by the chemokine decoy receptor D6," *Proceedings of the National Academy of Sciences of the United States of America*, vol. 104, no. 7, pp. 2319–2324, 2007.

[19] G. S. Whitehead, T. Wang, L. M. DeGraff et al., "The chemokine receptor D6 has opposing effects on allergic inflammation and airway reactivity," *American Journal of Respiratory and Critical Care Medicine*, vol. 175, no. 3, pp. 243–249, 2007.

[20] M.-L. Berres, C. Trautwein, M. M. Zaldivar et al., "The chemokine scavenging receptor D6 limits acute toxic liver injury in vivo," *Biological Chemistry*, vol. 390, no. 10, pp. 1039–1045, 2009.

[21] S. Vetrano, E. M. Borroni, A. Sarukhan et al., "The lymphatic system controls intestinal inflammation and inflammation-associated colon cancer through the chemokine decoy receptor D6," *Gut*, vol. 59, no. 2, pp. 197–206, 2010.

[22] S. Zheng, W. T. Noonan, N. S. Metreveli et al., "Development of late-stage diabetic nephropathy in OVE26 diabetic mice," *Diabetes*, vol. 53, no. 12, pp. 3248–3257, 2004.

[23] S. Zheng, Y. Huang, L. Yang, T. Chen, J. Xu, and P. N. Epstein, "Uninephrectomy of diabetic OVE26 mice greatly accelerates albuminuria, fibrosis, inflammatory cell infiltration and changes in gene expression," *Nephron. Experimental Nephrology*, vol. 119, no. 1, pp. e21–e32, 2011.

[24] L. Yang, S. Brozovic, J. Xu et al., "Inflammatory gene expression in OVE26 diabetic kidney during the development of nephropathy," *Nephron: Experimental Nephrology*, vol. 119, no. 1, pp. e8–e20, 2011.

[25] M. S. Forbes, B. A. Thornhill, and R. L. Chevalier, "Proximal tubular injury and rapid formation of atubular glomeruli in mice with unilateral ureteral obstruction: a new look at an old model," *The American Journal of Physiology—Renal Physiology*, vol. 301, no. 1, pp. F110–F117, 2011.

[26] J. Xu, Y. Huang, F. Li, S. Zheng, and P. N. Epstein, "FVB mouse genotype confers susceptibility to OVE26 diabetic albuminuria," *American Journal of Physiology—Renal Physiology*, vol. 299, no. 3, pp. F487–F494, 2010.

[27] S. Mezzano, C. Aros, A. Droguett et al., "NF-κB activation and overexpression of regulated genes in human diabetic nephropathy," *Nephrology Dialysis Transplantation*, vol. 19, no. 10, pp. 2505–2512, 2004.

[28] S. Giunti, F. Barutta, P. C. Perin, and G. Gruden, "Targeting the MCP-1/CCR2 system in diabetic kidney disease," *Current Vascular Pharmacology*, vol. 8, no. 6, pp. 849–860, 2010.

[29] L. Bradford, H. Marshall, H. Robertson et al., "Cardiac allograft rejection: examination of the expression and function of the decoy chemokine receptor D6," *Transplantation*, vol. 89, no. 11, pp. 1411–1416, 2010.

[30] E. Bazzan, M. Saetta, G. Turato et al., "Expression of the atypical chemokine receptor D6 in human alveolar macrophages in COPD," *Chest*, vol. 143, no. 1, pp. 98–106, 2013.

[31] P. M. Garcia-Garcia, M. A. Getino-Melian, V. Dominguez-Pimentel, and J. F. Navarro-Gonzalez, "Inflammation in diabetic kidney disease," *World Journal of Diabetes*, vol. 5, no. 4, pp. 431–443, 2014.

[32] F. Chow, E. Ozols, D. J. Nikolic-Paterson, R. C. Atkins, and G. H. Tesch, "Macrophages in mouse type 2 diabetic nephropathy: correlation with diabetic state and progressive renal injury," *Kidney International*, vol. 65, no. 1, pp. 116–128, 2004.

[33] M. D. Singh, V. King, H. Baldwin et al., "Elevated expression of the chemokine-scavenging receptor D6 is associated with impaired lesion development in psoriasis," *American Journal of Pathology*, vol. 181, no. 4, pp. 1158–1164, 2012.

[34] X.-H. Zeng, Z.-L. Ou, K.-D. Yu et al., "Coexpression of atypical chemokine binders (ACBs) in breast cancer predicts better outcomes," *Breast Cancer Research and Treatment*, vol. 125, no. 3, pp. 715–727, 2011.

[35] G.-J. Lin, S.-H. Huang, Y.-W. Chen et al., "Transgenic expression of murine chemokine decoy receptor D6 by islets reveals the role of inflammatory CC chemokines in the development of autoimmune diabetes in NOD mice," *Diabetologia*, vol. 54, no. 7, pp. 1777–1787, 2011.

[36] L. Liu, G. J. Graham, A. Damodamn et al., "Cutting edge: the silent chemokine receptor D6 is required for generating T cell responses that mediate experimental autoimmune encephalomyelitis," *The Journal of Immunology*, vol. 177, no. 1, pp. 17–21, 2006.

[37] Y. Bordon, C. A. H. Hansell, D. P. Sester, M. Clarke, A. M. Mowat, and R. J. B. Nibbs, "The atypical chemokine receptor D6

contributes to the development of experimental colitis," *Journal of Immunology*, vol. 182, no. 8, pp. 5032–5040, 2009.

[38] A. R. Hajrasouliha, Z. Sadrai, H. K. Lee, S. K. Chauhan, and R. Dana, "Expression of the chemokine decoy receptor D6 mediates dendritic cell function and promotes corneal allograft rejection," *Molecular Vision*, vol. 19, pp. 2517–2525, 2013.

[39] B. Savino, M. G. Castor, N. Caronni et al., "Control of murine Ly6C^{high} monocyte traffic and immunosuppressive activities by atypical chemokine receptor D6," *Blood*, vol. 119, no. 22, pp. 5250–5260, 2012.

5

High Glucose and Lipopolysaccharide Prime NLRP3 Inflammasome via ROS/TXNIP Pathway in Mesangial Cells

Hong Feng,[1,2] Junling Gu,[3] Fang Gou,[1] Wei Huang,[1] Chenlin Gao,[1] Guo Chen,[1] Yang Long,[1] Xueqin Zhou,[1] Maojun Yang,[1] Shuang Liu,[1] Shishi Lü,[1] Qiaoyan Luo,[1] and Yong Xu[1]

[1]*Department of Endocrinology, Affiliated Hospital of Luzhou Medical College, Luzhou, Sichuan 646000, China*
[2]*Department of Internal Medicine, Nan'an District People's Hospital, Chongqing 400060, China*
[3]*Department of Endocrinology, The Fifth People's Hospital of Chongqing, Chongqing 400062, China*

Correspondence should be addressed to Yong Xu; xywyll@aliyun.com

Academic Editor: Paolo Fiorina

While inflammation is considered a central component in the development in diabetic nephropathy, the mechanism remains unclear. The NLRP3 inflammasome acts as both a sensor and a regulator of the inflammatory response. The NLRP3 inflammasome responds to exogenous and endogenous danger signals, resulting in cleavage of procaspase-1 and activation of cytokines IL-1β, IL-18, and IL-33, ultimately triggering an inflammatory cascade reaction. This study observed the expression of NLRP3 inflammasome signaling stimulated by high glucose, lipopolysaccharide, and reactive oxygen species (ROS) inhibitor N-acetyl-L-cysteine in glomerular mesangial cells, aiming to elucidate the mechanism by which the NLRP3 inflammasome signaling pathway may contribute to diabetic nephropathy. We found that the expression of thioredoxin-interacting protein (TXNIP), NLRP3, and IL-1β was observed by immunohistochemistry in vivo. Simultaneously, the mRNA and protein levels of TXNIP, NLRP3, procaspase-1, and IL-1β were significantly induced by high glucose concentration and lipopolysaccharide in a dose-dependent and time-dependent manner in vitro. This induction by both high glucose and lipopolysaccharide was significantly inhibited by N-acetyl-L-cysteine. Our results firstly reveal that high glucose and lipopolysaccharide activate ROS/TXNIP/ NLRP3/IL-1β inflammasome signaling in glomerular mesangial cells, suggesting a mechanism by which inflammation may contribute to the development of diabetic nephropathy.

1. Introduction

Diabetic nephropathy (DN) is one type of microvascular complication of diabetes and the leading cause of end-stage renal disease in the Western world [1]. A primary hallmark of DN is the progressive damage and death of glomerular podocytes, resulting in renal sclerosis and fibrosis and the leaking of proteins into the urine. The onset of diabetic nephropathy is insidious and while the mechanism remains unclear, it is widely accepted that inflammation plays an important role [2]. The disorder of renal hemodynamics and metabolism caused by chronic hyperglycemia as well as hyperlipidemia may stimulate the secretion of inflammatory factors, leading to infiltration of immune cells in early diabetic nephrosis. Such immune-mediated inflammation is the essence of the microinflammatory state associated with innate immunity [3].

The mammalian immune system consists of two different arms: innate and adaptive immunity. Innate immunity is an evolutionarily conserved system that provides the first line of protection against invading microbes [4]. The NLRP3 (nucleotide-binding domain and leucine-rich repeat-containing family, pyrin domain-containing-3) inflammasome (also known as the NALP3 inflammasome) is an important component of the innate immune system and is composed of NLRP3, ASC (apoptosis-associated speck-like protein containing a CARD), and procaspase-1 [5]. The NLRP3 inflammasome senses endogenous and exogenous danger signals, such as lipopolysaccharide (LPS) and high glucose (HG), resulting in the activation of caspase-1 followed by activation of cytokines interleukin- (IL-) 1β, IL-18, and IL-33. This cascade triggers sustained inflammation, which has been associated with metabolic diseases [6, 7]. However, the role of the NLRP3 inflammasome in diabetic nephropathy remains unclear.

Lipopolysaccharide (LPS), often referred to as endotoxin, is found on the cell wall of Gram-negative bacteria. A high-fat diet increases the proportion of Gram-negative bacteria in the gut and causes a dramatic rise in the circulating concentration of plasma LPS, resulting in metabolic endotoxemia. Metabolic endotoxemia appears to be associated with a host of conditions including inflammation, obesity, type 2 diabetes, and metabolic syndrome [8, 9].

Thioredoxin-interacting protein (TXNIP) is an early response gene highly induced by diabetes and hyperglycemia [10–12]. TXNIP was initially identified as one of the proteins that interacts with thioredoxin (TRX) and reduces its function which scavenges reactive oxygen species (ROS) [13, 14]. Recent findings demonstrate a potential role for TXNIP in innate immunity via the NLRP3 inflammasome activation and release of IL-1β in diabetes and oxidative stress [15, 16]. Meanwhile, it is well known that oxidative stress plays an important role in the pathophysiology of diabetic nephropathy. However, a beneficial role of N-acetylcysteine (NAC) supplementation is discovered in oxidative stress [17]. NAC is an antioxidant that acts as a free radical scavenger [18]; it also activates glutathione (GSH), which acts intra- and extracellularly as an antioxidant eliminating ROS [19]. Based on these findings, we favor a model that ROS activate the NLRP3 inflammasome through the dissociation of TRX and TXNIP, contributing to the progression of diabetic complications [20, 21]. Therefore, we detected the expression of TXNIP, NLRP3, procaspase-1, and IL-1β in glomerular mesangial cells of diabetic nephropathy and then observed the changes of the players using NAC blocked ROS that stimulated by high glucose and LPS, aiming to elucidate the role of oxidative stress and the NLRP3 inflammasome signaling pathway in glomerular mesangial cells of diabetic nephropathy.

2. Materials and Methods

2.1. Establishing the Animal Model. Male Wistar rats weighing 200 g were purchased from the Biotechnology Corporation of Teng Xing (Chongqing, China). The rats were randomly allocated into two groups: a control group (NC group, n = 20) and a diabetic control group (DC group, n = 20). Rats in the diabetic control group were rendered diabetic by intraperitoneal injection of Streptozocin (STZ, Sigma, USA), at a dose of 60 mg/kg. STZ was dissolved in 0.1 M citrate buffer at pH4.5. Meanwhile, rats in the NC group received an intraperitoneal injection of the same volume of citrate buffer. After 3 days following the STZ injection, fasting glycemic measurements were performed in blood samples from tail veins, and blood glucose levels of ⩾16.7 mmol/L lasting 3 days were confirmed as being "diabetic."

2.2. Sample Collection. All rats were weighed and 24-hour urinary microalbumin was collected every day. After 6 or 8 weeks, all rats were sacrificed and heart blood was collected to measure BUN levels and fasting blood glucose (FBG) levels, using an automatic biochemistry analyzer. Both kidneys were cut along the coronal plane; upper poles of the right kidneys were used for pathology, and the left renal tissues were preserved at −80°C until required for Western blot analysis and RT-PCR.

2.3. Immunohistochemistry. Sections were incubated with the following primary antibodies: TXNIP (rabbit; 1:200; Abcam), NLRP3 (rabbit; 1:500; Abcam), and IL-1β (rabbit; 1:200; Abcam) over night at 4°C. After sections were washed with PBS, they were incubated with horseradish peroxidase-conjugated secondary antibodies (1:200 dilution) for 2 h at room temperature. For visualizing the signals, sections were treated with peroxidase substrate DAB (3, 3-diaminobenzidine) and counterstained with hematoxylin.

2.4. Renal Mesangial Cell Culture. Rat glomerular mesangial cells were cultured in Dulbecco's Modified Eagle Medium (DMEM) containing 5.6 mmol/L glucose and 10% fetal bovine serum (FBS) at 37°C and 5% CO_2. The glomerular mesangial cells were used for all experiments and were randomly divided into the following six groups: (1) normal control group (group NC, 5.6 mmol/L glucose); (2) high glucose group (group HG, 10, 20, or 30 mmol/L glucose); (3) osmotic pressure group (group OP, 5.6 mmol/L glucose + 24.4 mmol/L mannitol); (4) NAC intervention in high glucose group (group HG + NAC, 10 μmol/L NAC in 30 mmol/L glucose medium); (5) LPS group (group LPS, 1, 5, or 10 μg/L LPS); and (6) NAC intervention in LPS group (group LPS + NAC, 10 μmol/L NAC in 10 μg/L LPS medium). The cells in each group were induced for 6, 12, or 24 h before NLRP3, procaspase-1, IL-1β, TXNIP protein, and mRNA levels were measured.

2.5. Western Blotting. Total protein was extracted from glomerular mesangial cells using a protein extraction kit (Kaiji, Shanghai, China). Proteins were separated by sodium dodecyl sulfate-polyacrylamide gel electrophoresis and transferred to a polyvinylidene difluoride (PVDF) membrane (Millipore). Immunoblotting was performed using anti-NLRP3 antibody (rabbit; 1:4,000; Abcam), anti-TXNIP antibody (rabbit; 1:800; Abcam), anti-procaspase-1 antibody (rabbit; 1:700; Cell Signaling Technology), and anti-β-actin antibody (mouse; 1:3,000; Beyotime).

2.6. Reverse-Transcription Polymerase Chain Reaction (RT-PCR). Total RNA was isolated from glomerular mesangial cells using an RNA extraction kit (Tiangen Biotech, Beijing, China). Total RNA was reverse-transcribed (RT) using a Takara RNA PCR kit (Baoshengwu, Dalian, China). cDNA was amplified in a gradient thermal cycler (Eppendorf, Germany) using polymerase chain reaction (PCR) Master Mix (Baoshengwu, Dalian, China). Gene expression was normalized to β-actin. The primer sequences were as follows:

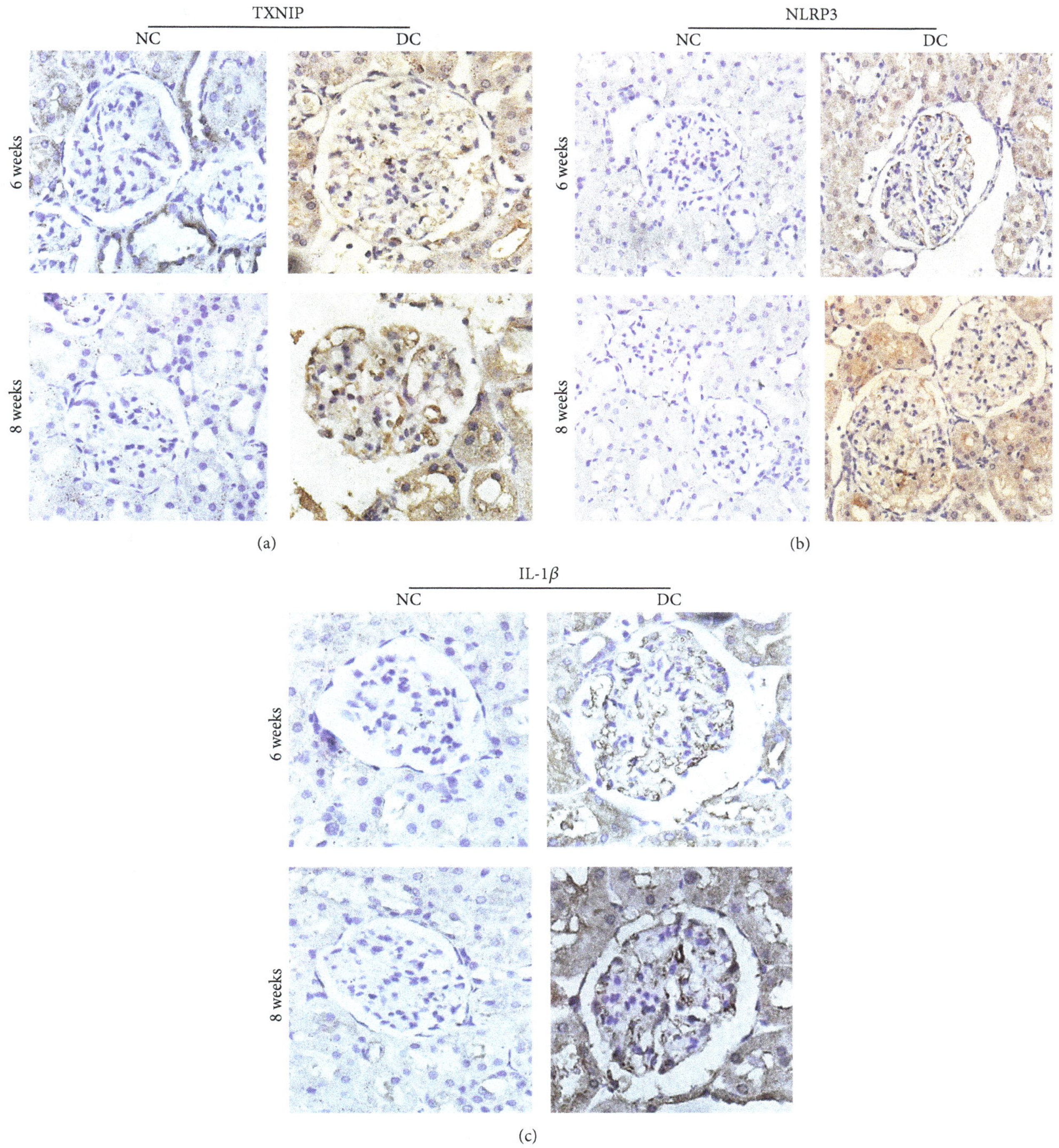

FIGURE 1: In the immunohistochemistry (×400 double), TXNIP, NLRP3, and IL-1β expression (a, b, and c) in the DC group were increased compared to the NC group.

NLRP3 (forward, 5′-CCA GGG CTC TGT TCA TTG -3′; reverse, 5′-CCT TCA CGT CTC GGT TC -3′), TXNIP (forward, 5′-CCA CGC TGA CTT TGA GAA CA -3′; reverse, 5′-GGA GCC AGG GAC ACT AAC ATA-3′), IL-1β (forward, 5′- CTT CAA ATC TCA CAG CAG CAT-3′; reverse, 5′- CAG GTC GTC ATC ATC CCA C-3′), and β-actin (forward, 5′-CGT TGA CAT CCG TAA AGA C-3′; reverse, 5′-TGG AAG GTG GAC AGT GAG -3′).

2.7. Data Analysis. All data obtained from at least three independent experiments were expressed as the mean ± standard deviation (SD) and analyzed using one-way analysis

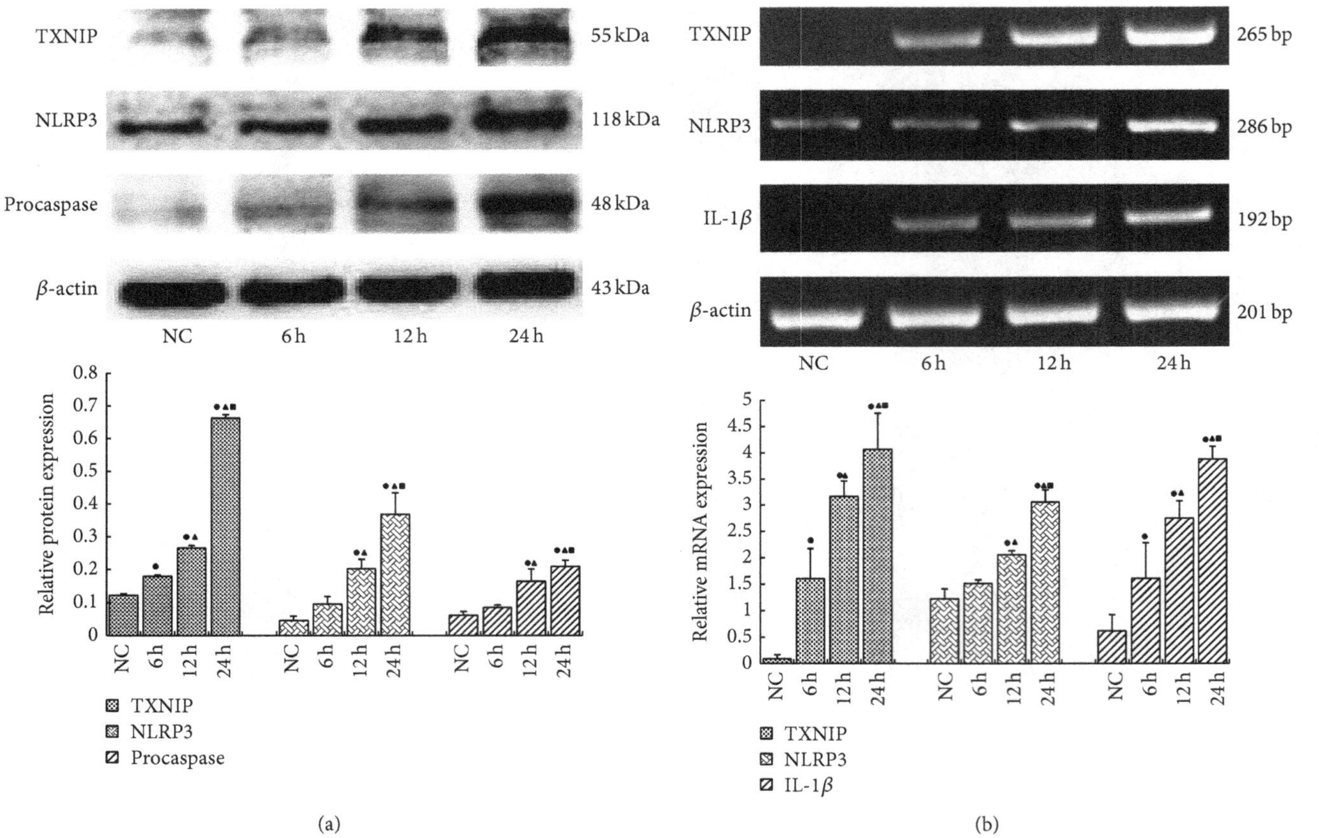

FIGURE 2: Compared to the normal control group, TXNIP, NLRP3, procaspase-1, and IL-1β were significantly induced at both the mRNA and protein levels following 6, 12, and 24 h of exposure to 30 mmol/L glucose. Moreover, protein and mRNA levels were highest at 24 h (a, b) (●$p < 0.05$ versus NC group, ▲$p < 0.05$ versus 6 h, and ■$p < 0.05$ versus 12 h).

of variance (ANOVA), followed by the LSD post hoc test for multiple comparisons (SPSS 11.5 statistical software). $p < 0.05$ was considered significant.

3. Results

3.1. STZ-Induced Changes in 24-Hour Urine Protein and Renal Function of Diabetic Rats. Compared to the NC group, fasting blood glucose (FBG) levels, 24-hour urine protein, urinary albumin-to-creatinine ratios (ACR), and BUN levels were increased in the DC group.

3.2. The Expression of TXNIP, NLRP3, and IL-1β Was Observed In Vivo. Renal tissue immunohistochemistry (Figures 1(a), 1(b), and 1(c)) showed that, compared with the NC group, there were increased *TXNIP, NLRP3, and IL-1β* expressions that were particularly evident in the DC group. The expression of those players in 8 weeks was stronger than that in 6 weeks.

3.3. TXNIP, NLRP3, Procaspase-1, and IL-1β Expression Is Induced by High Concentrations of Glucose. Compared to the normal control group, TXNIP, NLRP3, procaspase-1, and IL-1β were significantly induced at both the mRNA and protein levels following 6, 12, and 24 h of exposure to 30 mmol/L glucose ($p < 0.05$). Moreover, protein and mRNA levels were highest at 24 h (Figures 2(a) and 2(b)), suggesting that a high glucose concentration increased NLRP3 inflammasome levels in a time-dependent manner.

TXNIP, NLRP3, procaspase-1, and IL-1β were also significantly induced by several high concentrations of glucose at 24 h ($p < 0.05$). The highest relative expression of these factors was observed in the 30 mmol/L high glucose group (Figures 3(a) and 3(b)), suggesting that glucose increased NLRP3 inflammasome levels in a dose-dependent manner. No genes were significantly induced in the osmotic pressure group ($p > 0.05$).

3.4. TXNIP, NLRP3, Procaspase-1, and IL-1β Expression Is Induced by LPS. Compared to the normal control group, TXNIP, NLRP3, procaspase-1, and IL-1β were significantly induced at both the mRNA and protein levels following 6, 12, and 24 h of exposure to 10 μg/L LPS ($p < 0.05$). Protein and mRNA levels were highest at 12 h (Figures 4(a) and 4(b)).

TXNIP, NLRP3, procaspase-1, and IL-1β were also significantly induced by different concentrations of LPS at 12 h

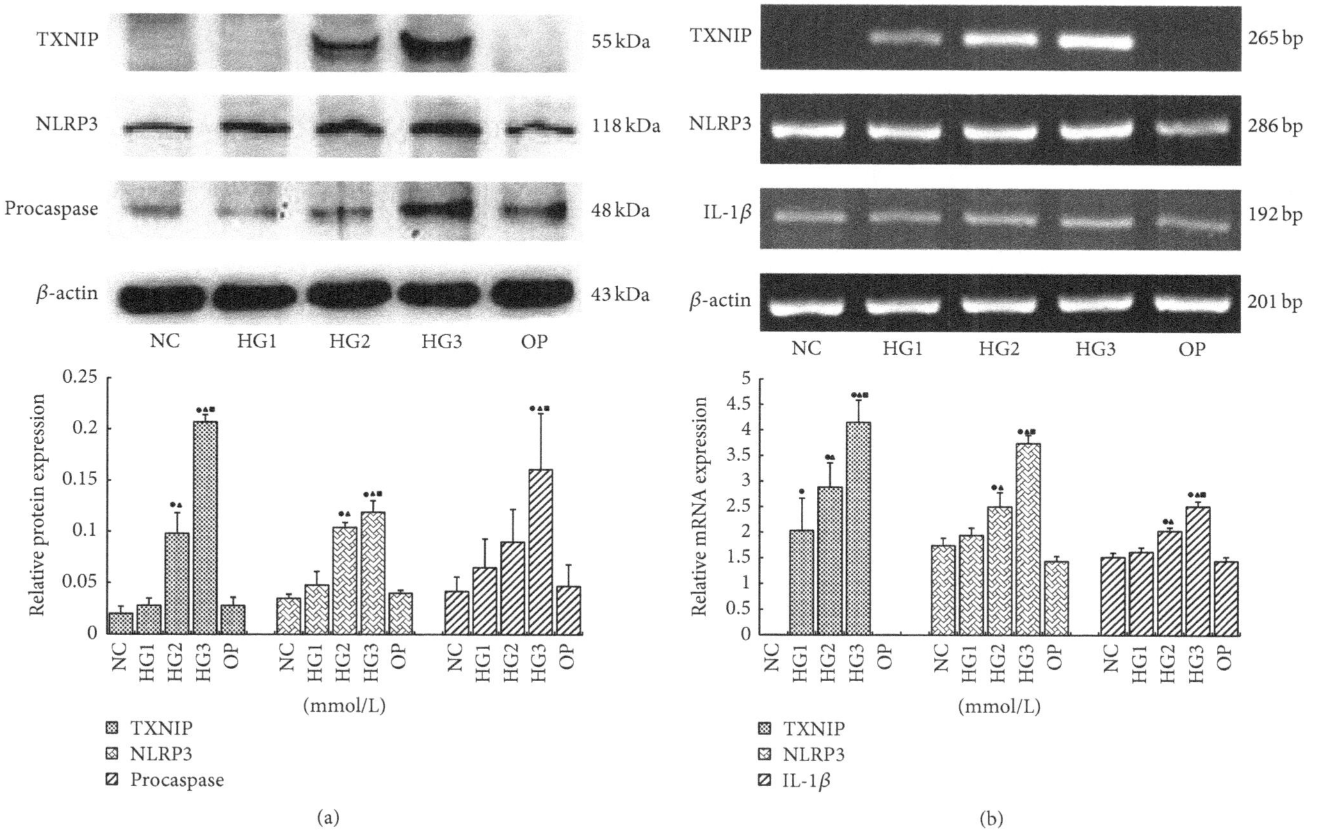

FIGURE 3: TXNIP, NLRP3, procaspase-1, and IL-1β were also significantly induced by several high concentrations of glucose at 24 h. The highest relative expression of these factors was observed in the 30 mmol/L high glucose group (a, b) (NC: 5.6 mmol/L glucose; HG1: 10 mmol/L glucose; HG2: 20 mmol/L glucose; HG3: 30 mmol/L glucose; OP: 5.6 mmol/L glucose + 24.4 mmol/L mannitol) ($^{\bullet}p < 0.05$ versus NC group or OP group, $^{\blacktriangle}p < 0.05$ versus HG1 group, and $^{\blacksquare}p < 0.05$ versus HG2 group).

($p < 0.05$). The highest relative expression of these factors was observed in the 10 μg/L LPS group (Figures 5(a) and 5(b)), suggesting that LPS increased NLRP3 inflammasome levels in a dose-dependent manner.

3.5. Induction of TXNIP, NLRP3, Procaspase-1, and IL-1β Is Inhibited by NAC. Compared with the high glucose group (30 mmol/L), mRNA and protein levels of TXNIP, NLRP3, procaspase-1, and IL-1β were significantly lower in the high glucose (30 mmol/L) plus NAC group ($p < 0.05$) (Figures 6(a) and 6(b)), suggesting that NAC inhibited induction by glucose.

Compared with the LPS (10 μg/L) group, mRNA and protein levels of TXNIP, NLRP3, procaspase-1, and IL-1β were significantly lower in the LPS (10 μg/L) plus NAC group ($p < 0.05$) (Figures 7(a) and 7(b)), suggesting that NAC inhibited induction by LPS.

4. Discussion

Diabetic nephropathy is characterized by chronic low-grade inflammation due to infiltration of immune cells and cytokines in kidney tissues. The immune-mediated inflammatory response is a key component of hyperglycemia and diabetic nephropathy. Inflammatory cytokines such as IL-1β, IL-18, TNF-α, MCP-1, and ICAM-1 are significantly increased in renal tissues during diabetic nephropathy and attenuating the expression of these cytokines may protect against diabetic renal injury [22].

IL-1β is not only a key contributor to obesity-induced inflammation and subsequent insulin resistance but also type 2 diabetes [6]. The level of IL-1β gradually increases from the development of normal glucose tolerance to impaired glucose tolerance to type 2 diabetes and is positively correlated with insulin resistance. Furthermore, IL-1β is also an instigator of the inflammation found in diabetic nephropathy. Hyperglycemia stimulates the secretion of macrophage-produced cytokine IL-1β, which induces inflammatory cytokine production and invasion into renal tissues [23]. Recent randomized clinical trials demonstrated that the level of IL-1β level was significantly increased in and positively correlated with renal function injury in patients with diabetic nephropathy [24, 25]. Here we showed that the IL-1β was significantly upregulated in the early stage of diabetic nephropathy, and the expression of IL-1β in glomerular mesangial cells was induced by high glucose and lipopolysaccharide in a dose-dependent and time-dependent manner. These results

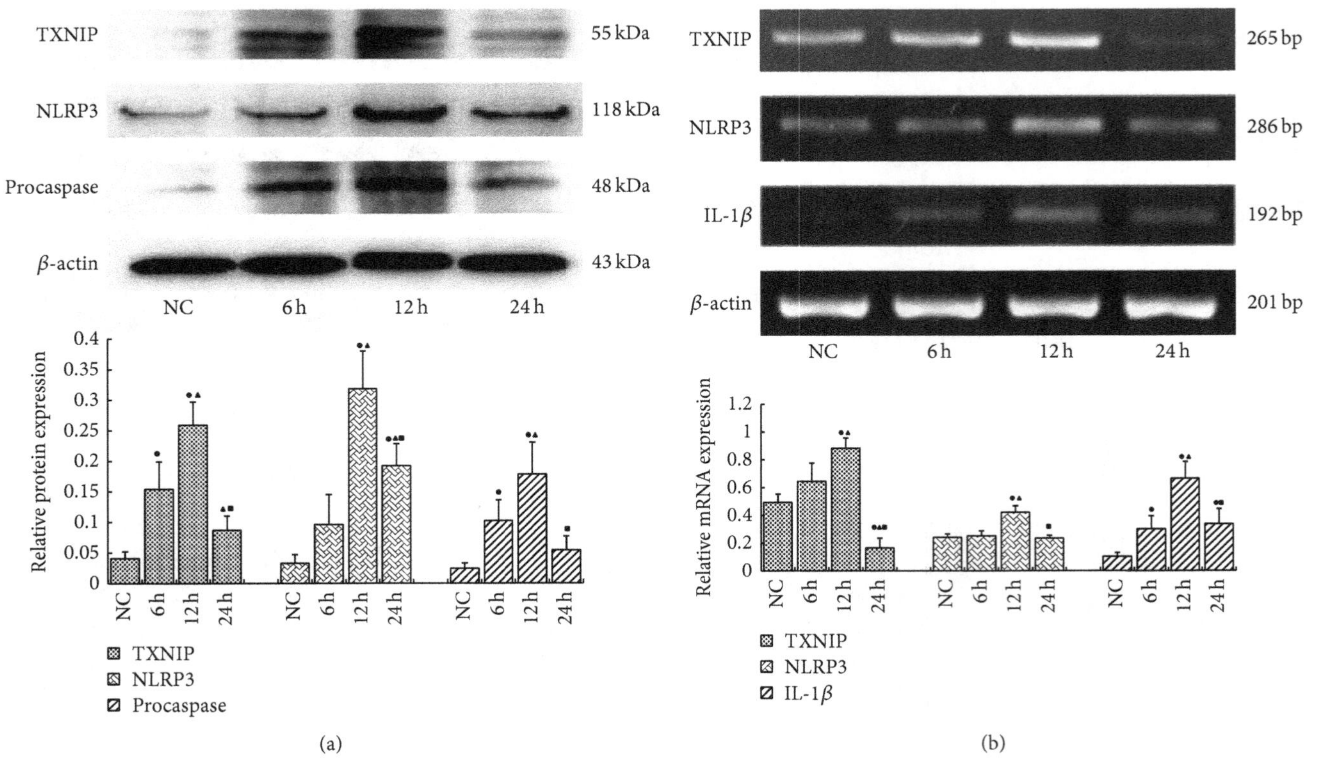

FIGURE 4: Compared to the normal control group, TXNIP, NLRP3, procaspase-1, and IL-1β were significantly induced at both the mRNA and protein levels following 6, 12, and 24 h of exposure to 10 μg/L LPS ($p < 0.05$). Protein and mRNA levels were highest at 12 h (a, b) (●$p < 0.05$ versus NC group, ▲$p < 0.05$ versus 6 h, and ■$p < 0.05$ versus 12 h).

suggest that high glucose and lipopolysaccharide induce a renal inflammatory reaction and IL-1β contributes to the pathogenesis of diabetic nephropathy, supporting the role of microinflammation in diabetic nephropathy.

The secretion of bioactive IL-1β is predominantly controlled by activation of caspase-1 through the assembly of a multiprotein scaffold inflammasome composed of NLRP3, ASC, and procaspase-1 [26]. NLRP3 is mainly responsible for the detection of infection-derived molecules such as lipopolysaccharide. Moreover, NLRP3 is unique in its ability to recognize molecular patterns associated with host-derived signals that are abundant in obese individuals, including excess ATP, glucose, ROS, and uric acid, as well as crystals of cholesterol [5]. ASC is the indispensable adaptor that connects NLRP3 and procaspase-1 [27]. Caspase-1 mediated cleavage is the limiting step for processing IL-1β into its secreted active forms. Inactive procaspase-1 molecules are recruited to the NLRP3 inflammasome [28]. The NLRP3 inflammasome is not only an important sensor of metabolic dysregulation, but also a molecular platform of procaspase-1 and IL-1β activation [26].

Mechanisms leading to NLRP3 inflammasome activation are a matter of debate. Several models are widely favored in the literature, including the K^+ channel model, lysosomal damage model, and ROS model, although they may not be mutually exclusive [16, 29, 30]. All NLRP3 agonists trigger the production of ROS, which leads to the activation of the NLRP3 inflammasome via the ROS-sensitive TXNIP protein [31].

However, the role and mechanism of NLRP3 inflammasome in diabetic nephropathy is not yet fully understood. Chen and colleagues discovered that ATP-P2X signaling mediates high glucose-induced activation of the NLRP3 inflammasome and IL-1 family cytokine secretion, causing the development of inflammation in renal tubular epithelial cells [24]. However, our results firstly demonstrate the activation of NLRP3 inflammasome following high glucose-induced expression of NLRP3 and procaspase-1 in mesangial cells in vivo and vitro. Taken together, these results reveal that high glucose activates the NLRP3 inflammasome and mediates inflammation in diabetic nephropathy. In addition, sustained hyperglycemia may increase uric acid and fatty acid levels in circulation. Hyperglycemia along with uric acid and fatty acid activates the NLRP3 inflammasome, which is involved in the occurrence and development of inflammation in diabetic nephropathy [32–34].

Endotoxin is associated with an increased risk for diabetes. Importantly, the risk is independent of other established risk factors like glucose and lipid levels [35]. Additionally, several clinical trials provide evidence that circulating lipopolysaccharide is higher in diabetic patients with kidney disease compared with nondiabetic nephropathy patients, and metabolic endotoxemia is also associated with the development of diabetic nephropathy [36, 37]. Endotoxemia

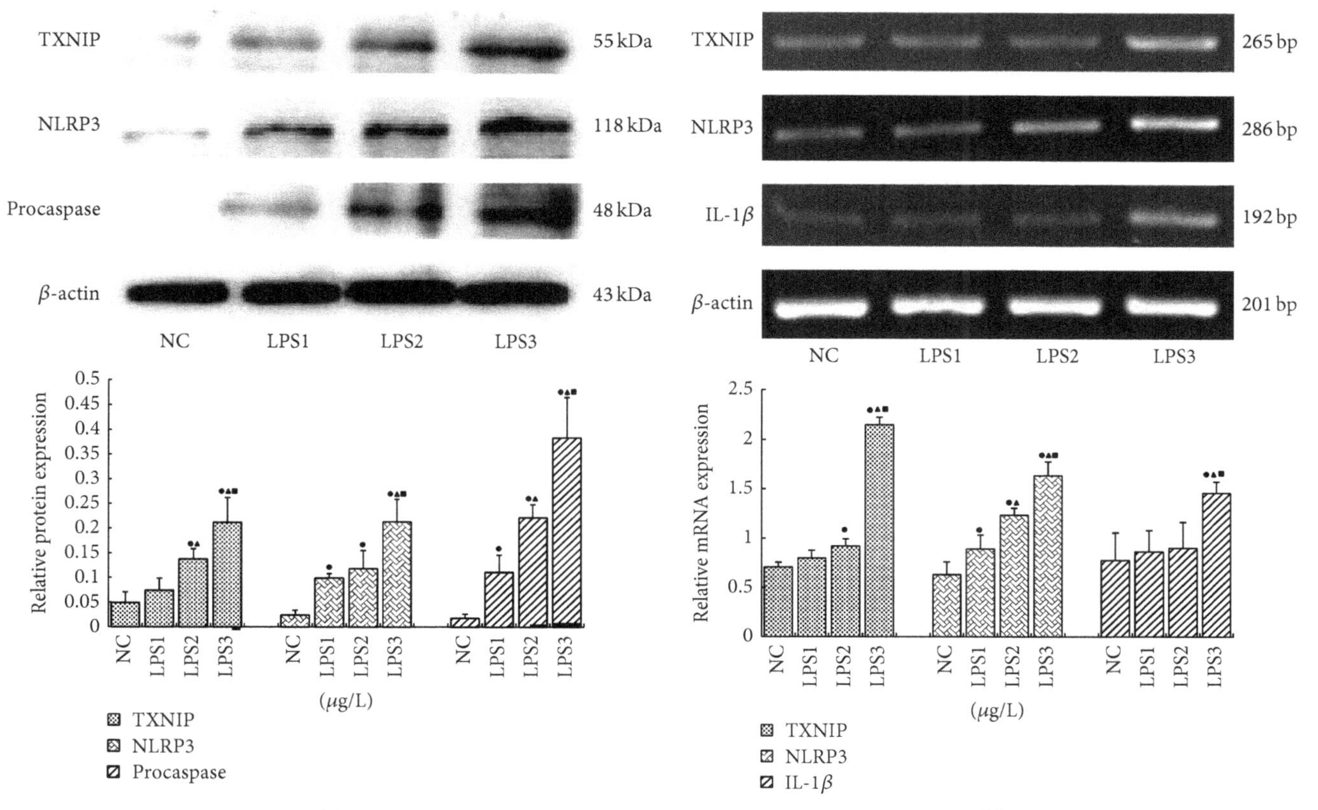

FIGURE 5: TXNIP, NLRP3, procaspase-1, and IL-1β were also significantly induced by different concentrations of LPS at 12 h. The highest relative expression of these factors was observed in the 10 μg/L LPS group (a, b) (NC: 0 μg/L LPS; LPS1: 1 μg/L; LPS2: 5 μg/L; LPS3: 10 μg/L) ($^{\bullet}p < 0.05$ versus NC group, $^{\blacktriangle}p < 0.05$ versus LPS1 group, and $^{\blacksquare}p < 0.05$ versus LPS2 group).

activates the innate immune system, characterized by a release of antibodies, cytokines, and other inflammatory mediators, which may promote kidney injury [38]. Our experimental results showed consistently increased expression of NLRP3 and procaspase-1 in mesangial cells treated with lipopolysaccharide. Thus, during metabolic endotoxemia, a large amount of lipopolysaccharide from the intestine that goes into the blood may activate the renal NLRP3 inflammasome, resulting in the release of IL-1β and promotion of kidney damage [39].

Oxidative stress created by hyperglycemia plays an important role in the pathology of diabetic nephropathy. Thioredoxin was initially identified as a protein that scavenges ROS and maintains cellular activity [40]. TXNIP is an endogenous inhibitor that interacts with thioredoxin, reducing its function to mediate oxidative stress. TXNIP is significantly increased in rats and humans with diabetic nephropathy and closely correlated with urinary albumin, renal fibrosis, and reactive oxygen species [41, 42]. We found that TXNIP was significantly induced by high glucose and LPS, even at 6 h, in our in vitro study. Our results suggest that TXNIP is an early response gene that is highly induced by hyperglycemia and diabetic nephropathy. Well, the expression of TXNIP, NLRP3, procaspase-1, and IL-1β was significantly increased by high glucose concentration and LPS in a dose-dependent and time-dependent manner in vitro. It indicated a subtle relationship between the players. Surprisingly, the induction of TXNIP, NLRP3, procaspase-1, and IL-1β by both high glucose and LPS was significantly inhibited by NAC intervention. It reveals a close connection between the players and an activation of ROS in the TXNIP pathway. ROS promotes the activation of TXNIP pathway; however, scavenging ROS may inhibit the activation of it. Additionally, in our previous studies, pathological changes in the kidney were obvious, followed by the upregulation of the proposed players in diabetic rats; the glomerular tuft and mesangial area were increased by HE staining [43]. There was a trend for an increase of glomerular volume in diabetic rats compared with normal rats. Collagen plays a critical structural role in renal fibrosis of DN. Observation with the light microscope, following Masson staining, demonstrated that accumulation of collagen in the kidney of the diabetic rats was greater than the normal rats in gross appearance [43]. These experiments and figures indicated that the proposed proteins in TXNIP pathway may play an important role in the inflammation of incipient diabetic nephropathy, renal sclerosis, and fibrosis. Based on our findings, we suggest a new model for the activation of the NLRP3 inflammasome and development of diabetic neuropathy. Exposure of the kidneys to high glucose and lipopolysaccharide results in

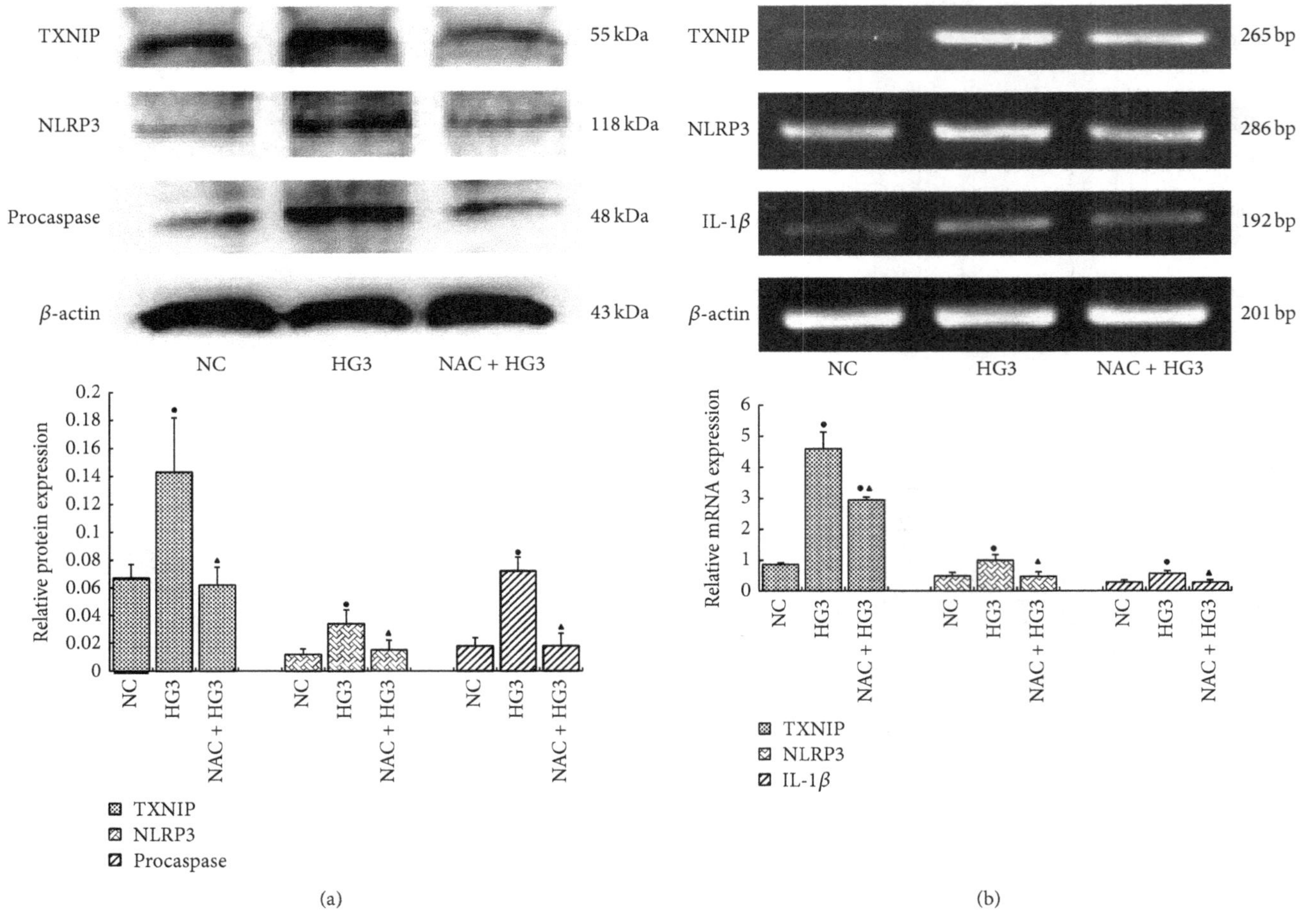

FIGURE 6: Compared with the high glucose group (30 mmol/L), mRNA and protein levels of TXNIP, NLRP3, procaspase-1, and IL-1β were significantly lower in the high glucose (30 mmol/L) plus NAC group (a, b) (NC: 5.6 mmol/L glucose; HG3: 30 mmol/L glucose; NAC + HG3: 10 μmol/L NAC + 30 mmol/L glucose) ($^{\bullet}p < 0.05$ versus NC group, $^{\blacktriangle}p < 0.05$ versus HG3 group).

the production of a massive amount of reactive oxygen species, which causes the TXNIP bound to thioredoxin to disassociate. TXNIP reduces the ROS scavenging capacity of thioredoxin and binds to NLRP3, mediating NLRP3 inflammasome assembly with ASC and procaspase-1. The subsequent autocleavage and activation of caspase-1 in turn results in the processing of pro-IL-1β to its mature form, which then leads to the induction of other proinflammatory genes, eventually promoting the oxidative stress and inflammation present in diabetic nephropathy [20, 44].

Although current treatments which concentrate on controlling hyperglycemia and hypertension reduce the risk of progressive kidney disease, diabetic kidney disease remains the leading cause of ESRD and the major risk amplifier for death in the population [45]. Therefore, novel therapeutic approaches are urgently needed, while a growing body of evidence from human, animal, and in vitro studies indicates that existing drugs, including the urate-lowering agent allopurinol, the anti-TNF agents etanercept, endothelin antagonist avosentan, and the immunomodulating drug abatacept, might be effective in preventing or slowing the progression of diabetic nephropathy to end-stage renal disease by targeting metabolic, inflammatory, and immunological pathways [45–47]. Rodrigues and colleagues showed that P2X7 receptor, which is also related to oxidative stress and induces tissue apoptosis or necrosis, was inhibited in diabetic rats treated with NAC [48]. They suggest that the maintenance of redox homeostasis could be useful as coadjuvant treatment to delay the progression of diabetic nephropathy. The P2 purinergic receptors, such as P2X7 receptor, modulate a variety of physiologic events upon the maintenance of a highly sensitive "set point," the derangement of which may lead to the development of key pathogenic mechanisms during acute and chronic diseases. Solini and colleagues suggest that extracellular ATP signaling via P2 purinergic receptors may be involved in different renal pathologic conditions [49]. This review summarizes that NAC is potential therapeutic options targeting due to inhibiting the activation of TXNIP signal and extracellular ATP signaling. Nevertheless, there is a contradiction that NAC in moderate doses given over a month did not have significant effect on the overall oxidative stress in patients with DN and did not reduce proteinuria

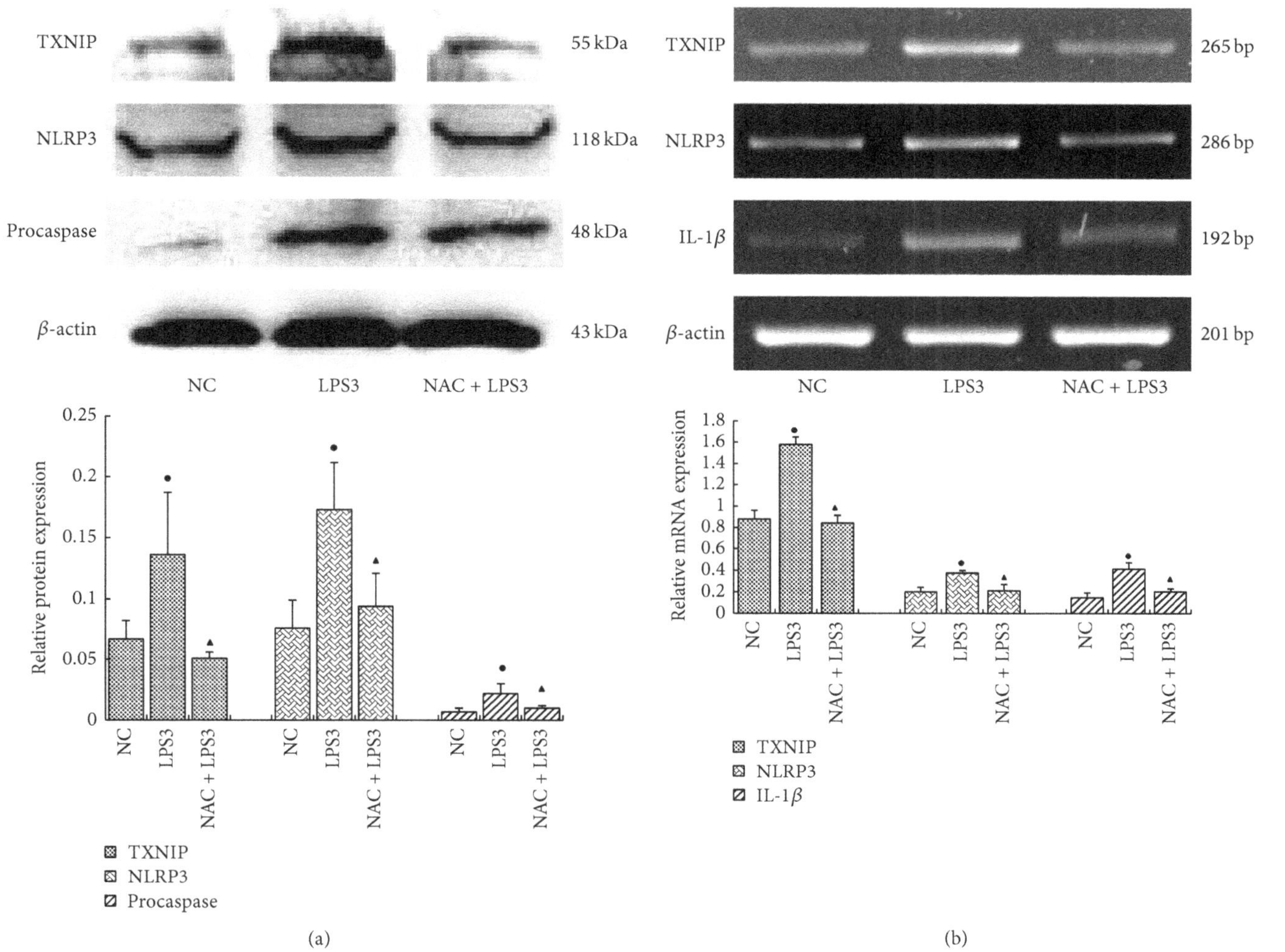

FIGURE 7: Compared with the LPS (10 μg/L) group, mRNA and protein levels of TXNIP, NLRP3, procaspase-1, and IL-1β were significantly lower in the LPS (10 μg/L) plus NAC group (a, b) (NC: 0 μg/L LPS; LPS3: 10 μg/L LPS; NAC + LPS3: 10 μmol/L NAC + 10 μg/L LPS) (● $p < 0.05$, versus NC group, ▲ $p < 0.05$ versus LPS3 group).

[50]. It shows that reactive oxygen species are not the only signal to induce oxidative stress in vivo. There must be else mechanisms such as inflammation, polyol pathway, and advanced glycation end products, involving in oxidative stress. Therefore, NAC do not completely inhibit the activation of oxidative stress. Moreover, NAC did not achieve the expected results in patients with DN, maybe due to not enough treatment time, not powerful reduction of oxidative stress, and so on.

5. Conclusion

Our study has firstly demonstrated that high glucose and lipopolysaccharide can activate the pathway of ROS/TXNIP/NLRP3 inflammasome signaling and results in the release of IL-1β in glomerular mesangial cells. These results help to clarify the cellular and molecular basis of the association between innate immunity and diabetic nephropathy, suggesting a new target for treatment of diabetic nephropathy. Future studies will focus on the interaction among pathogen-associated molecular patterns, damage-associated molecular patterns, and innate immunity in order to clarify the molecular mechanisms behind the development of metabolic diseases. Such findings have the potential which profoundly impact the prevention of diabetes and associated complications.

Disclosure

Junling Gu is a co-first author.

Conflict of Interests

The authors declare that they have no conflict of interests regarding the publication of this paper.

Acknowledgments

The authors gratefully acknowledge Neurobiology Laboratory and Clinical Center Laboratory for technical assistance.

The authors also thank BioMed Proofreading for English expression polished.

References

[1] C.-C. Wu, J.-S. Chen, K.-C. Lu et al., "Aberrant cytokines/chemokines production correlate with proteinuria in patients with overt diabetic nephropathy," *Clinica Chimica Acta*, vol. 411, no. 9-10, pp. 700–704, 2010.

[2] J. Wada and H. Makino, "Inflammation and the pathogenesis of diabetic nephropathy," *Clinical Science*, vol. 124, no. 3, pp. 139–152, 2013.

[3] J. M. Fernández-Real and J. C. Pickup, "Innate immunity, insulin resistance and type 2 diabetes," *Diabetologia*, vol. 55, no. 2, pp. 273–278, 2012.

[4] T. Kawai and S. Akira, "The roles of TLRs, RLRs and NLRs in pathogen recognition," *International Immunology*, vol. 21, no. 4, pp. 317–337, 2009.

[5] M. A. Mori, O. Bezy, and C. R. Kahn, "Metabolic syndrome: is Nlrp3 inflammasome a trigger or a target of insulin resistance?" *Circulation Research*, vol. 108, no. 10, pp. 1160–1162, 2011.

[6] Y.-H. Youm, A. Adijiang, B. Vandanmagsar, D. Burk, A. Ravussin, and V. D. Dixit, "Elimination of the NLRP3-ASC inflammasome protects against chronic obesity-induced pancreatic damage," *Endocrinology*, vol. 152, no. 11, pp. 4039–4045, 2011.

[7] M. Ganz, T. Csak, and G. Szabo, "High fat diet feeding results in gender specific steatohepatitis and inflammasome activation," *World Journal of Gastroenterology*, vol. 20, no. 26, pp. 8525–8534, 2014.

[8] P. D. Cani, M. Osto, L. Geurts, and A. Everard, "Involvement of gut microbiota in the development of low-grade inflammation and type 2 diabetes associated with obesity," *Gut Microbes*, vol. 3, no. 4, pp. 279–288, 2012.

[9] M. K. Piya, A. L. Harte, and P. G. McTernan, "Metabolic endotoxaemia: is it more than just a gut feeling?" *Current Opinion in Lipidology*, vol. 24, no. 1, pp. 78–85, 2013.

[10] L. Perrone, T. S. Devi, K.-I. Hosoya, T. Terasaki, and L. P. Singh, "Thioredoxin interacting protein (TXNIP) induces inflammation through chromatin modification in retinal capillary endothelial cells under diabetic conditions," *Journal of Cellular Physiology*, vol. 221, no. 1, pp. 262–272, 2009.

[11] J. Chen, G. Saxena, I. N. Mungrue, A. J. Lusis, and A. Shalev, "Thioredoxin-interacting protein: a critical link between glucose toxicity and β-cell apoptosis," *Diabetes*, vol. 57, no. 4, pp. 938–944, 2008.

[12] D. W. Cheng, Y. Jiang, A. Shalev, R. Kowluru, E. D. Crook, and L. P. Singh, "An analysis of high glucose and glucosamine-induced gene expression and oxidative stress in renal mesangial cells," *Archives of Physiology and Biochemistry*, vol. 112, no. 4-5, pp. 189–218, 2006.

[13] P. C. Schulze, J. Yoshioka, T. Takahashi, Z. He, G. L. King, and R. T. Lee, "Hyperglycemia promotes oxidative stress through inhibition of thioredoxin function by thioredoxin-interacting protein," *Journal of Biological Chemistry*, vol. 279, no. 29, pp. 30369–30374, 2004.

[14] M. T. Forrester, D. Seth, A. Hausladen et al., "Thioredoxin-interacting protein (Txnip) is a feedback regulator of S-nitrosylation," *Journal of Biological Chemistry*, vol. 284, no. 52, pp. 36160–36166, 2009.

[15] R. Zhou, A. Tardivel, B. Thorens, I. Choi, and J. Tschopp, "Thioredoxin-interacting protein links oxidative stress to inflammasome activation," *Nature Immunology*, vol. 11, no. 2, pp. 136–140, 2010.

[16] K. Schroder, R. Zhou, and J. Tschopp, "The NLRP3 inflammasome: a sensor for metabolic danger?" *Science*, vol. 327, no. 5963, pp. 296–300, 2010.

[17] G. B. Nogueira, A. M. Rodrigues, F. R. Maciel et al., "N-acetylcysteine and oxidative stress in the kidney of uninephrectomized rats with diabetes mellitus," in *Proceedings of the Annual Meeting on ASN Kidney Week*, vol. 1, Philadelphia, Pa, USA, 2011.

[18] E. P. Da Silva Jr. and R. H. Lambertucci, "Effects of N-acetylcysteine and L-arginine in the antioxidant system of C2C12 cells," *The Journal of Sports Medicine and Physical Fitness*, vol. 55, no. 6, pp. 691–699, 2015.

[19] C. K. Sen, "Antioxidant and redox regulation of cellular signaling: introduction," *Medicine and Science in Sports and Exercise*, vol. 33, no. 3, pp. 368–370, 2001.

[20] P. Gao, X. F. Meng, H. Su et al., "Thioredoxin-interacting protein mediates NALP3 inflammasome activation in podocytes duringdiabetic nephropathy," *Biochim Biophys Acta*, vol. 1843, no. 11, pp. 2448–2460, 2014.

[21] B. Luo, B. Li, W. Wang et al., "NLRP3 gene silencing ameliorates diabetic cardiomyopathy in a type 2 diabetes rat model," *PLoS ONE*, vol. 9, no. 8, Article ID e104771, 2014.

[22] H. Y. Chen, X. R. Huang, W. Wang et al., "The protective role of Smad7 in diabetic kidney disease: mechanism and therapeutic potential," *Diabetes*, vol. 60, no. 2, pp. 590–601, 2011.

[23] E. Sánchez-López, J. Rodriguez-Vita, C. Cartier et al., "Inhibitory effect of interleukin-1 beta on angiotensin II-induced connective tissue growth factor and type IV collagen production in cultured mesangial cells," *The American Journal of Physiology—Renal Physiology*, vol. 294, no. 1, pp. F149–F160, 2008.

[24] K. Chen, J. Zhang, W. Zhang et al., "ATP-P2X4 signaling mediates NLRP3 inflammasome activation: a novel pathway of diabetic nephropathy," *The International Journal of Biochemistry & Cell Biology*, vol. 45, no. 5, pp. 932–943, 2013.

[25] S. Maeda, "Do inflammatory cytokine genes confer susceptibility to diabetic nephropathy?" *Kidney International*, vol. 74, no. 4, pp. 413–415, 2008.

[26] R. W. Grant and V. D. Dixit, "Mechanisms of disease: inflammasome activation and the development of type 2 diabetes," *Frontiers in Immunology*, vol. 4, no. 4, article 50, 2013.

[27] A. Babelova, K. Moreth, W. Tsalastra-Greul et al., "Biglycan, a danger signal that activates the NLRP3 inflammasome via toll-like and P2X receptors," *The Journal of Biological Chemistry*, vol. 284, no. 36, pp. 24035–24048, 2009.

[28] T. Jourdan, G. Godlewski, R. Cinar et al., "Activation of the Nlrp3 inflammasome in infiltrating macrophages by endocannabinoids mediates β cell loss in type 2 diabetes," *Nature Medicine*, vol. 19, no. 9, pp. 1132–1140, 2013.

[29] S. Sun, S. Xia, Y. Ji, S. Kersten, and L. Qi, "The ATP-P2X 7 signaling axis is dispensable for obesity-associated inflammasome activation in adipose tissue," *Diabetes*, vol. 61, no. 6, pp. 1471–1478, 2012.

[30] Y. Yin, J. L. Pastrana, X. Li et al., "Inflammasomes: sensors of metabolic stresses for vascular inflammation," *Frontiers in Bioscience*, vol. 18, no. 8, pp. 638–649, 2013.

[31] M. S. Lee, "Role of innate immunity in diabetes and metabolism: recent progress in the study of inflammasomes," *Immune Network*, vol. 11, no. 2, pp. 95–99, 2011.

[32] C. Wang, Y. Pan, Q.-Y. Zhang, F.-M. Wang, and L.-D. Kong, "Quercetin and allopurinol ameliorate kidney injury in STZ-treated rats with regulation of renal NLRP3 inflammasome activation and lipid accumulation," *PLoS ONE*, vol. 7, no. 6, Article ID e38285, 2012.

[33] E. Benetti, F. Chiazza, N. S. A. Patel, and M. Collino, "The NLRP3 inflammasome as a novel player of the intercellular crosstalk in metabolic disorders," *Mediators of Inflammation*, vol. 2013, Article ID 678627, 9 pages, 2013.

[34] P. Duewell, H. Kono, K. J. Rayner et al., "NLRP3 inflammasomes are required for atherogenesis and activated by cholesterol crystals," *Nature*, vol. 464, no. 7293, pp. 1357–1361, 2010.

[35] P. J. Pussinen, A. S. Havulinna, M. Lehto, J. Sundvall, and V. Salomaa, "Endotoxemia is associated with an increased risk of incident diabetes," *Diabetes Care*, vol. 34, no. 2, pp. 392–397, 2011.

[36] M. I. Lassenius, K. H. Pietiläinen, K. Kaartinen et al., "Bacterial endotoxin activity in human serum is associated with dyslipidemia, insulin resistance, obesity, and chronic inflammation," *Diabetes Care*, vol. 34, no. 8, pp. 1809–1815, 2011.

[37] M. Nymark, P. J. Pussinen, A. M. Tuomainen, C. Forsblom, P.-H. Groop, and M. Lehto, "Serum lipopolysaccharide activity is associated with the progression of kidney disease in finnish patients with type 1 diabetes," *Diabetes Care*, vol. 32, no. 9, pp. 1689–1693, 2009.

[38] A. B. Hauser, A. E. M. Stinghen, S. M. Gonçalves, S. Bucharles, and R. Pecoits-Filho, "A gut feeling on endotoxemia: causes and consequences in chronic kidney disease," *Nephron Clinical Practice*, vol. 118, no. 2, pp. 165–172, 2011.

[39] M. Manco, L. Putignani, and G. F. Bottazzo, "Gut microbiota, lipopolysaccharides, and innate immunity in the pathogenesis of obesity and cardiovascular risk," *Endocrine Reviews*, vol. 31, no. 6, pp. 817–844, 2010.

[40] T. S. Devi, I. Lee, M. Hüttemann, A. Kumar, K. D. Nantwi, and L. P. Singh, "TXNIP links innate host defense mechanisms to oxidative stress and inflammation in retinal muller glia under chronic hyperglycemia: implications for diabetic retinopathy," *Experimental Diabetes Research*, vol. 2012, Article ID 438238, 19 pages, 2012.

[41] S. M. Tan, Y. Zhang, A. J. Cox, D. J. Kelly, and W. Qi, "Tranilast attenuates the up-regulation of thioredoxin-interacting protein and oxidative stress in an experimental model of diabetic nephropathy," *Nephrology Dialysis Transplantation*, vol. 26, no. 1, pp. 100–110, 2011.

[42] A. Advani, R. E. Gilhert, K. Thai et al., "Expression, localization, and function of the thioredoxin system in diabetic nephropathy," *Journal of the American Society of Nephrology*, vol. 20, no. 4, pp. 730–741, 2009.

[43] W. Huang, C. Yang, Q. Nan et al., "The proteasome inhibitor, MG132, attenuates diabetic nephropathy by inhibiting SnoN degradation in vivo and in vitro," *BioMed Research International*, vol. 2014, Article ID 684765, 11 pages, 2014.

[44] R. Stienstra, C. J. Tack, T.-D. Kanneganti, L. A. B. Joosten, and M. G. Netea, "The inflammasome puts obesity in the danger zone," *Cell Metabolism*, vol. 15, no. 1, pp. 10–18, 2012.

[45] R. Z. Alicic and K. R. Tuttle, "Novel therapies for diabetic kidney disease," *Advances in Chronic Kidney Disease*, vol. 21, no. 2, pp. 121–133, 2014.

[46] P. Fiorina, A. Vergani, R. Bassi et al., "Role of podocyte B7-1 in diabetic nephropathy," *Journal of the American Society of Nephrology*, vol. 25, no. 7, pp. 1415–1429, 2014.

[47] A. Doria, M. A. Niewczas, and P. Fiorina, "Can existing drugs approved for other indications retard renal function decline in patients with type 1 diabetes and nephropathy?" *Seminars in Nephrology*, vol. 32, no. 5, pp. 437–444, 2012.

[48] A. M. Rodrigues, C. T. Bergamaschi, M. J. S. Fernandes et al., "$P2x_7$ receptor in the kidneys of diabetic rats submitted to aerobic training or to N-acetylcysteine supplementation," *PLoS ONE*, vol. 9, no. 6, Article ID e97452, 2014.

[49] A. Solini, V. Usuelli, and P. Fiorina, "The dark side of extracellular ATP in kidney diseases," *Journal of the American Society of Nephrology*, vol. 26, no. 5, pp. 1007–1016, 2015.

[50] M. G. Saklayen, J. Yap, and V. Vallyathan, "Effect of month-long treatment with oral N-acetylcysteine on the oxidative stress and proteinuria in patients with diabetic nephropathy: a pilot study," *Journal of Investigative Medicine*, vol. 58, no. 1, pp. 28–31, 2010.

6

Type 2 Diabetes and ADP Receptor Blocker Therapy

Matej Samoš,[1] Marián Fedor,[2] František Kovář,[1] Michal Mokáň,[1] Tomáš Bolek,[1] Peter Galajda,[1] Peter Kubisz,[2] and Marián Mokáň[1]

[1]*Department of Internal Medicine I, Jessenius Faculty of Medicine in Martin, Comenius University in Bratislava, 036 59 Martin, Slovakia*
[2]*National Center of Hemostasis and Thrombosis, Department of Hematology and Blood Transfusion, Jessenius Faculty of Medicine in Martin, Comenius University in Bratislava, 036 59 Martin, Slovakia*

Correspondence should be addressed to Matej Samoš; matej.samos@gmail.com

Academic Editor: Andreas Melidonis

Type 2 diabetes (T2D) is associated with several abnormalities in haemostasis *predisposing* to thrombosis. Moreover, T2D was recently connected with a failure in antiplatelet response to clopidogrel, the most commonly used ADP receptor blocker in clinical practice. Clopidogrel high on-treatment platelet reactivity (HTPR) was repeatedly associated with the risk of ischemic adverse events. Patients with T2D show significantly higher residual platelet reactivity on ADP receptor blocker therapy and are more frequently represented in the group of patients with HTPR. This paper reviews the current knowledge about possible interactions between T2D and ADP receptor blocker therapy.

1. Introduction

Type 2 diabetes (T2D) is associated with several abnormalities in haemostasis, such as higher platelet reactivity [1, 2], endothelial dysfunction [3], and hypercoagulation and abnormalities in fibrinolysis [4], predisposing to thrombosis. ADP receptor blocker therapy is crucial in acute coronary syndrome (ACS) and postpercutaneous coronary intervention (PCI) patients to prevent future thrombotic events. According to current European Society of Cardiology and American Heart Association Clinical Practice Guidelines [5–7] ADP receptor blocker therapy should be administrated in all ST-elevation myocardial infarction (STEMI) and non-ST-elevation myocardial infarction (NSTEMI)/unstable angina (UA) patients, while in STEMI patients undergoing primary PCI new ADP receptor blockers (prasugrel, ticagrelor) should be preferred; in patients with NSTEMI/UA prasugrel should be used just when coronary anatomy is already known and a decision to perform PCI has been already established. Otherwise, ticagrelor or clopidogrel should be administrated. Moreover, these recommendations should be fully applicable in patients with as well as without T2D. Nevertheless, T2D was recently associated with a failure in antiplatelet response to clopidogrel [8, 9] which remains the most commonly used ADP receptor blocker in clinical practice [10]. Importantly, clopidogrel high on-treatment platelet reactivity (HTPR) was consistently associated with the risk of ischemic adverse events. This paper reviews the current approaches of ADP receptor blocker therapy in T2D patients.

2. Clopidogrel and Its Resistance in T2D Patients

Thienopyridine clopidogrel is an oral irreversible P2Y12 ADP receptor blocker. This prodrug requires oxidation by the hepatic cytochrome P450 system to generate an active metabolite. After absorption, an estimated 85% of the prodrug is hydrolysed by esterases into an inactive form, leaving only 15% of clopidogrel available for transformation to the active metabolite, which irreversibly and selectively inactivates P2Y12 ADP receptor and inhibits ADP-induced platelet aggregation [11]. The introduction of clopidogrel by the CURE study in patients with ACS [12] significantly improved the clinical outcome compared with patients treated with aspirin alone. Similar outcome was subsequently obtained in post-PCI patients [13, 14]. However, the antiplatelet effect of clopidogrel varies among individuals.

TABLE 1: ADP receptor blockers in current clinical practice.

Drug	Route of administration	Bioavailability	Receptor inhibition	Time to peak platelet inhibition	Clinical application	Interactions with T2D
Clopidogrel	Oral	Prodrug	Irreversible	Highly variable	PCI, arterial interventions, ACS, stroke, and secondary prevention	Repeatedly proven
Prasugrel	Oral	Prodrug	Irreversible	2 hours	ACS with PCI	Not explicitly proven
Ticagrelor	Oral	Direct-acting	Reversible	2 hours	ACS	Probably none
Cangrelor	Intravenous	Direct-acting	Reversible	30 minutes	PCI	Not studied

ACS: acute coronary syndromes, PCI: percutaneous coronary intervention, T2D: type 2 diabetes.

As mentioned previously, there are a growing number of data pointing to the failure in antiplatelet responses to clopidogrel which is specifically associated with insulin resistance and T2D [8, 9, 15]. These reports are based on ex vivo testing of platelet reactivity on clopidogrel therapy, as well as on subanalysis of clinical trials with clopidogrel. In these trials patients with T2D on clopidogrel therapy had worse clinical course and increased incidence of stent thrombosis [8, 9, 15–19]. The exact mechanism of this phenomenon remains currently unknown. However, the mechanism of poor clopidogrel response in T2D patients is probably multifactorial. T2D per se increases the platelet reactivity to ADP. Insulin could reduce the platelet aggregation by inhibiting the P2Y12 pathway through insulin receptors [20]. Insulin resistance might upregulate the P2Y12 ADP receptor, which is associated with clopidogrel resistance [21, 22]. An absolute or a relative lack of insulin was previously associated with increased P2Y12 signalling capacity. Moreover, this pathway appears to be in patients with T2D less sensitive to P2Y12 inhibition [23]. On the other hand, T2D may also interact with clopidogrel metabolism. T2D is already known to modulate cytochrome P450 activity in humans and in animal models [24–26]. Erlinge et al. [8] studied the prevalence and mechanism of antiplatelet failure to clopidogrel in T2D patients and in nondiabetic individuals. This double blinded study randomized totally 110 patients already treated with aspirin to clopidogrel (600 mg loading dose followed by a maintenance dose of 75 mg) or prasugrel (60 mg loading dose followed by daily maintenance dose of 10 mg) for a period of 28 days. Results of the study showed significantly higher incidence of HTPR in patients treated with clopidogrel compared to prasugrel. Diabetic patients were more frequently represented in the group with HTPR. Moreover, the HTPR was in T2D patients connected to the administration of clopidogrel. When compared with nondiabetic patients, patients with diabetes had significantly lower concentrations of clopidogrel active metabolite measured two hours after a loading dose administration ($p < 0.01$) and also on 29th day of maintenance dose usage ($p < 0.01$). It is interesting that, in this study, platelets of diabetic patients with HTPR responded well to ex vivo administration of the active clopidogrel metabolite. This observation indicates a low level of resistance on platelet P2Y12 ADP receptor and supports a potential interaction between T2D and pharmacokinetic processes of clopidogrel metabolism.

Angiolillo et al. [9] studied platelet function in diabetic and nondiabetic patients treated with aspirin and clopidogrel. Blood samples were taken after loading dose administration and on chronic therapy. The authors found significantly higher residual platelet reactivity in T2D patients both prior to clopidogrel administration and 24 hours after clopidogrel loading dose administration. In addition, the authors found a significantly higher number of patients with clopidogrel HTPR among patients with T2D. It is already known that HTPR is an independent predictor of cardiovascular events [9] and platelet reactivity on clopidogrel therapy higher than 50% was repeatedly associated with higher risk of coronary events after PCI [17, 18, 27].

The worse clinical outcome and an increased risk of ischemic events in clopidogrel-treated T2D patients were consistently demonstrated in the subanalysis of the CURE [12], CREDO [28], and Current-OASIS 7 [29] trials. These data indirectly support an incomplete response to clopidogrel associated with T2D. Additionally, Iakovou et al. [19] in an analysis of data from a prospective observational study showed that T2D is an independent predictor of stent thrombosis, despite dual antiplatelet therapy in patients after successful implantation of drug eluting stents. High frequency of clopidogrel HTPR led to the introduction of new ADP receptor blockers with more favourable pharmacodynamic profile to clinical practice.

3. Prasugrel: New ADP Receptor Blocker in T2D Patients

Prasugrel (Table 1) is a new thienopyridine P2Y12 ADP receptor blocker, recently introduced to clinical practice in patients with ACS and planned PCI. Prasugrel compared to clopidogrel offers more consistent inhibition of P2Y12 ADP receptor and has a lower intraindividual variability in efficacy. Prasugrel was extensively tested in the TRITON-TIMI 38 trial [30] which randomized 13 608 patients with ACS to clopidogrel or prasugrel. These patients were treated from 6 to 15 months. In this trial 3146 of patients had T2D; 776 patients were treated with insulin. The primary "endpoint" of this study was significantly decreased by prasugrel in nondiabetic group (9.2%

versus 10.6%, $p < 0.05$), as well as in those with T2D (12.2% versus 17.0%, $p < 0.001$). Benefit of prasugrel administration was observed consistently in insulin-treated patients (14.3% versus 22.2%, $p < 0.01$), as well as in T2D patients without insulin therapy (11.5% versus 15.3%, $p < 0.01$). Prasugrel significantly reduced the incidence of myocardial infarction (MI) by 18% in nondiabetic subjects and by 40% in subjects with T2D. Moreover, this study showed a significant reduction of stent thrombosis by prasugrel in the overall group (0.9% versus 2.0%), as well as in T2D patients (2.0% versus 3.5%). Nevertheless, major bleeding events not associated with coronary artery bypass graft surgery occurred overall significantly more often in patients treated with prasugrel, compared to clopidogrel (2.4 versus 1.8%). In summary, throughout the study, the greatest benefit of prasugrel therapy was observed preferentially in T2D patients, in whom prasugrel significantly reduced the risk of ischemic events, including the risk of recurrent MI and the risk of stent thrombosis, without increasing the risk of serious bleeding.

On the other hand, the efficacy of prasugrel is not so convincing in patients who do not undergo invasive coronary revascularization. The TRIOLOGY ACS study [31]—a double blind, randomized prospective trial involving 7243 patients—failed to proof the significant reduction of the primary endpoint with prasugrel (10 mg daily) compared to clopidogrel (75 mg daily). Similar bleeding risk was observed in both groups of patients. In this study, 37.7% of prasugrel-treated and 38.3% of clopidogrel-treated patients had a history of T2D. Although the subanalysis of T2D patients was not reported specifically, generally there was no significant difference in the hazard ratio for primary endpoint in T2D patients compared to nondiabetic individuals (17.8% versus 11.5% in clopidogrel-treated patients, 20.4% versus 13.2% in prasugrel-treated patients, resp.; $p = 0.71$). Nevertheless, in this study, reduced ADP blocker loading doses (30 mg of prasugrel and 300 mg of clopidogrel) were administrated only in patients who underwent randomization within first 72 hours after the first medical contact and were not previously pretreated with ADP receptor blocker. Patients who did not undergo randomization within first 72 hours were treated with daily maintenance dose administration (i.e., loading dose was not administrated). This fact could influence the reduction of the primary endpoint of this study.

4. Prasugrel Resistance: A New Phenomenon in Diabetic Patients with ACS?

Prasugrel was repeatedly described as an effective drug for overcoming clopidogrel resistance [27, 32]. However, several recently published data reported an incomplete response to prasugrel. Prasugrel resistance might therefore become another problem in patients requiring ADP receptor blocker therapy. Silvano et al. described a rare case of resistance to both clopidogrel and prasugrel in nondiabetic patient with acute STEMI due to stent thrombosis [33]. In addition, results of recently published studies [34, 35] suggest that real prevalence of HTPR in prasugrel-treated patients may be higher than that which is traditionally considered. Bonello et al. [35] pointed out the fact that up to 25% of patients with ACS did not reach effective antiplatelet response even after 6–12 hours from prasugrel loading dose administration. There is no definite answer to the question of a possible relationship between T2D and the phenomenon of "prasugrel resistance." We have previously described a delayed antiplatelet response to prasugrel in two T2D patients undergoing primary PCI for acute STEMI [36]. Consequently, Alexopoulos et al. [37] reported in an observational study involving 77 patients with ACS undergoing PCI that platelet reactivity in prasugrel-treated patients differed significantly by T2D status. By multivariable analysis, insulin-treated T2D was identified as the only predictor of high platelet reactivity ($p < 0.01$). The authors concluded that patients with insulin-treated T2D treated with prasugrel post-PCI have higher platelet reactivity than patients without T2D or noninsulin-treated diabetic patients. This observation supports the possible interaction between T2D and prasugrel HTPR. However, this possible interaction remains inadequately explained and further studies will be needed for the final clarification of this issue.

5. Cangrelor: The New Member of the ADP Receptor Blockers Family

Cangrelor (Table 1) is an intravenously administrated adenosine triphosphate analogue that binds reversibly and with high affinity to P2Y12 ADP receptor. It offers a highly effective inhibition of ADP-induced platelet aggregation immediately after administration and allows the restoration of platelet function within 1-2 hours of its discontinuation [38]. Cangrelor has been investigated in three clinical trials including a total of 24 910 patients [39–41]. A meta-analysis of these studies [42] observed a 19% risk reduction rate in periprocedural death, MI, ischemia-driven revascularization, and stent thrombosis, with a 39% risk reduction rate in stent thrombosis alone. The TIMI major and minor bleeds were increased, but there was no increase in the rate of transfusions. This new agent may be considered in ADP receptor blocker naïve patients undergoing PCI for ACS [6]. Recently, there is no study specifically investigating possible interactions between T2D and antiplatelet response to cangrelor.

6. Ticagrelor: A Safe and Effective ADP Receptor Blocker in T2D Patients?

Ticagrelor (Table 1) is a new oral, direct reversible P2Y12 ADP receptor blocker which achieves a higher range of inhibition of platelet aggregation compared to clopidogrel [43]. The PLATO study [44] tested the efficacy of ticagrelor and clopidogrel in the prevention of cardiovascular events in patients with ACS (totally 18.624 patients enrolled). The incidence of the primary endpoint after 12 months of follow-up was significantly lower in patients treated with ticagrelor (10.2% versus 12.3%, $p < 0.001$); there was also a significant reduction of cardiovascular deaths and stent thrombosis in the subgroup of ticagrelor-treated post-PCI patients. Ticagrelor administration was not associated with an increased risk of serious bleeding. In the group of diabetic patients ticagrelor reduced the incidence of the primary endpoint, all-cause mortality, and the risk of stent thrombosis. Similar benefit of

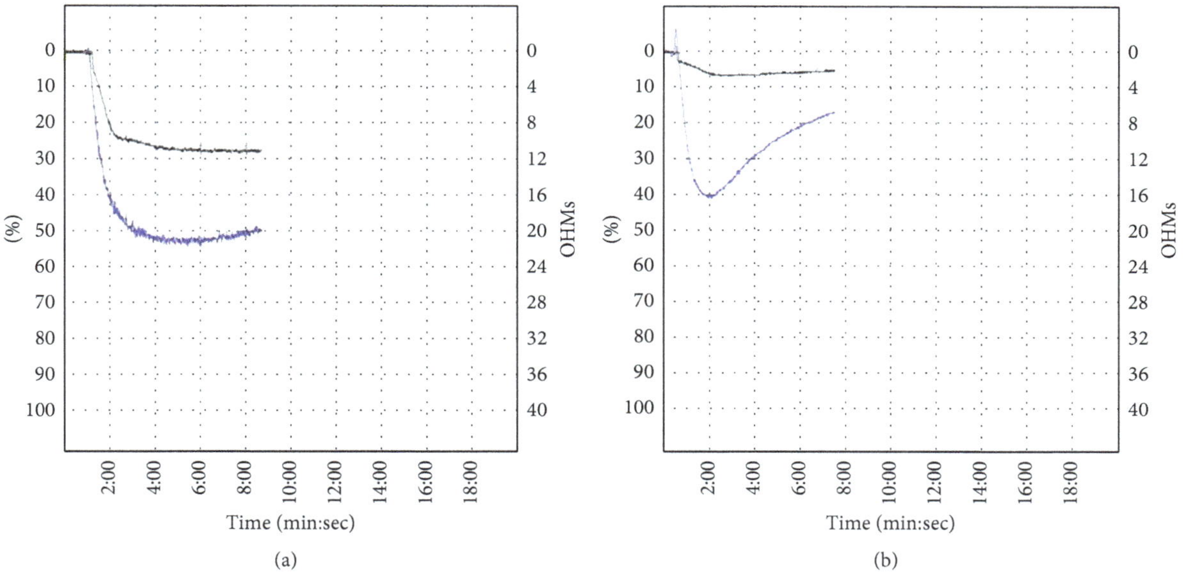

FIGURE 1: LTA with specific inducers (arachidonic acid: black curve, adenosine diphosphate: blue curve) showing difference between HTPR (a) and sufficient antiplatelet response (b) in T2D patient with acute ST-elevation myocardial infarction.

ticagrelor therapy was seen in insulin-treated T2D patients, as well as in diabetic patients without insulin therapy. In addition, Alexopoulos et al. [45] showed significantly lower platelet reactivity in ticagrelor-treated T2D patients compared to T2D patients treated with prasugrel. Moreover, in this single-center prospective randomized study none of the T2D patients was identified as a nonresponder for ticagrelor. Consistently, ticagrelor treatment was demonstrated to be effective and even superior to prasugrel [46] in high risk diabetic patients with ACS. These data suggest that ticagrelor may be a safe and effective ADP receptor blocker in T2D patients, which can ensure consistent platelet inhibition, without the risk of HTPR, together with a good safety profile.

7. Detection of HTPR in Clinical Practice

Assessing the individual level of platelet inhibition by implementing platelet function testing might help to identify patients with HTPR and therefore to reduce ischemic events. To assess the predictive level of platelet reactivity on ADP receptor blockers, numerous platelet function tests are currently available. Light transmission aggregometry (LTA) with specific inducer (adenosine diphosphate (ADP)) represents nowadays a "golden standard" in antiplatelet response testing. Maximal aggregation in response to ADP with LTA testing > 50% (Figure 1) had been associated with higher risk of ischemic events [47]. Second, vasodilator-stimulated phosphoprotein (VASP) phosphorylation flow cytometry assay represents a specific method for the assessment of ADP receptor blocker activity [48]. We have previously demonstrated that this assay is suitable for monitoring the ADP receptor blocker therapy in acute STEMI patients with primary PCI of culprit coronary lesion [49]. The advantage of this assay is its specificity for ADP receptor intracellular signaling pathway and sample stability. Nevertheless, instrumental and financial requirements may represent a possible limitation for the application of this assay in clinical practice. Third, several point-of-care assays are recently available. PFA-100 (Siemens Healthcare Diagnostics, Tarrytown, New York, USA) and Verify Now (Accumetries, San Diego, California, USA) assay methods—both based on modified aggregometry—allow quick platelet function testing in the setting of the intensive care units. Verify Now allows rapid assessment of platelet response on aspirin, P2Y12 ADP receptor antagonist, and glycoprotein IIb/IIIa antagonist treatment in one blood sample [50]. Bed site ADP receptor blockers testing may provide a rough guiding on how to proceed with treatment drugs and dosages, especially when both LTA and VASP phosphorylation assays are not available.

Although monitoring of ADP receptor blocker therapy is nowadays not generally recommended, this testing can significantly help to identify patients with HTPR. On the other hand, recently there is no definite answer to the question whether HTPR is a modifiable phenomenon. Several randomized studies trying to overcome HTPR with modified clopidogrel therapy guided by platelet function testing [51, 52] brought negative results. However, new antiplatelet agents were rarely used in these trials. Modified (increased) clopidogrel dosing, which was mostly used in these trials for overcoming the HPTR, failed to reduce the rate of major adverse cardiac events (cardiovascular death, nonfatal myocardial infarction, or stent thrombosis). The results of these randomized studies predominantly do not support a treatment strategy of high-dose clopidogrel in patients with HTPR and question the need of monitoring the on-treatment platelet reactivity in clinical practice. Nevertheless, a recently published observational study, which tested patients with planned PCI for stable angina or NSTE ACS [53], showed a reduced risk of adverse clinical events in HTPR patients with tailored intensified antiplatelet therapy. Thus, monitoring and tailoring the antiplatelet therapy might be beneficial in selected patients and deserve further investigation.

In summary, T2D seems to be associated with HTPR especially in clopidogrel-treated patients. Moreover, we have previously confirmed the association between HTPR and stent thrombosis in post-PCI patient with T2D [27]. Therefore, it is probably reasonable to routinely prefer new ADP receptor blockers over clopidogrel in T2D patients in order to ensure more effective platelet inhibition and prevent these serious thrombotic adverse events. Additionally, the subanalysis of T2D patients treated with new ADP receptor blockers did not reveal higher risk of serious bleeding. This indicates that the benefit/risk ratio is in favour of new antiplatelet agents. In case of choosing clopidogrel therapy in T2D patients, it seems to be reasonable to perform platelet function testing for the approval of sufficient on-treatment response. If this response is inadequate, the switch to new ADP receptor blocker therapy should be considered immediately. In addition, ticagrelor, in T2D patients with ACS, was demonstrated as more effective and superior even to prasugrel [46]. Thus this agent should be preferred especially in case of diabetics with acute coronary events. Nevertheless, the higher cost of medication, patient compliance, higher risk of bleeding, and other side effects should be also considered for a decision of ADP receptor blocker therapy strategy.

8. Conclusion

The above-mentioned evidence suggests that T2D is associated with clopidogrel HTPR. Patients with T2D show significantly higher residual platelet reactivity on clopidogrel therapy and are more frequently represented in the group of patients with clopidogrel HTPR. Moreover, several data reported that patients with insulin-treated T2D have higher residual platelet reactivity even on prasugrel therapy than patients without T2D or noninsulin-treated diabetic patients. On the other hand, ticagrelor treatment was demonstrated to be effective and even superior to prasugrel in high risk diabetic patients with ACS and ticagrelor may be a safe and effective ADP receptor blocker in these patients. However, the relationship between T2D and ADP receptor blocker therapy is not fully explained and deserves further investigation.

Disclosure

Formal consent for this type of study is not required.

Conflict of Interests

The authors have no conflict of interests to declare.

Acknowledgments

This study was supported by the APVV Project (Slovak Research and Development Agency) 0222-11 and the research project of the Slovak Society of Cardiology 2012–2015.

References

[1] D. Aronson, Z. Bloomgarden, and E. J. Rayfield, "Potential mechanisms promoting restenosis in diabetic patients," *Journal of the American College of Cardiology*, vol. 27, no. 3, pp. 528–535, 1996.

[2] D. Tschoepe, P. Roesen, L. Kaufmann et al., "Evidence for abnormal platelet glycoprotein expression in diabetes mellitus," *European Journal of Clinical Investigation*, vol. 20, no. 2, pp. 166–170, 1990.

[3] P. Kubisz, P. Chudý, J. Staško et al., "Circulating vascular endothelial growth factor in the normo- and/or microalbuminuric patients with type 2 diabetes mellitus," *Acta Diabetologica*, vol. 47, no. 2, pp. 119–124, 2010.

[4] P. Chudý, D. Kotuličová, J. Staško, and P. Kubisz, "The relationship among TAFI, t-PA, PAI-1 and F1 + 2 in type 2 diabetic patients with normoalbuminuria and microalbuminuria," *Blood Coagulation & Fibrinolysis*, vol. 22, no. 6, pp. 493–498, 2011.

[5] E. A. Amsterdam, N. K. Wenger, R. G. Brindis et al., "2014 AHA/ACC guideline for the management of patients with non-ST-elevation acute coronary syndromes: executive summary: a report of the American College of Cardiology/American Heart Association Task Force on Practice Guidelines," *Circulation*, vol. 130, no. 25, pp. 2354–2394, 2014.

[6] M. Roffi, C. Patrono, J.-P. Collet et al., "2015 ESC guidelines for the management of acute coronary syndromes in patients presenting without persistent ST-segment elevation," *European Heart Journal*, 2015.

[7] P. G. Steg, S. K. James, D. Atar et al., "ESC Guidelines for the management of acute myocardial infarction in patients presenting with ST-segment elevation," *European Heart Journal*, vol. 33, no. 20, pp. 2569–2619, 2012.

[8] D. Erlinge, C. Varenhorst, O. Ö. Braun et al., "Patients with poor responsiveness to thienopyridine treatment or with diabetes have lower levels of circulating active metabolite, but their platelets respond normally to active metabolite added ex vivo," *Journal of the American College of Cardiology*, vol. 52, no. 24, pp. 1968–1977, 2008.

[9] D. J. Angiolillo, E. Bernardo, M. Sabaté et al., "Impact of platelet reactivity on cardiovascular outcomes in patients with type 2 diabetes mellitus and coronary artery disease," *Journal of the American College of Cardiology*, vol. 50, no. 16, pp. 1541–1547, 2007.

[10] J. Tang, M. P. Li, H. H. Zhou, and X. P. Chen, "Platelet inhibition agents: current and future P2Y12 receptor antagonists," *Current Vascular Pharmacology*, vol. 13, no. 5, pp. 566–577, 2015.

[11] P. Savi and J.-M. Herbert, "Clopidogrel and ticlopidine: $P2Y_{12}$ adenosine diphosphate-receptor antagonists for the prevention of atherothrombosis," *Seminars in Thrombosis and Hemostasis*, vol. 31, no. 2, pp. 174–183, 2005.

[12] S. Yusuf, F. Zhao, S. R. Mehta, S. Chrolavicius, G. Tognoni, and K. K. Fox, "Effects of clopidogrel in addition to aspirin in patients with acute coronary syndromes without ST-segment elevation," *The New England Journal of Medicine*, vol. 345, no. 7, pp. 494–502, 2001.

[13] G. Patti, G. Colonna, V. Pasceri, L. L. Pepe, A. Montinaro, and G. Di Sciascio, "Randomized trial of high loading dose of clopidogrel for reduction of periprocedural myocardial infarction in patients undergoing coronary intervention: results from the ARMYDA-2 (Antiplatelet therapy for Reduction of MYocardial Damage during Angioplasty) Study," *Circulation*, vol. 111, no. 16, pp. 2099–2106, 2005.

[14] E. I. Lev, R. Kornowski, H. Vaknin-Assa et al., "Effect of clopidogrel pretreatment on angiographic and clinical outcomes in patients undergoing primary percutaneous coronary intervention for ST-elevation acute myocardial infarction," *The American Journal of Cardiology*, vol. 101, no. 4, pp. 435–439, 2008.

[15] D. J. Angiolillo, P. Capranzano, B. Desai et al., "Impact of $P2Y_{12}$ inhibitory effects induced by clopidogrel on platelet procoagulant activity in type 2 diabetes mellitus patients," *Thrombosis Research*, vol. 124, no. 3, pp. 318–322, 2009.

[16] T. Cuisset, C. Frere, J. Quilici et al., "High post-treatment platelet reactivity identified low-responders to dual antiplatelet therapy at increased risk of recurrent cardiovascular events after stenting for acute coronary syndrome," *Journal of Thrombosis and Haemostasis*, vol. 4, no. 3, pp. 542–549, 2006.

[17] P. A. Gurbel, K. P. Bliden, K. Guyer et al., "Platelet reactivity in patients and recurrent events post-stenting: results of the PREPARE POST-STENTING study," *Journal of the American College of Cardiology*, vol. 46, no. 10, pp. 1820–1826, 2005.

[18] P. A. Gurbel, K. P. Bliden, W. Samara et al., "Clopidogrel effect on platelet reactivity in patients with stent thrombosis: results of the CREST study," *Journal of the American College of Cardiology*, vol. 46, no. 10, pp. 1827–1832, 2005.

[19] I. Iakovou, T. Schmidt, E. Bonizzoni et al., "Incidence, predictors, and outcome of thrombosis after successful implantation of drug-eluting stents," *The Journal of the American Medical Association*, vol. 293, no. 17, pp. 2126–2130, 2005.

[20] I. A. Ferreira, K. L. Eybrechts, A. I. M. Mocking, C. Kroner, and J.-W. N. Akkerman, "IRS-1 mediates inhibition of Ca2 mobilization by insulin via the inhibitory G-protein Gi," *The Journal of Biological Chemistry*, vol. 279, no. 5, pp. 3254–3264, 2004.

[21] D. J. Angiolillo, E. Bernardo, C. Ramírez et al., "Insulin therapy is associated with platelet dysfunction in patients with type 2 diabetes mellitus on dual oral antiplatelet treatment," *Journal of the American College of Cardiology*, vol. 48, no. 2, pp. 298–304, 2006.

[22] D. J. Angiolillo, A. Fernandez-Ortiz, E. Bernardo et al., "Platelet function profiles in patients with type 2 diabetes and coronary artery disease on combined aspirin and clopidogrel treatment," *Diabetes*, vol. 54, no. 8, pp. 2430–2450, 2005.

[23] I. A. Ferreira, A. I. M. Mocking, M. A. H. Feijge et al., "Platelet inhibition by insulin is absent in type 2 diabetes mellitus," *Arteriosclerosis, Thrombosis, and Vascular Biology*, vol. 26, no. 2, pp. 417–422, 2006.

[24] S. Goldstein, A. Simpson, and P. Saenger, "Hepatic drug metabolism is increased in poorly controlled insulin-dependent diabetes mellitus," *Acta Endocrinologica*, vol. 123, no. 5, pp. 550–556, 1990.

[25] T. Kudo, T. Shimada, T. Toda et al., "Altered expression of CYP in TSOD mice: a model of type 2 diabetes and obesity," *Xenobiotica*, vol. 39, no. 12, pp. 889–902, 2009.

[26] D. Patoine, M. Petit, S. Pilote, F. Picard, B. Drolet, and C. Simard, "Modulation of CYP3a expression and activity in mice models of type 1 and type 2 diabetes," *Pharmacology Research & Perspectives*, vol. 2, no. 6, 2014.

[27] M. Samoš, R. Šimonová, F. Kovář et al., "Clopidogrel resistance in diabetic patient with acute myocardial infarction due to stent thrombosis," *The American Journal of Emergency Medicine*, vol. 32, no. 5, pp. 461–465, 2014.

[28] S. R. Steinhubl, P. B. Berger, J. Tift Mann III et al., "Early and sustained dual oral antiplatelet therapy following percutaneous coronary intervention: a randomized controlled trial," *The Journal of the American Medical Association*, vol. 288, no. 19, pp. 2411–2420, 2002.

[29] S. R. Mehta, J.-P. Bassand, S. Chrolavicius et al., "Dose comparisons of clopidogrel and aspirin in acute coronary syndromes," *The New England Journal of Medicine*, vol. 363, no. 10, pp. 930–942, 2010.

[30] S. D. Wiviott, E. Braunwald, C. H. McCabe et al., "Prasugrel versus clopidogrel in patients with acute coronary syndromes," *The New England Journal of Medicine*, vol. 357, no. 20, pp. 2001–2015, 2007.

[31] M. T. Roe, P. W. Armstrong, K. A. A. Fox et al., "Prasugrel versus clopidogrel for acute coronary syndromes without revascularization," *The New England Journal of Medicine*, vol. 367, no. 14, pp. 1297–1309, 2012.

[32] D. Alexopoulos, G. Dimitropoulos, P. Davlouros et al., "Prasugrel overcomes high on-clopidogrel platelet reactivity post-stenting more effectively than high-dose (150-mg) clopidogrel: the importance of cyp2c19*2 genotyping," *JACC: Cardiovascular Interventions*, vol. 4, no. 4, pp. 403–410, 2011.

[33] M. Silvano, C. F. Zambon, G. De Rosa et al., "A case of resistance to clopidogrel and prasugrel after percutaneous coronary angioplasty," *Journal of Thrombosis and Thrombolysis*, vol. 31, no. 2, pp. 233–234, 2011.

[34] G. Cayla, T. Cuisset, J. Silvain et al., "Prasugrel monitoring and bleeding in real world patients," *The American Journal of Cardiology*, vol. 111, no. 1, pp. 38–44, 2013.

[35] L. Bonello, M. Pansieri, J. Mancini et al., "High on-treatment platelet reactivity after prasugrel loading dose and cardiovascular events after percutaneous coronary intervention in acute coronary syndromes," *Journal of the American College of Cardiology*, vol. 58, no. 5, pp. 467–473, 2011.

[36] M. Samoš, M. Fedor, F. Kovář et al., "Prasugrel loading dose in diabetic patients with acute STEMI—always sufficiently effective? Observation in two cases and review of current knowledge," *Cor et Vasa*, vol. 56, no. 5, pp. e388–e395, 2014.

[37] D. Alexopoulos, C. Vogiatzi, K. Stavrou et al., "Diabetes mellitus and platelet reactivity in patients under prasugrel or ticagrelor treatment: an observational study," *Cardiovascular Diabetology*, vol. 14, article 68, 2015.

[38] R. F. Storey, K. G. Oldroyd, and R. G. Wilcox, "Open multicentre study of the P2T receptor antagonist AR-C69931MX assessing safety, tolerability and activity in patients with acute coronary syndromes," *Thrombosis and Haemostasis*, vol. 85, no. 3, pp. 401–407, 2001.

[39] R. A. Harrington, G. W. Stone, S. McNulty et al., "Platelet inhibition with cangrelor in patients undergoing PCI," *The New England Journal of Medicine*, vol. 361, no. 24, pp. 2318–2329, 2009.

[40] D. L. Bhatt, A. M. Lincoff, C. M. Gibson et al., "Intravenous platelet blockade with cangrelor during PCI," *The New England Journal of Medicine*, vol. 361, no. 24, pp. 2330–2341, 2009.

[41] D. L. Bhatt, G. W. Stone, K. W. Mahaffey et al., "Effect of platelet inhibition with cangrelor during PCI on ischemic events," *The New England Journal of Medicine*, vol. 368, no. 14, pp. 1303–1313, 2013.

[42] P. G. Steg, D. L. Bhatt, C. W. Hamm et al., "Effect of cangrelor on periprocedural outcomes in percutaneous coronary interventions: a pooled analysis of patient-level data," *The Lancet*, vol. 382, no. 9909, pp. 1981–1992, 2013.

[43] R. F. Storey, S. Husted, R. A. Harrington et al., "Inhibition of platelet aggregation by AZD6140, a reversible oral $P2Y_{12}$

receptor antagonist, compared with clopidogrel in patients with acute coronary syndromes," *Journal of the American College of Cardiology*, vol. 50, no. 19, pp. 1852–1856, 2007.

[44] L. Wallentin, R. C. Becker, A. Budaj et al., "Ticagrelor versus clopidogrel in patients with acute coronary syndromes," *The New England Journal of Medicine*, vol. 361, no. 11, pp. 1045–1057, 2009.

[45] D. Alexopoulos, I. Xanthopoulou, E. Mavronasiou et al., "Randomized assessment of ticagrelor versus prasugrel antiplatelet effects in patients with diabetes," *Diabetes Care*, vol. 36, no. 8, pp. 2211–2216, 2013.

[46] M. Laine, C. Frère, R. Toesca et al., "Ticagrelor versus prasugrel in diabetic patients with an acute coronary syndrome. A pharmacodynamic randomised study," *Thrombosis and Haemostasis*, vol. 111, no. 2, pp. 273–278, 2013.

[47] A. R. Harper and M. J. Price, "Platelet function monitoring and clopidogrel," *Current Cardiology Reports*, vol. 15, article 321, 2013.

[48] J. Geiger, J. Brich, P. Hönig-Liedl et al., "Specific impairment of human platelet $P2Y_{AC}$ ADP receptor-mediated signaling by the antiplatelet drug clopidogrel," *Arteriosclerosis, Thrombosis, and Vascular Biology*, vol. 19, no. 8, pp. 2007–2011, 1999.

[49] M. Fedor, M. Samoš, R. Šimonová et al., "Monitoring the efficacy of ADP inhibitor treatment in patients with acute STEMI post-PCI by VASP-P flow cytometry assay," *Clinical and Applied Thrombosis/Hemostasis*, vol. 21, no. 4, pp. 334–338, 2015.

[50] J. W. Smith, S. R. Steinhubl, A. M. Lincoff et al., "Rapid platelet-function assay: an automated and quantitative cartridge-based method," *Circulation*, vol. 99, no. 5, pp. 620–625, 1999.

[51] M. J. Price, P. B. Berger, P. S. Teirstein et al., "Standard- vs high-dose clopidogrel based on platelet function testing after percutaneous coronary intervention: the GRAVITAS randomized trial," *The Journal of the American Medical Association*, vol. 305, no. 11, pp. 1097–1105, 2011.

[52] J.-P. Collet, T. Cuisset, G. Rangé et al., "Bedside monitoring to adjust antiplatelet therapy for coronary stenting," *The New England Journal of Medicine*, vol. 367, no. 22, pp. 2100–2109, 2012.

[53] N. Paarup Dridi, P. I. Johansson, J. T. Lønborg et al., "Tailored antiplatelet therapy to improve prognosis in patients exhibiting clopidogrel low-response prior to percutaneous coronary intervention for stable angina or non-ST elevation acute coronary syndrome," *Platelets*, vol. 26, no. 6, pp. 521–529, 2015.

7

Vitamin D Deficiency Is Not Associated with Diabetic Retinopathy or Maculopathy

Uazman Alam,[1] Yasar Amjad,[1] Anges Wan Shan Chan,[2] Omar Asghar,[1] Ioannis N. Petropoulos,[2] and Rayaz A. Malik[1,3]

[1] *Centre for Endocrinology and Diabetes, Institute of Human Development, University of Manchester and the Manchester Royal Infirmary, Central Manchester Hospital Foundation Trust, Manchester M13 9NT, UK*
[2] *Department of Medicine, Barts and the London School of Medicine and Dentistry, London E1 2AD, UK*
[3] *Weill Cornell Medical College in Qatar, Doha, Qatar*

Correspondence should be addressed to Rayaz A. Malik; rayaz.a.malik@manchester.ac.uk

Academic Editor: Roberto Mallone

Background. Experimental and clinical studies suggest a possible association between vitamin D deficiency and both diabetic retinopathy and maculopathy. *Methods.* We have performed a cross-sectional study in adults with types 1 and 2 diabetes mellitus. The relationship between the presence and severity of diabetic retinopathy and maculopathy with serum 25-hydroxyvitamin D concentration was evaluated using logistic regression analyses in the presence of demographic and clinical covariates. *Results.* 657 adults with diabetes were stratified based on retinopathy grading: No Diabetic Retinopathy (39%), Background Diabetic Retinopathy (37%), Preproliferative Diabetic Retinopathy (21%), and Proliferative Diabetic Retinopathy (3%), respectively. There were no differences in serum 25-hydroxyvitamin D concentrations (25(OH)D) between the groups (15.3 ± 9.0 versus 16.4 ± 10.5 versus 15.9 ± 10.4 versus 15.7 ± 8.5 ng/mL, P = NS). Logistic regression analysis demonstrated no statistically significant relationship between the severity of retinopathy and serum 25(OH)D. Furthermore, there was no difference in serum 25(OH)D between those with ($n = 94$, 14%) and those without ($n = 563$, 86%) Diabetic Maculopathy (16.2 ± 10.0 versus 15.8 ± 9.8, P = NS) and no relationship was demonstrated by logistic regression analyses between the two variables. *Conclusions.* This study has found no association between serum 25(OH)D and the presence and severity of diabetic retinopathy or maculopathy.

1. Introduction

The prevalence of diabetic retinopathy (DR) approaches 93 million people worldwide [1] and is one of the leading causes of premature visual loss in the UK and worldwide [2]. Indeed, the World Health Organization estimates that whilst diabetic retinopathy accounts for approximately 5% of the global prevalence of blindness, the prevalence rises sharply to 15–17% in developed countries [3]. Several risk factors are implicated in the aetiology of DR with hyperglycemia and hypertension showing the strongest association [4], yet interventions aimed at correcting these risk factors have demonstrated moderate success [5, 6]. Therefore, the interactions between neural and retinal vascular dysfunction and the mechanisms resulting in retinal pathology including neovascularisation have been questioned recently [7]. Furthermore, micronutrients including vitamin C, vitamin E, and magnesium have been postulated to play a role in DR [8].

Vitamin D deficiency has been linked to a host of cardiovascular diseases including diabetes and hypertension [9, 10]. Vitamin D receptor (VDR) genotypes have been associated with the cumulative prevalence of diabetic retinopathy [11]. In two separate studies of the VDR gene in the French population, FokI and TaqI single nucleotide polymorphisms have been associated with DR [12, 13]. In a study of Caucasians with C-peptide-negative type 1 diabetes, there was a novel association between the functional *Fok*I VDR polymorphism and severe DR [12]. VDR dependent calcium binding proteins have been isolated in the human retina, particularly in the photoreceptor layer of the cones [14], and immunostaining in animal models has shown that VDR is expressed in the ganglion cells, the inner and outer plexiform layer, and the photoreceptor layer [15]. In an in vitro study of retinoblastoma tissue expressing VDR, supplementation with vitamin D resulted in a reduction of growth and apoptosis of the retinoblastoma cells [16]. 1,25-Dihydroxyvitamin D_3 ($1,25(OH)_2D_3$) closely regulates Vascular Endothelial Growth Factor in experimental models [17] and there is an inverse correlation of 25(OH)D with Vascular Endothelial Growth Factor, postulated to be related to tissue hypoxia [18]. In a mouse model of ischaemic retinopathy, $1,25(OH)_2D_3$ was shown to inhibit neovascularisation in retinal tissue [19]. Vitamin D may also have a direct effect on the renin-angiotensin-aldosterone-system and the renin-angiotensin-aldosterone-system is known to be overexpressed in patients with type 1 diabetes and retinopathy [20] and blockade of this system reduces DR progression [21]. A Vitamin D analogue (paricalcitol) has shown an improvement in microalbuminuria through a mechanism related to inhibition of renin-angiotensin-aldosterone-system [22].

Aksoy et al. demonstrated an inverse correlation in a Turkish cohort between worsening diabetic retinopathy and lower 1,25-dihydroxyvitamin D_3 (active vitamin D) in a population of 66 subjects [23]. Furthermore, severe vitamin D deficiency has been shown to predict not only mortality but the development of nephropathy and retinopathy in type 1 diabetes mellitus [4]. In a recent cross-sectional study of children and adolescents with type 1 diabetes, retinopathy prevalence was higher in children and adolescents with lower levels of vitamin D [24]. Other cross-sectional studies which have assessed vitamin D status in relation to DR in adults either have had small numbers [25] or have been based on retrospective analysis of data collected from the National Health and Nutrition Examination Survey between 1988 and 1994 [26]. However, since then, the targets for glycaemia, blood pressure, and lipids have changed and also this study made no assessment of Diabetic Maculopathy [26]. Therefore, we have undertaken a study to establish the relationship between vitamin D status and the severity of DR and maculopathy in a large adult population with type 1 and type 2 diabetes.

2. Method

All patients attending clinics were assessed for the level of 25(OH)D, irrespective of a history suggestive of vitamin D deficiency. Written informed consent and ethical approval were not required as the data were extracted retrospectively and did not extend beyond standard clinical practice. All patient records and information were anonymised and deidentified prior to analysis. 25(OH)D was added as a standard routine test from June 2009 due to the high levels of deficiency noted. This was a retrospective analysis of data which had been collected already in our clinic for clinical rather than research reasons; that is, the patients with diabetes attending clinic underwent assessment of vitamin D as the clinical practice was to assess vitamin D in all patients and subsequently treat those who are deficient. These same patients were also undergoing retinal assessment as part of the annual review under the English retinal screening programme. The data (vitamin D and retinopathy grade) were not collected specifically for this analysis. There were a sample of 657 subjects in this retrospective study and prospective sample size analyses were inappropriate as all data available were assessed.

3. Subjects

All participants were aged ≥ 18 years attending clinics at the Central Manchester Foundation Trust, Manchester, and the assessment was conducted from August 2009 to May 2011. Those with renal impairment (eGFR <30 mL/min/1.73 m^2 (CKD stages 4 and 5)), granulomatous diseases (tuberculosis, sarcoidosis, etc.), and malabsorption syndromes (coeliac disease, bacterial overgrowth, and concomitant orlistat treatment), pregnant and lactating women, and those currently on vitamin D supplementation were excluded from the analysis. Biases were limited by using an unselected cohort of subjects, not based on symptomatology of vitamin D deficiency.

3.1. Blood Pressure and Anthropometric Measurements. Body Mass Index (BMI) was measured as per the standard equation mass (kg)/$(\text{height(m)})^2$. Weight was measured with a digital scale (Seca 701, Seca, Hamburg, Germany) to the nearest 0.1 kg and height was measured to the nearest 0.1 cm. Blood pressure measurements were obtained with the use of an automated device (Dinamap pro 100v2, GE Medical Systems, Freiburg, Germany) with an appropriate cuff size. A minimum of two measurements of systolic and diastolic blood pressures were made five minutes apart with the lowest reading recorded and the mean of the preceding 2-year blood pressure results was used. Metabolic variables were also recorded with a mean of 2-year retrospective readings for glycosylated haemoglobin A1c (HbA1c) and components of the lipid profile (total cholesterol (CHL), high-density lipoprotein cholesterol [HDL-C], and triglycerides). The following measurements were taken as "spot readings" at the same date as baseline 25(OH)D measurements: Body Mass Index (BMI), bone profile markers such as corrected calcium (CCa), alkaline phosphatase (ALP), and estimated glomerular filtration rate (eGFR).

3.2. Assessment of Demographics, Cardiovascular Disease, and Medications. An assessment of patient demographics, previous cardiovascular events, and medications were made through analysis of medical records and an in-hospital medical record database (Diamond database, Hicom, Surrey, UK). Subject demographics extracted were age, sex, ethnicity (Caucasian, South Asian, Far East Asian, and Afro-Caribbean descent), smoking status (never, previous, and current), and type (types 1 and 2 diabetes) and duration of diabetes. Dates of baseline 25(OH)D were used to obtain respective retinopathy screening data. Only retinopathy screening data within 1 year of the baseline 25(OH)D and prior to vitamin D supplementation were included.

Baseline 25(OH)D status and retinopathy data were collected for 657 patients who had attended their retinopathy screening appointments. The retinopathy data were collected according to the grading criteria of the National Screening Committee [27]. Previous studies have shown acceptable level of quality and accuracy of grading compared to expert graders within the English National Screening Committee [28]. The national guidelines do not contain R1.5 or M0.5 grades and are categorised as Preproliferative Diabetic Retinopathy and Diabetic Maculopathy, respectively. These subgradings were used locally in screening centres and have been included. Retinopathy was graded as follows:

R0: No Diabetic Retinopathy (NDR).

R1: Background Diabetic Retinopathy (BDR): microaneurysms, retinal haemorrhages, and exudates.

R1.5: moderate numbers of intraretinal haemorrhages, hard exudates >1 disc diameter (DD) from fovea, and 3–6 cotton wool spots visible.

R2: Preproliferative Diabetic Retinopathy (PPDR): venous beading or looping, deep haemorrhages visible, and other microvascular anomalies visible.

R3: Proliferative Diabetic Retinopathy (PDR): new vessel formation, vitreous haemorrhage, preretinal haemorrhage or fibrosis, and/or retinal detachment.

M0: no maculopathy.

M0.5: hard exudates within the arcades >1DD from the centre of the fovea.

M1: exudates <1DD from the centre of the fovea; retinal thickening <1DD from the centre of the fovea.

P0: no photocoagulation scarring.

P1: photocoagulation scarring.

3.3. 25(OH)D Assay. Serum was separated from whole blood and stored at −20°C until assay. The assay used was an automated platform assay (ImmunoDiagnostic Systems Ltd., Bolden, Tyne and Wear, UK) and is based on chemiluminescence technology. The assay was performed exactly as per the manufacturer's instructions. Briefly, samples were subjected to a pretreatment step to denature the vitamin D binding protein. The treated samples were then neutralised in assay buffer and a specific anti-25(OH)D antibody labelled with acridinium was added. Following an incubation step, magnetic particles linked to 25(OH)D were added. Following a further incubation step, the magnetic particles were "captured" using a magnet. After a washing step and addition of trigger reagents, the light emitted by the acridinium label was inversely proportional to the concentration of 25(OH)D in the original sample. Concentration of 25(OH)D was calculated automatically using a 4-point logistic curve. The reportable range of the assay was 5–140 ng/mL. Inter- and intra-assay variation of the in-house control were 5.6% and 9.7%, respectively.

3.4. Statistical Analysis. Data were analysed using StatsDirect (StatsDirect, Altringham, Cheshire, UK). The data were stratified according to retinopathy (NDR, BDR, PPDR, and PDR) and maculopathy (no maculopathy and maculopathy) status and a comparison of means was undertaken using either ANOVA or Krus-Kal Wallis for DR data and Unpaired t-test or Mann-Whitney U test for maculopathy data. Chi-squared test was used for aetiology of diabetes, ethnicity, gender, and smoking status. Logistic regression analyses were undertaken to assess the association between serum 25(OH)D levels and retinopathy and maculopathy status (either present (1) or not present (0)), adjusting for mean values of duration of diabetes, smoking status, HbA1c, total cholesterol, HDL, triglycerides, and systolic and diastolic blood pressure. Further assessment of the results comparing vitamin D categories (severely deficient (<10 ng/mL), deficient (10–<20 ng/mL), insufficient (20–<30 ng/mL), and sufficient (>30 ng/mL)) and retinopathy (NDR, BDR, PPDR, and PDR), maculopathy (no maculopathy and maculopathy), and photocoagulation status (no photocoagulation and photocoagulation) was performed using Chi-squared testing. Appropriate statistical analyses were employed depending on the normality of the data. Overall, the P value was maintained at 0.05 for multiple comparison tests (Bonferoni adjustment or Dwass-Steel-Chritchlow-Fligner pairwise comparison). Statistically significant results were deemed at a P value ≤0.05.

4. Results

657 subjects were stratified according to their retinopathy status: No Diabetic Retinopathy (NDR) (n = 257, 39%), Background Diabetic Retinopathy (BDR) (n = 243, 37%), Preproliferative Diabetic Retinopathy (PPDR) (n = 135, 21%), and Proliferative Diabetic Retinopathy (PDR) (n = 22, 3%); No Diabetic Maculopathy (n = 563, 86%) and Diabetic Maculopathy (n = 94, 14%). 206 (31%) of the patients had severe vitamin D deficiency with 25(OH)D levels below 10 ng/mL, 284 (43%) were deficient with 25(OH)D of 10–<20 ng/mL, and 101 (14%) were insufficient with 25(OH)D of 20–<30 ng/mL. Only 65 (10%) individuals had "adequate" levels of 25(OH)D at >30 ng/mL. The mean 25(OH)D for the population was 15.8 ± 9.4 ng/mL.

Table 1 shows demographic and metabolic data based on retinopathy grading: NDR, BDR, PPDR, and PDR, respectively. There were no differences in 25(OH)D status between the groups (15.3 ± 9.0 versus 16.4 ± 10.5 versus 15.9 ± 10.4 versus 15.7 ± 8.5, P = NS). Subjects were matched for age (59.8 ± 13.8 versus 58.8 ± 13.3 versus 60.8 ± 10.9 versus 55.1 ± 13.6 years); however, the duration of diabetes was significantly lower in NDR (11.3 ± 8.7 versus 18.7 ± 11.7 versus 21.0 ± 9.8 versus 19.7 ± 10.0 years, $P < 0.0001$). The median number of metabolic and anthropometric measurements over the preceding two-year period from the baseline 25(OH)D result was 4 (interquartile range of 3–5). Two-year mean HbA1c (%) (8.2 ± 1.6 versus 8.6 ± 1.7 versus 8.9 ± 1.6 versus 8.9 ± 1.5, $P < 0.0006$) showed a significantly lower HbA1c, lower systolic blood pressure (129 ± 13 versus 131 ± 15 versus 134 ± 15 versus 134 ± 11 mmHg, P = 0.007), and higher eGFR (76.3 ± 16.9 versus 75.9 ± 17.5 versus 70.9 ± 16.9 versus 69.0 ± 21.6, P = 0.02) in NDR (Table 1). There was no difference for aetiology of diabetes, ethnicity, sex, smoking status, BMI, lipid and bone parameters, and diastolic blood pressure between the grades of DR.

Table 1: Demographic and metabolic parameters in subgroups based on severity of retinopathy.

	No Diabetic Retinopathy (NDR) (n = 257)	Background Diabetic Retinopathy (BDR) (n = 243)	Preproliferative Diabetic Retinopathy (PPDR) (n = 135)	Proliferative Diabetic Retinopathy (PDR) (n = 22)	P value
Age (years)	59.8 ± 13.8	58.8 ± 13.3	60.8 ± 10.9	55.1 ± 13.6	NS
Duration of diabetes (years)	11.3 ± 8.7†	18.7 ± 11.7†	21.0 ± 9.8†	19.7 ± 10.0†	**<0.0001**
Type 2 DM (%)	88	75	80	77	NS
Ethnicity (White European/South Asian (%))	48/45	55/38	50/45	52/48	NS
Sex (male (%))	51	50	48	53	NS
Current smokers/past smokers/never smoked (%)	14/25/61	14/33/53	14/26/60	4/23/71	NS
BMI (kg/m^2)	31.6 ± 10.6	31.1 ± 7.1	31.9 ± 6.4	31.1 ± 6.9	NS
25(OH)D (ng/mL)	15.3 ± 9.0	16.4 ± 10.5	15.9 ± 10.4	15.7 ± 8.5	NS
HbA1c (%)	8.2 ± 1.6*	8.6 ± 1.7*	8.9 ± 1.6*	8.9 ± 1.5	**<0.0001**
TC (mmol/L)	4.1 ± 1.0	4.2 ± 1.1	4.2 ± 1.3	4.3 ± 1.1	NS
HDL (mmol/L)	1.3 ± 0.5	1.4 ± 0.5	1.4 ± 0.7	1.3 ± 0.4	NS
Trig (mmol/L)	1.8 ± 0.9	1.8 ± 1.5	1.8 ± 0.9	2.5 ± 2.9	NS
eGFR (mL/min/L)	76.3 ± 16.9**	75.9 ± 17.5	70.9 ± 16.9**	69 ± 21.6	**0.02**
Systolic BP (mmHg)	129 ± 13***	131 ± 14.6	134 ± 15***	134 ± 11	**0.007**
Diastolic BP (mmHg)	70 ± 7	69 ± 7	70 ± 8	71 ± 8	NS
ALP (u/L)	87 ± 39	83 ± 34	84 ± 32	93 ± 43	NS
CCa (mmol/L)	2.4 ± 0.1	2.4 ± 0.1	2.3 ± 0.1	2.4 ± 0.2	NS

Duration of diabetes: †NDR versus BDR (P < 0.0001) versus PPDR (P < 0.0001) versus PDR (P = 0.001).
HbA1c: *NDR versus BDR (P = 0.01) versus PPDR (P < 0.0001).
eGFR: **NDR versus PPDR (P = 0.04).
Systolic BP: ***NDR versus PPDR (P = 0.008).
BMI: Body Mass Index, BP: blood pressure, TC: total cholesterol, HDL: high-density lipoprotein cholesterol, Trig: triglycerides, ALP; alkaline phosphatase, CCa; corrected calcium, and eGFR: estimated glomerular filtration rate.

There were no significant differences in the season of assessment in this study (Summer (32%) compared to Spring (22%), Autumn (24%), and Winter (22%)). However, there was a lower level of 25(OH)D in those who had their assessment in Winter (13.7 ± 8.4 ng/mL) compared to Spring (17.3±9.0 ng/mL, P = 0.002) and Summer (16.4±10.4 ng/mL, P = 0.04) with no difference compared to Autumn (16.0 ± 10.9 ng/mL). Mean value for all seasons was categorised as deficient (10–19.9 ng/mL) and a 3.6 ng/mL difference at most is unlikely to represent any clinical significance.

Table 2 shows logistic regression analyses for DR status with Odds Ratios (OR) and 95% CI. There was no correlation of DR with 25(OH)D (OR 1.00 (95% CI 0.98–1.02), P = NS), gender, or ethnicity. However, lower age (OR 0.97 (95% CI 0.96–0.99), P = 0.01), longer duration of diabetes (OR 1.09 (95% CI 1.06–1.13), P < 0.0001), higher HbA1c (OR 1.22 (95% CI 1.07–1.39), P = 0.003), and systolic blood pressure (OR 1.02 (95% CI 1.00–1.04), P = 0.02) were all associated with DR.

Table 3 shows demographic and metabolic data in patients with diabetes with (n = 94, 14%) and without (n = 563, 86%) maculopathy. There were no differences in 25(OH)D status between patients with and without maculopathy (16.2±10.0 versus 15.8±9.8 ng/mL, P = NS). Subjects were matched for age (59.1 ± 11.5 versus 59.5 ± 13.3 years); however, the duration of diabetes was significantly longer in patients with maculopathy (15.9 ± 11.1versus 19.2 ± 9.7 years, P = 0.0003). Two-year mean HbA1c (%) (8.4 ± 1.6 versus 9.1 ± 1.5, P < 0.0001) and systolic blood pressure (130 ± 14 versus 134 ± 14 mmHg, P = 0.01) were significantly higher in patients with diabetes and maculopathy. There were

Table 2: Logistic regression analyses for the relationship between retinopathy, 25(OH)D status, and other confounding variables.

	Odds Ratio	95% CI	P
25(OH)D	1.00	0.98–1.02	NS
Age (years)	**0.97**	**0.96–0.99**	**0.01**
Duration of diabetes (years)	**1.09**	**1.06–1.13**	**<0.0001**
Never smoked	0.48	0.21–1.09	NS
HbA1c (%)	**1.22**	**1.07–1.39**	**0.003**
TC (mmol/L)	1.09	0.88–1.36	NS
HDL (mmol/L)	0.88	0.55–1.41	NS
Triglycerides (mmol/L)	0.98	0.77–1.25	NS
Systolic BP (mmHg)	**1.02**	**1.00–1.04**	**0.02**
Diastolic BP (mmHg)	0.98	0.94–1.01	NS
eGFR (mL/min/L)	0.99	0.98–1.00	NS

BMI: Body Mass Index, BP: blood pressure, TC: total cholesterol, HDL: high-density lipoprotein cholesterol, ALP: alkaline phosphatase, CCa: corrected calcium, and eGFR: estimated glomerular filtration rate.

Table 3: Demographic and metabolic parameters in subgroups based on maculopathy.

	No Diabetic Maculopathy (n = 563)	Diabetic Maculopathy (n = 94)	P
Age (years)	59.5 ± 13.3	59.1 ± 11.5	NS
Duration of diabetes (years)	15.9 ± 11.1	19.2 ± 9.7	**0.0003**
Type 2 DM (%)	82	80	NS
Ethnicity (White European/South Asian (%))	40/50	49/48	NS
Sex (male (%))	51	47	NS
Current smokers/past smokers/never smoked (%)	15/28/57	16/27/57	NS
BMI	31.4 ± 8.8	31.3 ± 6.2	NS
25(OH)D (ng/mL)	15.8 ± 9.8	16.2 ± 10.0	NS
HbA1c (%)	8.4 ± 1.6	9.1 ± 1.5	**<0.0001**
TC (mmol/L)	4.1 ± 1.1	4.4 ± 1.4	NS
HDL (mmol/L)	1.3 ± 0.5	1.4 ± 0.8	NS
Trig (mmol/L)	1.8 ± 1.2	1.9 ± 1.6	NS
eGFR	75 ± 18	73 ± 20	NS
Systolic BP (mmHg)	130 ± 14	134 ± 14	**0.01**
Diastolic BP (mmHg)	71 ± 7	70 ± 7	NS
ALP (u/L)	87 ± 53	100 ± 129	NS
CCa (mmol/L)	2.3 ± 0.1	2.4 ± 0.1	NS

BMI: Body Mass Index, BP: blood pressure, TC: total cholesterol, HDL: high-density lipoprotein cholesterol, Trig: triglycerides, ALP: alkaline phosphatase, CCa: corrected calcium, and eGFR: estimated glomerular filtration rate.

Table 4: Logistic regression analyses for the relationship between maculopathy, 25(OH)D status, and other confounding variables.

	OR	95% CI	P
25(OH)D	1.00	0.98–1.03	NS
Age (years)	0.99	0.97–1.02	NS
Duration of diabetes (years)	**1.03**	**1.00–1.05**	**0.01**
Never smoked	1.24	0.73–2.12	NS
HbA1c (%)	**1.22**	**1.05–1.43**	**0.009**
TC (mmol/L)	1.05	0.84–1.33	NS
HDL (mmol/L)	1.12	0.73–1.73	NS
Triglycerides (mmol/L)	1.19	0.77–1.25	NS
Systolic BP (mmHg)	1.01	0.99–1.04	NS
Diastolic BP (mmHg)	1.03	0.98–1.07	NS
eGFR (mL/min/L)	0.99	0.97–1.00	NS

BMI: Body Mass Index, BP: blood pressure, TC: total cholesterol, HDL: high-density lipoprotein cholesterol, ALP: alkaline phosphatase, CCa: corrected calcium, and eGFR: estimated glomerular filtration rate.

no differences for type of diabetes, ethnicity, sex, smoking status, BMI, lipid and bone parameters, and diastolic blood pressure between patients with and without maculopathy. Table 4 shows logistic regression analyses for Diabetic Maculopathy status with Odds Ratios and 95% CI. There was no relationship of maculopathy status with 25(OH)D (OR 1.00 (95% CI 0.98–1.03), P = NS), age, gender, ethnicity, systolic blood pressure, or lipid fractions. However, a longer duration of diabetes (OR 1.03 (95% CI 1.00–1.05), $P = 0.01$) and higher HbA1c (OR 1.22 (95% CI 1.05–1.43), $P = 0.009$) were associated with maculopathy status.

The frequencies for severity of retinopathy, maculopathy, and photocoagulation were similar between the four vitamin D categories (severely deficient (<10 ng/mL), deficient (10–<20 ng/mL), insufficient (20–<30 ng/mL), and sufficient (>30 ng/mL)) (Figure 1).

Categorising the data based on vitamin D status (severely deficient (<10 ng/mL), deficient (10–<20 ng/mL), insufficient (20–<30 ng/mL), and sufficient (>30 ng/mL)), there were no differences in smoking status, sex, total cholesterol, and triglycerides. However, the Chi^2 analysis for ethnicity was significant ($P < 0.0001$) with a higher proportion of those with severe deficiency (n = 189, <10 ng/mL) being of South Asian origin (58%) and those with normal vitamin D status (n = 52, >30 ng/mL) being mainly of White European origin (75%). A further Chi^2 analysis of the aetiology of diabetes was significant ($P = 0.003$) with a greater proportion of type 2 diabetes in the severely deficient group (87%) (<10 ng/mL) compared to those who had a normal vitamin D status (66%) (>30 ng/mL). This reflects our previously published data [29]. BMI was higher in those with severe deficiency (32.1 ± 11.6 kg/m^2, $P = 0.02$) (<10 ng/mL) and deficiency (31.8 ± 6.7 kg/m^2, $P = 0.002$) (10–<20 ng/mL) compared to those with adequate vitamin D status (28.6 ± 5.2 kg/m^2) (>30 ng/mL). Corrected calcium status was marginally higher in those with a normal vitamin D status (2.38 ± 0.12 mmol/L, $P = 0.02$) (>30 ng/mL) compared with those who were deficient (2.33 ± 0.12 mmol/L) (<10 ng/mL) but still within the normal range for serum calcium status.

5. Discussion

Vitamin D deficiency has wide ranging implications for insulin resistance, beta cell dysfunction, and hypertension and therefore provides a potential link with diabetic complications. Experimental studies have postulated an important link between vitamin D deficiency and retinopathy [30]

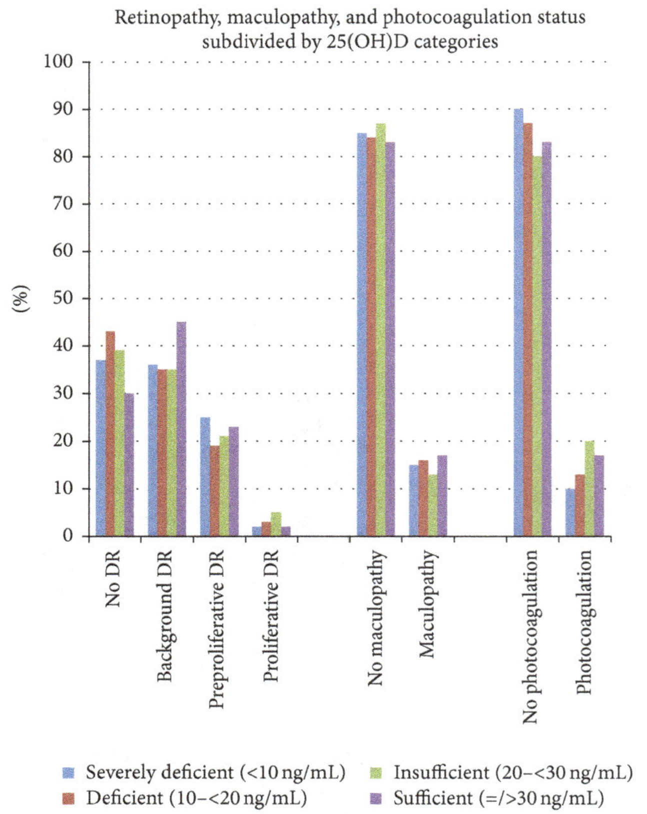

FIGURE 1: Frequencies of retinopathy, maculopathy, and photocoagulation scarring categorised by 25(OH)D status.

and an increased risk of diabetic retinopathy has been demonstrated in the presence of VDR polymorphisms [12].

However, our study has shown no relationship between the vitamin D status and the severity of diabetic retinopathy or maculopathy in a large cohort of patients with predominantly type 2 diabetes, after correcting for glycaemic control, blood pressure, and lipids. We confirm that the "usual culprits" of longer duration of diabetes, higher HbA1c, and systolic blood pressure are directly related to retinopathy and maculopathy [1], thereby providing confidence in the validity of our data. Furthermore, the metabolic and anthropometric measurements used in the regression analysis were taken over an extended period of time as opposed to "spot" readings taken in other studies [23, 25]. A possible explanation for the lack of relationship between vitamin D deficiency and retinopathy could be the striking extent of vitamin D deficiency in this population, although this is consistent with our previous data [29]. Thus, the majority of patients demonstrated deficiency (~90%) and indeed severe deficiency (~31%). Therefore, any relationship between retinopathy and adequacy of vitamin D could not be explored adequately. Furthermore, there were only a small number of patients with Diabetic Maculopathy ($n = 94$, 14%) in this study, which ultimately limits the power of the analysis. Only a limited number of clinical studies have investigated the role of vitamin D deficiency in DR. In one of the earliest studies, Aksoy et al. showed an inverse relationship between $1,25(OH)_2D_3$ and worsening retinopathy, although the short half-life of $1,25(OH)_2D_3$ may limit the interpretation of any such relationship [23]. Another smaller North American study has shown that subjects with DR, in particular PDR, have lower levels of 25(OH)D [25]. Whilst in a recent study the percentage of individuals with vitamin D deficiency increased with the severity of retinopathy, regression analysis did not demonstrate a statistically significant relationship between retinopathy severity and serum 25(OH)D concentration [26]. In a prospective observational follow-up study of a cohort of patients with type 1 diabetes, although severe vitamin D deficiency independently predicted all-cause mortality, it was not related to the development of either retinopathy or nephropathy [4]. In a recently published study of 715 patients with type 2 diabetes, serum 25(OH)D levels decreased significantly in relation to the severity of either retinopathy or nephropathy or both [31]. However, in the prospective EURODIAB study conducted in subjects with type 1 diabetes, both higher $25(OH)D_2$ and $25(OH)D_3$ were associated with a lower prevalence of macroalbuminuria, but not retinopathy and cardiovascular disease [32].

This large cross-sectional study found no association of vitamin D status with diabetic retinopathy or maculopathy. A population with a larger spread of vitamin D levels may provide further insight into a possible association, but this may not be possible due to the high prevalence of vitamin D deficiency. In the long term, randomised controlled trials of adequate vitamin D intervention and diabetic microvascular outcomes are required to truly assess any potential therapeutic benefit.

Conflict of Interests

The authors declare no conflict of interests regarding the publication of this paper.

References

[1] J. W. Y. Yau, S. L. Rogers, R. Kawasaki et al., "Global prevalence and major risk factors of diabetic retinopathy," *Diabetes Care*, vol. 35, no. 3, pp. 556–564, 2012.

[2] C. Bunce and R. Wormald, "Leading causes of certification for blindness and partial sight in England & Wales," *BMC Public Health*, vol. 6, article 58, 2006.

[3] S. Resnikoff, D. Pascolini, D. Etya'ale et al., "Global data on visual impairment in the year 2002," *Bulletin of the World Health Organization*, vol. 82, no. 11, pp. 844–851, 2004.

[4] C. Joergensen, P. Hovind, A. Schmedes, H.-H. Parving, and P. Rossing, "Vitamin D levels, microvascular complications, and mortality in type 1 diabetes," *Diabetes Care*, vol. 34, no. 5, pp. 1081–1085, 2011.

[5] F. Ismail-Beigi, T. Craven, M. A. Banerji et al., "Effect of intensive treatment of hyperglycaemia on microvascular outcomes in type 2 diabetes: an analysis of the ACCORD randomised trial," *The Lancet*, vol. 376, no. 9739, pp. 419–430, 2010.

[6] F. Ismail-Beigi, T. E. Craven, P. J. O'Connor et al., "Combined intensive blood pressure and glycemic control does not produce an additive benefit on microvascular outcomes in type 2

diabetic patients," *Kidney International*, vol. 81, no. 6, pp. 586–594, 2012.

[7] H.-P. Hammes, Y. Feng, F. Pfister, and M. Brownlee, "Diabetic retinopathy: targeting vasoregression," *Diabetes*, vol. 60, no. 1, pp. 9–16, 2011.

[8] C.-T. C. Lee, E. L. Gayton, J. W. J. Beulens, D. W. Flanagan, and A. I. Adler, "Micronutrients and diabetic retinopathy a systematic review," *Ophthalmology*, vol. 117, no. 1, pp. 71–78, 2010.

[9] M. F. Holick, "Medical progress: vitamin D deficiency," *The New England Journal of Medicine*, vol. 357, no. 3, pp. 266–281, 2007.

[10] T. J. Wang, M. J. Pencina, S. L. Booth et al., "Vitamin D deficiency and risk of cardiovascular disease," *Circulation*, vol. 117, no. 4, pp. 503–511, 2008.

[11] K. Bućan, M. Ivanišević, T. Zemunik et al., "Retinopathy and nephropathy in type 1 diabetic patients—association with polymorphysms of vitamin D-receptor, TNF, Neuro-D and Il-1 receptor 1 genes," *Collegium Antropologicum*, vol. 33, supplement 2, pp. 99–105, 2009.

[12] M. J. Taverna, J.-L. Selam, and G. Slama, "Association between a protein polymorphism in the start codon of the vitamin D receptor gene and severe diabetic retinopathy in C-peptide-negative type 1 diabetes," *Journal of Clinical Endocrinology and Metabolism*, vol. 90, no. 8, pp. 4803–4808, 2005.

[13] M. J. Taverna, A. Sola, C. Guyot-Argenton et al., "Taq I polymorphism of the vitamin D receptor and risk of severe diabetic retinopathy," *Diabetologia*, vol. 45, no. 3, pp. 436–442, 2002.

[14] A. Verstappen, M. Parmentier, M. Chirnoaga, D. E. Lawson, J. L. Pasteels, and R. Pochet, "Vitamin D-dependent calcium binding protein immunoreactivity in human retina," *Ophthalmic Research*, vol. 18, no. 4, pp. 209–214, 1986.

[15] T. A. Craig, S. Sommer, C. R. Sussman, J. P. Grande, and R. Kumar, "Expression and regulation of the vitamin D receptor in the zebrafish, *Danio rerio*," *Journal of Bone and Mineral Research*, vol. 23, no. 9, pp. 1486–1496, 2008.

[16] N. Wagner, K.-D. Wagner, G. Schley, L. Badiali, H. Theres, and H. Scholz, "1,25-Dihydroxyvitamin D_3-induced apoptosis of retinoblastoma cells is associated with reciprocal changes of Bcl-2 and bax," *Experimental Eye Research*, vol. 77, no. 1, pp. 1–9, 2003.

[17] A. Cardus, S. Panizo, M. Encinas et al., "1,25-Dihydroxyvitamin D3 regulates VEGF production through a vitamin D response element in the VEGF promoter," *Atherosclerosis*, vol. 204, no. 1, pp. 85–89, 2009.

[18] N. Panou, S. Georgopoulos, T. N. Sergentanis, A. Papalampros, M. Maropoulos, and N. Tentolouris, "Serum 25(OH)D and VEGF in diabetes mellitus type 2: gender-specific associations," *International Journal of Collaborative Research on Internal Medicine & Public Health*, vol. 3, pp. 790–795, 2011.

[19] D. M. Albert, E. A. Scheef, S. Wang et al., "Calcitriol is a potent inhibitor of retinal neovascularization," *Investigative Ophthalmology & Visual Science*, vol. 48, no. 5, pp. 2327–2334, 2007.

[20] O. Kordonouri, A. Wladimirowa, and T. Danne, "High total serum renin concentrations are associated with the development of background retinopathy in adolescents with type 1 diabetes," *Diabetes Care*, vol. 23, no. 7, pp. 1025–1026, 2000.

[21] T. Harindhanavudhi, M. Mauer, R. Klein, B. Zinman, A. Sinaiko, and M. L. Caramori, "Benefits of renin-angiotensin blockade on retinopathy in type 1 diabetes vary with glycemic control," *Diabetes Care*, vol. 34, no. 8, pp. 1838–1842, 2011.

[22] R. Ireland, "Diabetic nephropathy: paricalcitol lowers residual albuminuria in type 2 diabetes," *Nature Reviews Nephrology*, vol. 7, article 62, 2011.

[23] H. Aksoy, F. Akçay, N. Kurtul, O. Baykal, and B. Avci, "Serum 1,25 dihydroxy vitamin D ($1,25(OH)_2D_3$), 25 hydroxy vitamin D (25(OH)D) and parathormone levels in diabetic retinopathy," *Clinical Biochemistry*, vol. 33, no. 1, pp. 47–51, 2000.

[24] H. Kaur, K. C. Donaghue, A. K. Chan et al., "Vitamin D deficiency is associated with retinopathy in children and adolescents with type 1 diabetes," *Diabetes Care*, vol. 34, no. 6, pp. 1400–1402, 2011.

[25] J. F. Payne, R. Ray, D. G. Watson et al., "Vitamin D insufficiency in diabetic retinopathy," *Endocrine Practice*, vol. 18, no. 2, pp. 185–193, 2012.

[26] P. A. Patrick, P. F. Visintainer, Q. Shi, I. A. Weiss, and D. A. Brand, "Vitamin D and retinopathy in adults with diabetes mellitus," *Archives of Ophthalmology*, vol. 130, no. 6, pp. 756–760, 2012.

[27] P. H. Scanlon, "The English national screening programme for sight-threatening diabetic retinopathy," *Journal of Medical Screening*, vol. 15, no. 1, pp. 1–4, 2008.

[28] S. Patra, E. M. W. Gomm, M. Macipe, and C. Bailey, "Interobserver agreement between primary graders and an expert grader in the Bristol and Weston diabetic retinopathy screening programme: a quality assurance audit," *Diabetic Medicine*, vol. 26, no. 8, pp. 820–823, 2009.

[29] U. Alam, O. Najam, S. Al-Himdani et al., "Marked vitamin D deficiency in patients with diabetes in the UK: ethnic and seasonal differences and an association with dyslipidaemia," *Diabetic Medicine*, vol. 29, no. 10, pp. 1343–1345, 2012.

[30] H. F. Deluca and M. T. Cantorna, "Vitamin D: its role and uses in immunology," *The FASEB Journal*, vol. 15, no. 14, pp. 2579–2585, 2001.

[31] G. Zoppini, A. Galletti, G. Targher et al., "Lower levels of 25-hydroxyvitamin D_3 are associated with a higher prevalence of microvascular complications in patients with type 2 diabetes," *BMJ Open Diabetes Research & Care*, vol. 3, no. 1, Article ID e000058, 2015.

[32] L. Engelen, C. G. Schalkwijk, S. J. Eussen et al., "Low 25-hydroxyvitamin D2 and 25-hydroxyvitamin D3 levels are independently associated with macroalbuminuria, but not with retinopathy and macrovascular disease in type 1 diabetes: the EURODIAB prospective complications study," *Cardiovascular Diabetology*, vol. 14, article 67, 2015.

8

Diabetes Mellitus and Increased Tuberculosis Susceptibility: The Role of Short-Chain Fatty Acids

Ekta Lachmandas, Corina N. A. M. van den Heuvel, Michelle S. M. A. Damen, Maartje C. P. Cleophas, Mihai G. Netea, and Reinout van Crevel

Department of Internal Medicine and Radboudumc Center for Infectious Diseases, Radboud University Medical Center, Internal Postal Code 463, P.O. Box 9101, 6500 HB Nijmegen, Netherlands

Correspondence should be addressed to Ekta Lachmandas; ekta.lachmandas@radboudumc.nl

Academic Editor: Francisco J. Ruperez

Type 2 diabetes mellitus confers a threefold increased risk for tuberculosis, but the underlying immunological mechanisms are still largely unknown. Possible mediators of this increased susceptibility are short-chain fatty acids, levels of which have been shown to be altered in individuals with diabetes. We examined the influence of physiological concentrations of butyrate on cytokine responses to *Mycobacterium tuberculosis* (Mtb) in human peripheral blood mononuclear cells (PBMCs). Butyrate decreased Mtb-induced proinflammatory cytokine responses, while it increased production of IL-10. This anti-inflammatory effect was independent of butyrate's well-characterised inhibition of HDAC activity and was not accompanied by changes in Toll-like receptor signalling pathways, the eicosanoid pathway, or cellular metabolism. In contrast blocking IL-10 activity reversed the effects of butyrate on Mtb-induced inflammation. Alteration of the gut microbiota, thereby increasing butyrate concentrations, can reduce insulin resistance and obesity, but further studies are needed to determine how this affects susceptibility to tuberculosis.

1. Introduction

Tuberculosis (TB) is the second leading cause of death from an infectious disease worldwide [1]. Susceptibility to TB can be increased by several comorbidities, one of which is type 2 diabetes mellitus (DM) [2]. DM patients present with an overall threefold increased risk of developing active TB [3]. Globally, 15% of TB cases are estimated to be attributable to DM [4] and thus with a predicted increase of DM by 155% over the next 20 years, DM will become an increasingly important factor challenging TB control [5–7].

DM patients exhibit alterations in the immune response against *Mycobacterium tuberculosis* (Mtb), making them more susceptible to infection or progression towards active TB disease and less responsive to treatment [8–11]. However, the underlying biological mechanisms remain largely unknown [12, 13]. DM patients have been associated with dysregulated cytokine responses to Mtb [14–17]. Whilst proinflammatory cytokines are necessary for protection against Mtb, anti-inflammatory cytokines may counteract these effects. Possible factors that may impact the host response in patients with DM are short-chain fatty acids (SCFAs), the main metabolic products of fermentation of nondigestible dietary fibres by the gut microbiota. Numerous reports have demonstrated that DM patients present with an altered composition of their gut microbiota, which subsequently alters their SCFA levels [18–24]. SCFAs strongly modulate immune and inflammatory responses [22, 25–31], thereby influencing the host response to Mtb. SCFAs, of which butyrate (C4) is the most thoroughly studied, act on immune and endothelial cells via at least two mechanisms: activation of G-protein coupled receptors (GPCRs) and inhibition of histone deacetylase (HDAC) [32]. They affect the function of various cell types such as lymphocytes [33, 34], neutrophils [25, 31, 35], and macrophages [28, 36–38]. In light of the emerging role of the microbiota in inflammation and immunity, we hypothesized that SCFAs, and in particular butyrate, may affect the immune response and susceptibility to Mtb in type 2 DM patients.

In this study we investigated the role of physiological concentrations of SCFAs on the cytokine response against

Mtb in human peripheral blood mononuclear cells (PBMCs). We subsequently examined a number of possible mechanisms via which altered concentrations of one particular SCFA, C4, might affect the host immune response to Mtb in DM patients. To this purpose, we studied the influence of physiological concentrations of C4 on HDAC activity, immune signalling pathways, the eicosanoid pathway, and cellular metabolism. To our knowledge, this is the first study reporting on the effects of physiological plasma concentrations of C4 on Mtb-induced cellular responses. Physiological plasma concentrations of C4 are in the micromolar range [39], whilst in previous studies C4 has been used in the millimolar range. Thus, this study substantially adds to our knowledge of SCFAs as possible mediators of altered immune responses to Mtb in DM patients.

2. Materials and Methods

2.1. Human Samples. PBMCs were isolated from buffy coats donated after written informed consent by healthy volunteers to the Sanquin Blood Bank (http://www.sanquin.nl/en/) in Nijmegen. Experiments were conducted according to the principles expressed in the Declaration of Helsinki. Since blood donations were anonymous no tuberculosis skin test or IFN-γ release assay was performed. However, the incidence of TB in the Dutch population is extremely low (4/100,000), and Bacillus Calmette-Guérin (BCG) vaccination is not part of the routine vaccination program. Blood donors were not screened for DM as prevalence of DM among people under 45 years of age (median age of blood donors) is about 1.5% and therefore DM is unlikely to be a confounding factor [34].

2.2. H37Rv Lysates and Culture. H37Rv Mtb was grown to mid-log phase in Middlebrook 7H9 liquid medium (Difco, Becton Dickinson) supplemented with oleic acid/albumin/dextrose/catalase (OADC) (BBL, Becton Dickinson), washed three times in sterile saline, heat killed, and then disrupted using a bead beater, after which the concentration was measured using a bicinchoninic acid (BCA) assay (Pierce, Thermo Scientific).

2.3. Cell Stimulation Experiments. Isolation of PBMCs was performed by differential centrifugation over Ficoll-Paque (GE Healthcare). Cells were adjusted to 5×10^6 cells/mL (Beckman Coulter) and suspended in RPMI 1640 (Gibco) supplemented with 10 μg/mL gentamicin (Lonza), 10 mM L-glutamine (Life Technologies), and 10 mM pyruvate (Life Technologies). 100 μL of PBMCs was incubated in round-bottom 96-well plates (Greiner), pretreated with SCFAs for 1 h, and stimulated with 1 μg/mL of H37Rv lysate or 10 ng/mL LPS (Sigma-Aldrich, *E. coli* serotype 055:B5). Cells were incubated for 24 h or 7 days at 37°C in a 5% CO_2 environment (n = 6 to 11). Alternatively, PBMCs were pretreated for 1 hour (37°C, 5% CO_2) with ranolazine (ITK Diagnostics), trimetazidine (Sigma), pertussis toxin (Enzo Life Sciences), etomoxir (Sigma) (inhibitors of β-oxidation, n = 3), aspirin (Aspégic injection powder, n = 3), cycloheximide (Sigma, n = 6 to 7), anti-IL-10 antibody IgG2a (BioLegend, n = 10 to 12), or IgG2a isotype control (BioLegend, n = 10 to 12) prior to stimulation. Cell culture supernatants were collected and stored at −20°C for cytokine measurements, performed by ELISA: TNF-α, IL-1β, IL-17A, IL-22, and IL-1Ra (R&D Systems) and IL-6, IFN-γ, and IL-10 (Sanquin).

2.4. Quantification of Gene Expression. For quantitative real-time PCR (qPCR) analysis RNA was isolated from PBMCs using TRIzol reagent (Invitrogen Life Technologies) according to the manufacturer's protocol. RNA was transcribed into complementary DNA (cDNA) by reverse transcription using iScript cDNA synthesis kit (Bio-Rad, Hercules, CA). Primer sequences (Biolegio) are given in Table 1. Power SYBR Green PCR Master Mix (Applied Biosystems) was used for qPCR on an AB StepOnePlus real-time PCR system (Applied Biosystems). qPCR data were normalized to the housekeeping gene human β2M (n = 3 to 10).

2.5. Protein Phosphorylation Measurements. Western blotting was carried out using a Trans-Blot Turbo system (Bio-Rad) according to manufacturer's instructions. 5×10^6 PBMCs were lysed in 100 μL lysis buffer. The resulting lysate was used for Western blot analysis. Equal amounts of protein were separated by SDS-PAGE on 4–15% polyacrylamide gels (Bio-Rad) and transferred to PVDF (Bio-Rad) membranes. Membranes were blocked for 1 h and then incubated overnight with primary antibody (dilution 1:1000) in 5% (w/v) BSA or milk in TBS-Tween buffer (TBS-T). Blots were washed in TBS-T 3 times and incubated with HRP-conjugated anti-rabbit antibody (1:5000; Sigma) in 5% (w/v) milk in TBS-T for 1 h at room temperature (RT). After washing, blots were developed with ECL (Bio-Rad) following manufacturer's instructions. Primary antibodies used were rabbit anti-p38 MAPK, rabbit anti-phospho-p38 MAPK, rabbit anti-ERK1/2 (p44/p42 MAPK), rabbit anti-phospho-ERK1/2 (P44/42 MAPK, T202/Y204), and rabbit anti-phospho-JNK (T183/Y185) (all Cell Signalling) (n = 2).

2.6. Metabolite Measurements. Lactate was measured from cell culture supernatants using a coupled enzymatic assay in which lactate was oxidised and the resulting H_2O_2 was coupled to the conversion of Amplex Red reagent to fluorescent resorufin by HRP (horseradish peroxidase). 30 μL of lactate standard or 200x diluted sample was added to 30 μL of reaction mix. The 30 μL of reaction mix consisted of 0.6 μL of 10 U/mL HRP (Sigma), 0.6 μL of 100 U/mL lactate oxidase (Sigma), 0.3 μL of 10 mM Amplex Red reagent (Life Technologies), and 28.5 μL PBS. Samples were incubated for 20 min at RT and fluorescence (excitation/emission maxima = 570/585 nm) was measured on an ELISA reader (BioTek) (n = 3 to 5).

Measurements of the NAD^+/NADH redox ratio were adapted from Zhu and Rand [40]. Briefly, 1.5 million stimulated PBMCs were lysed in 75 μL of homogenization buffer (10 mM nicotinamide (Sigma), 10 mM Tris-Cl (Sigma), and 0.05% (w/v) Triton X-100 (Sigma), pH 7.4). The lysate was centrifuged at 12000 g for 1 min. From the resulting supernatants two 18 μL aliquots were removed and either

Table 1: Primer sequences used for gene expression measurements by qPCR.

Target	Forward 5′ → 3′	Reverse 5′ → 3′
h-β2M	ATGAGTATGCCTGCCGTGTG	CCAAATGCGGCATCTTCAAAC
h-COX-2	CTGGCGCTCAGCCATACAG	CGCACTTATACTGGTCAAATCCC
h-CS	GGTGGCATGAGAGGCATGAA	TAGCCTTGGGTAGCAGTTTCT
h-HDAC1	CCGCATGACTCATAATTTGCTG	ATTGGCTTTGTGAGGGCGATA
h-HDAC8	TCGCTGGTCCCGGTTTATATC	TACTGGCCCGTTTGGGGAT
h-HIF1-α	GAACGTCGAAAAGAAAAGTCTCG	CCTTATCAAGATGCGAACTCACA
h-IDH2	CGCCACTATGCCGACAAAAG	ACTGCCAGATAATACGGGTCA
h-IL-10	CAACCTGCCTAACATGCTTCG	TCATCTCAGACAAGGCTTGGC
h-IL-1β	GCCCTAAACAGATGAAGTGCTC	GAACCAGCATCTTCCTCAG
h-IL12p35	CCTTGCACTTCTGAAGAGATTGA	ACAGGGCCATCATAAAAGAGGT
h-IL23p19	CTCAGGGACAACAGTCAGTTC	ACAGGGCTATCAGGGAGC
h-MDH2	TCGGCCCAGAACAATGCTAAA	GCGGCTTTGGTCTCGATGT
h-SOCS1	TTTTCGCCCTTAGCGTGAAGA	GAGGCAGTCGAAGCTCTCG
h-SOCS3	TGCGCCTCAAGACCTTCAG	GAGCTGTCGCGGATCAGAAA
h-ST2	TTGTCTACCCACGGAACTACA	GCTCTTTCGTATGTTGGTTTCCA
h-TNF-α	CCTCTCTCTAATCAGCCCTCTG	GAGGACCTGGGAGTAGATGAG
h-Tollip	TGGGCCGACTGAACATCAC	GTGGATGACCTTATTCCAGCG

2 μL of 0.2 M HCl or 0.2 M NaOH was added to each aliquot. The samples were heated for 30 min at 65°C and after incubation 2 μL of opposite reagent (NaOH or HCl) was added to each aliquot. 5 μL of sample or NAD^+ (β-nicotinamide adenine dinucleotide hydrate; Sigma) standard was then mixed with 85 μL of reaction mix and 60 μL of fluorescence mix in a black 96-well plate. The reaction mix consisted of 100 mM bicine (N,N-bis(2-hydroxyethyl)glycine; Sigma), 0.6 mM ethanol (Sigma), and 5 mM EDTA (Life Technologies). The fluorescence mix consisted of 0.5 mM PMS (phenazine methosulfate; Sigma), 0.05 mM resazurin (Sigma), and 0.2 mg of ADH (alcohol dehydrogenase; Sigma). The reaction was incubated for 15 min at RT and fluorescence (excitation/emission maxima = 540/586 nm) was measured on an ELISA reader (BioTek) (n = 3 to 5).

2.7. HDAC Activity Assay. HDAC Fluorometric Cellular Activity Assay BML-AK503 (FLUOR DE LYS, Enzo Life Sciences, Inc., Farmingdale, NY) was used to determine HDAC activity in PBMCs pretreated with C4 (30 min) and then stimulated with H37Rv (30 min). Subsequently PBMCs were incubated with acetylated substrate for 2 hours, after which a developer was added to generate a fluorescent signal from the deacetylated substrate. Fluorescence was measured on a microplate reader (BioTek). Trichostatin A (TSA) was used as a positive control for HDAC inhibition (n = 5 to 6).

2.8. Flow Cytometry. PBMCs were treated with 50 μmol C4 for 1 h and stimulated with 1 μg/mL H37Rv or 10 ng/mL LPS for 7 days. Subsequently cells were restimulated with 200 μL RPMI supplemented with 10% serum, Golgi-plug inhibitor (GPI Brefeldin A; 1 μg/mL, BD Pharmingen), PMA (phorbol 12-myristate 13-acetate; 50 μg/mL, Sigma-Aldrich), and ionomycin (1 μg/mL, Sigma-Aldrich) for 4–6 h at 37°C and 5% CO_2. Cells were then washed with PBA (PBS 1% BSA (albumin from bovine serum)) and stained extracellularly for 30 min with CD4-PeCys7 (ITK) for T-helper 17 (Th17) cells at 4°C. Next, cells were washed and permeabilized by fix and perm buffer (eBioscience) according to the manufacturer's protocol for 45–60 min at 4°C. Finally cells were washed and resuspended in 300 μL PBA to be measured using the Cytomics FC500 (Beckman Coulter) (n = 8).

Cell death was measured by staining PBMCs with Annexin V-FITC (BioVision) and Propidium Iodide (PI) (Invitrogen Molecular Probes). Cells were incubated in the dark on ice with Annexin-V staining solution (RPMI supplemented with 5 mM $CaCl_2$ and 0.1 μL/mL Annexin-V) for 15 minutes. Subsequently PBMCs were stained with PI for 5 minutes. Cells were measured with the Cytomics FC500 (Beckman Coulter, Woerden, Netherlands), and data were analysed using CXP analysis software v2.2 (Beckman Coulter) (n = 3 to 5).

2.9. Statistical Analysis. All data were analysed using a paired nonparametric Wilcoxon signed-rank test, as the data were not normally distributed. Differences were considered statistically significant at p value < 0.05. Data are shown as cumulative results of levels obtained in all volunteers (means ± SEM).

3. Results

3.1. Short-Chain Fatty Acids Inhibit Mtb-Induced Cytokine Responses. DM is associated with altered gut microbiota and consequently altered SCFA levels [18–22]. In line with current literature [22, 25–31], we hypothesized that SCFAs have the potential to influence the host inflammatory response against Mtb. In particular we investigated the effects of varying doses of acetate (C2), propionate (C3), and butyrate (C4) on H37Rv-induced cytokine responses, with RPMI as negative control and LPS as positive control (Figure 1). SCFAs themselves did not induce cytokine production (results not shown) but significantly affected H37Rv-induced cytokine release. C2, C3, and C4 significantly, dose-dependently decreased H37Rv-induced production of proinflammatory cytokines TNF-α, IL-1β, and IL-17, while nonsignificant effects were found for IL-6, IFN-γ, and IL-22 production. In contrast, C3 and C4 induced a significant increase in H37Rv-induced production of the anti-inflammatory cytokine IL-10. Similarly, C3 and C4 but not C2 decreased LPS-induced production of TNF-α and IL-6, while the release of IL-1β was significantly decreased in response to all three SCFAs (results not shown). LPS did not induce production of IFN-γ, IL-17, or IL-22. Moreover, all three SCFAs incurred a dose-dependent, nonsignificant decrease in LPS-induced IL-10 production (results not shown).

Overall, C4 resulted in some of the most significant changes in cytokine responses (Figure 1(b)). Moreover, the potency of butyrate in reducing cytokine responses to H37Rv and LPS was greater than that for the other SCFAs. Importantly, changes in cytokine levels could not be explained by altered pH levels or cell death (Supplementary Figure 1 A and B in Supplementary Material available online at http://dx.doi.org/10.1155/2016/6014631). Therefore, following this screen, we continued our study with C4 at a concentration of 50 μM, which is physiologically relevant because it is comparable to human plasma concentrations [39].

3.2. Influence of Butyrate on HDAC Expression and Activity. Butyrate is reported to be a strong HDAC inhibitor. Since this might account for its anti-inflammatory effects [41–44], we examined the effect of C4 on HDAC expression and activity. C4 significantly decreased HDAC8 but not HDAC1 gene expression upon H37Rv stimulation of PBMCs (Figure 2(a)). Consistent with previous reports [36, 42–44], C4 at a high dose of 1 mM decreased HDAC activity upon both RPMI and H37Rv stimulation. However, different from its effect on gene expression, C4 at a physiological dose of 50 μM had no effect on actual HDAC activity (Figure 2(b)), while trichostatin A (TSA, positive control) strongly decreased HDAC activity. These data suggest that butyrate's inhibition of HDAC activity is unlikely to play a role in the effects of low doses of C4 on Mtb-induced inflammatory responses and stresses the importance of studying the effects of butyrate at physiologically relevant concentrations.

3.3. The Effects of Butyrate on TLR-Signalling Mediators and the Eicosanoid Pathway. Signalling of Toll-like receptors (TLRs), important receptors for Mtb recognition [45–47], is controlled by feedback mechanisms regulated by several intracellular kinases [48, 49]. Because impaired Mtb recognition and insufficient TLR signalling may account for the anti-inflammatory effects of C4, we examined whether C4 affected these feedback loops. However, C4 had no effect on phosphorylation of the MAP kinases p38, ERK (Figure 3(a)), or JNK (Supplementary Figure 2). C4 has also been reported to induce expression of inhibitors of TLR signalling pathways [50], but we found that C4 significantly decreased mRNA expression of TLR signalling inhibitors SOCS1 and Tollip and did not affect expression of SOCS3 or ST2 (Figure 3(b)). Of note, these results were not explained by cell death (Supplementary Figure 1 B).

Aside from TLR signalling, C4 possibly exerts its anti-inflammatory effects through modulation of the eicosanoid pathway. Eicosanoids, oxygenated metabolites of arachidonic acid, modulate the host immune response to Mtb [51–55]. C4 has been reported to upregulate key enzymes of the eicosanoid pathway upon LPS stimulation [30], but a reverse effect has also been described [56]. We did not observe a significant impact of C4 on transcript levels of cyclooxygenase 2 (COX-2), one of the main eicosanoid enzymes, upon H37Rv or LPS stimulation (Supplementary Figure 3 A). Alternatively, C4 has been described to induce release of the anti-inflammatory prostaglandin PGE_2 [26, 30, 57]. Inhibition of PGE_2 with aspirin could not counteract the inhibitory effects of C4 on TNF-α and IL-1β cytokine responses upon either H37Rv or LPS stimulation (Supplementary Figure 3 B). The eicosanoid pathway is therefore unlikely to be the mediator pathway through which C4 exerts its anti-inflammatory effects.

3.4. Influence of Butyrate on Cellular Metabolism. Another possible explanation for butyrate's anti-inflammatory effects is its influence on cellular metabolism. A recent paper described that microbiota have a strong effect on energy homeostasis in the mammalian colon and showed that C4 regulates different aspects of energy metabolism acting as an important energy source for colonocytes [58]. Contrary to this previous study, we observed no effects of C4 on cellular lactate production, the NAD^+/NADH redox ratio, TCA cycle gene expression (Figure 4), or β-oxidation (Supplementary Figure 4). These data strongly suggest that C4 modulates the immune response to Mtb independently of cellular metabolism.

3.5. Butyrate Transcriptionally Influences Cytokine Responses to Mtb, Possibly Mediated through IL-10 Induction. We next examined whether the inhibitory effect of C4 on Mtb-induced proinflammatory cytokine responses, with a concomitant increase in anti-inflammatory IL-10 production (Figure 1) and decrease in Th17 proliferation (Supplementary Figure 5 A), was also present at the level of gene transcription. C4 led to a decrease in TNF-α, IL-12, and IL-23 mRNA levels upon H37Rv stimulation and a parallel increase in IL-10 mRNA (Figure 5(a)), while no effect on production of the anti-inflammatory cytokine IL-1Ra was observed (Supplementary Figure 5 B). These data point to IL-10 as a possible intermediary mediator of the anti-inflammatory effects of C4. We therefore assessed whether removing IL-10 protein from the cellular environment could counteract the inhibitory effects of C4. To this end, we pretreated PBMCs with cycloheximide (CHX), an inhibitor of translation. Stimulation of PBMCs with H37Rv in the presence of C4 in combination with CHX resulted in higher TNF-α responses, as compared to incubation with H37Rv and C4 alone. Upon LPS stimulation, this effect was not present (Figure 5(b)). We subsequently examined whether

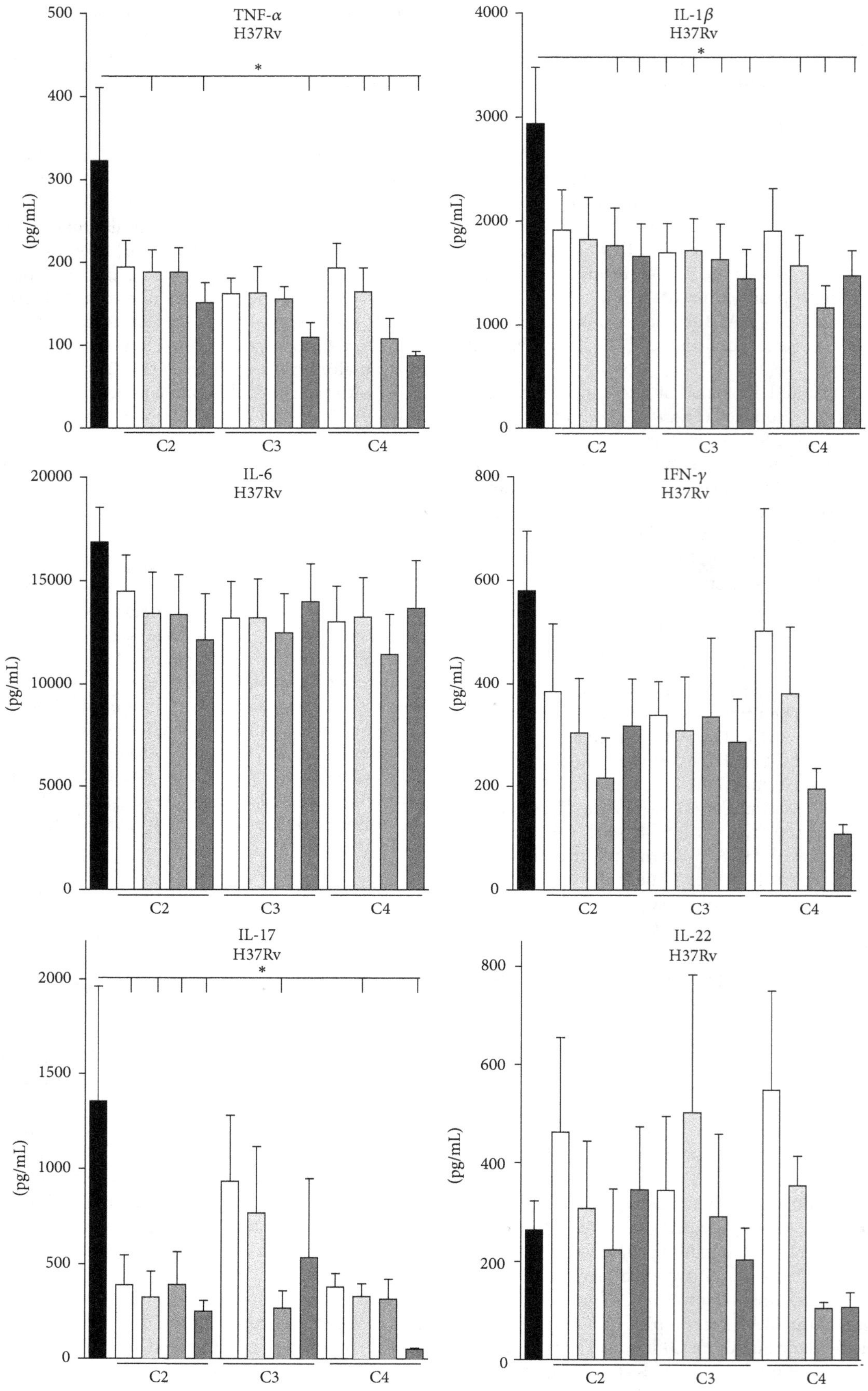

FIGURE 1: Continued.

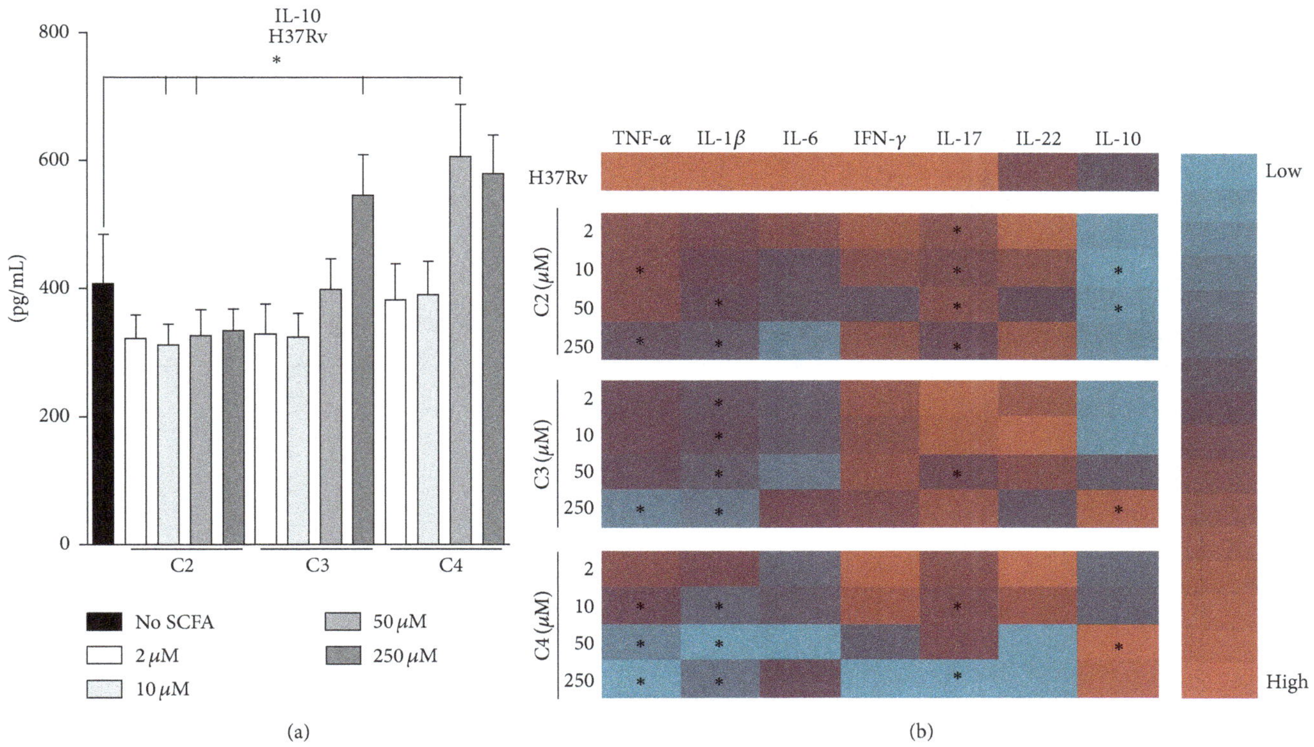

FIGURE 1: Short-chain fatty acids inhibit Mtb-induced cytokine responses. (a) PBMCs were preincubated with 2–250 μM SCFAs for 1 h prior to stimulation with Mtb lysate for 24 h and 7 d. Hereafter TNF-α, IL-6, IL-10, IFN-γ, IL-17, and IL-22 were measured in supernatants by ELISA. Data are means ± SEM ($n = 6$), using Wilcoxon signed-rank test, representative of 2 independent experiments. $^*p < 0.05$. (b) Heat map of log-transformed mean cytokine responses as measured by ELISA, showing cytokines upregulated (red) and downregulated (blue) upon H37Rv stimulation in the presence of different doses of SCFAs. Cytokine responses are shown as compared to H37Rv stimulation alone. $^*p < 0.05$.

blocking IL-10 specifically using an anti-IL-10 antibody could counteract the inhibitory effects of C4 on proinflammatory cytokine response. Blocking IL-10 completely restored IL-6 cytokine responses in response to H37Rv and C4, while TNF-α and IL-1β production was partly restored (Figure 5(c)). This suggests an important role for intermediary protein synthesis, specifically IL-10, in mediating the anti-inflammatory effects of C4.

4. Discussion

DM is associated with a threefold increased risk of active TB, but the underlying immunological mechanisms remain largely unknown [3, 12, 13]. Alterations in the gut microbiota of DM patients are associated with changes in plasma SCFA concentrations. Multiple papers have reported a decrease in C4-producing bacteria in type 2 DM patients [18, 19, 21, 23, 24]. We here show that SCFAs, especially C4, exhibit anti-inflammatory properties; low doses of C4 decreased Mtb-induced proinflammatory cytokine responses on both the transcriptional level and the translational level, while production of IL-10 was increased. This anti-inflammatory effect was independent of HDAC activity, Toll-like receptor signalling, the eicosanoid pathway, or cellular metabolism.

We observed a general anti-inflammatory effect of C2, C3, and C4 on Mtb-induced cytokine production. C4 induced some of the most significant and most potent changes in cytokine responses, which is in line with published results [29], although our study is the first to examine the effects of physiological concentrations of SCFAs on Mtb-induced cytokine responses *in vitro*. Several observations were made regarding the effect of SCFA on cytokines. Firstly, the inhibitory effect of all three SCFAs on production of TNF-α and IL-1β was comparable for Mtb and LPS stimulation. However, while C3 and C4 had a clear effect on LPS-induced IL-6 release, this was not found for Mtb. This suggests that SCFAs do not affect Mtb-induced IL-6, although IL-6 has been assigned an important role in Mtb host responses [59–62]. Secondly, C2, C3, and C4 had a much stronger inhibitory effect on T-cell derived cytokine IL-17 than on T-cell derived cytokines IFN-γ and IL-22. Because C4 also strongly decreased Th17 proliferation (Supplementary Figure 5 A), SCFAs may affect Th17 subsets more than other T-cell subsets. This may be of great relevance since Th17 cells, and IL-17 in particular, have been reported to be essential in protective immunity against Mtb [63, 64] but inversely associated with DM complications [65–67]. Lastly, the stimulatory effect of C3 and C4 on anti-inflammatory IL-10 release was Mtb-specific and was not seen with LPS stimulation. IL-10 has

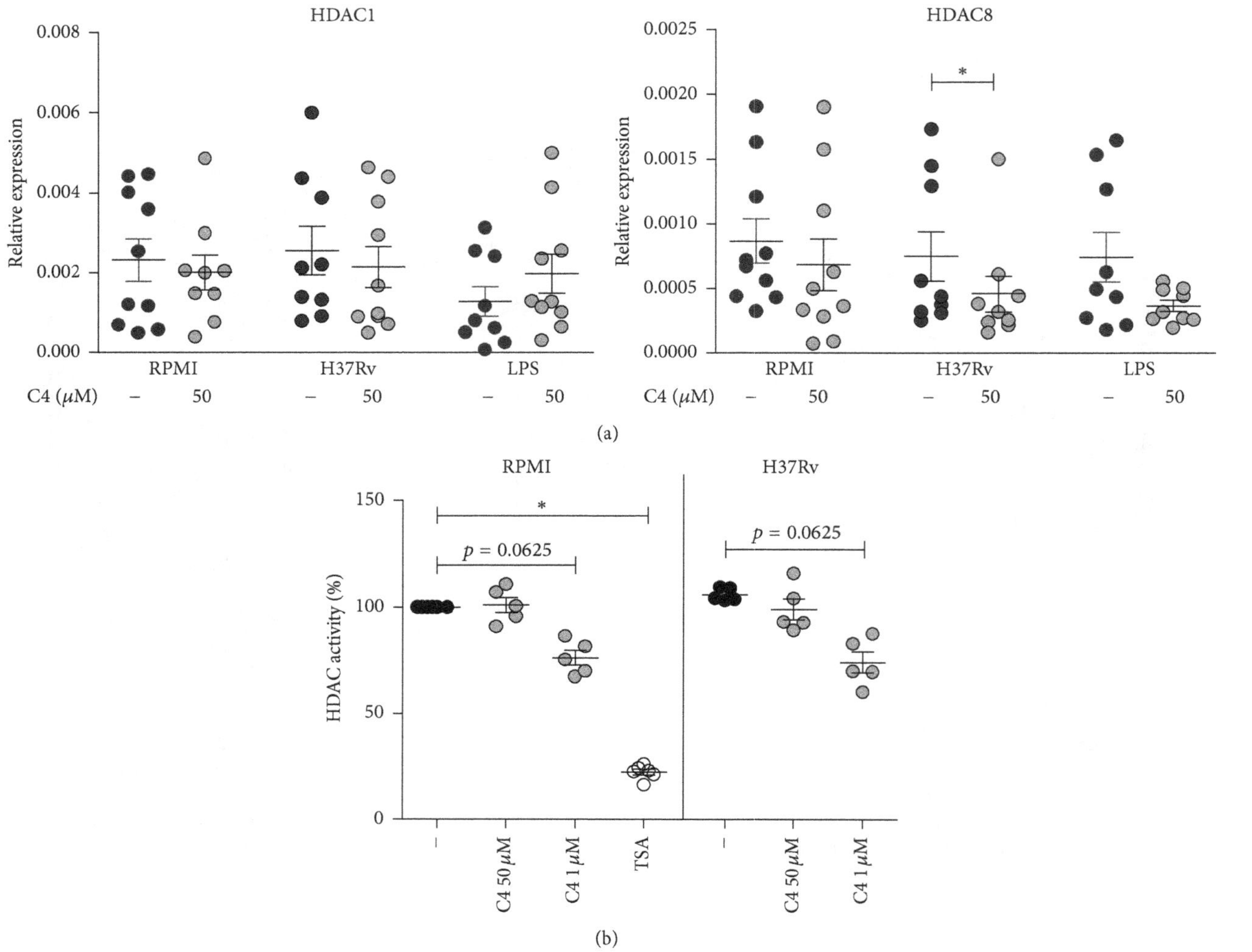

FIGURE 2: Influence of butyrate on HDAC expression and activity. (a) PBMCs were preincubated with 50 μM C4 for 1 h prior to stimulation with Mtb lysate or LPS for 4 h. Gene expression levels of HDAC1 and HDAC8 were measured by qPCR. Data are means ± SEM ($n = 10$), using Wilcoxon signed-rank test, representative of 3 independent experiments. $^{*}p < 0.05$. (b) Percentage of general HDAC activity relative to RPMI stimulated PBMCs, as measured by levels of substrate deacetylation after 30 min of preincubation with C4 (50 μM) and 30 min of stimulation with Mtb lysate. Data are means ± SEM ($n = 5$ to 6), using Wilcoxon signed-rank test, representative of 3 independent experiments. $^{*}p < 0.05$.

been delineated as an important mediator in Mtb infection: it has been reported to block bacterial killing in Mtb-infected macrophages, suppress multinucleated giant cell formation and cytokine production, and inhibit the development of protective immunity [68–74]. In contrast to TB, IL-10 may have a protective role in type 2 DM by reducing insulin resistance and obesity [75–77]. Therefore, the increase in IL-10 production we see as induced by C4 is very relevant for the course of both DM and TB disease.

We examined several possible mechanisms underlying the effect of C4 on cytokine production, starting with HDAC activity, which is known to be inhibited by SCFAs. C4 at a physiological low dose of 50 μM had little effect, while millimolar concentrations of C4 (as used in other studies [36, 41–44]) decreased HDAC activity upon H37Rv stimulation. This is expected as IC_{50} values of HDAC inhibition by C4 are >100 μM, depending on the class of HDAC [43]. The strongest effect was noted for HDAC8, which is reported to be most sensitive to C4 [43]. This argues that physiological C4 concentrations in human plasma do not exert HDAC inhibition and underlines the importance of using physiological concentrations within *in vitro* experimental models.

In contrast to a previous study [50], we observed a decreased gene expression of the TLR modulatory factors SOCS1 and Tollip when PBMCs were stimulated in the presence of C4, which thus cannot explain the inhibitory effects on cytokine production. This, together with our data showing that C4 does not affect MAP kinase activity, suggests that C4 does not act at the level of TLR signalling, as shown previously [36].

As a third possible mechanism, we assessed whether C4 exerts its effects through eicosanoid metabolism. The eicosanoid pathway is under influence of SCFAs [30, 56] and may modulate the host response to Mtb [51–55]. C4 did not

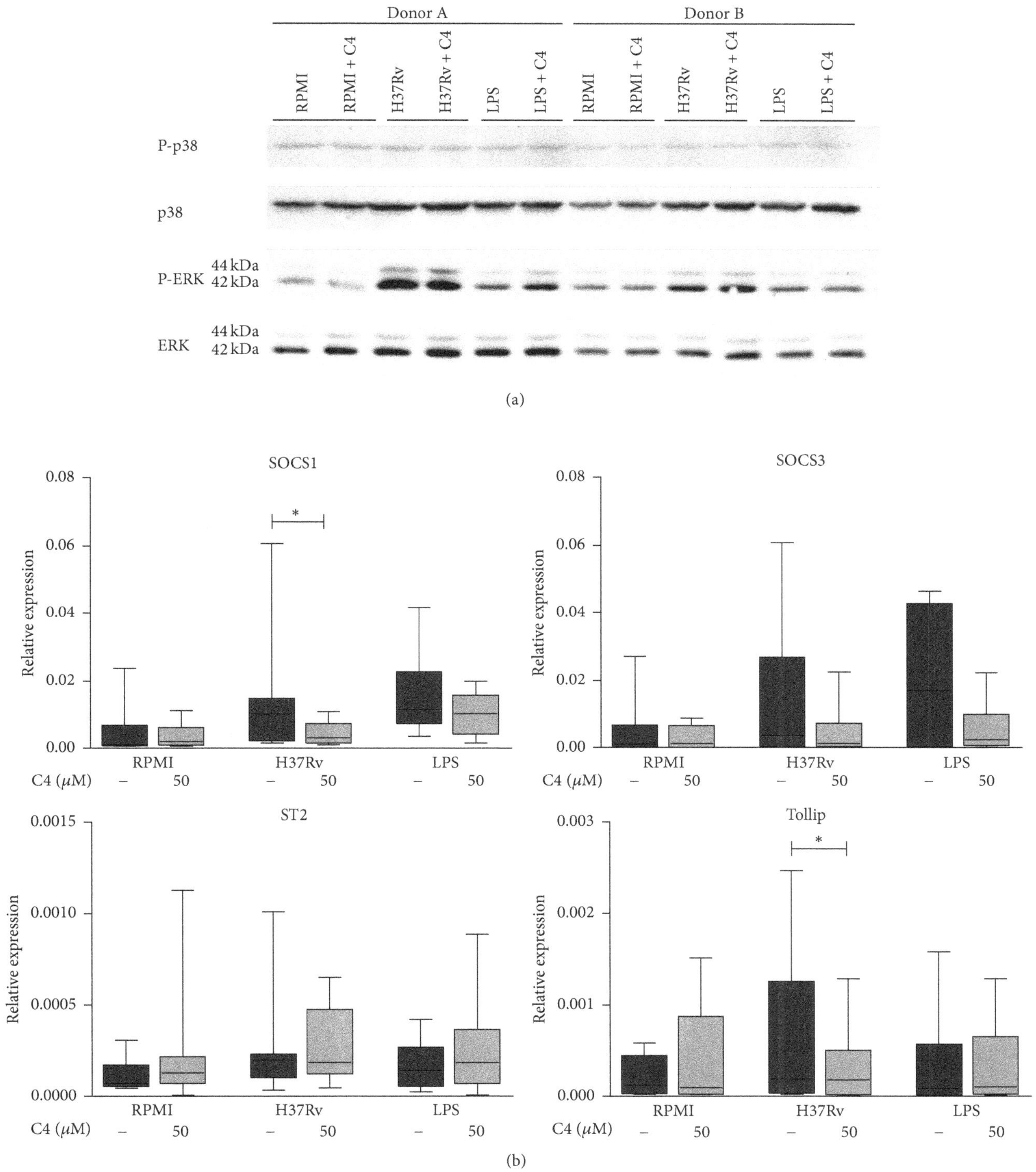

FIGURE 3: The effects of butyrate on TLR signalling mediators. (a) PBMCs were preincubated with 50 μM C4 (1 h) and stimulated with Mtb lysate or LPS. Cell lysates were harvested at 30 min after stimulation. Phospho-p38, p38, phospho-ERK, and ERK protein levels were determined by Western blot using specific antibodies ($n = 2$). (b) Gene expression levels of SOCS1, SOCS3, ST2, and Tollip in PBMCs preincubated with 50 μM C4 (1 h) and stimulated with Mtb lysate or LPS (4 h) as measured by qPCR. The box plot represents median with first and third quartiles; the whiskers represent minimum and maximum values. $n = 10$, using Wilcoxon signed-rank test, representative of 3 independent experiments. $^{*}p < 0.05$.

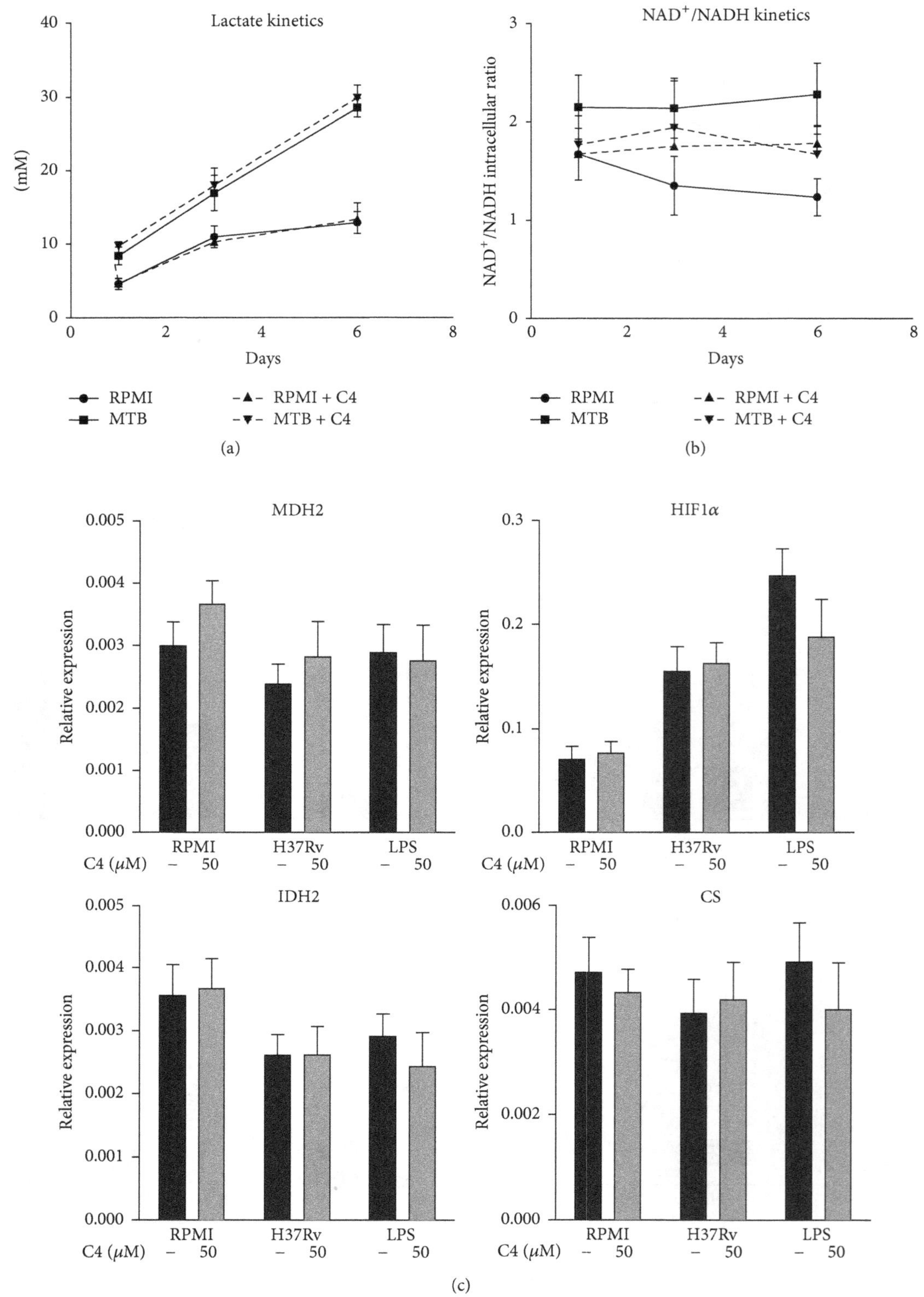

FIGURE 4: Influence of butyrate on cellular metabolism. (a and b) Kinetics of lactate production (a) and intracellular NAD^+/NADH ratios (b) from days 1, 3, and 7 of PBMCs preincubated with 50 μM C4 (1 h) with and without stimulation with Mtb lysate. Data are means ± SEM (n = 3 to 5), using Wilcoxon signed-rank test, representative of 1-2 independent experiments. (c) Expression levels of glycolysis and TCA cycle genes in PBMCs preincubated with 50 μM C4 (1 h) and stimulated with Mtb lysate or LPS (4 h) as measured by qPCR. Data are means ± SEM (n = 6), using Wilcoxon signed-rank test, representative of 2 independent experiments.

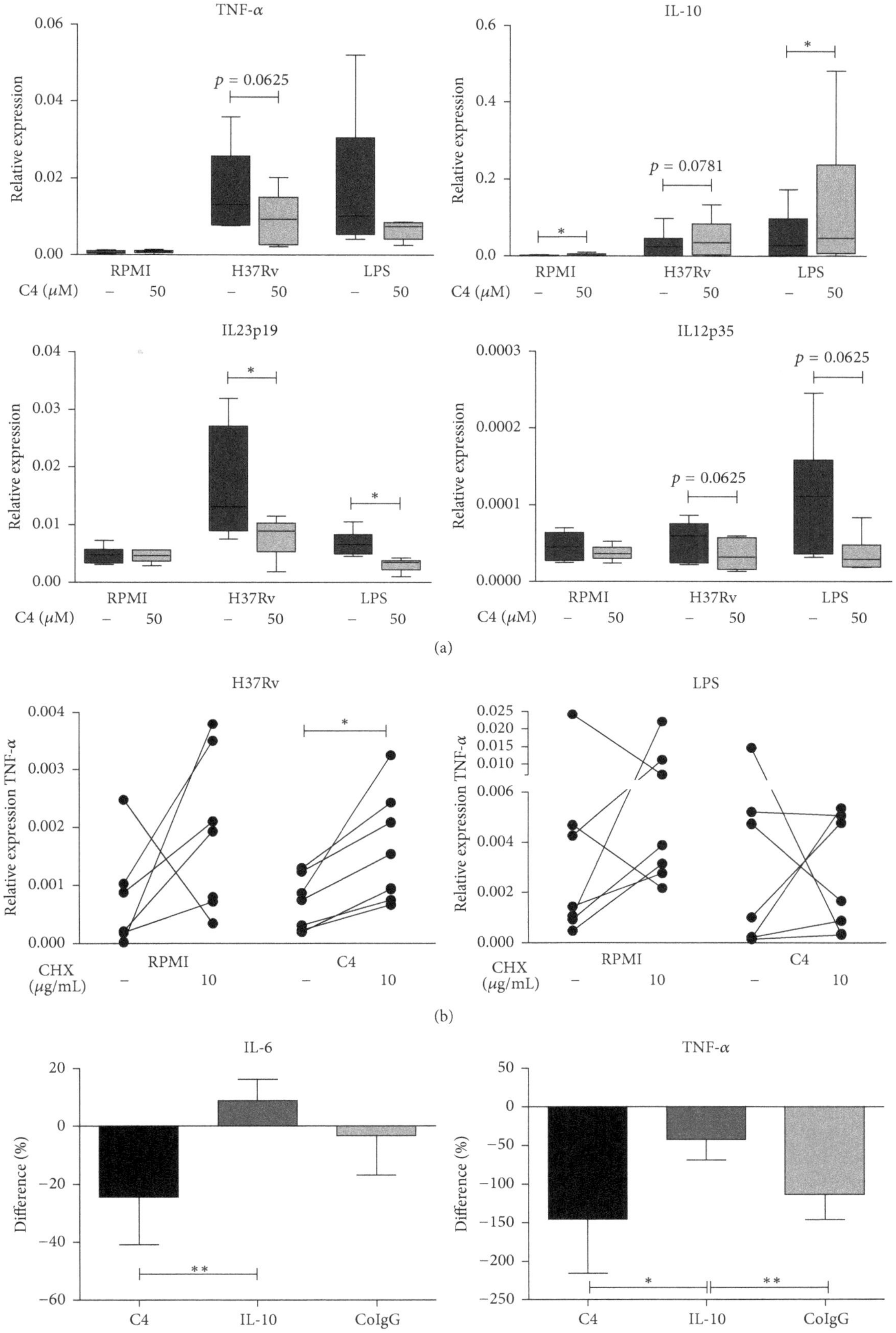

FIGURE 5: Continued.

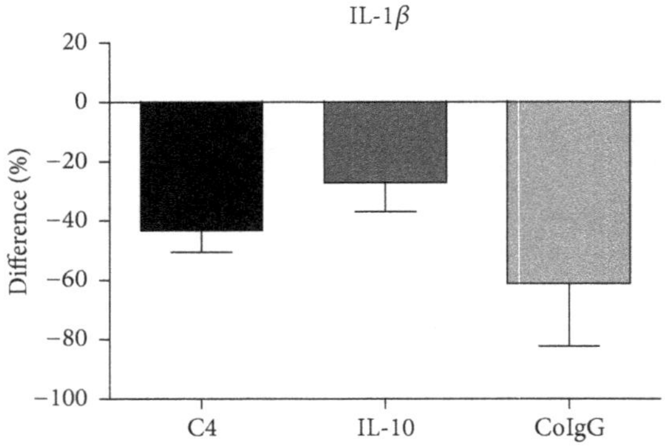

(c)

FIGURE 5: Butyrate transcriptionally influences cytokine responses to Mtb, possibly mediated through IL-10. (a) Cytokine gene expression levels in PBMCs preincubated with 50 μM C4 for 1 h prior to stimulation with Mtb lysate or LPS for 4 h, as measured by qPCR. The box plot represents median with first and third quartiles; the whiskers represent minimum and maximum values. $n = 6$ to 10, using Wilcoxon signed-rank test, representative of 2+ independent experiments. $^*p < 0.05$. (b) To block translation, PBMCs were preincubated with cycloheximide (CHX) for 1 h prior to 1 h incubation with C4 (50 μM). TNF-α transcript levels were measured by qPCR 4 h after stimulation with Mtb lysate or LPS. Data are single values ($n = 6$ to 7), using Wilcoxon signed-rank test, representative of 3 independent experiments. $^*p < 0.05$. (c) To block IL-10 activity, PBMCs were preincubated with IL-10 and C4 (50 μM) for 1 h. IL-6, TNF-α, and IL-1β production was measured by ELISA after 24 h of stimulation with Mtb lysate. Data are means ± SEM ($n = 10$ to 12), using Wilcoxon signed-rank test, representative of 4 independent experiments.

affect expression of COX-2, a key enzyme in the eicosanoid pathway, in contrast to previous reports that used supraphysiological C4 concentrations [30, 56]. In addition, inhibition of the eicosanoid pathway using aspirin did not counteract the effects of C4. Therefore, the eicosanoid pathway is unlikely to be involved in mediating the effects of C4.

The effect of diabetes on the host immune response to Mtb might also be explained by altered cellular metabolism, with a possible role for SCFA. Cellular metabolism is increasingly linked to immunology [78–80]. One previous study noted that C4 influences metabolic processes in colonocytes [58], which use butyrate as their primary energy source [58]. However, we did not observe any effect of C4 on lactate production, the redox status, TCA cycle gene expression, or β-oxidation in PBMCs. We therefore conclude that cellular metabolism does not mediate the effect of C4 on Mtb-induced cytokine production.

Finally, we further examined the effect of C4 on the anti-inflammatory cytokine IL-10. IL-10 is detrimental to TB outcome, while it may improve DM symptoms [68–77]. In line with previous studies [33, 81, 82], we report an upregulation in IL-10 production induced by C4. Removal of all intermediary protein, including IL-10, from PBMCs stimulated with H37Rv and C4 led to a significant increase in TNF-α transcript, thereby counteracting the decrease in TNF-α production induced by C4. Moreover, blocking IL-10 specifically fully restored IL-6 responses in PBMCs stimulated with H37Rv and C4 and partly restored TNF-α and IL-1β responses. These data suggest that the anti-inflammatory cytokine IL-10 may play a role in the inhibitory effects of C4 on Mtb-induced inflammatory responses.

Currently, much research focuses on modulation of the gut microbiota in order to treat obesity and type 2 DM [83–86]. Administration of sodium butyrate or butyrate-inducing probiotics in mice significantly increased plasma insulin levels and insulin sensitivity and suppressed body weight gain [87–89]. The anti-inflammatory effects of C4 may attenuate the chronic inflammatory state associated with type 2 DM, thereby improving DM symptoms. If chronic inflammation is a causal factor of the impaired host response to Mtb in type 2 DM patients, attenuation of this hyperinflammatory state may improve not only DM but also TB outcome in patients with coincident DM and TB disease.

Some limitations of our study need to be addressed. Firstly, we studied the effects of C4 on Mtb-induced inflammation in PBMCs *in vitro*. SCFA levels have been shown to be altered in DM patients [18–22], but this *in vitro* model does not include other aspects of the pathophysiology of DM such as hyperglycemia, hyperinsulinemia, or dyslipidemia, phenomena which have also been reported to affect immunity [90–94]. Furthermore, DM medications possibly interfere with the intestinal microbiota and immune responses in patients [95–97]. It is therefore unclear how accurately our *in vitro* model reflects the *in vivo* situation in DM patients.

In conclusion, we show an anti-inflammatory effect of low, physiological doses of C4 on Mtb-induced inflammatory responses. The anti-inflammatory cytokine IL-10 may play a role in mediating the inhibitory effects of C4 on the host immune response to Mtb. Further studies are needed to precisely explore the pathways by which physiological concentrations of C4 exert their anti-inflammatory effects and to define the mechanism of increased TB sensitivity in type 2 DM patients. Moreover, current research on modulating gut microbiota in DM should include its possible effects on TB.

Conflict of Interests

The authors declare that there is no conflict of interests regarding the publication of this paper.

Acknowledgment

This study was supported by the TANDEM (Tuberculosis and Diabetes Mellitus) Grant of the ECFP7 (European Union's Seventh Framework Programme) under Grant Agreement no. 305279.

References

[1] WHO, *Global Tuberculosis Report 2014*, World Health Organization, Geneva, Switzerland, 2014, http://apps.who.int/iris/bitstream/10665/137094/1/9789241564809_eng.pdf?ua=1.

[2] IDF, *IDF Diabetes Atlas Update Poster*, IDF, 6th edition, 2014, http://www.idf.org/sites/default/files/EN_6E_Atlas_Full_0.pdf.

[3] C. Y. Jeon and M. B. Murray, "Diabetes mellitus increases the risk of active tuberculosis: a systematic review of 13 observational studies," *PLoS Medicine*, vol. 5, no. 7, article e152, 2008.

[4] R. Ruslami, R. E. Aarnoutse, B. Alisjahbana, A. J. A. M. Van Der Ven, and R. Van Crevel, "Implications of the global increase of diabetes for tuberculosis control and patient care," *Tropical Medicine and International Health*, vol. 15, no. 11, pp. 1289–1299, 2010.

[5] B. Dixon, "Diabetes and tuberculosis: an unhealthy partnership," *The Lancet Infectious Diseases*, vol. 7, no. 7, p. 444, 2007.

[6] B. I. Restrepo and L. S. Schlesinger, "Impact of diabetes on the natural history of tuberculosis," *Diabetes Research and Clinical Practice*, vol. 106, no. 2, pp. 191–199, 2014.

[7] C. R. Stevenson, N. G. Forouhi, G. Roglic et al., "Diabetes and tuberculosis: the impact of the diabetes epidemic on tuberculosis incidence," *BMC Public Health*, vol. 7, article 234, 2007.

[8] M. A. Baker, H.-H. Lin, H.-Y. Chang, and M. B. Murray, "The risk of tuberculosis disease among persons with diabetes mellitus: a prospective cohort study," *Clinical Infectious Diseases*, vol. 54, no. 6, pp. 818–825, 2012.

[9] C. Y. Jeon, M. B. Murray, and M. A. Baker, "Managing tuberculosis in patients with diabetes mellitus: why we care and what we know," *Expert Review of Anti-Infective Therapy*, vol. 10, no. 8, pp. 863–868, 2012.

[10] M. E. Jimenez-Corona, L. P. Cruz-Hervert, L. García-García et al., "Association of diabetes and tuberculosis: impact on treatment and post-treatment outcomes," *Thorax*, vol. 68, no. 3, pp. 214–220, 2013.

[11] B. Alisjahbana, E. Sahiratmadja, E. J. Nelwan et al., "The effect of type 2 diabetes mellitus on the presentation and treatment response of pulmonary tuberculosis," *Clinical Infectious Diseases*, vol. 45, no. 4, pp. 428–435, 2007.

[12] A. L. Riza, F. Pearson, C. Ugarte-Gil et al., "Clinical management of concurrent diabetes and tuberculosis and the implications for patient services," *The Lancet Diabetes and Endocrinology*, vol. 2, no. 9, pp. 740–753, 2014.

[13] K. Ronacher, S. A. Joosten, R. van Crevel, H. M. Dockrell, G. Walzl, and T. H. M. Ottenhoff, "Acquired immunodeficiencies and tuberculosis: focus on HIV/AIDS and diabetes mellitus," *Immunological Reviews*, vol. 264, no. 1, pp. 121–137, 2015.

[14] N. P. Kumar, V. V. Banurekha, D. Nair et al., "Coincident pre-diabetes is associated with dysregulated cytokine responses in pulmonary tuberculosis," *PLoS ONE*, vol. 9, no. 11, Article ID e112108, 2014.

[15] N. P. Kumar, P. J. George, P. Kumaran, C. K. Dolla, T. B. Nutman, and S. Babu, "Diminished systemic and antigen-specific type 1, type 17, and other proinflammatory cytokines in diabetic and prediabetic individuals with latent mycobacterium tuberculosis infection," *The Journal of Infectious Diseases*, vol. 210, no. 10, pp. 1670–1678, 2014.

[16] N. P. Kumar, R. Sridhar, V. V. Banurekha, M. S. Jawahar, T. B. Nutman, and S. Babu, "Expansion of pathogen-specific T-helper 1 and T-helper 17 cells in pulmonary tuberculosis with coincident type 2 diabetes mellitus," *Journal of Infectious Diseases*, vol. 208, no. 5, pp. 739–748, 2013.

[17] B. I. Restrepo, S. P. Fisher-Hoch, P. A. Pino et al., "Tuberculosis in poorly controlled type 2 diabetes: altered cytokine expression in peripheral white blood cells," *Clinical Infectious Diseases*, vol. 47, no. 5, pp. 634–641, 2008.

[18] J.-P. Furet, L.-C. Kong, J. Tap et al., "Differential adaptation of human gut microbiota to bariatric surgery-induced weight loss: links with metabolic and low-grade inflammation markers," *Diabetes*, vol. 59, no. 12, pp. 3049–3057, 2010.

[19] F. H. Karlsson, V. Tremaroli, I. Nookaew et al., "Gut metagenome in European women with normal, impaired and diabetic glucose control," *Nature*, vol. 498, no. 7452, pp. 99–103, 2013.

[20] N. Larsen, F. K. Vogensen, F. W. J. van den Berg et al., "Gut microbiota in human adults with type 2 diabetes differs from non-diabetic adults," *PLoS ONE*, vol. 5, no. 2, Article ID e9085, 2010.

[21] J. Qin, J. Wang, Y. Li et al., "A metagenome-wide association study of gut microbiota in type 2 diabetes," *Nature*, vol. 490, no. 7418, pp. 55–60, 2012.

[22] K. M. Maslowski, A. T. Vieira, A. Ng et al., "Regulation of inflammatory responses by gut microbiota and chemoattractant receptor GPR43," *Nature*, vol. 461, no. 7268, pp. 1282–1286, 2009.

[23] M. Remely, E. Aumueller, C. Merold et al., "Effects of short chain fatty acid producing bacteria on epigenetic regulation of FFAR3 in type 2 diabetes and obesity," *Gene*, vol. 537, no. 1, pp. 85–92, 2014.

[24] X. Zhang, D. Shen, Z. Fang et al., "Human gut microbiota changes reveal the progression of glucose intolerance," *PLoS ONE*, vol. 8, no. 8, Article ID e71108, 2013.

[25] U. Böcker, T. Nebe, F. Herweck et al., "Butyrate modulates intestinal epithelial cell-mediated neutrophil migration," *Clinical and Experimental Immunology*, vol. 131, no. 1, pp. 53–60, 2003.

[26] M. A. Cox, J. Jackson, M. Stanton et al., "Short-chain fatty acids act as antiinflammatory mediators by regulating prostaglandin E_2 and cytokines," *World Journal of Gastroenterology*, vol. 15, no. 44, pp. 5549–5557, 2009.

[27] L. Klampfer, J. Huang, T. Sasazuki, S. Shirasawa, and L. Augenlicht, "Inhibition of interferon gamma signaling by the short chain fatty acid butyrate," *Molecular Cancer Research*, vol. 1, no. 11, pp. 855–862, 2003.

[28] M.-C. Maa, M. Y. Chang, M.-Y. Hsieh et al., "Butyrate reduced lipopolysaccharide-mediated macrophage migration by suppression of Src enhancement and focal adhesion kinase activity," *Journal of Nutritional Biochemistry*, vol. 21, no. 12, pp. 1186–1192, 2010.

[29] K. Meijer, P. de Vos, and M. G. Priebe, "Butyrate and other short-chain fatty acids as modulators of immunity: what relevance for health?" *Current Opinion in Clinical Nutrition and Metabolic Care*, vol. 13, no. 6, pp. 715–721, 2010.

[30] J. J. Kovarik, M. A. Hölzl, J. Hofer et al., "Eicosanoid modulation by the short-chain fatty acid n-butyrate in human monocytes," *Immunology*, vol. 139, no. 3, pp. 395–405, 2013.

[31] S. Tedelind, F. Westberg, M. Kjerrulf, and A. Vidal, "Anti-inflammatory properties of the short-chain fatty acids acetate and propionate: a study with relevance to inflammatory bowel disease," *World Journal of Gastroenterology*, vol. 13, no. 20, pp. 2826–2832, 2007.

[32] M. A. R. Vinolo, H. G. Rodrigues, R. T. Nachbar, and R. Curi, "Regulation of inflammation by short chain fatty acids," *Nutrients*, vol. 3, no. 10, pp. 858–876, 2011.

[33] E. Bailón, M. Cueto-Sola, P. Utrilla et al., "Butyrate in vitro immune-modulatory effects might be mediated through a proliferation-related induction of apoptosis," *Immunobiology*, vol. 215, no. 11, pp. 863–873, 2010.

[34] T. Kurita-Ochiai, K. Ochiai, and K. Fukushima, "Butyric acid-induced T-cell apoptosis is mediated by caspase-8 and -9 activation in a Fas-independent manner," *Clinical and Diagnostic Laboratory Immunology*, vol. 8, no. 2, pp. 325–332, 2001.

[35] M. Aoyama, J. Kotani, and M. Usami, "Butyrate and propionate induced activated or non-activated neutrophil apoptosis via HDAC inhibitor activity but without activating GPR-41/GPR-43 pathways," *Nutrition*, vol. 26, no. 6, pp. 653–661, 2010.

[36] P. V. Chang, L. Hao, S. Offermanns, and R. Medzhitov, "The microbial metabolite butyrate regulates intestinal macrophage function via histone deacetylase inhibition," *Proceedings of the National Academy of Sciences of the United States of America*, vol. 111, no. 6, pp. 2247–2252, 2014.

[37] J.-S. Park, E.-J. Lee, J.-C. Lee, W.-K. Kim, and H.-S. Kim, "Anti-inflammatory effects of short chain fatty acids in IFN-gamma-stimulated RAW 264.7 murine macrophage cells: involvement of NF-kappaB and ERK signaling pathways," *International Immunopharmacology*, vol. 7, no. 1, pp. 70–77, 2007.

[38] S. M. Behar, C. J. Martin, M. G. Booty et al., "Apoptosis is an innate defense function of macrophages against *Mycobacterium tuberculosis*," *Mucosal Immunology*, vol. 4, no. 3, pp. 279–287, 2011.

[39] J. H. Cummings, E. W. Pomare, H. W. J. Branch, C. P. E. Naylor, and G. T. MacFarlane, "Short chain fatty acids in human large intestine, portal, hepatic and venous blood," *Gut*, vol. 28, no. 10, pp. 1221–1227, 1987.

[40] C.-T. Zhu and D. M. Rand, "A hydrazine coupled cycling assay validates the decrease in redox ratio under starvation in *Drosophila*," *PLoS ONE*, vol. 7, no. 10, Article ID e47584, 2012.

[41] E. P. M. Candido, R. Reeves, and J. R. Davie, "Sodium butyrate inhibits histone deacetylation in cultured cells," *Cell*, vol. 14, no. 1, pp. 105–113, 1978.

[42] J. R. Davie, "Inhibition of histone deacetylase activity by butyrate," *Journal of Nutrition*, vol. 133, no. 7, supplement, pp. 2485S–2493S, 2003.

[43] M. C. P. Cleophas, T. O. Crisan, H. Lemmers et al., "Suppression of monosodium urate crystal-induced cytokine production by butyrate is mediated by the inhibition of class I histone deacetylases," *Annals of the Rheumatic Diseases*, 2015.

[44] M. Kilgore, C. A. Miller, D. M. Fass et al., "Inhibitors of class 1 histone deacetylases reverse contextual memory deficits in a mouse model of Alzheimer's disease," *Neuropsychopharmacology*, vol. 35, no. 4, pp. 870–880, 2010.

[45] J. Kleinnijenhuis, M. Oosting, L. A. B. Joosten, M. G. Netea, and R. Van Crevel, "Innate immune recognition of *Mycobacterium tuberculosis*," *Clinical and Developmental Immunology*, vol. 2011, Article ID 405310, 12 pages, 2011.

[46] T. K. Means, S. Wang, E. Lien, A. Yoshimura, D. T. Golenbock, and M. J. Fenton, "Human Toll-like receptors mediate cellular activation by *Mycobacterium tuberculosis*," *Journal of Immunology*, vol. 163, no. 7, pp. 3920–3927, 1999.

[47] Y. Bulut, K. S. Michelsen, L. Hayrapetian et al., "*Mycobacterium tuberculosis* heat shock proteins use diverse Toll-like receptor pathways to activate pro-inflammatory signals," *The Journal of Biological Chemistry*, vol. 280, no. 22, pp. 20961–20967, 2005.

[48] L. A. J. O'Neill, D. Golenbock, and A. G. Bowie, "The history of Toll-like receptors—redefining innate immunity," *Nature Reviews Immunology*, vol. 13, no. 6, pp. 453–460, 2013.

[49] M. Y. Peroval, A. C. Boyd, J. R. Young, and A. L. Smith, "A critical role for MAPK signalling pathways in the transcriptional regulation of toll like receptors," *PLoS ONE*, vol. 8, no. 2, Article ID e51243, 2013.

[50] S.-M. Gao, C.-Q. Chen, L.-Y. Wang et al., "Histone deacetylases inhibitor sodium butyrate inhibits JAK2/STAT signaling through upregulation of SOCS1 and SOCS3 mediated by HDAC8 inhibition in myeloproliferative neoplasms," *Experimental Hematology*, vol. 41, no. 3, pp. 261.e4–270.e4, 2013.

[51] S. M. Behar, M. Divangahi, and H. G. Remold, "Evasion of innate immunity by *Mycobacterium tuberculosis*: is death an exit strategy?" *Nature Reviews Microbiology*, vol. 8, no. 9, pp. 668–674, 2010.

[52] M. Chen, M. Divangahi, H. Gan et al., "Lipid mediators in innate immunity against tuberculosis: opposing roles of PGE_2 and LXA_4 in the induction of macrophage death," *Journal of Experimental Medicine*, vol. 205, no. 12, pp. 2791–2801, 2008.

[53] M. Divangahi, M. Chen, H. Gan et al., "Mycobacterium tuberculosis evades macrophage defenses by inhibiting plasma membrane repair," *Nature Immunology*, vol. 10, no. 8, pp. 899–906, 2009.

[54] J. R. Moreno, I. E. García, M. D. L. L. G. Hernández, D. A. Leon, R. Marquez, and R. H. Pando, "The role of prostaglandin E_2 in the immunopathogenesis of experimental pulmonary tuberculosis," *Immunology*, vol. 106, no. 2, pp. 257–266, 2002.

[55] F. G. M. Snijdewint, P. Kaliński, E. A. Wierenga, J. D. Bos, and M. L. Kapsenberg, "Prostaglandin E2 differentially modulates cytokine secretion profiles of human T helper lymphocytes," *The Journal of Immunology*, vol. 150, no. 12, pp. 5321–5329, 1993.

[56] X. Tong, L. Yin, and C. Giardina, "Butyrate suppresses Cox-2 activation in colon cancer cells through HDAC inhibition," *Biochemical and Biophysical Research Communications*, vol. 317, no. 2, pp. 463–471, 2004.

[57] M. Usami, K. Kishimoto, A. Ohata et al., "Butyrate and trichostatin A attenuate nuclear factor kappaB activation and tumor necrosis factor alpha secretion and increase prostaglandin E2 secretion in human peripheral blood mononuclear cells," *Nutrition Research*, vol. 28, no. 5, pp. 321–328, 2008.

[58] D. R. Donohoe, N. Garge, X. Zhang et al., "The microbiome and butyrate regulate energy metabolism and autophagy in the mammalian colon," *Cell Metabolism*, vol. 13, no. 5, pp. 517–526, 2011.

[59] R. K. Dutta, M. Kathania, M. Raje, and S. Majumdar, "IL-6 inhibits IFN-gamma induced autophagy in *Mycobacterium tuberculosis* H37Rv infected macrophages," *International Journal of Biochemistry and Cell Biology*, vol. 44, no. 6, pp. 942–954, 2012.

[60] C. H. Ladel, C. Blum, A. Dreher, K. Reifenberg, M. Kopf, and S. H. E. Kaufmann, "Lethal tuberculosis in interleukin-6-deficient mutant mice," *Infection and Immunity*, vol. 65, no. 11, pp. 4843–4849, 1997.

[61] A. N. Martinez, S. Mehra, and D. Kaushal, "Role of interleukin 6 in innate immunity to *Mycobacterium tuberculosis* infection,"

The Journal of Infectious Diseases, vol. 207, no. 8, pp. 1253–1261, 2013.

[62] V. Nagabhushanam, A. Solache, L.-M. Ting, C. J. Escaron, J. Y. Zhang, and J. D. Ernst, "Innate inhibition of adaptive immunity: *Mycobacterium tuberculosis*-induced IL-6 inhibits macrophage responses to IFN-gamma," *Journal of Immunology*, vol. 171, no. 9, pp. 4750–4757, 2003.

[63] R. Gopal, L. Monin, S. Slight et al., "Unexpected role for IL-17 in protective immunity against hypervirulent *Mycobacterium tuberculosis* HN878 infection," *PLoS Pathogens*, vol. 10, no. 5, Article ID e1004099, 2014.

[64] S. A. Khader, G. K. Bell, J. E. Pearl et al., "IL-23 and IL-17 in the establishment of protective pulmonary CD4+ T cell responses after vaccination and during *Mycobacterium tuberculosis* challenge," *Nature Immunology*, vol. 8, no. 4, pp. 369–377, 2007.

[65] N. Afzal, S. Zaman, F. Shahzad, K. Javaid, A. Zafar, and A. H. Nagi, "Immune mechanisms in type-2 diabetic retinopathy," *Journal of Pakistan Medical Association*, vol. 65, no. 2, pp. 159–163, 2015.

[66] N. Afzal, K. Javaid, W. Sami et al., "Inverse relationship of serum IL-17 with type-II diabetes retinopathy," *Clinical Laboratory*, vol. 59, no. 11-12, pp. 1311–1317, 2013.

[67] N. Afzal, S. Zaman, A. Asghar et al., "Negative association of serum IL-6 and IL-17 with type-II diabetes retinopathy," *Iranian Journal of Immunology*, vol. 11, no. 1, pp. 40–48, 2014.

[68] J. C. Cyktor, B. Carruthers, R. A. Kominsky, G. L. Beamer, P. Stromberg, and J. Turner, "IL-10 inhibits mature fibrotic granuloma formation during *Mycobacterium tuberculosis* infection," *The Journal of Immunology*, vol. 190, no. 6, pp. 2778–2790, 2013.

[69] N. P. Kumar, V. Gopinath, R. Sridhar et al., "IL-10 dependent suppression of type 1, type 2 and type 17 cytokines in active pulmonary tuberculosis," *PLoS ONE*, vol. 8, no. 3, Article ID e59572, 2013.

[70] B. Liang, Y. Guo, Y. Li, and H. Kong, "Association between IL-10 gene polymorphisms and susceptibility of tuberculosis: evidence based on a meta-analysis," *PLoS ONE*, vol. 9, no. 2, Article ID e88448, 2014.

[71] F. W. McNab, J. Ewbank, A. Howes et al., "Type I IFN induces IL-10 production in an IL-27-independent manner and blocks responsiveness to IFN-γ for production of IL-12 and bacterial killing in *Mycobacterium tuberculosis*-infected macrophages," *Journal of Immunology*, vol. 193, no. 7, pp. 3600–3612, 2014.

[72] P. S. Redford, A. Boonstra, S. Read et al., "Enhanced protection to *Mycobacterium tuberculosis* infection in IL-10-deficient mice is accompanied by early and enhanced Th1 responses in the lung," *European Journal of Immunology*, vol. 40, no. 8, pp. 2200–2210, 2010.

[73] P. S. Redford, P. J. Murray, and A. O'Garra, "The role of IL-10 in immune regulation during M. tuberculosis infection," *Mucosal Immunology*, vol. 4, no. 3, pp. 261–270, 2011.

[74] P. Shrivastava and T. Bagchi, "IL-10 modulates in vitro multinucleate giant cell formation in human tuberculosis," *PLoS ONE*, vol. 8, no. 10, Article ID e77680, 2013.

[75] E.-G. Hong, J. K. Hwi, Y.-R. Cho et al., "Interleukin-10 prevents diet-induced insulin resistance by attenuating macrophage and cytokine response in skeletal muscle," *Diabetes*, vol. 58, no. 11, pp. 2525–2535, 2009.

[76] M. Straczkowski, I. Kowalska, A. Nikolajuk, A. Krukowska, and M. Gorska, "Plasma interleukin-10 concentration is positively related to insulin sensitivity in young healthy individuals," *Diabetes Care*, vol. 28, no. 8, pp. 2036–2037, 2005.

[77] E. van Exel, J. Gussekloo, A. J. M. De Craen, M. Frölich, A. B.-V. D. Wiel, and R. G. J. Westendorp, "Low production capacity of interleukin-10 associates with the metabolic syndrome and type 2 diabetes: the Leiden 85-plus study," *Diabetes*, vol. 51, no. 4, pp. 1088–1092, 2002.

[78] K. Ganeshan and A. Chawla, "Metabolic regulation of immune responses," *Annual Review of Immunology*, vol. 32, pp. 609–634, 2014.

[79] D. J. Kominsky, E. L. Campbell, and S. P. Colgan, "Metabolic shifts in immunity and inflammation," *The Journal of Immunology*, vol. 184, no. 8, pp. 4062–4068, 2010.

[80] E. Pearce and E. Pearce, "Metabolic pathways in immune cell activation and quiescence," *Immunity*, vol. 38, no. 4, pp. 633–643, 2013.

[81] M. D. Säemann, G. A. Böhmig, C. H. Osterreicher et al., "Anti-inflammatory effects of sodium butyrate on human monocytes: potent inhibition of IL-12 and up-regulation of IL-10 production," *The FASEB Journal*, vol. 14, no. 15, pp. 2380–2382, 2000.

[82] T. E. Weber and B. J. Kerr, "Butyrate differentially regulates cytokines and proliferation in porcine peripheral blood mononuclear cells," *Veterinary Immunology and Immunopathology*, vol. 113, no. 1-2, pp. 139–147, 2006.

[83] R. Burcelin, M. Serino, C. Chabo, V. Blasco-Baque, and J. Amar, "Gut microbiota and diabetes: from pathogenesis to therapeutic perspective," *Acta Diabetologica*, vol. 48, no. 4, pp. 257–273, 2011.

[84] A. M. Caricilli and M. J. A. Saad, "The role of gut microbiota on insulin resistance," *Nutrients*, vol. 5, no. 3, pp. 829–851, 2013.

[85] B. M. Carvalho and M. J. A. Saad, "Influence of gut microbiota on subclinical inflammation and insulin resistance," *Mediators of Inflammation*, vol. 2013, Article ID 986734, 13 pages, 2013.

[86] A. Puddu, R. Sanguineti, F. Montecucco, and G. L. Viviani, "Evidence for the gut microbiota short-chain fatty acids as key pathophysiological molecules improving diabetes," *Mediators of Inflammation*, vol. 2014, Article ID 162021, 9 pages, 2014.

[87] Z. Gao, J. Yin, J. Zhang et al., "Butyrate improves insulin sensitivity and increases energy expenditure in mice," *Diabetes*, vol. 58, no. 7, pp. 1509–1517, 2009.

[88] H. V. Lin, A. Frassetto, E. J. Kowalik Jr. et al., "Butyrate and propionate protect against diet-induced obesity and regulate gut hormones via free fatty acid receptor 3-independent mechanisms," *PLoS ONE*, vol. 7, no. 4, Article ID e35240, 2012.

[89] H. Yadav, J.-H. Lee, J. Lloyd, P. Walter, and S. G. Rane, "Beneficial metabolic effects of a probiotic via butyrate-induced GLP-1 hormone secretion," *The Journal of Biological Chemistry*, vol. 288, no. 35, pp. 25088–25097, 2013.

[90] S. Devaraj, S. K. Venugopal, U. Singh, and I. Jialal, "Hyperglycemia induces monocytic release of interleukin-6 via induction of protein kinase C-α and -β," *Diabetes*, vol. 54, no. 1, pp. 85–91, 2005.

[91] C. Sun, L. Sun, H. Ma et al., "The phenotype and functional alterations of macrophages in mice with hyperglycemia for long term," *Journal of Cellular Physiology*, vol. 227, no. 4, pp. 1670–1679, 2012.

[92] D. I. Gomez, M. Twahirwa, L. S. Schlesinger, and B. I. Restrepo, "Reduced *Mycobacterium tuberculosis* association with monocytes from diabetes patients that have poor glucose control," *Tuberculosis*, vol. 93, no. 2, pp. 192–197, 2013.

[93] J. M. Han, S. J. Patterson, M. Speck, J. A. Ehses, and M. K. Levings, "Insulin inhibits IL-10-mediated regulatory T cell function: implications for obesity," *The Journal of Immunology*, vol. 192, no. 2, pp. 623–629, 2014.

[94] A. T. Shamshiev, F. Ampenberger, B. Ernst, L. Rohrer, B. J. Marsland, and M. Kopf, "Dyslipidemia inhibits Toll-like receptor-induced activation of CD8alpha-negative dendritic cells and protective Thl type immunity," *The Journal of Experimental Medicine*, vol. 204, no. 2, pp. 441–452, 2007.

[95] K. A. Pyra, D. C. Saha, and R. A. Reimer, "Prebiotic fiber increases hepatic acetyl CoA carboxylase phosphorylation and suppresses glucose-dependent insulinotropic polypeptide secretion more effectively when used with metformin in obese rats," *Journal of Nutrition*, vol. 142, no. 2, pp. 213–220, 2012.

[96] N.-R. Shin, J.-C. Lee, H.-Y. Lee et al., "An increase in the *Akkermansia* spp. population induced by metformin treatment improves glucose homeostasis in diet-induced obese mice," *Gut*, vol. 63, no. 5, pp. 727–735, 2014.

[97] H. A. Hirsch, D. Iliopoulos, and K. Struhl, "Metformin inhibits the inflammatory response associated with cellular transformation and cancer stem cell growth," *Proceedings of the National Academy of Sciences of the United States of America*, vol. 110, no. 3, pp. 972–977, 2013.

9

Hypoxia Alters the Expression of Dipeptidyl Peptidase 4 and Induces Developmental Remodeling of Human Preadipocytes

Helena H. Chowdhury,[1,2] **Jelena Velebit,**[1,2] **Nataša Radić,**[1,2] **Vito Frančič,**[2] **Marko Kreft,**[1,2,3] **and Robert Zorec**[1,2]

[1]*Laboratory for Neuroendocrinology-Molecular Cell Physiology, Institute of Pathophysiology, Faculty of Medicine, University of Ljubljana, Zaloska 4, SI-1000 Ljubljana, Slovenia*
[2]*Celica Biomedical Center, Tehnološki Park 24, SI-1000 Ljubljana, Slovenia*
[3]*Department of Biology, Biotechnical Faculty, University of Ljubljana, Večna Pot 111, SI-1000 Ljubljana, Slovenia*

Correspondence should be addressed to Robert Zorec; robert.zorec@mf.uni-lj.si

Academic Editor: Lei Xi

Dipeptidyl peptidase 4 (DPP4), a transmembrane protein, has been identified in human adipose tissue and is considered to be associated with obesity-related type 2 diabetes. Since adipose tissue is relatively hypoxic in obese participants, we investigated the expression of DPP4 in human preadipocytes (hPA) and adipocytes in hypoxia, during differentiation and upon insulin stimulation. The results show that DPP4 is abundantly expressed in hPA but very sparsely in adipocytes. During differentiation *in vitro*, the expression of DPP4 in hPA is reduced on the addition of differentiation medium, indicating that this protein can be hPA marker. Long term hypoxia altered the expression of DPP4 in hPA. In *in vitro* hypoxic conditions the protease activity of shed DPP4 is reduced; however, in the presence of insulin, the increase in DPP4 expression is potentiated by hypoxia.

1. Introduction

Dipeptidyl peptidase 4 (DPP4) is a 110 kDa transmembrane glycoprotein. A soluble form of DPP4 (sDPP4) in the circulation is the result of proteolytic cleavage of the membrane bound form [1]. DPP4 has a rare protease activity, cleaving N-terminal x-Pro dipeptide from selected proteins. Besides enzymatic inactivation of incretins, DPP4 also mediates degradation of several growth factors, neuropeptides, chemokines, and vasoactive peptides, which results in alterations in their biological activity, often by altering their receptor specificity [2].

Altered DPP4 activity has been reported in a number of diseases, including type 2 diabetes [3, 4] and tumor biology [2, 5–7]. It is thought to be associated with sensitivity to anticancer agents in haematologic malignancies and is involved in the development of various chronic liver diseases [8]. DPP4 was considered as a therapeutic target for type 2 diabetes as it degrades incretins: glucagon-like peptide- (GLP-) 1 and gastric inhibitory peptide (GIP). Both hormones cause an increase in insulin secretion. DPP4 inhibitors target the enzyme activity of DPP4, thus prolonging the insulinotropic effects of incretins [9].

In patients with type 2 diabetes acute hypoxia increases the glucose uptake into the tissue [10, 11]; however, prolonged exposure to hypoxia has been associated with induction of insulin resistance in adipose tissue [12, 13]. More specifically, adipose tissue hypoxia, which develops with the onset of obesity [14, 15], has been linked to the development of insulin resistance and type 2 diabetes by decreasing insulin signaling pathways [13]. It was reported that DPP4 is expressed in preadipocytes and in adipocytes [16], indicating that adipose tissue might be a major source of circulating DPP4. Therefore, an altered expression of adipose tissue DPP4 could be linked to the development of type 2 diabetes; however the factors that alter the expression of DPP4 are poorly understood.

In the present study we developed a confocal microscopy assay to study the expression of DPP4 in human preadipocytes (hPA). We evaluated DPP4 expression during the differentiation of human preadipocytes into adipocytes and studied how insulin affects the expression and activity of released DPP4. The results show that in hypoxic conditions the protease activity of shed DPP4 is reduced. Interestingly, insulin increases DPP4 expression and this is potentiated by hypoxia.

2. Experimental Procedures

2.1. Chemicals. Dulbecco's modified Eagle's medium/Ham's F12 (DMEM/F12), l-glutamine, dexamethasone, isobutylmethylxanthine (IBMX), biotin, d-pantothenic acid hemicalcium salt, phosphate-buffered saline (PBS), bovine serum albumin (BSA), trypsin-EDTA, Trypan Blue, and goat serum were purchased from Sigma (St. Louis, MO). Insulin was purchased from Novo Nordisk (Bagsvaerd, Denmark). Fetal bovine serum (FBS) was obtained from Biochrom (Berlin, Germany). Rosiglitazone maleate was obtained from GlaxoSmithKline (Worthing, UK). Dimethyl sulfoxide (DMSO) was purchased from Merck Schuchardt (Hohenbrunn, Germany). Antibiotic-antimycotic mixture was purchased from Gibco (Invitrogen Corporation, NY). Paraformaldehyde was purchased from Thermo Scientific, USA.

2.2. Primary Preadipocyte Maintenance and Differentiation Procedure. Preadipocytes (human subcutaneous) were purchased from ZenBio, Inc. (Research Triangle Park, NC). Cells were cultured under standard conditions (at 37°C, humidified atmosphere, 5% CO_2) in PM medium. For each set of experiments, cells were seeded on coverslips in uniform density, which was provided by counting cells before seeding. For differentiation into adipocytes we used the protocol from ZenBio. The start of the differentiating procedure was marked as day 0. On indicated days the 16 h conditioned 1% BSA/PBS medium was collected, filtered (0.2 μm), and analyzed for enzymatic activity and quantification of sDPP4. On day 21 60–70% of cells were fully differentiated, indicated by the accumulation of lipid droplets (not shown). The cells were than subjected to immunolabeling protocol or trypsinized and counted using a hemocytometer (improved Neubauer type). Three separate samples were prepared for each time point.

2.3. Hypoxia Treatment In Vitro. For the study of DPP4 expression under hypoxic conditions, preadipocytes were cultured in a hypoxic chamber (Billups-Rothenberg, Dell Mar, CA), flushed twice at a 2 h interval for 4 min with a gas mixture consisting of 1% O_2, 5% CO_2, and 94% N_2, and incubated for the indicated time at 37°C in a humidified atmosphere.

2.4. Immunocytochemistry. To identify the expression of HIF-1α and DPP4 in the preadipocytes, primary monoclonal mouse anti-HIF-1α antibodies and primary monoclonal mouse anti-DPP4 antibodies (both Abcam, Cambridge, UK; ab8366 and ab3154) were used and secondary goat anti-mouse antibody conjugated to Alexa Fluor 546 and to Alexa Fluor 488, respectively (A11003 and A11001, Molecular Probes). Cells were washed with PBS and fixed in 2% paraformaldehyde for 20 min, which was sufficient to permeabilise the cell membrane and allow binding of antibody to a total cell protein. Cells were incubated at 37°C in blocking buffer (3% BSA, 10% goat serum in PBS) for 1 h, with primary antibodies for 2 h and with secondary antibodies for 45 min. Subsequently, they were mounted using a Light Antifade kit (Invitrogen).

2.5. Confocal Microscopy. Z-stacks of immunolabeled cells were acquired using a Zeiss LSM 510 confocal microscope through a Plan Apochromatic oil-immersion objective (63x, NA = 1.4), excited by the 488 nm argon laser line and filtered with the 505–560 nm low-pass emission filter and excited by the 543 nm He/Ne laser line and filtered with the 560 nm low-pass emission filter. Images were analyzed quantitatively using LSM 510 software (Carl Zeiss). Eight to 15 markers were manually set to the cell perimeter, and the software interpolated the curve between them. The area above the threshold (20% of the maximal fluorescence intensity) fluorescence intensity relative to the cell cross-sectional area was determined.

2.6. Enzymatic Activity. Peptidase activity of the sDPP4 released from nonpermeabilised cells from the cell surface was determined using the DPPIV/CD26 assay kit for biological samples (Enzo Life Sciences, Plymouth Meeting, PA) according to the manufacturer instructions. The relative fluorescence units for each sample were calculated by plotting the linear region of the change in fluorescence over time and calculating the slope of the line. This was then used with the conversion factor to calculate the activity expressed as pmol/min and divided by the number of cells in individual samples to obtain the values expressed as pmol/min/cell. Data are presented as means ± s.e.m. of all tests ($n = 9$).

2.7. ELISA. The amount of sDPP4 released by the cell at different stages of differentiation and at different oxygenation of the cell atmosphere was quantified by a Human DPPIV/CD26 Quantikine ELISA kit (R&D Systems, Minneapolis MN) following the manufacturer's recommendations.

3. Results

3.1. Hypoxia-Mediated Reduction in DPP4 Expression in Single hPA. hPA were cultured in a normoxic chamber (18% pO_2) and in a hypoxic chamber (1% pO_2). To confirm that these hPA responded to hypoxia, cells were immunolabeled with antibodies against hypoxia-inducible factor-1α (HIF1-α). The results show that exposure to 1% pO_2 induced a massive expression of transcriptional factor HIF1-α (Figure 1(b)) and are consistent with previously published data [17]. In cells cultured in 18% pO_2, the expression of HIF1-α was negligible (Figure 1(a)). Thus hPA incubated under hypoxic conditions responded physiologically to the lowered pO_2.

To examine the expression of DPP4 in a hypoxic environment *in vitro* and to get insights into short and long term effects of hypoxia, cells were incubated at 1% pO_2 for 2 and 9 days and labeled with the anti-DPP4 antibody. The images of the largest optical slice of hPA (Figure 2(a)) were analyzed by determining the percent area of DPP4-labelled

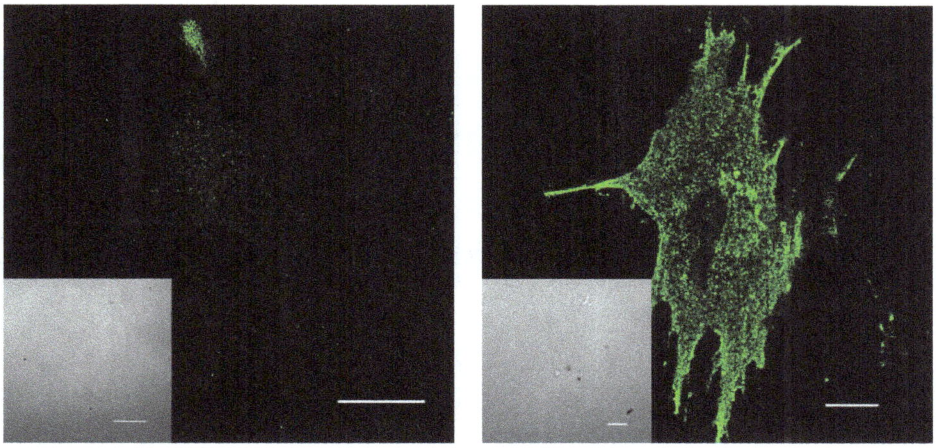

(a) (b)

FIGURE 1: Expression of HIF-1α, a hypoxia marker, in human preadipocytes cultured *in vitro*. Confocal images and transmission light images (insets) of human preadipocytes immunolabeled with antibody against HIF-1α. Preadipocytes were cultured for 2 days in normoxic conditions (a, 18% O_2) or hypoxic conditions (b, 1% O_2). Cells were fixed and immunolabeled with an antibody against HIF-1α. Inserts show transmission light microscopy images of the same cells as in the confocal fluorescent images. Scale bars indicate 20 μm.

part relative to the area of the entire optical slice of a cell. Note that the staining pattern of cells in Figure 2(a) is evenly distributed through the entire cell area. The 2-day exposure to hypoxia significantly reduced the expression density of DPP4 to 25.7 ± 2.7% compared with cells in normoxia (37.0 ± 2.9%; $P < 0.001$; Figure 2(b)). Prolonged incubation (9 days) had no further effect on DPP4 expression density in a hypoxic (28.3 ± 2.5%) or normoxic environment (41.8 ± 2.7%).

3.2. Time-Dependent Increase in the Protease Activity of sDPP4 Is Reduced by Hypoxia. DPP4 is a transmembrane protein; however, it is also active in its soluble form, after shedding the extracellular domain of the protein from the cell's surface. We investigated the protease activity of sDPP4 in conditioned medium of cells incubated in different oxygenation environments. Significant differences were detected between samples incubated in normoxia for 2 versus 9 days (Figure 2(c)). After 2 days, the activity of DPP4 was 2.0 ± 0.6 fmol/min/cell, increasing to 4.4 ± 0.7 fmol/min/cell after 9 days ($P < 0.05$). In samples incubated in hypoxia, the activity also appeared to increase from day 2 to day 9, from 0.9 ± 0.2 fmol/min/cell to 2.1 ± 0.3 fmol/min/cell ($P = 0.08$). In hypoxia on day 2, the DPP4 activity was similar to that in normoxia. However, in the 9-day samples, the activity of DPP4 significantly decreased with hypoxia ($P < 0.05$). We conclude that although the amount of DPP4 protein that is shed from the cell surface of hPA is insensitive to 2 or 9 days of culture under normoxic and hypoxic conditions, we detected a significant time-dependent increase in DPP4 protease activity in normoxic controls; the increase was relatively reduced by hypoxia.

3.3. Differentiation-Mediated Decrease in DPP4 Expression in Adipocytes Is Potentiated by Hypoxia. We studied the influence of the state of differentiation of adipocytes on the DPP4 expression pattern. In normoxia DPP4 expression is variable but tends to decline as a function of time (Figure 3(a)), especially at the induction of differentiation, and is barely detectable on mature adipocytes on day 21 (Figure 3(a)). In hypoxia (Figure 3(b)), the expression of DPP4 also decreased continuously. Comparison of differentiation-dependent DPP4 expression between both oxygenation conditions revealed that, with the exception of day 21, DPP4 expression density is significantly lower under hypoxic conditions at all stages of differentiation ($P < 0.05$), consistent with data in Figure 2.

We also studied the concentration of sDPP4 in conditioned medium of cells, which tended to decrease as a function of differentiation (Figure 4(a)). With only a few exceptions (see # on Figure 4(a)), the concentration of sDPP4 seemed to decrease at a similar rate under normoxic and hypoxic conditions during differentiation.

Investigation of the protease activity of sDPP4 in the culture medium revealed that as in Figure 4(a) a similar trend of decrease during differentiation was found (Figure 4(b)). To confirm that the protease activity of sDPP4 is significantly lower under hypoxic versus normoxic conditions, we correlated the concentration of sDPP4 protein and its protease activity in normoxic and hypoxic conditions (Figure 4(c)). The slopes of the regression lines are significantly different, indicating that hypoxic conditions significantly enhance the differentiation-dependent reduction of sDPP4 protease activity, relative to the protein content of DPP4.

3.4. Insulin Enhances the Shedding and Protease Activity of sDPP4 in Normoxic and Hypoxic Preadipocytes. Preadipocytes incubated for 2 days at 18% and 1% pO_2 were stimulated with insulin (100 nM) for 30 min. In normoxia, insulin significantly increased DPP4 expression in preadipocytes (42.2±2.5%; Figure 5(a)) versus stimulation with vehicle only (31.3 ± 4.7%; $P < 0.05$). A similar increase was observed

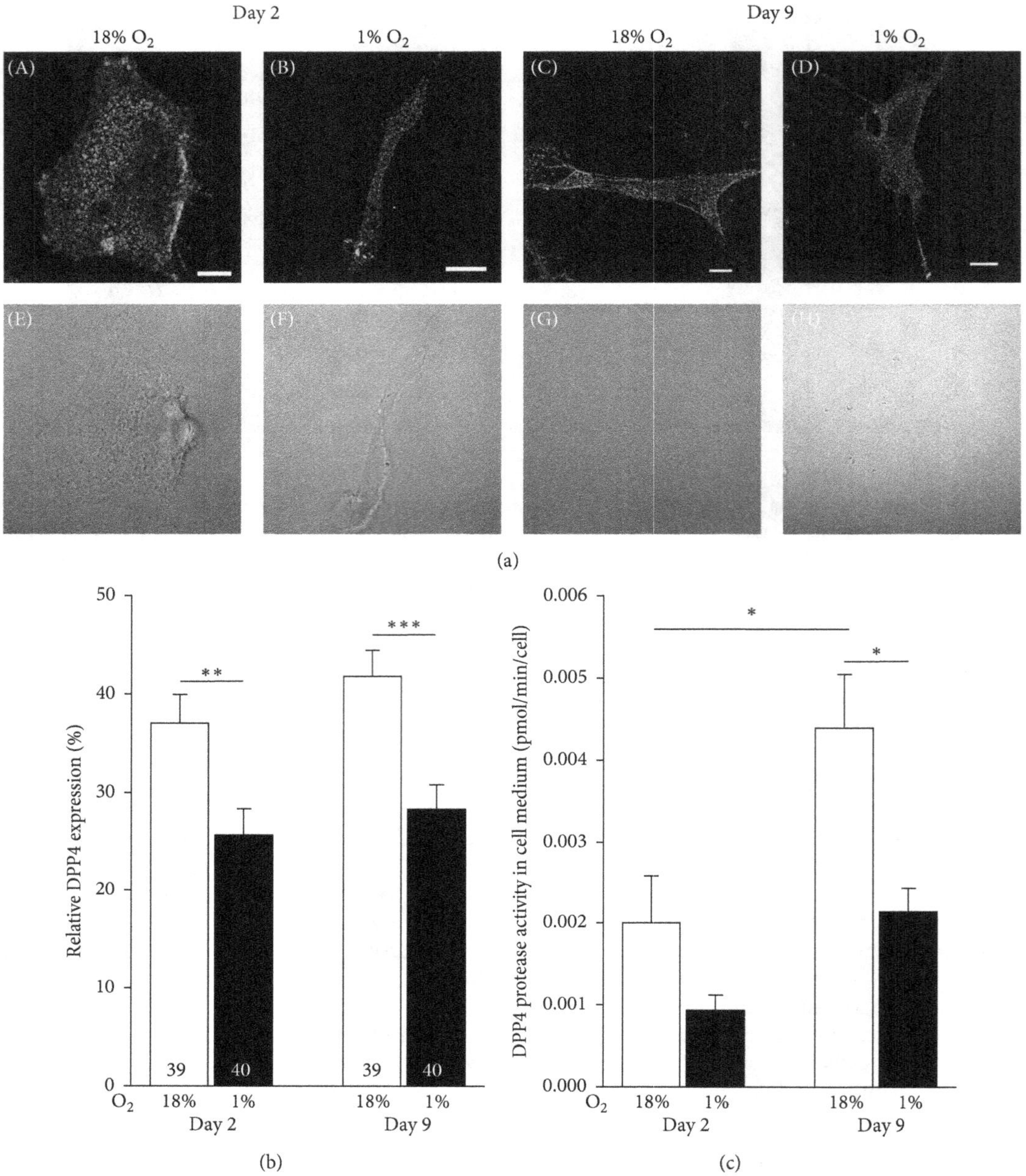

FIGURE 2: Oxygenation-dependent expression density and shedding of DPP4 in human preadipocytes cultured *in vitro*. (a) Confocal images (upper panels) and transmission light microscopy images (lower panels) of human preadipocytes (subconfluent cultures) immunolabeled with antibody against DPP4. Each panel shows representative confocal images of a cell incubated for 2 days (A, B, E, and F) and 9 days (C, D, G, and H) under normoxic (A, C, E, and G) and hypoxic (B, D, F, and H) environmental conditions. Scale bars indicate 10 μm. (b) Relative expression density of DPP4 in human preadipocytes cultured for 2 and 9 days in normoxic or hypoxic conditions. Numbers denote the number of cells imaged. (c) Normalized DPP4 protease activity in conditioned medium. Asterisks denote statistically significant difference ($^{*}P < 0.05$; $^{**}P < 0.01$; $^{***}P < 0.001$, two-way ANOVA).

in hypoxia; insulin significantly increased DPP4 expression (41.9 ± 2.7%) versus controls (23.2 ± 4.2%; $P < 0.001$).

To study shedding, we also examined the concentration of sDPP4 in the conditioned medium (Figure 5(b)) of cells stimulated with insulin. Hypoxia did not influence the sDPP4 concentration in controls or insulin-stimulated cells. However, insulin treatment significantly increased DPP4 protein shedding in normoxia ($P < 0.001$) and in hypoxia ($P < 0.01$). Under both oxygenation conditions, we recorded a pronounced effect of insulin treatment on sDPP4 protease activity in the culture medium (Figure 5(c)). In normoxia, insulin significantly increased protease activity (8.0 ± 1.4 fmol/min/cell) compared to nonstimulated cells (2.0 ± 0.6 fmol/min/cell; $P < 0.05$). In hypoxia, insulin stimulation also increased the activity of shed protein (13.1 ± 3.0 fmol/min/cell) compared to controls (0.9 ±

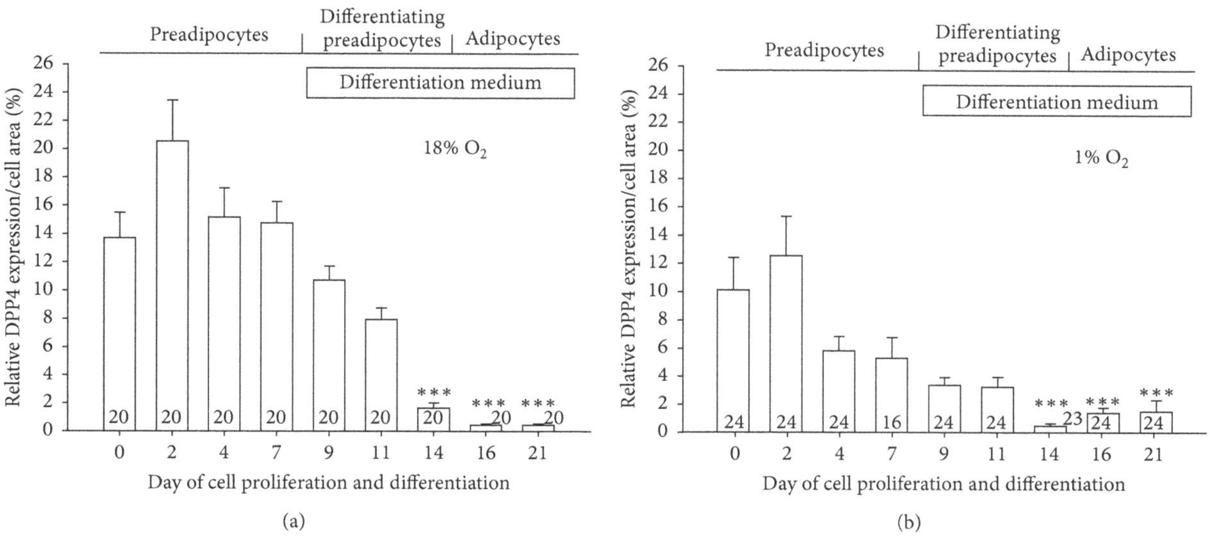

FIGURE 3: Differentiation-dependent expression density of membrane DPP4 of human preadipocytes and adipocytes cultured *in vitro* under different environmental conditions. Relative expression density of DPP4 in human preadipocytes in the course of differentiation to mature adipocytes cultured in normoxia (a) and hypoxia (b). Data are presented as mean values ± SE. Numbers denote the number of cells imaged ($^{***}P \leq 0.001$ versus preadipocytes on day 0; one-way ANOVA on ranks). On day 0, cells were already confluent.

0.2 fmol/min/cell; $P < 0.001$). These results indicate that hypoxic conditions increase insulin-mediated expression, shedding, and protease activity of DPP4 in preadipocytes.

4. Discussion

4.1. Is DPP4 a Marker for Differentiation Status of Adipocytes? DPP4 is abundantly expressed in hPA, while in mature adipocytes we found very modest, if any, expression of DPP4 (Figure 3). The significantly lower expression of DPP4 in mature adipocytes could not be explained with differences in cell size between both stages of differentiation, since the difference is not statistically significant (not shown). These results suggest that during differentiation from hPA into adipocytes cells gradually suppress the DPP4 expression. If this reduction in DPP4 in hPA is associated with differentiation into adipocytes *in vivo*, then DPP4 may well represent a marker for differentiation status. Therefore, like Pref-1, a stemness marker for preadipocytes, DPP4 is also robustly expressed in hPA: the higher the expression of DPP4 in preadipocytes, the higher the stem-like character of these cells. In support of this, DPP4 is abundantly expressed in cultured hPA (Figure 2), and during differentiation DPP4 expression declines (Figure 3). It is unlikely that DPP4 downexpression during differentiation is associated with a response to some of the factors in the differentiation medium added, as the DPP4 downexpression started prior to the addition of differentiation medium (Figures 3 and 4), at a stage when cells reached confluence. Although these results contrast with the report where cancer cells were studied by Abe et al. [18], the most probable explanation for the reduction of DPP4 in the (pre)adipocytes is the cell-to-cell contact-induced differentiation process into mature adipocytes that contain very modest amounts of DPP4.

DPP4 was found to be expressed in a variety of cell types [19, 20], from which it is also shed and sDPP4 may influence the shedding of membrane bound DPP4 from preadipocytes that were investigated in this study.

Current experiments revealed that the stage of differentiation of hPA into adipocytes can be assessed by monitoring the DPP4 density in cells, which can be considered as a developmental or differentiation marker, reporting the relatively undifferentiated stage of these cells. Consistent with this, it has recently been demonstrated that hypoxia inhibits adipogenesis through the HIF1α pathway [21, 22]. Hypoxia arrests preadipocytes in an undifferentiated state, thereby maintaining their stemness [23, 24].

The reduction in DPP4 in single differentiating cells is further supported by the determination of the concentration of sDPP4 and its enzymatic activity. Both parameters exhibit a differentiation-dependent decrease (Figures 4(a) and 4(b)) and this is consistent with the view that the soluble protein arises from the shedding of DPP4 from the plasma membrane. DPP4 has been shown to move from the cytoplasm to the cell surface rapidly and consequently the protein amount on the cell membrane is steadily proportional to the total cell protein [25]. The correlation between the concentration of sDPP4 and its activity (Figure 4(c)) shows that in hypoxia the activity is reduced by almost a factor of three relative to the concentration of soluble protein. One possible explanation would be that hypoxia lowers pH of cells. DPP4 enzymatic activity is pH dependent with the optimum at 7.8 [26]. A lower pH in hypoxic conditions would result in lower DPP4 activity. However, the activity assay was performed with buffered solution maintaining constant pH during the assay; therefore we can exclude the pH influence at the time of measurements of enzymatic activity. Although pH was not quantitatively measured during hypoxia it was observed qualitatively with pH indicator in the cell medium with no obvious changes during incubation in hypoxia, indicating that pH of the cell medium did not change significantly.

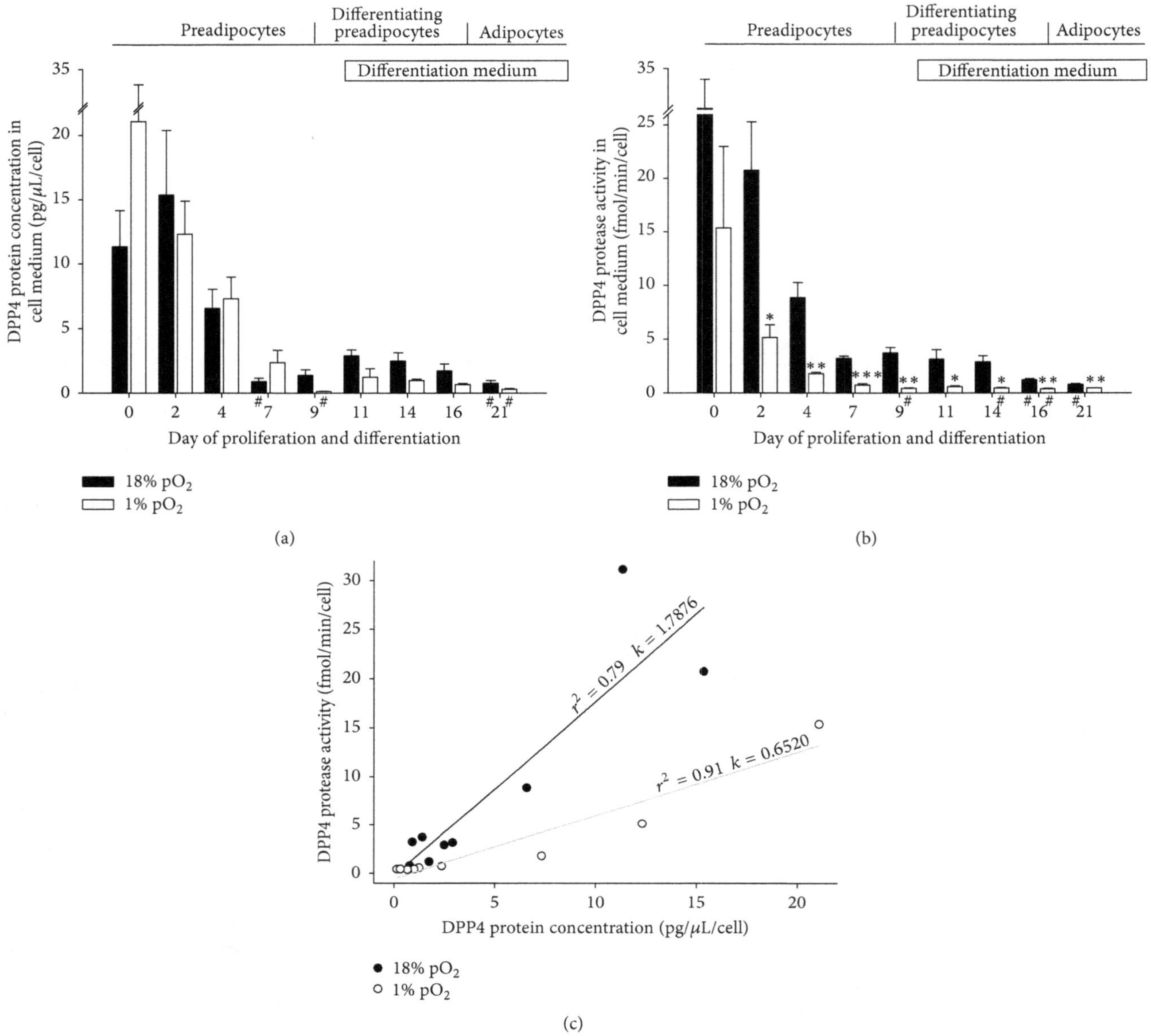

FIGURE 4: Differentiation and hypoxia reduce the shedding of DPP4 from human preadipocytes cultured *in vitro*. (a) Normalized DPP4 protein concentration in conditioned medium of cells at different stages of differentiation from preadipocytes to mature adipocytes cultured under normoxic (black bars) and hypoxic (white bars) environmental conditions. (b) Normalized DPP4 protease activity in conditioned medium of cells at different stages of differentiation from human preadipocytes to mature adipocytes cultured in normoxic (black bars) and hypoxic (white bars) environmental conditions. Data are normalized to the total cell number in the sample and presented as mean values ± SE. Asterisks above the white bars denote significant difference between hypoxic versus normoxic condition on the same differentiation day (Student's t-test; $^{*}P < 0.05$; $^{**}P < 0.01$; $^{***}P < 0.001$); # under the bars denotes significant difference compared with day 0 for respective oxygenation condition (one-way ANOVA; $^{\#}P \leq 0.01$). (c) Correlation between the concentration of DPP4 in the conditioned media and its activity under normoxic (black dots) and hypoxic (open dots) conditions (k, slope coefficient; r^2, correlation coefficient). The equation of regression lines is as follows: DPP4 activity [fmol/min/cell] = (1.79 ± 0.35) × DPP4 concentration [pg/μL/cell] − (0.2 ± 2.4) [fmol/min/cell] for the correlation in normoxia and DPP4 activity [fmol/min/cell] = (0.65 ± 0.08) × DPP4 concentration [pg/μL/cell] − (0.6 ± 0.7) [fmol/min/cell] for the correlation in hypoxia. The slopes are significantly different ($P < 0.001$), whereas the intercepts are similar and not different from 0.

Hypoxia-related increase of preadipocyte stemness could be an additional mechanism in the development of insulin resistance. The results imply that in obesity-related hypoxia DPP4 is abundantly expressed, contributing to the reduction in insulin activity and thereby to the onset of insulin resistance in these subjects.

4.2. Insulin Increases DPP4 Expression Density in hPA. Most gastrointestinal (GI) hormones involved in satiety regulation and glucose metabolism, especially through regulation of insulin secretion, are hydrolyzed and inactivated by DPP4 [27]. Thus DPP4 action reduces the amount of insulin secretion. This mechanism of action is well exploited by

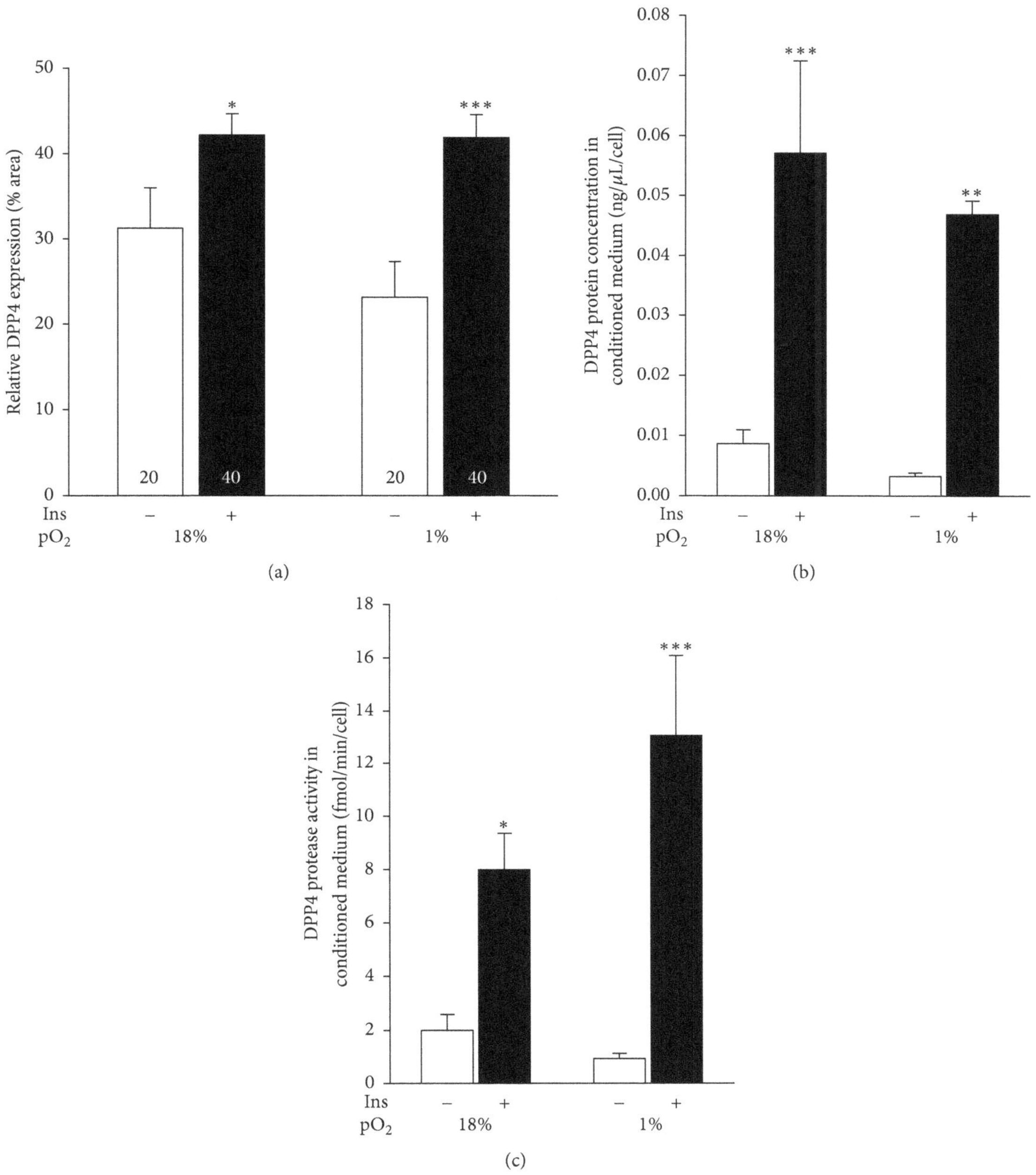

FIGURE 5: The effect of insulin on DPP4 expression and activity in human preadipocytes. (a) Human preadipocytes cultured for 2 days under normoxic (18% pO_2) and hypoxic (1% pO_2) conditions were treated for 30 min with 100 nM insulin (black bars). Control cells were treated with vehicle only for 30 min (white bars). Subsequently, the cells were immunolabeled with an antibody against DPP4 and imaged on a confocal microscope. The expression density of immunolabeled DPP4 was analyzed. Data are presented as means ± SE. Numbers denote the number of cells analyzed. The conditioned media were collected from cells treated for 30 min with insulin (Ins) and the protein concentration (b) and protease activity (c) of DPP4 were analyzed. Data are normalized to the number of cells in the sample and presented as means ± SE. Asterisks denote statistically significant differences compared with controls treated with vehicle only, as denoted ($^{*}P < 0.05$; $^{**}P < 0.01$; $^{***}P < 0.001$; ANOVA).

the development of a class of antidiabetic drugs that inhibit DPP4. But little is known about how insulin influences the expression of DPP4. The results of this study demonstrate that at single-cell level insulin significantly increases DPP4 expression in hPA in a rapid manner (30 min) by about 35%. Under hypoxic conditions, this increase was 63% relative to control (Figure 5(a)). These results indicate that DPP4 is also regulated by insulin but unlike hypoxia, which renders DPP4 expression, the rapid effect of insulin is most likely posttranscriptional.

Insulin induces DPP4 expression on cells which in turn deactivated GI hormones, thereby inhibiting the stimulation of insulin secretion. In agreement with this, incubation of cells with insulin for 5 and 24 h resulted in decreased DPP4 expression to baseline level (not shown). This is probably due to insulin receptor internalization and deactivation of insulin signaling. As expected, sDPP4 in culture medium and its protease activity also significantly increased after 30 min of insulin action in both oxygenation environments.

5. Conclusions

This study shows that human preadipocytes express DPP4 abundantly and this expression decreases in the course of differentiation into mature adipocytes. Therefore, DPP4 can be considered a differentiation marker highlighting the stemness properties of preadipocytes. The strong inhibition of DPP4 protease activity by hypoxia and the insulin-mediated increase in DPP4 indicate that DPP4 represents an important marker for early detection of insulin resistance.

Conflict of Interests

The authors declare that there is no conflict of interests regarding the publication of this paper.

Acknowledgments

The human preadipocytes cell line was a kind gift from Professor Jürgen Eckel, German Diabetes Center, Dusseldorf, Germany. The study was supported in part by the Slovenian Research Agency (Grants J3 3632 to Robert Zorec, J3 4051 to Robert Zorec, J3 4146 to Marko Kreft, and P3 310 to Robert Zorec).

References

[1] R. Yazbeck, G. S. Howarth, and C. A. Abbott, "Dipeptidyl peptidase inhibitors, an emerging drug class for inflammatory disease?" *Trends in Pharmacological Sciences*, vol. 30, no. 11, pp. 600–607, 2009.

[2] C. A. Abbott, D. M. T. Yu, E. Woollatt, G. R. Sutherland, G. W. McCaughan, and M. D. Gorrell, "Cloning, expression and chromosomal localization of a novel human dipeptidyl peptidase (DPP) IV homolog, DPP8," *European Journal of Biochemistry*, vol. 267, no. 20, pp. 6140–6150, 2000.

[3] B. Gallwitz, "The evolving place of incretin-based therapies in type 2 diabetes," *Pediatric Nephrology*, vol. 25, no. 7, pp. 1207–1217, 2010.

[4] L. K. Phillips and J. B. Prins, "Update on incretin hormones," *Annals of the New York Academy of Sciences*, vol. 1243, pp. E55–E74, 2011.

[5] P. A. Havre, M. Abe, Y. Urasaki, K. Ohnuma, C. Morimoto, and N. H. Dang, "The role of CD26/dipeptidyl peptidase IV in cancer," *Frontiers in Bioscience*, vol. 13, no. 5, pp. 1634–1645, 2008.

[6] M. Javidroozi, S. Zucker, and W.-T. Chen, "Plasma seprase and DPP4 levels as markers of disease and prognosis in cancer," *Disease Markers*, vol. 32, no. 5, pp. 309–320, 2012.

[7] A. Varona, L. Blanco, I. Perez et al., "Expression and activity profiles of DPP IV/CD26 and NEP/CD10 glycoproteins in the human renal cancer are tumor-type dependent," *BMC Cancer*, vol. 10, article 193, 2010.

[8] M. Itou, T. Kawaguchi, E. Taniguchi, and M. Sata, "Dipeptidyl peptidase-4: a key player in chronic liver disease," *World Journal of Gastroenterology*, vol. 19, no. 15, pp. 2298–2306, 2013.

[9] B. Ahrén, "DPP-4 inhibitors," *Best Practice & Research in Clinical Endocrinology and Metabolism*, vol. 21, no. 4, pp. 517–533, 2007.

[10] R. Mackenzie, N. Maxwell, P. Castle, G. Brickley, and P. Watt, "Acute hypoxia and exercise improve insulin sensitivity (S_I^{2*}) in individuals with type 2 diabetes," *Diabetes/Metabolism Research and Reviews*, vol. 27, no. 1, pp. 94–101, 2011.

[11] W. Schobersberger, P. Schmid, M. Lechleitner et al., "Austrian Moderate Altitude Study 2000 (AMAS 2000). The effects of moderate altitude (1,700 m) on cardiovascular and metabolic variables in patients with metabolic syndrome," *European Journal of Applied Physiology*, vol. 88, no. 6, pp. 506–514, 2003.

[12] N. Halberg, T. Khan, M. E. Trujillo et al., "Hypoxia-inducible factor 1α induces fibrosis and insulin resistance in white adipose tissue," *Molecular and Cellular Biology*, vol. 29, no. 16, pp. 4467–4483, 2009.

[13] C. Regazzetti, P. Peraldi, T. Grémeaux et al., "Hypoxia decreases insulin signaling pathways in adipocytes," *Diabetes*, vol. 58, no. 1, pp. 95–103, 2009.

[14] N. Hosogai, A. Fukuhara, K. Oshima et al., "Adipose tissue hypoxia in obesity and its impact on adipocytokine dysregulation," *Diabetes*, vol. 56, no. 4, pp. 901–911, 2007.

[15] M. E. Rausch, S. Weisberg, P. Vardhana, and D. V. Tortoriello, "Obesity in C57BL/6J mice is characterized by adipose tissue hypoxia and cytotoxic T-cell infiltration," *International Journal of Obesity*, vol. 32, no. 3, pp. 451–463, 2008.

[16] D. Lamers, S. Famulla, N. Wronkowitz et al., "Dipeptidyl peptidase 4 is a novel adipokine potentially linking obesity to the metabolic syndrome," *Diabetes*, vol. 60, no. 7, pp. 1917–1925, 2011.

[17] B. Wang, I. S. Wood, and P. Trayhurn, "Hypoxia induces leptin gene expression and secretion in human preadipocytes: differential effects of hypoxia on adipokine expression by preadipocytes," *Journal of Endocrinology*, vol. 198, no. 1, pp. 127–134, 2008.

[18] M. Abe, P. A. Havre, Y. Urasaki et al., "Mechanisms of confluence-dependent expression of CD26 in colon cancer cell lines," *BMC Cancer*, vol. 11, article 51, 2011.

[19] S. Mentzel, H. B. P. M. Dijkman, J. P. H. F. Van Son, R. A. P. Koene, and K. J. M. Assmann, "Organ distribution of aminopeptidase A and dipeptidyl peptidase IV in normal mice," *Journal of Histochemistry and Cytochemistry*, vol. 44, no. 5, pp. 445–461, 1996.

[20] M. D. Gorrell, "Dipeptidyl peptidase IV and related enzymes in cell biology and liver disorders," *Clinical Science*, vol. 108, no. 4, pp. 277–292, 2005.

[21] Z. Yun, H. L. Maecker, R. S. Johnson, and A. J. Giaccia, "Inhibition of PPARγ2 gene expression by the HIF-1-regulated gene DEC1/Stra13: a mechanism for regulation of adipogenesis by hypoxia," *Developmental Cell*, vol. 2, no. 3, pp. 331–341, 2002.

[22] Q. Lin, Y.-J. Lee, and Z. Yun, "Differentiation arrest by hypoxia," *The Journal of Biological Chemistry*, vol. 281, no. 41, pp. 30678–30683, 2006.

[23] Y. Yamamoto, M. Fujita, Y. Tanaka et al., "Low oxygen tension enhances proliferation and maintains stemness of adipose tissue-derived stromal cells," *BioResearch Open Access*, vol. 2, no. 3, pp. 199–205, 2013.

[24] P. Trayhurn, "Hypoxia and adipose tissue function and dysfunction in obesity," *Physiological Reviews*, vol. 93, no. 1, pp. 1–21, 2013.

[25] L. Baricault, J. A. M. Fransen, M. Garcia et al., "Rapid sequestration of DPP IV/CD26 and other cell surface proteins in an autophagic-like compartment in Caco-2 cells treated with forskolin," *Journal of Cell Science*, vol. 108, part 5, pp. 2109–2121, 1995.

[26] T. Yoshimoto, M. Fischl, R. C. Orlowski, and R. Walter, "Post-proline cleaving enzyme and post-proline dipeptidyl aminopeptidase. Comparison of two peptidases with high specificity for proline residues," *The Journal of Biological Chemistry*, vol. 253, no. 10, pp. 3708–3716, 1978.

[27] W. Kim and J. M. Egan, "The role of incretins in glucose homeostasis and diabetes treatment," *Pharmacological Reviews*, vol. 60, no. 4, pp. 470–512, 2008.

10

The Expression of miR-192 and Its Significance in Diabetic Nephropathy Patients with Different Urine Albumin Creatinine Ratio

Xiaoyu Ma,[1] Canlu Lu,[2] Chuan Lv,[3] Can Wu,[2] and Qiuyue Wang[2]

[1]*Geriatrics Department, The First Hospital of China Medical University, Shenyang, Liaoning, China*
[2]*Endocrine Department, The First Hospital of China Medical University, Shenyang, Liaoning, China*
[3]*Endocrine Department, The People Hospital of Liaoning Province, Shenyang, Liaoning, China*

Correspondence should be addressed to Qiuyue Wang; wqycmu123@163.com

Academic Editor: Carlos Martinez Salgado

Objective. To investigate the expression of miR-192 and its significance in diabetic nephropathy (DN) patients. *Methods.* 464 patients with type 2 diabetes mellitus (T2DM) were divided into normal albuminuria group (NA, $n = 157$), microalbuminuria group (MA, $n = 159$), and large amount of albuminuria group (LA, $n = 148$). 127 healthy persons were selected as the control group (NC, $n = 127$). The serum miR-192 levels were detected by Real-Time PCR and transforming growth factor-$\beta 1$ (TGF-$\beta 1$) and fibronectin (FN) were detected by enzyme-linked immunosorbent assay. The relationships among these parameters were analyzed by Pearson correlation analysis and multiple linear regression analysis. *Results.* The miR-192 in the LA group was significantly lower than other groups, which was lower in the MA group than in the NA group ($P < 0.01$). The TGF-$\beta 1$ and FN in the LA group were significantly higher than other groups, which were higher in the MA group than in the NA group ($P < 0.01$). The expression of miR-192 was negatively correlated with TGF-$\beta 1$, FN, and Ln (UACR) and miR-192, TGF-$\beta 1$, and FN were independent relevant factors affecting Ln (UACR) in T2DM ($P < 0.01$). *Conclusions.* These findings indicate that the levels of miR-192 were lower accompanied by the decrease of urine albumin creatinine ratio (UACR) and the association between miR-192 and nephritic fibrosis in DN.

1. Introduction

DN is one of the chronic complications of diabetes and it is the main cause of end-stage renal disease (ESRD). DN is characterized by glomerular basement membrane (GBM) and tubular basement membrane (TBM) thickening, extracellular matrix (ECM) of glomerular mesangial area accumulation, and renal tubule interstitial fibrosis, which cause glomerular sclerosis, proteinuria, and renal failure eventually.

TGF-$\beta 1$ belongs to transforming growth factor superfamily and it can promote renal fibrosis, increase the number of glomerular mesangial cells, and stimulate ECM accumulation in experimental and human DN [1–3]. ECM accumulation can induce further glomerular sclerosis and tubular endothelium fibrosis and cause glomerular filtration rate to progressively decrease and renal failure in DN. Miller et al. [4] found that the TGF-$\beta 1$ mRNA was higher in the glomerulus of DN patients and it is parallel with the glomerular sclerosis extents. Therefore TGF-$\beta 1$ is supposed to be a marker of glomerular sclerosis. FN is a noncollagenous glycoprotein which is the main component of ECM. The ECM consists of collagens, laminin, FN, and proteoglycans under physiologic conditions. Since FN is a main component of ECM, significant increases in FN can represent the fibrosis of ECM in many glomerulopathies including DN. TGF-$\beta 1$ and FN increase significantly in DN and lead to glomerular sclerosis and fibrosis finally. MicroRNAs (miRNAs) are endogenously produced short noncoding RNAs of 21–25 nucleotides; they can inhibit gene expression by mRNA degradation, translation, or transcriptional inhibition [5].

miRNAs have been shown to play important roles in many cellular and biologic processes such as cell proliferation and differentiation, cancer, stress response, and development [6–8]. Recent studies have showed that miR-192 participated in the renal fibrosis in DN induced by TGF-β1, but the results are inconsistent. Our study aimed to investigate the relationships among miR-192, TGF-β1, and FN in DN with microalbuminuria and large amount of albuminuria, to explore the significance of miR-192 expression in DN.

2. Materials and Methods

2.1. Subjects and Grouping. The subjects of experimental groups were type 2 diabetes patients admitted to the Endocrine Department of The First Hospital of China Medical University from January 2013 to October 2014. The subjects of control group were healthy persons whose age and gender were matched. Permissions were got from all the subjects before their enrollment and this paper was approved by the Ethics Institutional Review Board of China Medical University. The patients were asked about their medical history carefully including duration which indicated the time since T2DM diagnosis and their height (cm), weight (kg), and drugs.

Admission standards were as follows: type 2 diabetes patients diagnosed by OGTT according to the WHO diagnostic criteria in 1999. Patients with the following were excluded: heart diseases; hypertension; hepatic dysfunction; cancer; being pregnant; other kidney diseases (such as glomerulonephritis) or diseases of urinary system; having infection, surgery, or trauma; using agents that could affect glucose metabolism such as glucocorticoid; using agents that could affect urinary albumin excretion rate (UAER) such as ACE inhibitor or angiotensin receptor blocker.

Finally, 464 subjects were enrolled in the experimental group and they were divided into three groups according to the urine albumin creatinine ratio (UACR): normal albuminuria group (NA, UACR < 30 mg/g, $n = 157$), microalbuminuria group (MA, UACR: 30–300 mg/g, $n = 159$), and large amount of albuminuria group (LA, UACR > 300 mg/g, $n = 148$). 127 healthy persons whose age and gender were matched were selected as the control group (NC, $n = 127$).

2.2. Measurements of Some Parameters. All the subjects fasted at night for over 12 h. The venous blood about 5 mL of every research object was collected after 12-hour overnight fasting state and centrifuged for 15 min at 4°C with 1000 rounds/min. The supernatant was centrifuged for 5 min at 4°C with 2000 rounds/min. The supernatants were conserved at −80°C. The levels of fasting blood glucose (FBG), postprandial blood glucose (PBG), glycated hemoglobin (HbA1C), fasting insulin (FINS), postprandial insulin (PINS), fasting C peptides (FCPS), postprandial C peptides (PCPS), blood urea nitrogen (BUN), creatinine (Cr), low density lipoprotein cholesterol (LDL-C), high density lipoprotein cholesterol (HDL-C), triglyceride (TG), and cholesterol (CHO) were detected in the clinical laboratory and the endocrine experimental laboratory of The First Hospital of China Medical University.

MicroRNAs (miRNAs) were isolated from a serum volume of 400 μL using the miRcute miRNA isolation kit (TianGen Biotech, Beijing, China) according to the manufacturer's instructions. Before RNA extraction, *C. elegans* synthetic miRNA cel-miR-39 miRNA Mimic (Qiagen, Hilden, Germany) was added to serum samples to correct for variations in RNA isolation derived. 5 μL of miRNAs was used for reverse transcription using the miRcute miRNA First-Strand cDNA Synthesis Kit (TianGen Biotech, Beijing, China). miRcute miRNA qPCR Detection Kit (SYBR Green) (TianGen Biotech, Beijing, China) was performed using 3.0 μL cDNA template under the following conditions: 94°C for 2 minutes and 45 cycles of 94°C for 5 seconds and 60°C for 40 seconds. Data analysis based on measurements of the threshold cycle was performed using the $2^{-\Delta\Delta CT}$ method. $\Delta\Delta$CT values are defined as the raw CT value-average of raw CT values for syncel-miR-39. For each sample, quantitative Real-Time PCR was performed in triplicate.

TGF-β1 and FN were detected by enzyme-linked immunosorbent assay (Abcam Company from China and Technoclone Company from Austria, resp.).

2.3. Statistical Method. The gene expression level of miR-192 was calculated with $2^{-\Delta\Delta CT}$. Quantitative data that conformed to the normal distribution were reported as mean ± SDs and those that did not conform to the normal distribution were reported as median. Qualitative data were reported as percentage (%). Comparison among groups was as follows: Quantitative data that conformed to the normal distribution were compared with one-way ANOVA and those that did not conform to the normal distribution were compared with rank sum test. Qualitative data were compared with chi-square test. The correlations of any of two parameters which conformed to the normal distribution were analyzed by Pearson correlation analysis and those that did not conform to the normal distribution were analyzed by Spearman correlation analysis. The correlations of UACR and other indexes were analyzed by multiple linear regression analysis. Data were processed with the software package of SPSS 17.0. $P < 0.05$ by two-tailed test was considered to be significant.

3. Results

3.1. Clinical Characteristics of the Subjects (Table 1). There were significant differences in BMI, SBP, DBP, FBG, PBG, BUN, CHO, TG, LDL-C, HDL-C, and Ln (ACR) between NC group and T2DM groups (including NA, MA, and LA groups) ($P < 0.05$). Comparison among experimental groups was as follows: There were significant differences in duration, SBP, DBP, HbA1C, FBG, PBG, FINS, PINS, TG, LDL-C, HDL-C, Ln (ACR), miR-192, TGF-β1, and FN between NA group and MA group ($P < 0.05$). There were significant differences in duration, SBP, DBP, HbA1C, FBG, PBG, FINS, PINS, BUN, CHO, TG, LDL-C, HDL-C, Ln (ACR), miR-192, TGF-β1, and FN between NA group and LA group ($P < 0.05$). There were significant differences in duration, SBP, DBP, HbA1C, FCPS, BUN, CHO, TG, HDL-C, Ln (ACR), miR-192, TGF-β1, and FN between MA group and LA group ($P < 0.05$).

Table 1: Clinical characteristics of the subjects.

	NC	NA	MA	LA
Age (years)	51.33 ± 9.16	51.4 ± 8.57	55.40 ± 12.06	58.33 ± 9.04
Duration (years)	—	5.03 ± 1.27	8.21 ± 0.99b	11.53 ± 1.05bc
BMI (Kg/m^2)	23.76 ± 1.60	26.49 ± 1.36a	25.30 ± 1.81a	25.31 ± 1.81a
SBP (mmHg)	115.51 ± 3.22	125.72 ± 3.43a	130.43 ± 3.04ab	136.49 ± 4.78abc
DBP (mmHg)	75.13 ± 2.64	77.67 ± 3.35a	80.21 ± 2.17ab	82.84 ± 1.73abc
HbA1C (%)	5.16 ± 0.24	8.20 ± 0.12a	8.67 ± 0.21b	8.89 ± 0.22bc
FBG (mmol/L)	5.36 ± 0.47	8.03 ± 0.60a	9.50 ± 0.34ab	9.27 ± 0.63ab
PBG (mmol/L)	6.52 (6.33–6.83)	14.46 (14.17–14.66)a	18.66 (15.4621.69)ab	16.69 (14.15–19.48)ab
FINS (mIU/L)	8.98 (8.42–9.65)	6.20 (6.15–6.25)a	7.36 (6.32–7.93)ab	7.19 (6.37–7.66)ab
PINS (mIU/L)	17.04 ± 1.04	16.59 ± 1.37	18.12 ± 1.13b	17.62 ± 1.45b
FCPS (mmol/L)	588.26 ± 4.37	590.84 ± 2.89	531.14 ± 161.08	709.38 ± 284.56c
PCPS (mmol/L)	1305.48 (1298.32–1309.87)	1388.76 (1383.28–1393.87)a	1300.00 (1295.10–1305.80)b	1513.70 (1507.60–1517.30)abc
BUN (mmol/L)	5.57 ± 1.35	6.60 ± 0.85a	6.55 ± 0.72a	7.95 ± 0.33abc
Cr (μmol/L)	60.00 (54.00–72.00)	60.00 (51.00–73.00)	63.00 (57.00–70.00)	221.00 (208.00–241.00)abc
CHO (mmol/L)	4.62 ± 0.41	5.03 ± 0.40a	5.06 ± 0.33a	5.44 ± 0.44abc
TG (mmol/L)	1.39 ± 0.16	1.57 ± 0.05a	1.76 ± 0.14ab	2.11 ± 2.00abc
LDL-C (mmol/L)	2.24 ± 0.19	3.07 ± 0.22a	3.31 ± 0.21ab	3.30 ± 0.25ab
HDL-C (mmol/L)	1.20 ± 0.01	1.50 ± 0.02a	1.00 ± 0.01ab	0.80 ± 0.01abc
Ln (UACR) (mmol/L)	2.50 ± 0.06	2.87 ± 0.07a	4.88 ± 0.33ab	7.11 ± 0.91abc
miR-192 ($2^{-\Delta\Delta CT}$) (ng/mg)	1.00 ± 0.02	0.99 ± 0.01	0.63 ± 0.01ab	0.34 ± 0.01abc
TGF-β1 (ng/mL)	6.49 ± 0.24	11.61 ± 0.32e	20.35 ± 0.97ef	28.95 ± 1.28efg
FN (μg/mL)	85.67 ± 2.08	99.71 ± 2.65e	166.8 ± 13.42ef	245.83 ± 9.04efg

a: compared with NC group, $P < 0.05$; b: compared with NA group, $P < 0.05$; c: compared with MA group, $P < 0.05$; e: compared with NC group, $P < 0.01$; f: compared with MA group, $P < 0.01$; g: compared with MA group, $P < 0.01$. "—" presents no data.

BMI: body mass index; SBP: systolic blood pressure; DBP: diastolic blood pressure; HbA1C: glycated hemoglobin; FBG: fasting blood glucose; PBG: postprandial blood glucose; FINS: fasting insulin; PINS: postprandial insulin; FCPS: fasting C peptides; PCPS: postprandial C peptides; BUN: blood urea nitrogen; Cr: creatinine; CHO: cholesterol; TG: triglyceride; LDL-C: low density lipoprotein cholesterol; HDL-C: high density lipoprotein cholesterol; Ln (UACR): logarithm of urine albumin creatinine ratio; TGF-β1: transforming growth factor; FN: fibronectin.

3.2. Comparison of miR-192, TGF-β1, and FN (Table 1). There were no significant differences in miR-192, TGF-β1, and FN between NC group and NA group ($P > 0.05$). The expression of miR-192 in LA group was significantly lower than in MA and NA groups and the miR-192 was lower in MA group than in NA group ($P < 0.01$). The levels of TGF-β1 and FN in LA group were significantly higher than in MA and NA groups and those in MA group were higher in NA group than in NA group ($P < 0.01$).

3.3. Pearson/Spearman Correlation Analysis. In T2DM groups, the Pearson/Spearman correlation analysis showed that miR-192 ($2^{-\Delta\Delta CT}$) was negatively correlated with TGF-β1 and FN ($r = -0.902$, $P < 0.01$, and $r = -0.797$, $P < 0.01$, resp.); TGF-β1 was positively correlated with FN ($r = 0.824, P < 0.01$); Ln (ACR) was negatively correlated with miR-192 ($2^{-\Delta\Delta CT}$) ($r = -0.965, P < 0.01$), but Ln (ACR) was positively correlated with TGF-β1 ($r = 0.763, P < 0.01$), FN ($r = 0.726$, $P < 0.01$), duration ($r = 0.502$, $P < 0.01$), SBP ($r = 0.411$, $P < 0.001$), DBP ($r = 0.302$, $P < 0.05$), HbA1C ($r = 0.465$, $P < 0.01$), FBG ($r = 0.313$, $P < 0.05$), FINS ($r = 0.362$, $P < 0.05$), PCPS ($r = 0.470$, $P < 0.01$), BUN ($r = 0.401$, $P < 0.01$), Cr ($r = 0.700$, $P < 0.01$), CHO ($r = 0.554$, $P < 0.01$), TG ($r = 0.636$, $P < 0.01$), and HDL-C ($r = -0.493$, $P < 0.01$); Ln (ACR) was not correlated with age, BMI, PBG, PINS, FCPS, and LDL-C.

3.4. Multiple Linear Regression Analysis of Ln (UACR) and Other Parameters including miR-192, TGF-β1, and FN. We took Ln (UACR) as a dependent variable. Age, duration, BMI, SBP, DBP, FBG, PBG, HbA1C, FINS, PINS, FCPS, PCPS, BUN, Cr, LDL-C, HDL-C, TG, CHO, miR-192 ($2^{-\Delta\Delta CT}$), TGF-β1, and FN were selected as independent variables. The analysis showed that miR-192 ($2^{-\Delta\Delta CT}$), TGF-β1, FN, duration, and HbA1C were the independent relevant factors affecting Ln (UACR) in T2DM groups ($P < 0.01$). The regression equation is $Y = 3.297 - 1.573X1 + 1.988X2 + 0.897X3 + 0.572X4 + 0.038X5$ ($X1$ is miR-192 ($2^{-\Delta\Delta CT}$), $X2$ is TGF-β1, $X3$ is FN, $X4$ is duration, and $X5$ is HbA1C).

4. Discussion

The pathogenesis of DN is very complicated including glucose and lipid metabolism disorder, change of haemodynamics, oxidative stress, and cytokines, which can cause GBM thickening, ECM accumulation, glomerular sclerosis, filtration membrane damage, renal tubule atrophy, and renal interstitial fibrosis. These pathological changes cause urinary albumin excretion rate (UAER) increasing, slowly progressive proteinuria, and even renal dysfunction in clinical practice. Studies found recently that podocytopathy is an important cause of DN [9, 10]. Podocytes are a kind of highly differentiated cells with poor proliferation ability in glomerular basement membrane and they are an important component of glomerular filtration membrane. When the podocytes are damaged, the glomerular filtration charge barrier is weakened and albuminuria is induced. Albuminuria can increase the extracellular matrix (ECM) and accentuate renal fibrosis. Moreover, the regulation to the generation of ECM by the damaged podocytes is disordered and causes TGF-β1 and FN increase in DN.

TGF-β is a well-known cytokine that mediates the fibrosis and inflammation of kidney. TGF-β1 can promote the synthesis of ECM, prevent the degradation of ECM, and accumulate ECM by promoting the adhesion between cells and matrix [11]. TGF-β1 increase not only in the late stage, but also in the early stage of DN. Renal biopsy [4] from diabetes patients shows that the expression of TGF-β1 mRNA significantly increased. FN is a macromolecule glycoprotein which is the main component of ECM and it can be used to evaluate the extent of ECM accumulation [12]. FN is a main component of ECM; significant increases in FN can represent the fibrosis of ECM in many glomerulopathies including DN. Both of the synthesizing capacity of FN and the combining capacity of FN in combination with GBM increase in DM and the circulating fibronectin increased in the diabetic nephropathy [13, 14]. Basic studies found that high glucose concentration could stimulate the synthesis of FN in glomerular mesangial cells and this effect was mediated by TGF-β1 [15]. The FN mRNA increased in parallel with the endogenous TGF-β1 activity increase, and the neutralizing antibody of TGF-β1 could reverse this effect [16].

MicroRNAs (miRNAs) are endogenously produced short noncoding RNAs of 21–25 nucleotides. miRNAs are expressed with high tissue specificity, developmental stage specificity, and conservative property. miRNAs have been shown to play important roles in many cellular and biologic processes such as cell proliferation, differentiation and apoptosis, immune development, metabolism, virus infection, stress response, and cancer [17]. Moreover, miRNAs are expressed specifically in many diseases and different cancers such as diabetes, hepatic cancer, prostatic cancer, breast cancer, gastric cancer, squamous cell carcinoma, lymphoma, colon cancer, and lung cancer. The specific serum miRNAs phenotypes have the potential to become new kinds of diagnostic markers. miR-192 are expressed highly in kidney especially in renal cortex. Many studies have confirmed that miR-192 played important roles in the fibrosis of kidney and liver, but the conclusions are still controversial about the effect of miR-192 in DN.

Recent studies have showed that TGF-β1 could control the process of renal fibrosis by upregulating or downregulating several miRNAs including miR-192 [18–22]. Krupa et al. [23] found that TGF-β1 inhibited miR-192 expression in human proximal tubular cells (PTCs) and deficiency of miR-192 associates with renal fibrosis acceleration and GFR reduction in DN. Moreover, the expression of miR-192 was lower when the duration was longer. Wang et al. [24] also found that TGF-β1 decreased the expression of miR-192 in rat proximal tubular cells, mesangial cells, and human podocytes. The biopsy of diabetic patients showed that they had lower level of miR-192.

The zinc finger E-box binding homeobox-1 (Zeb1) and Zeb2 are two transcription factors located downstream of TGF-β1 signaling pathway which can repress E-cadherin and regulate renal fibrosis. Overexpression of miR-192 could inhibit the TGF-β1-mediated downregulation of E-cadherin by inhibiting the expression of Zeb1 and Zeb2 and then prevented the kidney from fibrosis. So it was reported that TGF-β1 inhibit the expression of miR-192, and miR-192 targeted Zeb1/2 to activate TGF-β1 signaling pathway and accentuated renal fibrosis in DN [23].

In our study, we found that there were no significant differences in miR-192, TGF-β1, and FN between NC group and NA group ($P > 0.05$). The expression of miR-192 in LA group was significantly lower than in MA and NA groups and the miR-192 was lower in MA group than in NA group ($P < 0.01$). The levels of TGF-β1 and FN in LA group were significantly higher than in MA and NA groups and those in MA group were higher in NA group than in NA group ($P < 0.01$). The results indicated that miR-192, TGF-β1, and FN could reflex the pathological progress of DN to some extent. The three parameters are significantly changed in early period of DN indicating that they may be worth for early diagnosis of DN. The multiple linear regression analysis showed that miR-192 ($2^{-\Delta\Delta CT}$), TGF-β1, and FN were the independent relevant factors affecting Ln (UACR) and also indicated that these three parameters were important factors affecting renal fibrosis process in DN. Our correlation analysis among Ln (UACR), miR-192, TGF-β1, and FN also showed that miR-192 was negatively correlated with TGF-β1, FN, and Ln (UACR); TGF-β1 was positively correlated with FN. These results indicated that TGF-β1 might downregulate miR-192, although we could not confirm the causality between them in this cross-sectional study.

However, there are several studies with opposite conclusions [25–30]. These studies find that the renal miR-192 are overexpressed in MCs and TECs of db/db mice as well as T2DM patients and miR-192 increase in parallel with increased TGF-β1. Deletion of inhibition of miR-192 can attenuate proteinuria and renal fibrosis and the renal function can be improved. The possible mechanisms include Smad and Akt signaling pathways. The discrepancy in these studies may be due to differences in animal species, cell types (including podocyte, mesangial cells, and renal tube cells), and experiment conditions.

5. Conclusions

We found that miR-192 was decreased in early DN and the levels of miR-192 were lower accompanied by the decrease of UACR. We also found that miR-192 was negatively correlated with TGF-β1 and FN—two parameters which represent the fibrosis extent of the kidney. These results provide us with the significance of serum miR-192 expression in clinical DN patients. The miR-192 may be the potential marker of DN diagnosis. More researches are needed to confirm the correlation of miR-192 and renal fibrosis in human DN and the underlying mechanisms.

Conflict of Interests

The authors confirm that there is no conflict of interests.

Acknowledgments

The authors thank The First Hospital of China Medical University for providing the data and for the use of the central experimental laboratory. This study is supported by Higher School "High-End Talent Team Construction" in Liaoning province (no. [2014] 187).

References

[1] S. L. Habib, "Alterations in tubular epithelial cells in diabetic nephropathy," *Journal of Nephrology*, vol. 26, no. 5, pp. 865–869, 2013.

[2] H. O. El Mesallamy, H. H. Ahmed, A. A. Bassyouni, and A. S. Ahmed, "Clinical significance of inflammatory and fibrogenic cytokines in diabetic nephropathy," *Clinical Biochemistry*, vol. 45, no. 9, pp. 646–650, 2012.

[3] S. Chen, B. Jim, and F. N. Ziyadeh, "Diabetic nephropathy and transforming growth factor-beta: transforming our view of glomerulosclerosis and fibrosis build-up," *Seminars in Nephrology*, vol. 23, no. 6, pp. 532–543, 2003.

[4] C. G. Miller, A. Pozzi, R. Zent, and J. E. Schwarzbauer, "Effects of high glucose on integrin activity and fibronectin matrix assembly by mesangial cells," *Molecular Biology of the Cell*, vol. 25, no. 16, pp. 2342–2350, 2014.

[5] X. Zhong, A. C. K. Chung, H.-Y. Chen, X.-M. Meng, and H. Y. Lan, "Smad3-mediated upregulation of miR-21 promotes renal fibrosis," *Journal of the American Society of Nephrology*, vol. 22, no. 9, pp. 1668–1681, 2011.

[6] Y. Zhang, D. Liu, X. Chen et al., "Secreted monocytic miR-150 enhances targeted endothelial cell migration," *Molecular Cell*, vol. 39, no. 1, pp. 133–144, 2010.

[7] A. A. Shah, P. Leidinger, N. Blin, and E. Meese, "miRNA: small molecules as potential novel biomarkers in cancer," *Current Medicinal Chemistry*, vol. 17, no. 36, pp. 4427–4432, 2010.

[8] N. Schöler, C. Langer, H. Döhner, C. Buske, and F. Kuchenbauer, "Serum microRNAs as a novel class of biomarkers: a comprehensive review of the literature," *Experimental Hematology*, vol. 38, no. 12, pp. 1126–1130, 2010.

[9] W. Liu, Y. Zhang, J. Hao et al., "Nestin protects mouse podocytes against high glucose-induced apoptosis by a Cdk5-dependent mechanism," *Journal of Cellular Biochemistry*, vol. 113, no. 10, pp. 3186–3196, 2012.

[10] R. Li, L. Zhang, W. Shi et al., "NFAT2 mediates high glucose-induced glomerular podocyte apoptosis through increased Bax expression," *Experimental Cell Research*, vol. 319, no. 7, pp. 992–1000, 2013.

[11] J. Winter, S. Jung, S. Keller, R. I. Gregory, and S. Diederichs, "Many roads to maturity: microRNA biogenesis pathways and their regulation," *Nature Cell Biology*, vol. 11, no. 3, pp. 228–234, 2009.

[12] F. P. Schena and L. Gesualdo, "Pathogenetic mechanisms of diabetic nephropathy," *Journal of the American Society of Nephrology*, vol. 16, supplement 1, pp. S30–S33, 2005.

[13] X. Huang, Y.-X. Su, H.-C. Deng, M.-X. Zhang, J. Long, and Z.-G. Peng, "Suppression of mesangial cell proliferation and extracellular matrix production in streptozotocin-induced diabetic mice by adiponectin in vitro and in vivo," *Hormone and Metabolic Research*, vol. 46, no. 10, pp. 736–743, 2014.

[14] C. Lv, Y. H. Zhou, C. Wu, Y. Shao, C. Lu, and Q. Wang, "The changes in miR-130b levels in human serum and the correlation with the severity of diabetic nephropathy," *Diabetes/Metabolism Research and Reviews*, vol. 31, no. 7, pp. 717–724, 2015.

[15] N. F. Van Det, N. A. M. Verhagen, J. T. Tamsma et al., "Regulation of glomerular epithelial cell production of fibronectin and transforming growth factor-β by high glucose, not by angiotensin II," *Diabetes*, vol. 46, no. 5, pp. 834–840, 1997.

[16] K. Sharma, Y. Jin, J. Guo, and F. N. Ziyadeh, "Neutralization of TGF-β by anti-TGF-β antibody attenuates kidney hypertrophy and the enhanced extracellular matrix gene expression in STZ-induced diabetic mice," *Diabetes*, vol. 45, no. 4, pp. 522–530, 1996.

[17] S. Saal and S. J. Harvey, "MicroRNAs and the kidney: coming of age," *Current Opinion in Nephrology and Hypertension*, vol. 18, no. 4, pp. 317–323, 2009.

[18] P. Kantharidis, B. Wang, R. M. Carew, and H. Y. Lan, "Diabetes complications: the microRNA perspective," *Diabetes*, vol. 60, no. 7, pp. 1832–1837, 2011.

[19] H. Y. Lan and A. C.-K. Chung, "TGF-β/Smad signaling in kidney disease," *Seminars in Nephrology*, vol. 32, no. 3, pp. 236–243, 2012.

[20] A. C. K. Chung, Y. Dong, W. Yang, X. Zhong, R. Li, and H. Y. Lan, "Smad7 suppresses renal fibrosis via altering expression of TGF-β/Smad3-regulated microRNAs," *Molecular Therapy*, vol. 21, no. 2, pp. 388–398, 2013.

[21] A. J. Kriegel, Y. Liu, B. Cohen, K. Usa, Y. Liu, and M. Liang, "MiR-382 targeting of kallikrein 5 contributes to renal inner medullary interstitial fibrosis," *Physiological Genomics*, vol. 44, no. 4, pp. 259–267, 2012.

[22] A. J. Kriegel, Y. Fang, Y. Liu et al., "MicroRNA-target pairs in human renal epithelial cells treated with transforming growth factor beta 1: a novel role of miR-382," *Nucleic Acids Research*, vol. 38, no. 22, pp. 8338–8347, 2010.

[23] A. Krupa, R. Jenkins, D. D. Luo, A. Lewis, A. Phillips, and D. Fraser, "Loss of microRNA-192 promotes fibrogenesis in diabetic nephropathy," *Journal of the American Society of Nephrology*, vol. 21, no. 3, pp. 438–447, 2010.

[24] B. Wang, M. Herman-Edelstein, P. Koh et al., "E-cadherin expression is regulated by miR-192/215 by a mechanism that is independent of the profibrotic effects of transforming growth factor-β," *Diabetes*, vol. 59, no. 7, pp. 1794–1802, 2010.

[25] S. Putta, L. Lanting, G. Sun, G. Lawson, M. Kato, and R. Natarajan, "Inhibiting microRNA-192 ameliorates renal fibrosis in diabetic nephropathy," *Journal of the American Society of Nephrology*, vol. 23, no. 3, pp. 458–469, 2012.

[26] A. C. K. Chung, X. R. Huang, X. Meng, and H. Y. Lan, "miR-192 mediates TGF-beta/Smad3-driven renal fibrosis," *Journal of the American Society of Nephrology*, vol. 21, no. 8, pp. 1317–1325, 2010.

[27] X. Zhong, A. C. K. Chung, H.-Y. Chen, X.-M. Meng, and H. Y. Lan, "Smad3-mediated upregulation of miR-21 promotes renal fibrosis," *Journal of the American Society of Nephrology*, vol. 22, no. 9, pp. 1668–1681, 2011.

[28] S. D. Deshpande, S. Putta, M. Wang et al., "Transforming growth factor-β-induced cross talk between p53 and a microRNA in the pathogenesis of diabetic nephropathy," *Diabetes*, vol. 62, no. 9, pp. 3151–3162, 2013.

[29] M. Kato, L. Arce, M. Wang, S. Putta, L. Lanting, and R. Natarajan, "A microRNA circuit mediates transforming growth factor-beta1 autoregulation in renal glomerular mesangial cells," *Kidney International*, vol. 80, no. 4, pp. 358–368, 2011.

[30] M. Kato, V. Dang, M. Wang et al., "TGF-β induces acetylation of chromatin and of Ets-1 to alleviate repression of miR-192 in diabetic nephropathy," *Science Signaling*, vol. 6, no. 278, article ra43, 2013.

11

Fyn Mediates High Glucose-Induced Actin Cytoskeleton Reorganization of Podocytes via Promoting ROCK Activation *In Vitro*

Zhimei Lv,[1] Mengsi Hu,[1] Xiaoxu Ren,[1] Minghua Fan,[2] Junhui Zhen,[3] Liqun Chen,[4] Jiangong Lin,[1] Nannan Ding,[1] Qun Wang,[1] and Rong Wang[1]

[1]*Department of Nephrology, Provincial Hospital Affiliated to Shandong University, Jinan 250021, China*
[2]*Department of Obstetrics and Gynecology, Second Hospital of Shandong University, Jinan 250033, China*
[3]*Department of Pathology, Medical School of Shandong University, Jinan 250012, China*
[4]*Department of Nephrology, First Affiliated Hospital of Chongqing Medical University, Chongqing 400042, China*

Correspondence should be addressed to Rong Wang; sdwangrong@sina.cn

Academic Editor: Jennifer L. Wilkinson-Berka

Fyn, a member of the Src family of tyrosine kinases, is a key regulator in cytoskeletal remodeling in a variety of cell types. Recent studies have demonstrated that Fyn is responsible for nephrin tyrosine phosphorylation, which will result in polymerization of actin filaments and podocyte damage. Thus detailed involvement of Fyn in podocytes is to be elucidated. In this study, we investigated the potential role of Fyn/ROCK signaling and its interactions with paxillin. Our results presented that high glucose led to filamentous actin (F-actin) rearrangement in podocytes, accompanied by paxillin phosphorylation and increased cell motility, during which Fyn and ROCK were markedly activated. Gene knockdown of Fyn by siRNA showed a reversal effect on high glucose-induced podocyte damage and ROCK activation; however, inhibition of ROCK had no significant effects on Fyn phosphorylation. These observations demonstrate that *in vitro* Fyn mediates high glucose-induced actin cytoskeleton remodeling of podocytes via promoting ROCK activation and paxillin phosphorylation.

1. Introduction

Advanced albuminuria, one of the signatures of diabetic nephropathy, causes progressive loss of renal function and leads to terminal renal impairment. Damage to podocytes, which is considered to be a possible early pathological marker for diabetic nephropathy, is important due to its role in causing albuminuria and glomerular damage [1–3]. In diabetic nephropathy, it is necessary to study the regulation of the actin cytoskeleton directly in podocytes because the dysregulation of the highly specialized podocyte actin cytoskeleton is closely associated with albuminuria [4, 5]. Fyn is a member of the Src family of kinases, and it responds to many stimuli to facilitate downstream signaling that regulates cell growth, adhesion, and motility [6, 7]. Earlier reports have demonstrated that Fyn associates with multiple intracellular substrates, such as focal adhesion kinase (FAK), paxillin, and β-adducin, to regulate cytoskeletal architecture and cell-cell interactions [8, 9]. It resides in podocytes and binds directly to and phosphorylates nephrin during podocyte differentiation and in response to injury, and this phosphorylation event results in polymerization of actin filaments [10–12]. Rho-associated coiled-coil forming protein kinase (ROCK) is a downstream effector of the small G protein Rho, which has been implicated in a variety of biological functions including cell contraction, migration, adhesion, and gene expression. The ROCK kinases phosphorylate a variety of substrates, which collectively lead to increased myosin ATPase activity and inhibition of the depolymerisation of actin and the assembly of stress fibers and focal adhesions; these events contribute to the reorganization of the actin cytoskeleton [11, 13]. Furthermore, it has been shown that ROCK may be a pivotal downstream target of Fyn for F-actin formation in fibroblasts exposed to lysophosphatidic acid [14].

The activation of ROCK in the kidney has been confirmed in models of diabetes both *in vitro* and *in vivo* [15–17], whereas inhibition of ROCK ameliorated the structural changes in the diabetic kidney together with a modest antiproteinuric effect [18]. In this study, we aimed to reveal the role of the Fyn/ROCK signaling pathway in podocyte injury that was induced by high glucose and its interactions with paxillin. We found that exposure of podocytes to high glucose led to a rearrangement of the filamentous actin (F-actin), accompanied by paxillin phosphorylation and increased cell motility. Both knockdown of Fyn by siRNA and inhibition of ROCK by Y27632 suppressed high glucose-induced F-actin rearrangement and paxillin phosphorylation. These findings demonstrated that high glucose-induced podocyte F-actin rearrangement was associated with the activation of Fyn/ROCK signaling pathway and the axis-mediated phosphorylation of paxillin.

2. Materials and Methods

2.1. Cell-Culture and Pharmacological Treatments. Conditionally immortalized mouse podocytes (a kind gift from Professor Peter Mundel) were cultured on type I collagen-coated dishes in RPMI1640 (HyClone, Logan, Utah, USA) supplemented with 10% fetal bovine serum (HyClone, Logan, Utah, USA), 100 U/mL penicillin, and 100 mg/mL streptomycin (HyClone, Logan, Utah, USA) under permissive conditions 33°C plus 10 U/mL mouse recombinant γ-interferon (Pepro Technology, London, UK). Podocyte differentiation was induced by maintaining podocytes on type I collagen-coated dishes at 37°C without γ-interferon for at least 14 days. Differentiated podocytes between passages 15 and 20 were incubated in serum-free RPMI1640 medium for 24 hours before being subjected to different treatments.

To investigate the effect of high glucose stimulation on podocytes, cells were exposed to low glucose medium (RPMI1640 medium containing 5.5 mM glucose and 10% fetal bovine serum) or high glucose medium (RPMI1640 medium containing 30 mM glucose and 10% fetal bovine serum) for 48 hours. Podocytes incubated in RPMI1640 with 5.5 mM glucose plus 24.5 mM mannitol and 10% fetal bovine serum for 48 hours were considered as the control for osmolarity. Podocytes were pretreated with 10 μM Y27632 (Merck Chemicals Ltd., Nottingham, UK), an inhibitor reported to be specific for ROCK, for 30 minutes, and then incubated in high glucose medium for 48 hours to investigate whether ROCK is involved in high glucose-induced podocyte injury.

2.2. Fyn Gene Knockdown. RNA interfering technology was used during the investigation of Fyn as described below. Podocytes were prepared the day prior to transfection. Following incubation with Fyn siRNA or Cont-siRNA for 24 hours, podocytes were then either incubated in standard-glucose medium or high glucose medium for an additional 48 hours. Cells that were not transfected which were exposed to standard-glucose medium were considered to be controls. SiRNA oligonucleotides with the following sequences were designed: siRNA, 5′-CCTGTATGGAAGGTTCACAAT-3′; negative Cont-siRNA, 5′-TTCTCCGAACGTGTCACGT-3′. Transfection was performed in 24-well plates using 40 nM siRNAs in Lipofectamine 2000 (Invitrogen, Carlsbad, CA, USA). Fyn gene knockdown was confirmed by western blotting and quantitative real-time PCR.

2.3. Fyn Kinase Activity Assay. Podocytes were lysed in radioimmunoprecipitation assay (RIPA) buffer at 4°C for 10 minutes. Equal amounts of podocyte lysate were incubated with anti-Fyn antibody (Santa Cruz Biotechnology, CA, USA) at room temperature for 2 hours. Immunocomplexes were isolated using Protein A/G PLUS-Agarose (Santa Cruz Biotechnology, CA, USA) and recovered by boiling for 3 minutes in 1x electrophoresis buffer. Proteins were eluted with SDS-PAGE sample buffer and immunoblotted with anti-Src [PY418] (Invitrogen, CA, USA).

2.4. Measurement of ROCK Activity. The activity of ROCK was assessed by determining the phosphorylation state of myosin phosphatase targeting subunit 1 (MYPT1), a downstream target of ROCK, using anti-MYPT1 [PY853] antibody (Santa Cruz Biotechnology, CA, USA) and an appropriate secondary antibody (Jackson ImmunoResearch Laboratories, West Grove, PA) for immunoblotting.

2.5. Protein Isolation and Western Blotting Analyses. Cells were washed with PBS and lysed with 2x SDS-PAGE sample buffer. Next, 50 μg of total protein was separated by SDS-PAGE and transferred to nitrocellulose membranes; the membranes were then blocked with 1% polyvinylalcohol in PBS containing 0.2% Tween 20 for 10 minutes and incubated at 4°C overnight with primary antibodies diluted to various concentrations in blocking buffer (5% or 1% skim milk in PBS-Tween (0.2% Tween 20)) targeted against the following target proteins: Fyn (1:100), Src [PY418] (1:500), paxillin [PY31] (1:5000), desmin (1:500), vimentin (1:500), synaptopodin (1:200), MYPT1 [PY853] (1:200), or β-actin (1:200). The membranes were then washed three times with PBS-Tween for 10 minutes and incubated with specific peroxidase-conjugated secondary antibodies diluted in blocking buffer (5% skim milk in PBS-Tween) for 2 hours at room temperature. Specific bands were detected using the ECL system and the Bio-Rad electrophoresis image analyzer (Bio-Rad Laboratories, Hercules, CA).

2.6. RNA Extraction and Quantitative Real-Time PCR. Total RNA was extracted from cells using the TRIpure Reagent (Takara, Dalian, China) according to the manufacturer's instructions. RNA samples were quantified by measuring optical absorbance at 260 and 280 nm. A260/A280 ratios ranged from 1.8 to 2.0, which indicated a high purity of the extracted RNA. The concentration of total RNA was calculated based on A260. Aliquots of total RNA (1.0 μg each) from each sample were reverse-transcribed into cDNA according to the instructions of the PrimeScript RT Reagent Kit (Takara, Dalian, China). Quantitative real-time PCR was used to detect the specificity and knockdown efficiency of the Fyn siRNA and to determine the steady-state mRNA levels of synaptopodin and desmin and vimentin. Briefly, after reverse transcription of total RNA, cDNA was used as a template for the PCR reactions using gene-specific primer pairs. Amplification was performed using SYBR Premix Ex Taq Kit (Takara, Dalian, China) in the LightCycler 480 Real-Time PCR system (Roche Applied Science, Penzberg, Germany). The primers were purchased from Sangon Biotech Co., Ltd. (Shanghai, China). The designed sequences were as follows: synaptopodin: sense, 5′-CGGAGAATCAAAACCCTCAG-3′, antisense, 5′-CAGGACACTGCCATCAGACT-3′; desmin: sense, 5′-GTGAAGATGGCCTTGGATGT-3′, antisense, 5′-GCTGGTTTCTCGGAAGTTGA-3′; vimentin: sense, 5′-GATCAGCTCACCAACGACAA-3′, antisense, 5′-GCTTTCGGCTTCCTCTCTCT-3′; Fyn: sense, 5′-AAGGATAAAGAAGCAGCGAAAC-3′, antisense, 5′-TGCGTGGAAGTTGTTGTAGTTC-3′; β-actin: sense, 5′-GTGGGCCGCTCTAGGCACCAA-3′, antisense, 5′-CTCTTTGATGTCACGCACGATTTC-3′.

2.7. Immunofluorescence. Cells growing on glass slides were pretreated with different conditions and then fixed in 4% paraformaldehyde for 20 minutes followed by permeabilization in 0.3% Triton X-100 for 10 minutes. After preincubation with 5% bovine serum albumin to block nonspecific binding, cells were individually incubated with primary antibodies against synaptopodin (ProteinTech Group, Chicago, IL, USA), desmin (ImmunoWay, Newark, USA), vimentin (ProteinTech, Chicago, IL, USA), or paxillin [PY31] (Abcam Inc., Cambridge, MA, USA) at 4°C overnight. After washing, the slides were stained with Dylight 649-conjugated secondary antibodies (ZSGB-Bio, Beijing, China) and double-stained with DAPI to visualize nuclei. Cells were observed and images captured at randomly selected fields using an inverted phase fluorescence microscope (Leica, Wetzlar, Germany).

F-actin staining was in accordance with the procedure recommended by the dye manufacturer, and images were taken at randomly selected fields using an LSM780 confocal microscope (Carl Zeiss, Jena, Germany).

2.8. Transwell Migration Assay. Transwell cell-culture inserts (pore size 8 μm; Corning Costar Corp., Cambridge, MA, USA) were rinsed once with PBS and placed in RPMI1640 with 10% fetal bovine serum in the lower compartment. The heights of the medium in the upper and lower compartments were maintained at similar levels; thus, bulk flow was not due to a hydrostatic pressure gradient. Podocytes pretreated with different conditions were harvested with trypsin and resuspended in serum-free RPMI1640 medium; the upper chambers were seeded with $1 \times 10^4\ mL^{-1}$ cells, which were then allowed to attach for 6 hours. After incubation for 12 hours at 37°C, nonmigratory cells were removed from the upper surface of the membrane using cotton-tipped applicators, and migrating cells were fixed with 4% paraformaldehyde and stained with Hematoxylin. The number of migrating cells in the center of a membrane (one field) was counted using phase contrast microscopy (Leica, Wetzlar, Germany). The data presented denote the mean ± SD of 6 independent experiments.

2.9. Wound-Healing Assay. Confluent monolayers of podocytes seeded onto type I collagen-coated six-well plates were pretreated with different conditions and scraped with a 20 μL pipette and then allowed to migrate for 12 hours. The percentage of wound closure was captured using an inverted phase contrast microscope (Leica, Wetzlar, Germany) and calculated using NIH ImageJ. Migratory rates were calculated as $(A - B)/A \times 100\%$, where A and B reflect the width of the wound at 0 or 12 hours, respectively. The data denote the mean ± SD of 6 independent experiments.

2.10. Statistical Analyses. The experiments were repeated at least three times. SPSS13.0 software was used for data analysis. Values are presented as the mean ± SD. Statistical significance was assessed using LSD t-tests and ANOVAs, and values of $P < 0.05$ were considered statistically significant.

3. Results

3.1. High Glucose Causes F-Actin Cytoskeleton Rearrangements and Injury to Podocytes. Podocyte foot processes (PFPs) are characterized by a podocome-like cortical network of branched actin filaments, which are linked to the glomerular basement membrane at focal contacts to modulate the permeability of the filtration barrier via changes in PFP morphology [19, 20]. In this study, morphological changes of podocytes under different conditions were captured using a confocal microscope. Podocytes under low glucose conditions demonstrated that F-actin is distributed as obvious homogenous bundles that traverse the cell along the axis of the podocyte (Figure 1). Exposure to high osmotic pressure for 48 hours caused no significant effect compared with incubation in a low glucose concentration. Podocytes stimulated with high glucose for 48 hours showed an assembly of F-actin in cortical regions, agminated F-actin along the cell periphery, and a slightly diffuse cytoplasmic distribution (Figure 1).

To fully characterize the changes in podocytes stimulated by high glucose, we further examined the expression of synaptopodin, desmin, and vimentin. Synaptopodin is an important actin-associated protein, a decrease of which has been confirmed as a remarkable phenomenon during podocytopathy [21–23]. Vimentin and desmin, which are known markers of podocyte injury [24, 25], were also assessed in this study. We observed that podocytes cultured for 48 hours in high glucose demonstrated a significant downregulation of synaptopodin compared with podocytes cultured in low glucose conditions, at both the protein and mRNA levels (Figure 2), whereas high osmotic pressure showed no obvious effects. The effects of high glucose on synaptopodin expression were further confirmed by immunofluorescence, where reduced fluorescence staining was observed (Figure 2). Moreover, significant increases in desmin and vimentin expression were also detected, at both the protein and mRNA levels following 48 hours of incubation in high glucose, compared with incubation with low glucose (Figures 3 and 4). Increased fluorescent staining further confirmed the high glucose-induced overexpression of desmin and vimentin in podocytes (Figures 3 and 4).

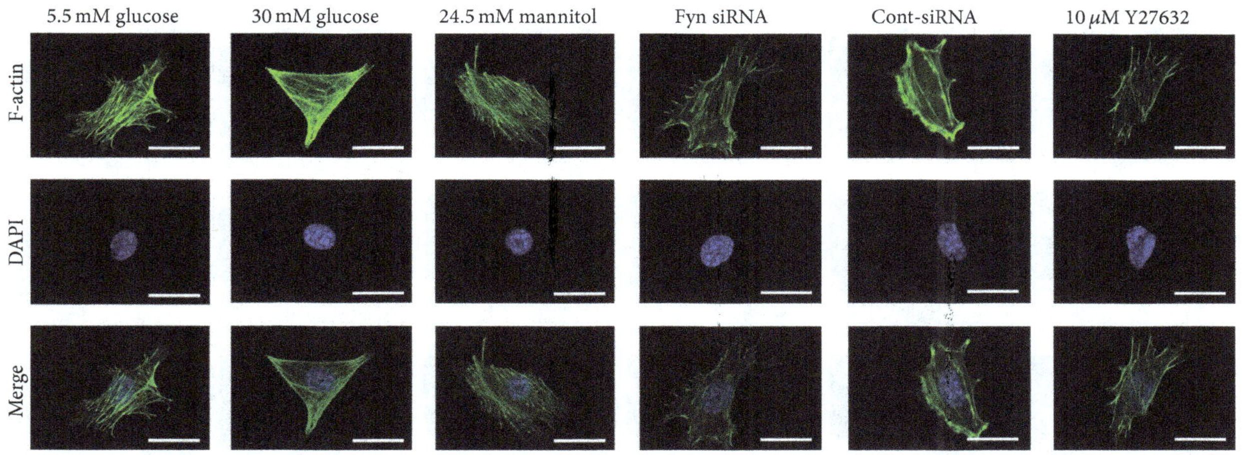

FIGURE 1: Reorganization of the F-actin cytoskeleton in podocytes by confocal microscopy. Podocytes under 5.5 mM glucose conditions (column 1) demonstrated that F-actin is distributed as obvious homogenous bundles that traverse the cell along the axis of the podocyte. 30 mM glucose stimulation for 48 hours (column 2) showed an assembly of F-actin in cortical regions, agminated F-actin along the cell periphery, and a slightly diffuse cytoplasmic distribution. Podocytes transfected with Fyn siRNA and then stimulated by 30 mM glucose for 48 hours (column 4) showed reversed F-actin distribution. Pretreatment with 10 μM Y27632 for 30 minutes revealed similar F-actin amelioration (column 6). Podocytes that were exposed to high osmotic pressure (column 3) or transfected with Cont-siRNA (column 6) were considered as controls.

3.2. Fyn Is Involved in High Glucose-Induced Podocyte F-Actin Cytoskeleton Remodeling. As a member of the Src family of kinases, Fyn is known as a nonreceptor tyrosine kinase that responds to many stimuli to regulate the cytoskeleton and process formation. The activity of Fyn is regulated by intramolecular interactions and depends upon the phosphorylation state of two tyrosine residues, Y529 and Y418. Dephosphorylation of Y529 results in autophosphorylation at Y418 in the activation loop of the catalytic domain of Fyn, thereby stabilizing it in the active conformation [9, 26]. To detect activated Fyn, podocyte lysates were immunoprecipitated with anti-Fyn antibody followed by western blotting with anti-Src [PY418] antibody. As demonstrated by the western blotting (Figure 5), high glucose promoted Fyn activation in podocytes compared with cells incubated in low glucose conditions, with no alterations in total Fyn expression noted. To gain insight into the mechanism of the high glucose-induced podocyte F-actin cytoskeleton reorganization, we utilized a small interfering RNA (siRNA) to knock Fyn expression down. To validate the efficiency of the Fyn siRNA, podocytes were transfected with Fyn siRNA for 24 hours and then incubated in low glucose medium for another 48 hours. A significant reduction of Fyn at both the protein and mRNA levels was detected (Figure 6). Podocytes transfected with Fyn siRNA for 24 hours and then incubated under high glucose conditions for 48 hours were used to perform further experiments. The high glucose-induced F-actin cytoskeleton reorganization was markedly ameliorated by Fyn gene knockdown (Figure 1). Furthermore, after silencing Fyn expression with siRNA, the alterations to synaptopodin, desmin, and vimentin were also ameliorated (Figures 2, 3, and 4).

3.3. ROCK Is Involved in High Glucose-Induced Podocyte F-Actin Cytoskeleton Remodeling. ROCK is a critical Rho effector in the regulation of F-actin, focal adhesion formation, cell morphology, and cell motility. The activation of Rho/ROCK in the kidney has been confirmed in models of diabetes both *in vitro* and *in vivo* [15–17]. Here, we demonstrated that podocytes cultured in high glucose for 48 hours showed increased ROCK activity compared with podocytes incubated in low glucose conditions, shown by the increase in phosphorylation of MYPT1 [27], a downstream target of ROCK (Figure 7). Knocking down Fyn with siRNA reversed the upregulation of ROCK activity stimulated by high glucose. Pretreatment with 10 μM Y27632, an inhibitor specific to ROCK, for 30 minutes, inhibited effectively the high glucose-induced ROCK activation (Figure 7), with no significant alteration to total Fyn expression noted (Figure 5). The F-actin reorganization induced by high glucose was remarkably ameliorated by pretreatment with Y27632 (Figure 1). Moreover, the high glucose-induced alterations to synaptopodin, desmin, and vimentin were also partially reversed in the presence of Y27632, at both protein and mRNA levels (Figures 2, 3, and 4).

3.4. Under High Glucose Conditions, Paxillin Is Phosphorylated in Podocytes. Paxillin is a phosphorylation-dependent protein that links the intracellular actin cytoskeleton to integrin-rich adhesion sites. The phosphorylation of paxillin tyrosine residue 31 (Y31) is particularly important and prevalent in regulating downstream signaling and causes profound effects on the cytoskeleton, cell adhesion, and movement [28–30]. In this study, an increase in tyrosine phosphorylation of paxillin at Y31, which has been shown to be an effector of high glucose, was detected. Incubation with high glucose medium for 48 hours enhanced tyrosine phosphorylation of paxillin at Y31 compared with podocytes incubated in low glucose conditions or exposed to high osmotic pressure,

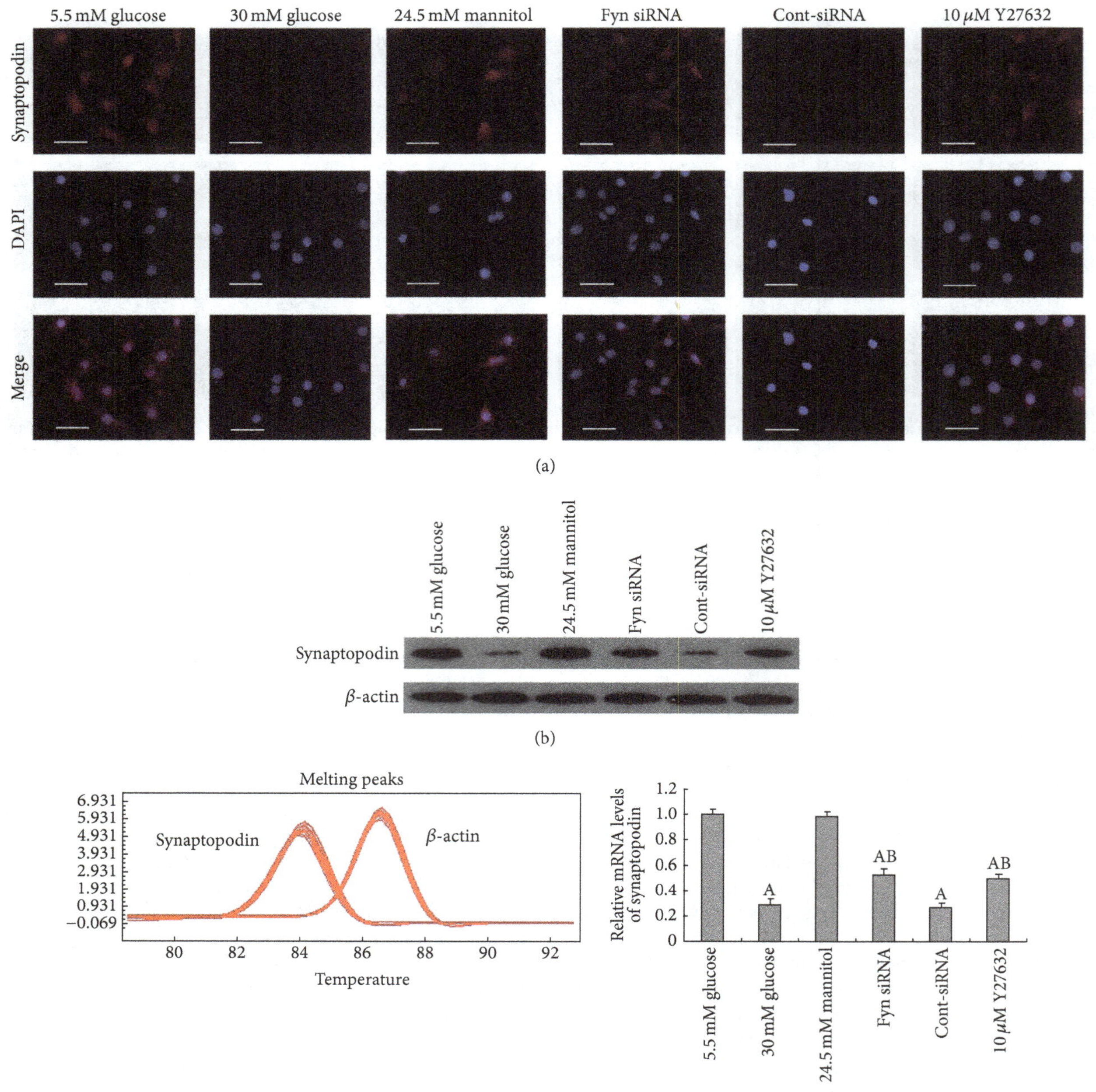

FIGURE 2: Alterations of protein and mRNA levels of synaptopodin in podocytes. Immunofluorescence (a), western blot (b), and real-time PCR (c) revealed that synaptopodin expression was markedly decreased following 48-hour incubation with 30 mM glucose (column 2) when compared with cells incubated in 5.5 mM glucose (column 1) on both protein and mRNA levels. Transfection with Fyn siRNA (column 4) or pretreatment with 10 μM Y27632 for 30 minutes (column 6) partially reversed these alterations. Control podocytes were treated with 5.5 mM glucose plus 24.5 mM mannitol (column 3) or transfected with Cont-siRNA (column 5). Magnification: 400x. Values denote the mean ± SD; ${}^{A}P < 0.05$ versus 5.5 mM glucose and ${}^{B}P < 0.05$ versus 30 mM glucose.

without alterations of total paxillin expression; high glucose promoted paxillin phosphorylation at Y31 was markedly decreased by both Fyn knockdown and ROCK inhibition (Figure 8). Moreover, the immunofluorescence data showed that the distribution of phosphorylated paxillin was predominantly along the cell periphery and was associated with reorganized F-actin (Figure 9). These findings suggested that the Fyn/ROCK signaling pathway potentially interacted with paxillin in podocytes under high glucose conditions.

3.5. High Glucose Promotes Podocyte Spreading and Migration. To examine coordinated sheet migration, we next performed a scrap-wound-healing assay on a monolayer of podocytes. Compared with podocytes in standard-glucose conditions,

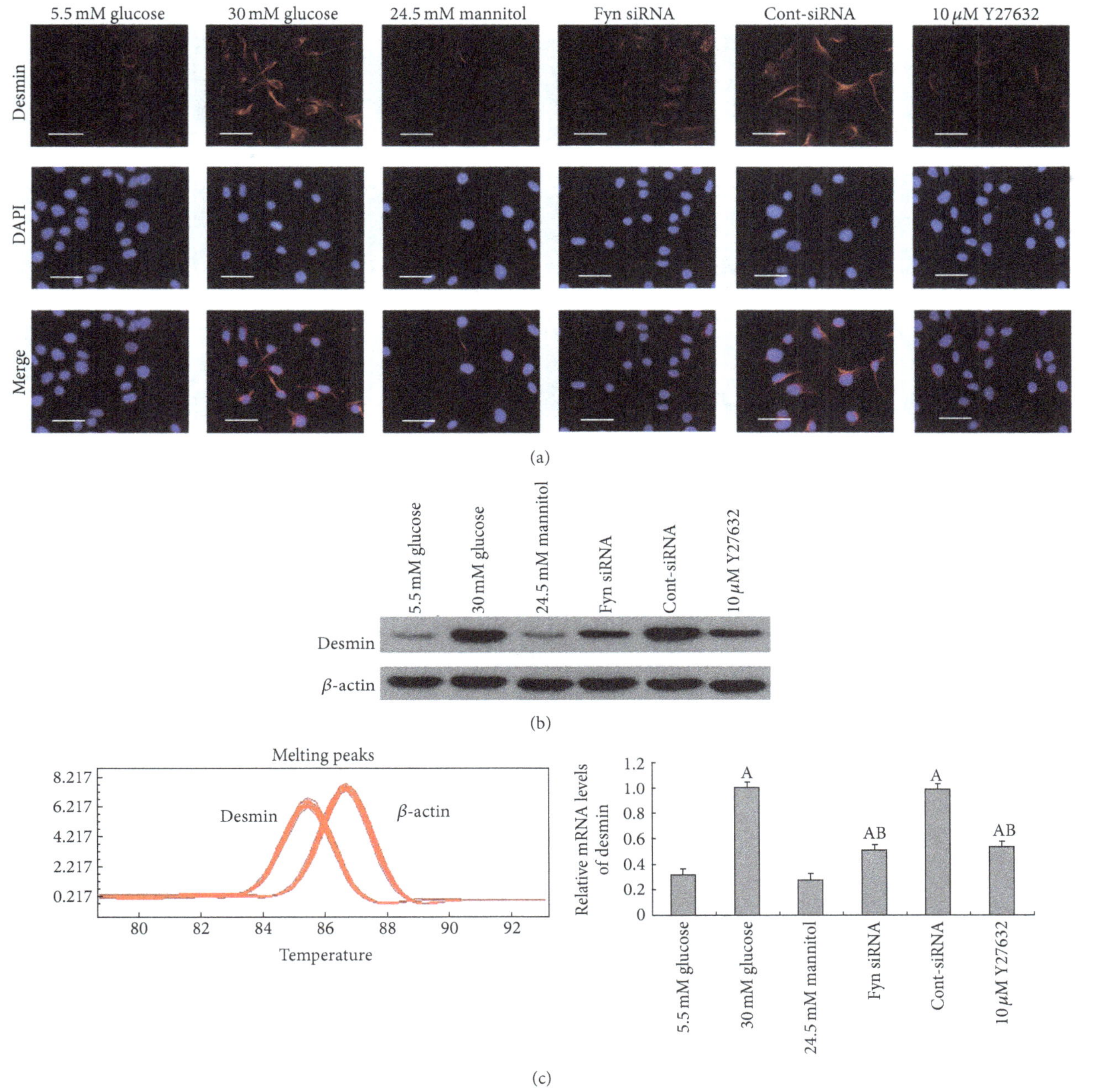

FIGURE 3: Changes of desmin on protein and mRNA levels in podocytes under different stimulations. Immunofluorescence (a), western blot (b), and real-time PCR (c) presented that desmin protein was increased markedly following incubation with 30 mM glucose for 48 hours (column 2), and the increase was partially inhibited by transfection with Fyn siRNA for 24 hours (column 4) or pretreatment with 10 μM Y27632 for 30 minutes (column 6). Control podocytes were treated with Cont-siRNA (column 5) or 5.5 mM glucose plus 24.5 mM mannitol (column 3). Magnification: 400x. Values denote the mean ± SD; $^{A}P < 0.05$ versus 5.5 mM glucose and $^{B}P < 0.05$ versus 30 mM glucose.

high glucose increased the speed at which the podocyte monolayer filled a uniform-width scratch wound in. Both Fyn gene knockdown and inhibition of ROCK slowed high glucose podocyte wound healing (Figures 10(a) and 10(c)). Next, we used the modified transwell migration assay and wound-healing assay to test the motility of cultured podocytes in different conditions. Podocytes subjected to high glucose showed significantly increased cell migration through the transwell filters compared with those incubated in low glucose or high osmotic pressure conditions. This effect was reversed partially by both Fyn gene knockdown and inhibition of ROCK (Figures 10(b) and 10(d)).

4. Discussion

Podocytes possess a contractile structure, composed of abundant microfilaments that modulate glomerular filtration,

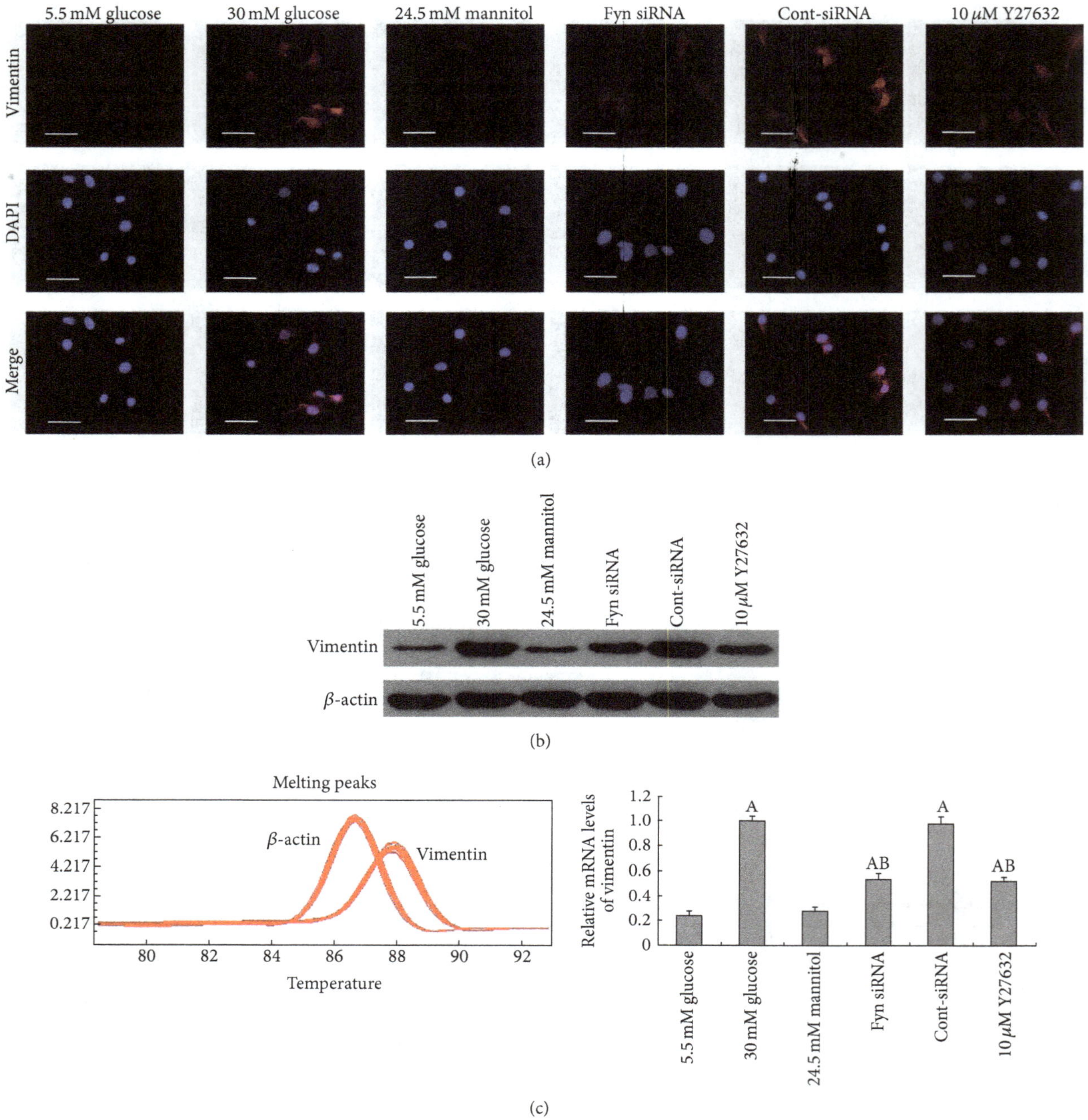

FIGURE 4: Alterations of vimentin on protein and mRNA levels in podocytes under different stimulations. Immunofluorescence (a), western blot (b), and real-time PCR (c) presented that vimentin expression was increased markedly following incubation with 30 mM glucose for 48 hours (column 2), and the increase was partially inhibited by transfection with Fyn siRNA for 24 hours (column 4) or pretreatment with 10 μM Y27632 for 30 minutes (column 6). Control podocytes were treated with Cont-siRNA (column 5) or 5.5 mM glucose plus 24.5 mM mannitol (column 3). Magnification: 400x. Values denote the mean ± SD; $^{A}P < 0.05$ versus 5.5 mM glucose and $^{B}P < 0.05$ versus 30 mM glucose.

and their structure is based on an actin cytoskeleton [4, 5]. Interference with cytoskeleton interactions with the slit diaphragm or defects in cytoskeletal components will cause foot process effacement, alterations in cell motility, and disruption of kidney filtration. Accumulating evidence has indicated that podocyte damage is a prerequisite for diabetic nephropathy, which, characterized by advanced albuminuria, has become one of the leading cause of end-stage renal disease [31]. It has been recently shown that effacement of podocyte foot processes occurs in diabetic nephropathy and that it is accompanied by a rearrangement of the actin cytoskeleton [3, 5, 32]. The podocyte cytoskeletal system includes actin regulatory proteins, such as α-actinin-4, synaptopodin, and the most important component called F-actin [4].

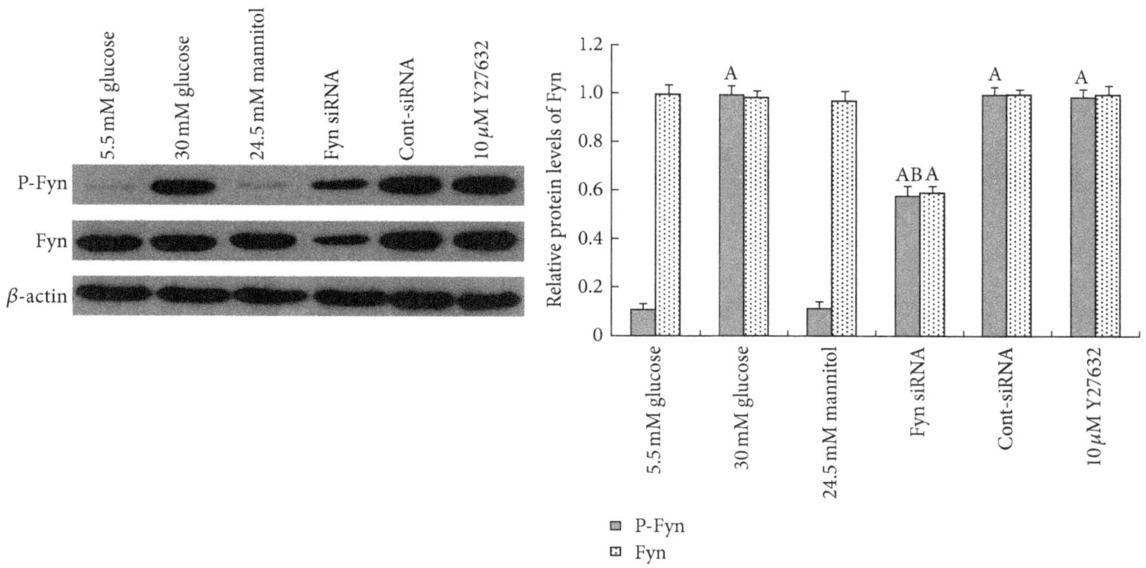

FIGURE 5: Western blot analysis of alterations to Fyn expression and Fyn activation in podocytes. Levels of activated Fyn exhibited a remarkable upregulation after 48-hour incubation with 30 mM glucose (lane 2) compared with cells incubated with 5.5 mM glucose (lane 1). Fyn siRNA significantly downregulated Fyn expression and activity (lane 4), whereas pretreatment with 10 μM Y27632 for 30 minutes showed little effects on Fyn activation (lane 5). Control podocytes were treated with 5.5 mM glucose plus 24.5 mM mannitol for 48 hours (lane 3) or transfected with Cont-siRNA (lane 5). Values denote the mean ± SD; $^{A}P < 0.05$ versus 5.5 mM glucose and $^{B}P < 0.05$ versus 30 mM glucose.

The actin cytoskeleton plays a crucial role in regulating the movement of cells via the highly dynamic and reversible polymerization of actin filaments, which provides the internal mechanical support that drives cell motility [4, 5]. In this study, under normal glucose conditions, podocytes showed obvious homogenous F-actin bundle distribution along the axis. Exposure to high glucose conditions for 48 hours led to the assembly of F-actin into cortical regions. And modified transwell migration assays and wound-healing assays revealed an increase in spreading and migration of podocytes cultured in high glucose conditions. Podocytes stimulated with high glucose showed significantly increased cell migration through transwell filters compared with cells subjected to normal glucose and high osmotic pressure conditions. Much work has demonstrated that increased podocyte motility may be an important aspect of podocytes depletion [4, 33, 34]. Therefore, it appeared that high glucose-induced dynamic rearrangement of the podocyte actin cytoskeleton, which subsequently promoted podocyte migration, which may initiate the depletion of podocytes and a vicious cycle of progressive glomerular damage.

Synaptopodin is an important marker of podocyte foot processes necessary for the maintenance of appropriate process structure and function in podocytes. A decrease in synaptopodin has been confirmed as an important phenomenon in podocytopathy [21, 22]. The results of this study demonstrate a significant decrease in synaptopodin expression at both mRNA and protein levels in podocytes cultured in high glucose conditions. Increased expression of desmin and vimentin, both observed in the present study, is associated with damage to podocytes in diabetic nephropathy [23, 24] and several other renal disease models [25, 35]. These observations revealed that high glucose-induced podocyte injury, characterized by a significant downregulation of synaptopodin together with an upregulation of desmin and vimentin at both mRNA and protein levels.

Fyn tyrosine kinase, a member of the Src family protein tyrosine kinases, has been suggested to be involved in cytoskeletal regulation and cell-process branching in a variety of cell types [6–9, 12]. Fyn is necessary for neuronal synaptic regulation, and overexpression of Fyn exacerbates neurodegeneration [36]. Since podocytes and neurons share many structural and molecular features, a similar mechanism may be involved in the modulation of podocyte processes [37]. Previous studies have shown that, in podocytes, Fyn directly binds to nephrin and phosphorylates the latter at tyrosine residues during podocyte differentiation [12]. In our study, we found that the high glucose stimulation led to the activation of Fyn, accompanied by a rearrangement of F-actin bundles. Gene knockdown of Fyn by its specific siRNA ameliorated this high glucose-induced Fyn activation and F-actin remodeling, suggesting that Fyn is a triggering factor for F-actin cytoskeletal rearrangement under high glucose conditions.

ROCK, the best studied downstream target of RhoA, is involved in a myriad of signaling cascades including the regulation of stress fibers, focal adhesion formation, and cell motility. It is also a pivotal controller of the actin cytoskeleton during cell morphogenesis and migration [11, 13, 14, 16]. In the kidney, ROCK activation was found in models of diabetes both *in vitro* and *in vivo* [15–17]. And inhibition of ROCK helped ameliorate structural changes in the kidney together with a modest antiproteinuric effect [18]. Our results presented that ROCK could be activated

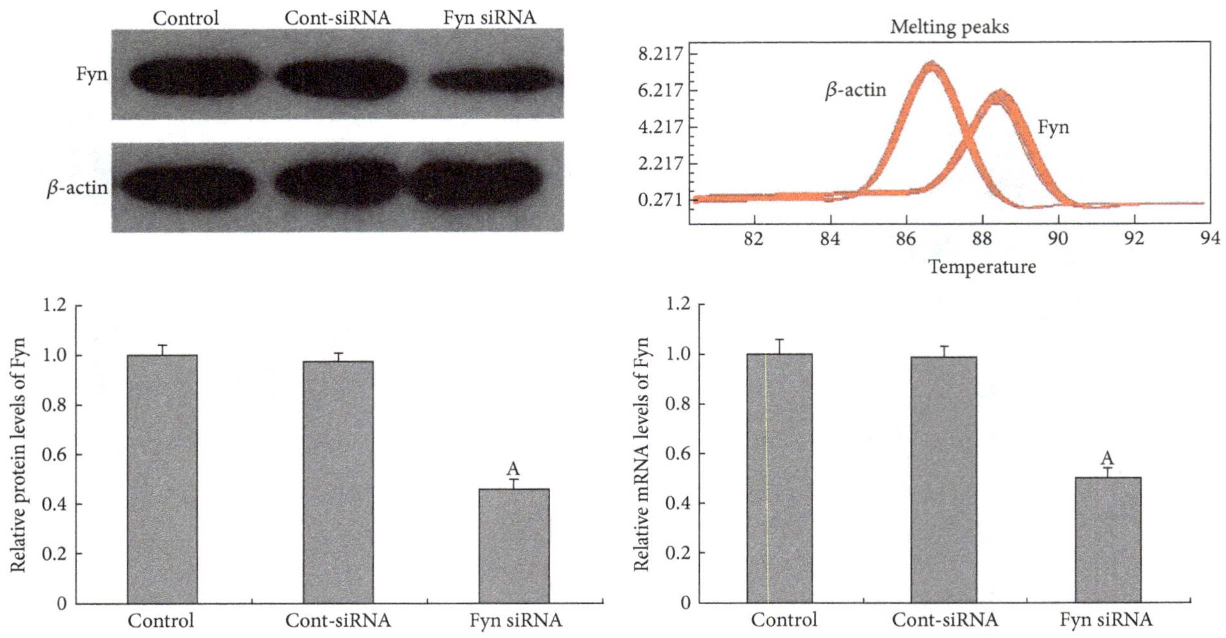

FIGURE 6: Fyn siRNA gene knockdown effects on Fyn expression in podocytes by western blotting and quantitative real-time PCR. A 24-hour transfection with Fyn siRNA notably reduced the expression of Fyn in cells treated with 5.5 mM glucose on both protein and mRNA levels (lane 3). Fyn expression was not significantly altered in podocytes transfected with Cont-siRNA for 24 hours (lane 2) compared with untransfected cells treated with 5.5 mM glucose (lane 1). Values denote the mean ± SD; $^{A}P < 0.05$ versus 5.5 mM glucose.

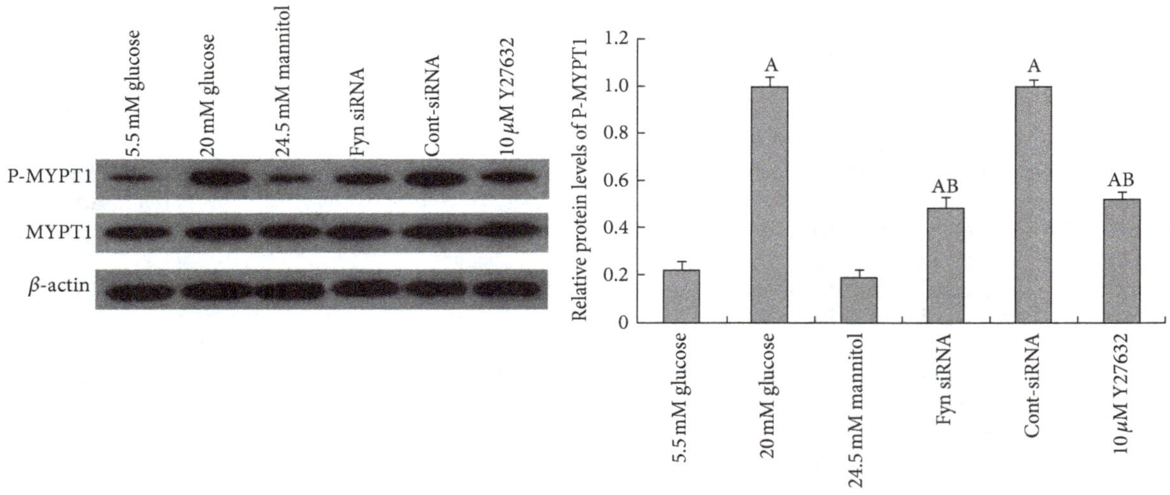

FIGURE 7: Western blotting analysis of alterations to ROCK activity in podocytes. ROCK activity was analyzed by determining the phosphorylation state of MYPT1, a downstream target of ROCK. The phosphorylation status of MYPT1 was significantly enhanced after 48-hour incubation with 30 mM glucose (lane 2) compared with cells incubated with 5.5 mM glucose (lane 1). Transfection with Fyn siRNA for 24 hours (lane 4) or pretreatment with 10 μM Y27632 for 30 minutes (lane 6) decreased MYPT1 phosphorylation. Control podocytes were treated with Cont-siRNA (lane 5) or 5.5 mM glucose plus 24.5 mM mannitol (lane 3). Values denote the mean ± SD; $^{A}P < 0.05$ versus 5.5 mM glucose and $^{B}P < 0.05$ versus 30 mM glucose.

by high glucose stimulation, which occurred concomitantly with the rearrangement of F-actin. Pretreatment of Y27632, the ROCK inhibitor, showed decreased activity of ROCK and partially reversed F-actin remodeling. Prior studies have suggested that, in fibroblasts, Fyn kinase may act as an upstream factor of ROCK in the pathway governing the cytoskeletal changes and process remodeling [14, 38]. In our study, we found that gene knockdown of Fyn remarkably inhibited ROCK activation, with reversed F-actin remodeling, whereas pretreatment of Y27632 showed no significant effects on total Fyn or phosphorylated Fyn expression, suggesting that, under high glucose conditions, Fyn

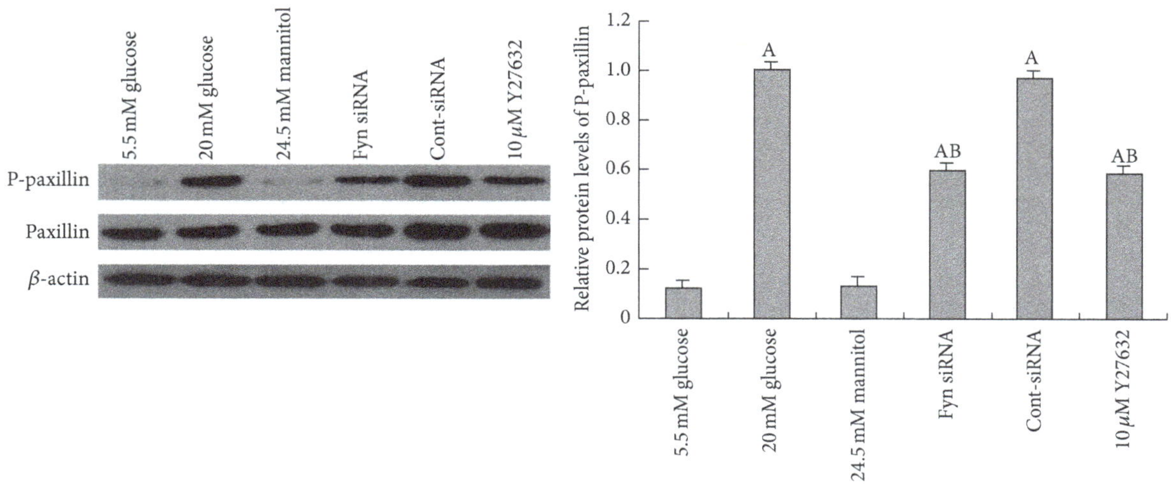

FIGURE 8: Western blotting analysis of the phosphorylation levels of paxillin in podocytes. The phosphorylation of paxillin (PY31) was significantly increased after a 48-hour incubation with 30 mM glucose (lane 2) compared with cells incubated with 5.5 mM glucose (lane 1), and no alterations in total paxillin expression were noted. Transfection with Fyn siRNA for 24 hours (lane 4) or pretreatment with 10 μM Y27632 for 30 minutes (lane 6) partially decreased high glucose-induced paxillin phosphorylation. Control podocytes were treated with Cont-siRNA (lane 5) or 5.5 mM glucose plus 24.5 mM mannitol (lane 3). Values denote the mean ± SD; $^{A}P < 0.05$ versus 5.5 mM glucose and $^{B}P < 0.05$ versus 30 mM glucose.

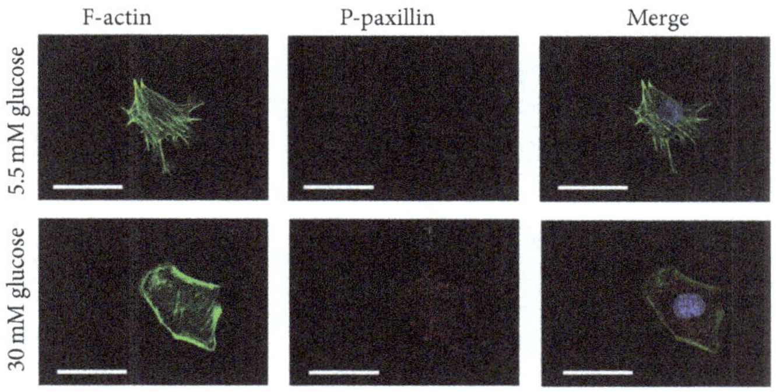

FIGURE 9: F-actin and paxillin expression by immunofluorescence. Under low glucose conditions (column 1), paxillin phosphorylation was undetectable and F-actin was distributed along the cell axis. After 48 hours of 30 mM glucose stimulation (column 2), the activation of paxillin was markedly upregulated with F-actin expressed at the cortical regions of the podocytes. Magnification: 400x.

promoted F-actin cytoskeletal remodeling via activation of ROCK.

Paxillin serves as a phosphorylation-dependent signaling scaffold, functioning in integrating and disseminating signals that affect cell adhesion, motility, and actin cytoskeletal remodeling [27]. A recent study suggested that lipopolysaccharide-induced podocyte injury was accompanied by increased paxillin phosphorylation and cell spreading [39]. In this study, we observed significantly upregulated paxillin phosphorylation in podocytes after high glucose treatment, which occurred concomitantly with F-actin bundles redistribution. Extensive research on cancer has documented that Fyn associates with intracellular substrates like FAK, paxillin, and β-adducin to regulate cytoskeletal architecture and cell-cell interactions [8, 40, 41]. In human umbilical vein endothelial cells, the activation of the ROCK signaling pathway was followed by tyrosine phosphorylation of paxillin, which further led to actin reorganization [42]. Inhibition of ROCK, however, could attenuate bombesin-induced increase in tyrosine phosphorylation of paxillin in Swiss 3T3 cells [43]. Our findings provided credible data that the upregulation of paxillin activity by high glucose was markedly abolished by Fyn gene knockdown or pretreatment of ROCK inhibitor, demonstrating that high glucose-stimulated phosphorylation of paxillin was in close association with Fyn/ROCK signaling pathway in cultured podocytes. Kleveta et al. found that LPS-induced phosphorylation of paxillin was responsible for the actin reassembly in macrophage and reassembly-associated cell motility. It is hypothesized that reorganization of F-actin may be regulated by phosphorylated paxillin under high glucose conditions, which was triggered by the activation of Fyn/ROCK signaling pathway.

The dynamic regulation of the podocyte cytoskeleton is paramount for the appropriate function of kidney filtration

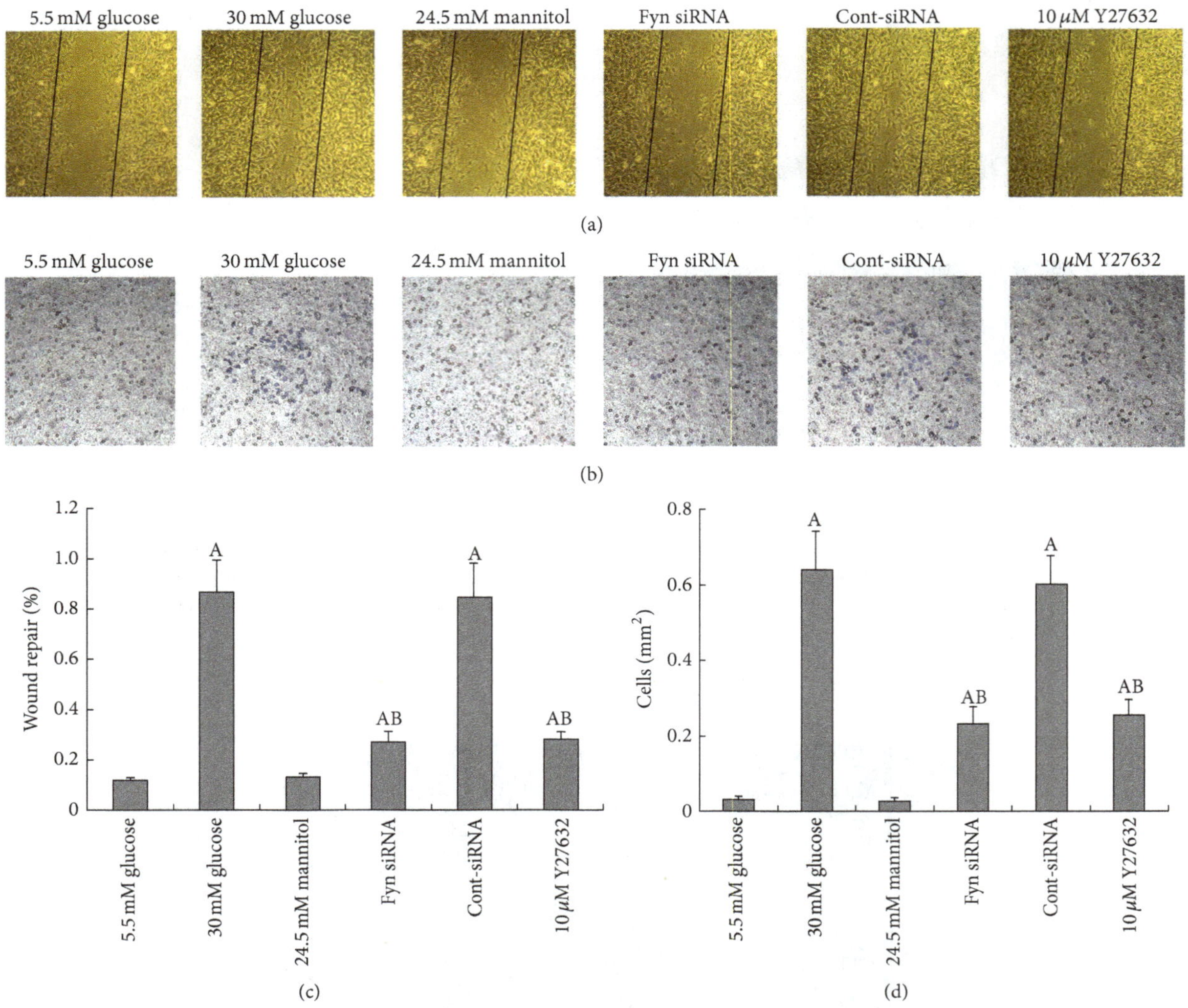

FIGURE 10: Podocyte motility by wound-healing assay and transwell migration assay. The wound-healing assay (a) and the modified transwell migration assay (b) were performed. Podocytes showed little migration when incubated in 5.5 mM glucose (column 1). Stimulation with 30 mM glucose-induced increased migration of podocytes (column 2), which was partially decreased by transfection with Fyn siRNA for 48 hours (column 4) or pretreatment with 10 μM Y27632 for 30 minutes (column 6). Control podocytes were treated with Cont-siRNA (column 5) or 5.5 mM glucose plus 24.5 mM mannitol (column 3). Magnification: 200x.

barrier. In the current study, we sought further confirmation that the reorganization of the F-actin cytoskeleton, along with paxillin phosphorylation and increased cell motility, is a consequence of Fyn/ROCK signaling pathway activation in high glucose-induced podocyte injury, represented by alterations to synaptopodin, desmin, and vimentin expression. These observations shed light on one possible mechanism responsible for podocyte dysfunction in diabetes mellitus and may facilitate the development of novel strategies for treating diabetic nephropathy by targeting cytoskeletal rearrangement in podocytes.

Conflict of Interests

The authors declare that there is no conflict of interests regarding the publication of this paper.

Acknowledgments

This study was supported by the National Natural Science Foundation of China (Grant nos. 81370834 and 81400732), Shandong Young Scientists Award Fund (2010BSB14076), and Chinese Society of Nephrology Scientific Fund (14050480585). The authors thank Dr. Wan Qiang for the review and suggestions for the paper.

References

[1] K. Susztak, A. C. Raff, M. Schiffer, and E. P. Böttinger, "Glucose-induced reactive oxygen species cause apoptosis of podocytes and podocyte depletion at the onset of diabetic nephropathy," *Diabetes*, vol. 55, no. 1, pp. 225–233, 2006.

[2] G. Wolf, S. Chen, and F. N. Ziyadeh, "From the periphery of the glomerular capillary wall toward the center of disease: podocyte

injury comes of age in diabetic nephropathy," *Diabetes*, vol. 54, no. 6, pp. 1626–1634, 2005.

[3] E. J. Weil, K. V. Lemley, C. C. Mason et al., "Podocyte detachment and reduced glomerular capillary endothelial fenestration promote kidney disease in type 2 diabetic nephropathy," *Kidney International*, vol. 82, no. 9, pp. 1010–1017, 2012.

[4] C. Faul, K. Asanuma, E. Yanagida-Asanuma, K. Kim, and P. Mundel, "Actin up: regulation of podocyte structure and function by components of the actin cytoskeleton," *Trends in Cell Biology*, vol. 17, no. 9, pp. 428–437, 2007.

[5] S. J. Shankland, "The podocyte's response to injury: role in proteinuria and glomerulosclerosis," *Kidney International*, vol. 69, no. 12, pp. 2131–2147, 2006.

[6] D. Smyth, V. Phan, A. Wang, and D. M. McKay, "Interferon-γ-induced increases in intestinal epithelial macromolecular permeability requires the Src kinase Fyn," *Laboratory Investigation*, vol. 91, no. 5, pp. 764–777, 2011.

[7] J. W. Um, H. B. Nygaard, J. K. Heiss et al., "Alzheimer amyloid-β oligomer bound to postsynaptic prion protein activates Fyn to impair neurons," *Nature Neuroscience*, vol. 15, no. 9, pp. 1227–1235, 2012.

[8] E. M. Posadas, H. Al-Ahmadie, V. L. Robinson et al., "FYN is overexpressed in human prostate cancer," *BJU International*, vol. 103, no. 2, pp. 171–177, 2009.

[9] Y. D. Saito, A. R. Jensen, R. Salgia, and E. M. Posadas, "Fyn: a novel molecular target in cancer," *Cancer*, vol. 116, no. 7, pp. 1629–1637, 2010.

[10] H. Li, S. Lemay, L. Aoudjit, H. Kawachi, and T. Takano, "Src-family kinase Fyn phosphorylates the cytoplasmic domain of nephrin and modulates its interaction with podocin," *Journal of the American Society of Nephrology*, vol. 15, no. 12, pp. 3006–3015, 2004.

[11] M. Maekawa, T. Ishizaki, S. Boku et al., "Signaling from Rho to the actin cytoskeleton through protein kinases ROCK and LIM-kinase," *Science*, vol. 285, no. 5429, pp. 895–898, 1999.

[12] R. Verma, B. Wharram, I. Kovari et al., "Fyn binds to and phosphorylates the kidney slit diaphragm component Nephrin," *The Journal of Biological Chemistry*, vol. 278, no. 23, pp. 20716–20723, 2003.

[13] S. Narumiya, M. Tanji, and T. Ishizaki, "Rho signaling, ROCK and mDia1, in transformation, metastasis and invasion," *Cancer and Metastasis Reviews*, vol. 28, no. 1-2, pp. 65–76, 2009.

[14] D. Xu, H. Kishi, H. Kawamichi, K. Kajiya, Y. Takada, and S. Kobayashi, "Involvement of Fyn tyrosine kinase in actin stress fiber formation in fibroblasts," *FEBS Letters*, vol. 581, no. 27, pp. 5227–5233, 2007.

[15] A. Gojo, K. Utsunomiya, K. Taniguchi et al., "The Rho-kinase inhibitor, fasudil, attenuates diabetic nephropathy in streptozotocin-induced diabetic rats," *European Journal of Pharmacology*, vol. 568, no. 1–3, pp. 242–247, 2007.

[16] Y. Kikuchi, M. Yamada, T. Imakiire et al., "A Rho-kinase inhibitor, fasudil, prevents development of diabetes and nephropathy in insulin-resistant diabetic rats," *Journal of Endocrinology*, vol. 192, no. 3, pp. 595–603, 2007.

[17] F. Peng, D. Wu, B. Gao et al., "RhoA/Rho-kinase contribute to the pathogenesis of diabetic renal disease," *Diabetes*, vol. 57, no. 6, pp. 1683–1692, 2008.

[18] R. Komers, T. T. Oyama, D. R. Beard et al., "Rho kinase inhibition protects kidneys from diabetic nephropathy without reducing blood pressure," *Kidney International*, vol. 79, no. 4, pp. 432–442, 2011.

[19] P. Mundel, J. Reiser, A. Z. M. Borja et al., "Rearrangements of the cytoskeleton and cell contacts induce process formation during differentiation of conditionally immortalized mouse podocyte cell lines," *Experimental Cell Research*, vol. 236, no. 1, pp. 248–258, 1997.

[20] H. Pavenstädt, W. Kriz, and M. Kretzler, "Cell biology of the glomerular podocyte," *Physiological Reviews*, vol. 83, no. 1, pp. 253–307, 2003.

[21] S. Doublier, G. Salvidio, E. Lupia et al., "Nephrin expression is reduced in human diabetic nephropathy: evidence for a distinct role for glycated albumin and angiotensin II," *Diabetes*, vol. 52, no. 4, pp. 1023–1030, 2003.

[22] P. Mundel and S. J. Shankland, "Podocyte biology and response to injury," *Journal of the American Society of Nephrology*, vol. 13, no. 12, pp. 3005–3015, 2002.

[23] Z. Lv, M. Hu, J. Zhen, J. Lin, Q. Wang, and R. Wang, "Rac1/PAK1 signaling promotes epithelial-mesenchymal transition of podocytes in vitro via triggering β-catenin transcriptional activity under high glucose conditions," *The International Journal of Biochemistry & Cell Biology*, vol. 45, no. 2, pp. 255–264, 2013.

[24] M. Herman-Edelstein, M. C. Thomas, V. Thallas-Bonke, M. Saleem, M. E. Cooper, and P. Kantharidis, "Dedifferentiation of immortalized human podocytes in response to transforming growth factor-β: a model for diabetic podocytopathy," *Diabetes*, vol. 60, no. 6, pp. 1779–1788, 2011.

[25] J. Zou, E. Yaoita, Y. Watanabe et al., "Upregulation of nestin, vimentin, and desmin in rat podocytes in response to injury," *Virchows Archiv*, vol. 448, no. 4, pp. 485–492, 2006.

[26] L. S. Laursen, C. W. Chan, and C. Ffrench-Constant, "An integrin–contactin complex regulates CNS myelination by differential Fyn phosphorylation," *The Journal of Neuroscience*, vol. 29, no. 29, pp. 9174–9185, 2009.

[27] V. Kolavennu, L. Zeng, H. Peng, Y. Wang, and F. R. Danesh, "Targeting of RhoA/ROCK signaling ameliorates progression of diabetic nephropathy independent of glucose control," *Diabetes*, vol. 57, no. 3, pp. 714–723, 2008.

[28] M. D. Schaller, "Paxillin: a focal adhesion-associated adaptor protein," *Oncogene*, vol. 20, no. 44, pp. 6459–6472, 2001.

[29] D. J. Webb, K. Donais, L. A. Whitmore et al., "FAK-Src signalling through paxillin, ERK and MLCK regulates adhesion disassembly," *Nature Cell Biology*, vol. 6, no. 2, pp. 154–161, 2004.

[30] Z.-M. Lv, Q. Wang, Q. Wan et al., "The role of the p38 MAPK signaling pathway in high glucose-induced epithelial-mesenchymal transition of cultured human renal tubular epithelial cells," *PLoS ONE*, vol. 6, no. 7, Article ID e22806, 2011.

[31] M. Lin, W. H. Yiu, H. J. Wu et al., "Toll-like receptor 4 promotes tubular inflammation in diabetic nephropathy," *Journal of the American Society of Nephrology*, vol. 23, no. 1, pp. 86–102, 2012.

[32] J. J. Li, S. J. Kwak, D. S. Jung et al., "Podocyte biology in diabetic nephropathy," *Kidney International*, vol. 72, no. 106, pp. S36–S42, 2007.

[33] K. Asanuma, E. Yanagida-Asanuma, C. Faul, Y. Tomino, K. Kim, and P. Mundel, "Synaptopodin orchestrates actin organization and cell motility via regulation of RhoA signalling," *Nature Cell Biology*, vol. 8, no. 5, pp. 485–491, 2006.

[34] C. Wei, C. C. Möller, M. M. Altintas et al., "Modification of kidney barrier function by the urokinase receptor," *Nature Medicine*, vol. 14, no. 1, pp. 55–63, 2008.

[35] A. Kuhlmann, C. S. Haas, M.-L. Gross et al., "1,25-Dihydroxyvitamin D_3 decreases podocyte loss and podocyte

hypertrophy in the subtotally nephrectomized rat," *American Journal of Physiology—Renal Physiology*, vol. 286, no. 3, pp. F526–F533, 2004.

[36] J. Chin, J. J. Palop, G.-Q. Yu, N. Kojima, E. Masliah, and L. Mucke, "Fyn kinase modulates synaptotoxicity, but not aberrant sprouting, in human amyloid precursor protein transgenic mice," *Journal of Neuroscience*, vol. 24, no. 19, pp. 4692–4697, 2004.

[37] N. Kobayashi, "Mechanism of the process formation; podocytes vs. neurons," *Microscopy Research and Technique*, vol. 57, no. 4, pp. 217–223, 2002.

[38] A. S. Baer, Y. A. Syed, S. U. Kang et al., "Myelin-mediated inhibition of oligodendrocyte precursor differentiation can be overcome by pharmacological modulation of Fyn-RhoA and protein kinase C signalling," *Brain*, vol. 132, no. 2, pp. 465–481, 2009.

[39] H. Ma, A. Togawa, K. Soda et al., "Inhibition of podocyte FAK protects against proteinuria and foot process effacement," *Journal of the American Society of Nephrology*, vol. 21, no. 7, pp. 1145–1156, 2010.

[40] K. Azuma, M. Tanaka, T. Uekita et al., "Tyrosine phosphorylation of paxillin affects the metastatic potential of human osteosarcoma," *Oncogene*, vol. 24, no. 30, pp. 4754–4764, 2005.

[41] X. Li, Y. Yang, Y. Hu et al., "$\alpha v\beta 6$-Fyn signaling promotes oral cancer progression," *Journal of Biological Chemistry*, vol. 278, no. 43, pp. 41646–41653, 2003.

[42] M. Hirakawa, M. Oike, Y. Karashima, and Y. Ito, "Sequential activation of RhoA and FAK/paxillin leads to ATP release and actin reorganization in human endothelium," *The Journal of Physiology*, vol. 558, no. 2, pp. 479–488, 2004.

[43] J. Sinnett-Smith, J. A. Lunn, D. Leopoldt, and E. Rozengurt, "Y-27632, an inhibitor of Rho-associated kinases, prevents tyrosine phosphorylation of focal adhesion kinase and paxillin induced by bombesin: dissociation from tyrosine phosphorylation of $p130^{cas}$," *Experimental Cell Research*, vol. 266, no. 2, pp. 292–302, 2001.

Knowledge and Lifestyle-Associated Prevalence of Obesity among Newly Diagnosed Type II Diabetes Mellitus Patients Attending Diabetic Clinic at Komfo Anokye Teaching Hospital, Kumasi, Ghana: A Hospital-Based Cross-Sectional Study

Yaa Obirikorang,[1] Christian Obirikorang,[2] Enoch Odame Anto,[2,3] Emmanuel Acheampong,[2] Nyalako Dzah,[1] Caroline Nkrumah Akosah,[1] and Emmanuella Batu Nsenbah[2]

[1]*Department of Nursing, Faculty of Health and Allied Sciences, Garden City University College (GCUC), Kenyasi, Kumasi, Ghana*
[2]*Department of Molecular Medicine, School of Medical Science, Kwame Nkrumah University of Science and Technology (KNUST), Kumasi, Ghana*
[3]*Royal Ann College of Health, Department of Medical Laboratory Technology, Atwima Manhyia, Kumasi, Ghana*

Correspondence should be addressed to Emmanuel Acheampong; emmanuelachea1990@yahoo.com

Academic Editor: Raffaele Marfella

This study aimed to determine the knowledge and prevalence of obesity among Ghanaian newly diagnosed type 2 diabetics. This cross-sectional study was conducted among diagnosed type 2 diabetics. Structured questionnaire was used to obtain data. Anthropometric measurements and fasting blood sugar levels were also assessed. Participants had adequate knowledge about the general concept of obesity (72.0%) and method of weight measurement (98.6%) but were less knowledgeable of ideal body weight (4.2%). The commonly known cause, complication, and management of obesity were poor diet (76.9%), hypertension (81.8%), and diet modification (86.7%), respectively. The anthropometric measures were higher among females compared to males. Prevalence of obesity was 61.3% according to WHR classification, 40.8% according to WHtR classification, 26.1% according to WC, and 14.8% according to BMI classification. Being female was significantly associated with high prevalence of obesity irrespective of the anthropometric measure used ($p < 0.05$). Taking of snacks in meals, eating meals late at night, physical inactivity, excessive fast food intake, and alcoholic beverage intake were associated with increased prevalence of obesity ($p < 0.05$). Prevalence of obesity is high among diabetic patient and thus increasing effort towards developing and making education programs by focusing on adjusting to lifestyle modifications is required.

1. Introduction

Diabetes is now recognized as a major chronic public health problem throughout the world and affecting a large number of people in a wide range of ethnic and economic levels in both developed and developing countries. However, it is estimated that the developing countries will bear the brunt of this epidemic in the 21st century, with 80% of all new cases of diabetes expected to appear in the developing countries like Ghana by 2025 [1] including South Asian countries. The risk of diabetes mellitus is independently associated with increasing age, modifiable factors related to rapid urban growth and changing lifestyle (i.e., obesity, sedentary lifestyle, lack of physical activity, diet, smoking, and physical and emotional stress), and nonmodifiable factors such as family history of diabetes, age, and race/ethnicity [2, 3].

Obesity in persons with diabetes is associated with poorer control of blood glucose levels, blood pressure, and cholesterol [4, 5], placing patients at higher risk for both cardiovascular and microvascular disease [6]. Obesity is a complex disorder involving appetite regulation and energy metabolism, as the excess of body fat results from an imbalance of intake and expenditure [7]. Obesity is considered a major risk factor for type 2 diabetes [8]. It has been found that the incidence of diabetes increases by a 2-3-fold factor in obese individuals when obesity is defined as 120% of ideal weight [9]. It does interfere with not only effective treatment of hyperglycemia, but also hypertension and dyslipidemia [10], cardiovascular disease, cerebrovascular disease, hyperlipidemia, increased incidence of arthritis of the hands and knees, gallbladder disease, and sleep apnea [11]. In addition to the increased risk of morbidity and mortality, obesity leads to various psychological stresses that vary from emotional distress to social stigmatization [12]. The rising prevalence of obesity in type 2 diabetes in Ghana is though not known but may be attributed to rapid urbanization and associated changes in lifestyle, such as sedentary lifestyle, higher-calorie food intake, and stressful life. However, evidence suggests that lifestyle related interventions targeting modifiable risk factors can either prevent or delay the onset of type 2 diabetes and future risk of obesity [13]. Management of obesity largely depends on patient motivation and education. These in turn can be greatly facilitated by adequate baseline data on the knowledge of patients about obesity. Knowledge is influenced by socioeconomic and cultural factors, attitude, readiness to learn, family support, and barriers to care. However, knowledge and prevalence of obesity among Ghanaian diabetic patients have received very little or no attention. This study was therefore conducted to assess the knowledge and prevalence of obesity among diabetic patients attending the diabetic clinic at the Komfo Anokye Teaching Hospital (KATH).

2. Materials and Methods

2.1. Study Design/Settings. This hospital-based cross-sectional descriptive study was conducted at the Komfo Anokye Teaching Hospital (KATH), Ghana. Komfo Anokye Teaching Hospital (KATH) is located in Kumasi, the regional capital of the Ashanti Region in Ghana with a total projected population of 4,780,380 (Ghana statistical service, 2010). It is the second largest hospital in Ghana with trained doctors, nurses, anaesthetists, health care assistants, and specialties in surgery internal medicine, obstetrical and gynaecological, child health, oncology, family medicine, and emergency medicine. The geographical location of the thousand-(1000-) bed capacity, the road network of the country, and commercial nature of Kumasi make the hospital accessible to all the areas that share the boundaries with Ashanti Region and others that are further away. The diabetic centre of the KATH is situated beneath the medicine block (D block) just between the chest clinic and diagnostic centre and behind the emergency unit of the hospital.

2.2. Study Population/Selection of Participants. Using a purposive sampling technique a total of 543 newly diagnosed type II diabetes (T2DM) patients have reported at the diabetic clinic from the period of October 2014 to May 2015. Diabetic patients who have been previously diagnosed as having T2DM before the study period and patients who are unable to give informed consent were excluded from the study. Quantitative research approach was the research method used to determine knowledge and prevalence of obesity among newly diagnosed T2DM patients. Structured questionnaire was used to obtain information from all study respondents. A structured questionnaire divided into four sections with open- and close-ended questions was used for this study. Section A involved questions that elicited information on sociodemographic variables of the diabetic patient such as age, occupation, marital status, economic income, levels of education, ethnicity, family type, and religion. Section B included questions on the knowledge T2DM patients have about obesity. Section C contained items that elicited information on dietary lifestyle, physical activity, and others such as alcohol intake and smoking. In Section D, questions were designed to obtain information relating to obesity measurements such as height, weight, waist circumference, and hip circumference of studied subjects.

2.3. Criteria for Scoring on the Knowledge of Obesity. Participants were said to have "adequate" knowledge of obesity if they responded to at least three correct answers each about causes, complication, management of obesity, and method of weight measurement, "inadequate" knowledge if they responded to at most one correct answer each to causes, complications, management of obesity, and method of weight measurement, and "no" knowledge (do not know) if they did not know anything about causes, complication, management of obesity, and method of weight measurement.

2.4. Anthropometric Measurements. Participants were made to stand without their sandals, bags, or anything of significant weight on the weighing scale (Seca, Hamburg, Deutschland) and against the stadiometer (Seca, Hamburg, Deutschland). The weight was read to the nearest 0.1 kilograms and recorded. The value for the height was recorded to the nearest 0.1 centimeters and then converted to meters. The body mass index (BMI) was calculated using formula (weight/height squared) and expressed in kg/m^2. Gulick II spring-loaded measuring tape (Gays Mills, WI) was used to measure waist circumference midway between the inferior angle of the ribs and the suprailiac crest, whereas hip circumference was measured at the outermost points of the greater trochanters [14]. WHR and WHtR were recorded to the nearest 2 decimal places. WHR and WHtR were measured during first phase of sample collection.

BMI (kg/m^2) was categorized, using the current World Health Organization (WHO) definitions. BMI of $<18.5\,kg/m^2$, $18.5–24.9\,kg/m^2$, $25–29.9\,kg/m^2$, and $30\,kg/m^2$ were used to define underweight, normal, overweight, and obese cases, respectively. Waist circumference (WC) was defined for both males and females with WC <94, 94–101.9, and ≥ 102 cm defined as normal, overweight, and obese, respectively for males and <80, 80–87.9, and ≥ 88 cm defined as normal, overweight, and obese, respectively, for females. WHR was also defined for both males and females with WHR <0.90, 0.90–0.99, and ≥1.0 defined as normal, overweight, and obese, respectively, for males and <0.80, 0.80–0.84, and ≥0.85 defined as normal, overweight, and underweight, respectively, for females. With WHtR <0.5 is considered normal and ≥0.5 is considered obese [14, 15].

2.5. Statistical Methods. The data entry and analysis were performed using IBM statistical package for social science (SPSS) version 20. Descriptive statistics such as frequencies, percentage, and charts were used. Chi-square or Fischer's exact test statistical methods were used as appropriate. All results were confirmed at 5% level of significance. *p* value less than 0.05 was considered statistically significant difference.

2.6. Ethical Consideration. Approval for this study was obtained from the Committee on Human Research, Publication and Ethics of the School of Medical Sciences (SMS), Kwame Nkrumah University of Science and Technology (KNUST), and the Research and Development (R & D) Unit at KATH and the Head of Department of the Diabetes Unit (Ref-CHRPE/RC/157/13). Participation was voluntary and written informed consent was obtained from each participant.

3. Results

Table 1 shows general sociodemographic characteristics of type 2 diabetic patients. A total of five hundred and forty-three (543) type 2 diabetic (T2D) patients were recruited for this study. The mean age of the general type 2 diabetic (T2D) participants in this study was 51.14 ± 14.45 years. Higher proportions (42.7%) of them were between the ages of 40 and 59 years. Among the T2D participants, there were more females (57.3%) than males (42.7%). Three hundred and four (304) of them representing 55.9% were self-employed while 399 (73.4%) were married. Out of a total of 543 participants, higher proportions (53.8%) of them had low socioeconomic income, 38.4% had completed primary education, and 88.1% were Akans (Table 1).

As shown in Table 2, out of 543 participants, 391 representing 72.0% had adequate knowledge on the general understanding of obesity. Approximately, 26.0% of them had inadequate knowledge and a very few (2.1%) had no knowledge of the meaning of obesity. For ideal body weight, most (56.6%) of them had inadequate knowledge and 39.2% of them did not know about it though a very few (4.2%) of the participants had adequate knowledge. A higher proportion (98.6%) of the participants had adequate knowledge on the methods used in measuring weight while 1.4% had inadequate knowledge. Table 2 also shows the knowledge on understanding of obesity, ideal body weight, and methods of weight measurements among type 2 diabetic patients. Higher proportion (76.9%) of the participants responded that poor diet was a common cause of obesity followed by physical inactivity (67.1%), family history of obesity (56.6%), and insufficient sleep and stress (0.7%) The common known complications by the type 2 diabetic patients were hypertension (81.8%), followed by stroke (34.3%) and cancer (1.4%).

Table 1: Sociodemographic characteristics of type 2 diabetic patients.

Variable	Frequency	Percentage
Age (years) (mean ± SD)	51.14 ± 14.45	
<19	7	1.4%
20–39	91	16.8%
40–59	232	42.7%
60–79	198	36.4%
80–99	15	2.8%
Gender		
Male	232	42.7%
Female	311	57.3%
Occupation		
None	167	30.8%
Self-employed	304	55.9%
Govt employed	72	13.3%
Marital status		
Single	49	9.1%
Married	399	73.4%
Divorced	49	9.1%
Widowed	46	8.4%
Socioeconomic income (GHS)		
<500 (low)	292	53.8%
500–1000 (moderate)	205	37.8%
>1000 (high)	46	8.4%
Highest level of education		
None	61	11.2%
Primary	208	38.4%
Secondary	194	35.7%
Tertiary	80	14.7%
Ethnicity		
Akan	478	88.1%
Ga-Adangbe	4	0.7%
Ewe	15	2.8%
Mole-Dagbani	46	8.4%

Four hundred and seventy-one (471) of the participants representing 86.7% knew that adjusting to dietary modification is the best mode of managing obesity while 68.6% and 28.7% of them knew that doing regular physical activity and health check-up, respectively, could help manage obesity (Table 2).

Table 3 shows lifestyle characteristic of type 2 diabetic patients on the nutritional lifestyles, most (74.8%) of the participants ate thrice a day, 16.8% of them took snacks in between meals, and 13.3% ate at late hours. Most (62.2%) of the participants took their meals around 6 pm. Four hundred and ten (410) representing 75.5% of the participants were not physically active. Only 133 (24.5%) do regular exercise. The common type of exercise among the participants was walking (57.1%) followed by jogging (42.9%). Most (48.6%) of them did their exercise daily per week, though a very few (2.9%) did exercise once per week. Out of 543 participants four (4) participants (0.7%) were smoker while 15 (2.8%) of them had history of alcoholic beverage intake. A higher proportion

Table 2: Knowledge on understanding of obesity, ideal body weight, and methods of weight and knowledge on causes, complications, and management of obesity among type 2 diabetic patients.

(a)

General knowledge	Adequate	Inadequate	Do not know
Understanding the meaning of obesity	391 (72.0%)	141 (25.9%)	11 (2.1%)
Ideal body weight	23 (4.2%)	307 (56.6%)	213 (39.2%)
Method of weight measurement	535 (98.6%)	8 (1.4%)	—

(b)

Knowledge on causes and complications	N	Frequency
Causes of obesity		
Poor diet	418	76.9%
Physical inactivity	364	67.1%
Insufficient sleep/stress	4	0.7%
Family history of obesity	307	56.6%
Complications on obesity		
Hypertension	444	81.8%
Stroke	186	34.3%
Cancer	8	1.4%
Knowledge about management		
Dietary modification	471	86.7%
Physical activity	372	68.6%
Regular health check-up/medication	156	28.7%
Other lifestyle (alcohol intake, smoking, and sedentary activity)	—	—

Variables presented as frequency (percentages).

(56.6%) of the participants prefer eating butter, cheese, and cream, 53.1% prefer soft drinks, 40.6% prefer fast foods, and 30.7% prefer fiber rich foods (30.7%) while 21.7% and 11.9% prefer to eat red meat and egg yolk, respectively (Table 3).

Table 4 shows the anthropometric, clinical, and FBS levels characteristic of type 2 diabetic patients. The mean weight, BMI, WC, HC, WHR, and WHtR were higher among females compared to males. There was statistically significant difference between mean BMI levels ($p = 0.0038$). Meanwhile males were significantly ($p < 0.0001$) taller (1.69 ± 0.01 m) than the female (1.61 ± 0.01 m) participants. There was no statistically significant difference in levels of SBP and DBP between males and females ($p > 0.05$). Mean levels of FBS were significantly higher in males (13.52 ± 0.93 mmol/L) compared to females (10.50 ± 0.58 mmol/L) ($p = 0.0044$) (Table 4).

Table 5 shows the prevalence of obesity according the gender. There was a significantly higher proportion of obesity among females compared to male participants. Prevalence of obesity in male compared to females was 14.3% versus 85.7% using BMI classification, 13.5% versus 86.5% using WC, 14.9% versus 85.1% using WHR, and 37.9% versus 62.1% using WHtR. The difference in proportion was statistically significant irrespective of the method used ($p < 0.05$) (Table 5).

Tables 6 and 7 show the lifestyle characteristic features in relation to prevalence of obesity classified by BMI, WC, WHR, and WHtR. For participants who took snacks in between meals the prevalence of obesity was 33.3% using BMI, 25.0% using WC, 62.5% using WHR, and 54.2% using WHtR classification. The prevalence of obesity using BMI was 31.5% for those who ate late at night, 31.6% using WC, 73.7% using WHR, and 52.6% using WHtR. Approximately, eighteen percent (17.6%) of participants who were physically inactive were obese according to the BMI classification while 27.8%, 62.0%, and 40.8% were obese when WC, WHR, and WHtR, respectively, were used. The prevalence of obesity among participants who eat fast foods was 17.2% using BMI, 29.3% using WC, 64.3% using WHR, and 55.4% using WHtR. Twenty-five percent (25.0%) of participants with history of alcohol intake were obese using the BMI, WC, and WHR whereas 75.0% were obese using WHtR (Tables 6 and 7).

Table 8 shows the association between level of knowledge of obesity and the prevalence among type 2 diabetics. Using BMI as an indicator, 21.2% of participants who had adequate knowledge, 17.7% who had inadequate knowledge, and 54.5% who had no knowledge were obese ($p = 0.1282$) while 23.3% of participants with adequate knowledge, 36.2% with inadequate knowledge, and 81.8% of those with no knowledge of obesity were obese using WC ($p < 0.0001$). Using WHR as an indicator, 19.7% of participants with adequate knowledge, 29.1% with inadequate knowledge, and 45.5% with no knowledge of obesity were obese ($p = 0.0101$) while 22.5% of participants with adequate knowledge, 39.3% with inadequate knowledge, and 72.2% with no knowledge of obesity were obese ($p < 0.0001$).

TABLE 3: Lifestyle characteristic of type 2 diabetic patients.

Lifestyle characteristics features	Frequency	Response
Diet		
Number of times meals are taken per day		
Twice	107	19.6%
Thrice	406	74.8%
Four	30	5.6%
Snack in between meals		
Yes	91	16.8%
No	452	83.2%
Taking meals late at night		
Yes	72	13.3%
No	471	86.7%
Time for taking late meal		
5 pm	69	12.6%
6 pm	338	62.2%
7 pm	125	23.1%
8 pm	11	2.1%
Physical activity		
Regular exercise		
Yes	133	24.5%
No	410	75.5%
Type of exercise		
Walking	310	57.1%
Jogging	233	42.9%
Gym	0	—
Number of weekly exercises		
Once	16	2.9%
Twice	186	34.3%
Thrice	31	5.7%
Daily	264	48.6%
Smoking lifestyle		
Yes	4	0.7%
No	539	99.3%
Alcohol intake		
Yes	15	2.8%
No	528	97.2%
Food preferences		
Soft drinks	288	53.1%
Fast food (burger, deep fried foods, and pizza)	213	39.2%
Red meat	118	21.7%
Butter, cheese, and cream	307	56.6%
Egg yolk	65	11.9%
Fiber rich foods	167	30.7%

4. Discussion

Globally, over 300 million and 1.1 billion cases of adult obesity and overweight are reported annually [8]. For the first time, this study assessed the knowledge and prevalence of obesity among newly diagnosed type 2 diabetic patients at the Komfo Anokye Teaching Hospital, Kumasi, Ghana. In this study, 72.0% of the respondents had adequate knowledge about general concept of obesity and 98.6% were knowledgeable of the weight measurement technique while only 4.2% had adequate knowledge of their ideal body weight. In a study by Qidwai and Azam [16] majority of the participants were well informed on the general concept of obesity which is consistent with the finding of this study. Again, the findings that participants had adequate knowledge of weight measurement techniques are not consistent with findings by Saleh et al. [17].

Table 4: Anthropometric, clinical, and FBS levels characteristic of type 2 diabetic patients.

Parameters	Total	Male	Female	p value
Anthropometric index				
Weight (Kg)	64.37 ± 1.18	64.56 ± 1.77	64.24 ± 1.59	0.8959
Height (m)	1.65 ± 0.01	1.69 ± 0.01	1.61 ± 0.01	**<0.0001**
BMI (Kg/m^2)	23.72 ± 0.42	22.31 ± 0.53	24.76 ± 0.60	**0.0038**
WC (cm)	74.85 ± 1.91	73.49 ± 2.82	75.84 ± 2.59	0.5452
HC (cm)	80.35 ± 2.05	77.90 ± 2.96	82.15 ± 2.81	0.3073
WHR	0.93 ± 0.01	0.93 ± 0.01	0.95 ± 0.01	0.1204
WHtR	0.46 ± 0.01	0.43 ± 0.02	0.47 ± 0.02	0.1001
Clinical characteristics				
SBP (mmHg)	130.8 ± 1.78	130.7 ± 2.39	131.0 ± 2.54	0.9319
DBP (mmHg)	79.30 ± 1.06	79.50 ± 1.45	79.15 ± 1.49	0.8693
FBS (mmol/l)	11.78 ± 0.53	13.52 ± 0.93	10.50 ± 0.58	**0.0044**

Mean ± SD. SD: standard deviation; BMI: body mass index; WC: waist circumference; HC: hip circumference; WHR: waist to hip ratio; WHtR: waist to height ratio; SBP: systolic blood pressure; DBP: diastolic blood pressure; FBS: fasting blood sugar.

Table 5: Prevalence of obesity according the gender.

Anthropometrics	Total (n = 543)	Male (n = 235)	Females (n = 308)	p value (χ^2, df)
BMI classification				0.003 (13.90, 3)
Underweight	77 (14.1%)	106 (45.0%)	169 (55.0%)	
Normal	260 (47.9%)	131 (55.9%)	136 (44.1%)	
Overweight	126 (23.2%)	71 (30.3%)	215 (69.7%)	
Obese	80 (14.8)	34 (14.3%)	264 (85.7%)	
WC				<0.0001 (27.56, 2)
Normal	325 (59.9%)	141 (60.0%)	123 (40.0%)	
Overweight	77 (14.1%)	47 (20.0%)	246 (80.0%)	
Obese	142 (26.1)	32 (13.5%)	266 (86.5%)	
WHR				<0.0001 (76.57, 2)
Normal	46 (8.5%)	118 (50.0%)	154 (50.0%)	
Overweight	165 (30.3%)	224 (95.3%)	15 (4.7%)	
Obese	333 (61.3%)	35 (14.9%)	262 (85.1%)	
WHtR				0.0386 (0.7508, 1)
Normal	84 (59.2%)	38 (45.2%)	169 (54.8%)	
Obese	58 (40.8%)	22 (37.9%)	191 (62.1%)	

Values are presented in frequency with percentages in parenthesis. χ^2: Chi-square value; df: degree of freedom. $p < 0.05$ showed statistically significant difference. BMI: body mass index; WC: waist circumference; WHR: waist to hip ratio; WHtR: waist to height ratio.

Conversely, 56.6% had inadequate knowledge about ideal body weight which is consistent with Saleh et al. [17].

Moreover, when knowledge of diabetic patients was assessed on causes, complications, and management of obesity, most of the participants knew that poor dietary habit is a major cause obesity and also hypertension and stroke were the commonly known complications of obesity. Dietary modification and regular physical activity were the common management approaches of obesity known by participants.

Furthermore, participants were asked about the kind of food they considered healthy. Majority of them considered butter, cheese, and cream (56.6%), soft drinks (53.1%), fast foods (40.6%), fiber rich foods (30.7%), red meat (21.7%), and egg yolk (11.9%) as healthier food. This is in agreement with a study by Saleh et al. [17] who reported that majority of the diabetic patients preferred fast food, soft drinks, and mayonnaise as they considered them healthy food. Such eating preferences result in the development of overweight and obesity among patients and evidence suggests that reduction in the intake of fat and sugar leads to body weight control and prevents overweight and obesity [18]. Similar study conducted in Karachi, Pakistan, also showed that a large proportion of participants preferred oily and fried food [16]. The need for education in these areas is required. Badruddin et al. reported that dietary advice should be given to individuals with clear view of its purpose, so that they can understand and follow it in practice [19]. Therefore the role of appropriate dietary measures to control bodyweight is extremely important. It is encouraging to note that majority of the respondents believe that dietary modification is the

TABLE 6: Association between lifestyle characteristic and obesity using BMI as an indicator.

Lifestyle	BMI Underweight $n = 76$	Normal $n = 258$	Overweight $n = 125$	Obese $n = 84$	χ^2, df (p value)
Snack in between meals					30.13, 3 (<0.0001)
Yes ($n = 95$)	8 (8.3%)	40 (41.7%)	16 (16.7%)	31 (33.3%)	
No ($n = 448$)	69 (15.3%)	238 (53.1%)	92 (20.5%)	49 (11.0%)	
Taking meals late at night					23.39, 3 (<0.0001)
Yes ($n = 76$)	12 (15.8%)	32 (42.1%)	8 (10.5%)	24 (31.5%)	
No ($n = 467$)	64 (13.8%)	228 (48.8%)	118 (25.2%)	57 (12.2%)	
Regular exercise					43.60, 3 (<0.0001)
Yes ($n = 133$)	15 (11.4%)	95 (71.4%)	15 (11.4%)	7 (5.4%)	
No ($n = 410$)	61 (14.8%)	163 (39.8%)	110 (26.9%)	72 (17.6%)	
Fast food intake					3.074, 3 (0.3804)
Yes ($n = 220$)	30 (13.8%)	113 (51.7%)	46 (20.7%)	38 (17.2%)	
No ($n = 323$)	45 (14.1%)	144 (44.7%)	80 (24.7%)	42 (12.9%)	
Alcohol intake					51.08, 3 (<0.0001)
Yes ($n = 15$)	11 (75.0%)	0 (0)	0 (0)	4 (25.0%)	
No ($n = 523$)	64 (12.2%)	256 (48.9%)	124 (23.7%)	75 (14.4%)	

Values are presented in frequency with percentages in parenthesis. BMI: body mass index.

TABLE 7: Association between lifestyle characteristic and obesity using WC, WHR, and WHtR as indicators.

Lifestyles features	WC Normal $n = 325$	WC Overweight $n = 76$	WC Obese $n = 142$	WHR Normal $n = 46$	WHR Overweight $n = 165$	WHR Obese $n = 330$	WHtR Normal $n = 323$	WHtR Obese $n = 220$
Snack in between meals	0.6843, 2 ($p = 0.7102$)			12.84, 2 ($p = 0.0016$)			4.803, 1 ($p = 0.0284$)	
Yes ($n = 95$)	55 (58.3%)	16 (16.7%)	24 (25.0%)	16 (16.7%)	20 (20.8%)	59 (62.5%)	43 (45.8%)	13 (54.2%)
No ($n = 448$)	270 (60.2%)	61 (13.6%)	118 (26.3%)	30 (6.7%)	145 (32.2%)	273 (61.0%)	277 (61.9%)	171 (38.1%)
Taking meals late at night	1.929, 2 ($p = 0.3812$)			8.719, 2 ($p = 0.0128$)			4.882, 1 ($p = 0.0271$)	
Yes ($n = 76$)	40 (52.6%)	12 (15.8%)	24 (31.6%)	8 (10.5%)	12 (15.8%)	56 (73.7%)	36 (47.3%)	40 (52.6%)
No ($n = 467$)	284 (60.9%)	64 (13.8%)	118 (25.2%)	38 (8.1%)	152 (32.5%)	277 (59.3%)	284 (60.9%)	183 (39.1%)
Regular exercise	10.26, 2 ($p = 0.0059$)			1.486, 2 ($p = 0.4757$)			0.08455, 1 ($p = 0.7712$)	
Yes ($n = 133$)	95 (71.4%)	11 (8.6%)	27 (20.0%)	11 (8.6%)	46 (34.3%)	76 (57.1%)	80 (60.0%)	53 (40.0%)
No ($n = 410$)	228 (55.6%)	64 (15.7%)	114 (27.8%)	34 (8.3%)	118 (28.7%)	254 (62.0%)	239 (58.3%)	168 (40.7%)
Fast food intake	3.435, 2 ($p = 0.1795$)			17.27, 2 ($p = 0.0002$)			25.01, 1 ($p < 0.0001$)	
Yes ($n = 220$)	121 (55.2%)	34 (15.5%)	64 (29.3%)	31 (14.3%)	55 (25.0%)	141 (64.3%)	106 (48.2%)	122 (55.4%)
No ($n = 323$)	201 (62.3%)	42 (12.9%)	76 (23.5%)	15 (4.7%)	110 (34.1%)	194 (60.0%)	217 (67.1%)	103 (31.8%)
Alcohol intake	2.629, 2 ($p = 0.2686$)			8.748, 2 ($p = 0.0126$)			2.037, 1 ($p = 0.1535$)	
Yes ($n = 15$)	11 (75.0%)	—	4 (25.0%)	4 (25.0%)	7 (50.0%)	4 (25.0%)	1 (25.0%)	3 (75.0%)
No ($n = 528$)	314 (58.9%)	76 (14.4%)	138 (25.9%)	417 (7.9%)	156 (29.5%)	327 (61.9%)	315 (59.7%)	209 (39.6%)

Values are presented in frequency with percentages in parenthesis. Chi-square value (χ^2), df (p value). BMI: body mass index; WC: waist circumference; WHR: waist to hip ratio; WHtR: waist to height ratio.

first line of management to obesity. If such belief could be transformed into practice, then a reduced future risk of cardiovascular disease will be an achievable target.

This study also assessed several lifestyle characteristics of diabetic patients. The common lifestyle behaviours were taking snacks in between meals (16.8%), eating at late hours in the night (13.3%), regular physical exercise (24.5%), smoking (0.7%), and alcoholic intake (2.8%). From this study, less than 30% of the diabetic patients did regular physical exercise and the most common forms were walking (57.1%) and jogging (42.9%). This proportion of participants in this study who did regular exercise is low compared to 59% reported by Qidwai and Azam [16]. It has been shown that reduced levels of physical activity play a predominant role in the development of obesity [20]. Therefore there is need for education on the importance of exercise and also on the need to exercise for certain duration and at the optimum frequency. Several studies conducted in urbanizing rural community of Bangladesh showed that there is a significant association between higher body mass index (BMI) and

TABLE 8: Association between level of knowledge of obesity and prevalence of obesity among type 2 diabetic patients.

Anthropometric indicators	General knowledge of obesity Adequate ($n = 391$)	Inadequate ($n = 141$)	Do not know ($n = 11$)	χ^2, df (p value)
BMI classification				9.917, 6 (0.1282)
Underweight	9 (2.3)	5 (3.5)	0 (0.0)	
Normal	101 (25.8)	38 (27.0)	3 (27.3)	
Overweight	198 (50.6)	73 (51.8)	2 (18.2)	
Obese	83 (21.2)	25 (17.7)	6 (54.5)	
WC				42.77, 4 (<0.0001)
Normal	113 (28.9)	57 (40.4)	2 (18.2)	
Overweight	187 (47.8)	33 (23.4)	0 (0.0)	
Obese	91 (23.3)	51 (36.2)	9 (81.8)	
WHR				13.26, 4 (0.0101)
Normal	121 (30.9)	51 (36.2)	3 (27.3)	
Overweight	193 (49.4)	49 (34.8)	3 (27.3)	
Obese	77 (19.7)	41 (29.1)	5 (45.5)	
WHtR				26.37, 2 (<0.0001)
Normal	303 (77.5)	85 (60.3)	3 (27.3)	
Obese	88 (22.5)	56 (39.3)	8 (72.7)	

Values are presented in frequency with percentages in parenthesis. Chi-square value (χ^2), df (p value). BMI: body mass index; WC: waist circumference; WHR: waist to hip ratio; WHtR: waist to height ratio.

incidence of diabetes mellitus [2–4]. However, in Ghana, published data showing the relationship between obesity and newly diagnosed diabetic patient is scarce. Aside the paucity of data, majority of these studies focus on using only BMI as a measure of obesity. In this study, obesity was assessed by BMI, WC, WHR, and WHtR classification. The results indicated that the prevalence of obesity among type 2 diabetic patients was 61.3% according to WHR classification, 40.8% according to WHtR classification, 26.1% according to WC, and 14.8% according to BMI classification.

The prevalence of obesity using WC, WHR, and WHtR (Table 6) was significantly higher compared to using BMI. Previous studies have also reported increased prevalence of obesity by WHR and WC [21, 22] and WHtR [23] which is inconsistent with findings of this study. Another study reported both WC and BMI as having equal diagnostic accuracy for obesity, and they are also components for metabolic syndrome [24]. Discrepancies in results suggest that prognostic ability of each index of obesity may differ by age, gender, and ethnic group. It is therefore believed that the discrete criteria to select a particular obesity index should be age, gender, and ethnic group specific. In this study, we observed that using WHR followed by WHtR yielded the highest prevalence of obesity compared to using BMI. It is with no doubt that the use of BMI alone may underutilize other equally obesity indicators such as WC, WHR, and WHtR.

Prevalence of obesity irrespective of the anthropometric measure used was higher among female than male participants. Being male or a female was significantly associated with obesity. Some authors [25–28] but not Gopalakrishnan et al. [29] have consistently reported that increased prevalence of obesity is associated with females than male participants. Findings of this study concur with the earlier authors. The proportion of obesity in females was extremely high in this study compared to current study by Mogre et al. [28]. The higher rate of obesity and overweight among the females is expected because there is a social perception which encourages fatness in the females in Ghanaian population. Females prefer being fat which is considered as a sign of good living in a society than having a slender body. Contraceptives usage is also known to cause the body to produce increased amount of fat in the females due to its appetite inducing nature, Reid et al. [30]. All these factors may account for the high prevalence of obesity among the women compared to the men.

The prevalence of obesity was also assessed in relation to the lifestyle characteristics of study participants. Interestingly, participants who ate snacks in between meals and ate late at night and those who were physically inactive and preferred fast foods were obese irrespective of the anthropometric measures used. However, among participants who had history of high alcoholic intake, the prevalence of obesity was significantly high when WHtR was used compared to WC, WHR, and BMI. This clearly shows that these lifestyle behaviours could be independent risk factors of obesity and thus early health advice on the need for diabetic patient to adjust to lifestyle modification may help prevent future risk of cardiovascular disease and cerebrovascular accidents (stroke).

The major limitation of this study is the use of hospital-based cross-sectional study design and thus the findings of this study cannot conclusively represent the general diabetic patients in Ghana. However, some findings of this study concur well with other previous studies.

5. Conclusion

There is an increased prevalence of obesity among diabetic patients. Being a female was significantly associated with increased risk of obesity. Taking of snacks in between meals, eating meals late at night, physical inactivity, excessive fast food intake, and alcoholic beverage intake were common causes of obesity among diabetic patients. Physical exercise and dietary measures to control body weight are lacking despite the desire to have appropriate body weight. There is a need and we strongly recommend patient education programs for the control of obesity among our patients. Again, public health awareness especially hospital-based awareness on healthy lifestyle and nutrition is essential in early management of diabetes. Using other anthropometric measurements such as WC, WHR, and WHtR in conjunction with BMI would be useful for better diagnosis of obesity condition.

Conflict of Interests

The authors declare that there is no conflict of interests regarding the publication of this paper.

Acknowledgments

Gratitude goes to workers at diabetic clinic and authorities of Komfo Anokye Teaching Hospital and Nursing Departments in GCUC and Department of Molecular Medicine, KNUST, Kumasi, Ghana.

References

[1] S. J. Mumu, F. Saleh, F. Ara, M. R. Haque, and L. Ali, "Awareness regarding risk factors of type 2 diabetes among individuals attending a tertiary-care hospital in Bangladesh: a cross-sectional study," *BMC Research Notes*, vol. 7, article 599, 2014.

[2] A. Hussain, B. Claussen, A. Ramachandran, and R. Williams, "Prevention of type 2 diabetes: a review," *Diabetes Research and Clinical Practice*, vol. 76, no. 3, pp. 317–326, 2007.

[3] H. S. Buttar, T. Li, and N. Ravi, "Prevention of cardiovascular diseases: role of exercise, dietary interventions, obesity and smoking cessation," *Experimental & Clinical Cardiology*, vol. 10, no. 4, pp. 229–249, 2005.

[4] C. Merlotti, A. Morabito, and A. E. Pontiroli, "Prevention of type 2 diabetes; a systematic review and meta-analysis of different intervention strategies," *Diabetes, Obesity and Metabolism*, vol. 16, no. 8, pp. 719–727, 2014.

[5] J. W. Anderson, "Whole grains protect against atherosclerotic cardiovascular disease," *Proceedings of the Nutrition Society*, vol. 62, no. 1, pp. 135–142, 2003.

[6] J. B. Buse, H. N. Ginsberg, G. L. Bakris et al., "Primary prevention of cardiovascular diseases in people with diabetes mellitus: a scientific statement from the American Heart Association and the American Diabetes Association," *Diabetes Care*, vol. 30, no. 1, pp. 162–172, 2007.

[7] K. Ashrafi, "Obesity and the regulation of fat metabolism," in *WormBook*, pp. 1–20, 2007.

[8] WHO, *Obesity: Preventing and Managing the Global Epidemic*, World Health Organization, Geneva, Switzerland, 2000.

[9] K. M. Mugharbel and M. A. Al-Mansouri, "Prevalence of obesity among type 2 diabetic patients in Al-Khobar primary health care centers," *Journal of Family & Community Medicine*, vol. 10, no. 2, pp. 49–53, 2003.

[10] S. M. Grundy, I. J. Benjamin, G. L. Burke et al., "Diabetes and cardiovascular disease: a statement for healthcare professionals from the American Heart Association," *Circulation*, vol. 100, no. 10, pp. 1134–1146, 1999.

[11] S. S. Habib, "Cardiovascular disease in diabetes: an enigma of dyslipidemia, thrombosis and inflammation," *Basic Research Journals of Medicine and Clinical Science*, vol. 1, pp. 33–42, 2012.

[12] T. L. S. Visscher and J. C. Seidell, "The public health impact of obesity," *Annual Review of Public Health*, vol. 22, pp. 355–375, 2001.

[13] K. G. M. M. Alberti, P. Zimmet, and J. Shaw, "International Diabetes Federation: a consensus on Type 2 diabetes prevention," *Diabetic Medicine*, vol. 24, no. 5, pp. 451–463, 2007.

[14] WHO, "Physical status: the use of and interpretation of anthropometry," Report of a WHO Expert Committee, World Health Organization, Geneva, Switzerland, 1995.

[15] M. de Onis and J.-P. Habicht, "Anthropometric reference data for international use: recommendations from a World Health Organization Expert Committee," *The American Journal of Clinical Nutrition*, vol. 64, no. 4, pp. 650–658, 1996.

[16] W. Qidwai and S. I. Azam, "Knowledge, attitude and practice regarding obesity among patients, at Aga Khan University Hospital, Karachi," *Journal of Ayub Medical College, Abbottabad*, vol. 16, no. 3, pp. 32–34, 2004.

[17] F. Saleh, S. J. Mumu, F. Ara, L. Ali, S. Hossain, and K. R. Ahmed, "Knowledge, attitude and practice of type 2 diabetic patients regarding obesity: study in a tertiary care hospital in Bangladesh," *Journal of Public Health in Africa*, vol. 3, article 8, p. 8, 2012.

[18] W. H. M. Saris, "Sugars, energy metabolism, and body weight control," *The American Journal of Clinical Nutrition*, vol. 78, no. 4, pp. 850S–857S, 2003.

[19] N. Badruddin, A. Basit, M. Z. I. Hydrie, and R. Hakeem, "Knowledge, attitude and practices of patients visiting a diabetes care unit," *Pakistan Journal of Nutrition*, vol. 1, no. 2, pp. 99–102, 2002.

[20] J. Webber, "Energy balance in obesity," *Proceedings of the Nutrition Society*, vol. 62, no. 2, pp. 539–543, 2003.

[21] E. Akpinar, I. Bashan, N. Bozdemir, and E. Saatci, "Which is the best anthropometric technique to identify obesity: body mass index, waist circumference or waist-hip ratio?" *Collegium Antropologicum*, vol. 31, no. 2, pp. 387–393, 2007.

[22] T. Bhurosy and R. Jeewon, "Overweight and obesity epidemic in developing countries: a problem with diet, physical activity, or socioeconomic status?" *The Scientific World Journal*, vol. 2014, Article ID 964236, 7 pages, 2014.

[23] M. Ashwell, P. Gunn, and S. Gibson, "Waist-to-height ratio is a better screening tool than waist circumference and BMI for adult cardiometabolic risk factors: systematic review and meta-analysis," *Obesity Reviews*, vol. 13, no. 3, pp. 275–286, 2012.

[24] T. S. Han, K. Williams, N. Sattar, K. J. Hunt, M. E. J. Lean, and S. M. Haffner, "Analysis of obesity and hyperinsulinemia in the development of metabolic syndrome: San Antonio Heart Study," *Obesity Research*, vol. 10, no. 9, pp. 923–931, 2002.

[25] U. A. Onyechi and A. C. Okolo, "Prevalence of obesity among undergraduate students, living in halls of residence, University of Nigeria, Nsukka Campus, Enugu State," *Animal Research International*, vol. 5, no. 3, pp. 928–931, 2008.

[26] K. E. Oghagbon, V. U. Odili, E. K. Nwangwa, and K. E. Pender, "Body mass index and blood pressure pattern of students in a Nigerian University," *International Journal of Health Research*, vol. 2, no. 2, pp. 177–182, 2009.

[27] D. L. van der A, A. C. Nooyens, F. J. van Duijnhoven, M. M. Verschuren, and J. M. Boer, "All–cause mortality risk of metabolically healthy abdominal obese individuals: the EPIC–MORGEN study," *Obesity*, vol. 22, no. 2, pp. 557–564, 2014.

[28] V. Mogre, R. Nyaba, and S. Aleyira, "Lifestyle risk factors of general and abdominal obesity in students of the School of Medicine and Health Science of the University of Development Studies, Tamale, Ghana," *ISRN Obesity*, vol. 2014, Article ID 508382, 10 pages, 2014.

[29] S. Gopalakrishnan, P. Ganeshkumar, M. V. S. Prakash, and A. V. Christopher, "Prevalence of overweight/obesity among the medical students, Malaysia," *The Medical Journal of Malaysia*, vol. 67, no. 4, pp. 442–444, 2012.

[30] I. R. Reid, L. D. Plank, and M. C. Evans, "Fat mass is an important determinant of whole body bone density in premenopausal women but not in men," *The Journal of Clinical Endocrinology & Metabolism*, vol. 75, no. 3, pp. 779–782, 1992.

13

Inability of Some Commercial Assays to Measure Suppression of Glucagon Secretion

Nicolai J. Wewer Albrechtsen,[1,2] Simon Veedfald,[1,2] Astrid Plamboeck,[1,2] Carolyn F. Deacon,[1,2] Bolette Hartmann,[1,2] Filip K. Knop,[1,2,3] Tina Vilsboll,[3] and Jens J. Holst[1,2]

[1] *Department of Biomedical Sciences, Faculty of Health and Medical Sciences, University of Copenhagen, 2200 Copenhagen, Denmark*
[2] *Novo Nordisk Foundation Center for Basic Metabolic Research, Faculty of Health and Medical Sciences, University of Copenhagen, 2200 Copenhagen, Denmark*
[3] *Center for Diabetes Research, Gentofte Hospital, University of Copenhagen, 2900 Hellerup, Denmark*

Correspondence should be addressed to Jens J. Holst; jjholst@sund.ku.dk

Academic Editor: Raffaele Marfella

Glucagon levels are increasingly being included as endpoints in clinical study design and more than 400 current diabetes-related clinical trials have glucagon as an outcome measure. The reliability of immune-based technologies used to measure endogenous glucagon concentrations is, therefore, important. We studied the ability of immunoassays based on four different technologies to detect changes in levels of glucagon under conditions where glucagon levels are strongly suppressed. To our surprise, the most advanced technological methods, employing electrochemiluminescence or homogeneous time resolved fluorescence (HTRF) detection, were not capable of detecting the suppression induced by a glucose clamp (6 mmol/L) with or without atropine in five healthy male participants, whereas a radioimmunoassay and a spectrophotometry-based ELISA were. In summary, measurement of glucagon is challenging even when state-of-the-art immune-based technologies are used. Clinical researchers using glucagon as outcome measures may need to reconsider the validity of their chosen glucagon assay. The current study demonstrates that the most advanced approach is not necessarily the best when measuring a low-abundant peptide such as glucagon in humans.

1. Introduction

Glucagon, a 29-amino-acid peptide secreted from the pancreatic alpha cells in response to hypoglycemia [1], is derived from the proglucagon molecule, which is also expressed in the intestine and brain [2]. Glucagon has stimulatory effect on hepatic glucose production, and dysregulation of its secretion may contribute to the development of diabetes [3–6]. Glucagon measurements are, therefore, often an important study outcome; according to clinicaltrials.gov, it is included as an endpoint in more than 400 clinical studies. However, measurement of glucagon is a delicate matter and the validity of the data relies on sufficient specificity and sensitivity of the assay. Differential tissue-specific processing of proglucagon results in molecular heterogeneity, meaning that assay specificity with respect to the different molecular forms is important. Thus, in addition to glucagon itself, proglucagon gives rise to several peptides containing the glucagon sequence, including oxyntomodulin, glicentin, and proglucagon 1–61, as well as molecules with some sequence homology to glucagon, including glucagon-like peptide-1 (GLP-1) and glucagon-like peptide-2 (GLP-2) and major proglucagon fragment [7]. Furthermore, each of these molecular forms may occur in extended or truncated forms, which may or may not be biologically active [2]. The immediate specificity problem is therefore of considerable magnitude. Sensitivity is equally important, since glucagon occurs in low picomolar concentrations in the circulation. Its concentration rises in response to hypoglycemia and falls in response to rising glucose (e.g., after carbohydrate meals), with the rate of as well as the absolute magnitude of the decrease being of considerable importance for the resulting glucose tolerance. The ability of assays to register these decreases from already low levels is, therefore, critical [8].

In the current study, we investigated assays based on four widely applied immune-based technologies: a radioimmunoassay (RIA), a spectrophotometric enzyme-linked immunoassay (ELISA), and ELISAs based on electrochemiluminescence (ECL), and homogeneous time-resolved fluorescence (HTRF) detection. We hypothesized that the assay type might influence measured glucagon concentrations. To address this, we analyzed glucagon levels during a glucose clamp with or without atropine (atropine blocks cholinergic signaling through the muscarinic receptors and leads to further suppression of glucagon secretion) in five healthy male participants using these four different approaches; previous measurements indicated that the clamp + atropine protocol resulted in pronounced suppression of glucagon levels [9].

2. Methods

2.1. Participants, Procedures, and Samples. Samples were derived from a previously published study by Plamboeck et al. [9]. The study was conducted in accordance with the Helsinki Declaration II and was approved by the Scientific-Ethical Committee of the Capital Region of Denmark (registration number: H-2-2011-062) and by the Danish Data Protection Agency (journal number: 2011-41-6381) and registered at clinicaltrials.gov (ID: NCT01534442). Oral and written informed consent was obtained from all participants. Glucose clamps (6 mmol/L) were performed in five healthy male participants (age: 25 ± 1 years, body mass index: 24 ± 0.5 kg/m^2, and HbA_{1c}: 5.1±1%) with or without blocking efferent muscarinic activity by infusion of atropine (1 mg bolus + an 80 ng/kg/min infusion). Samples were collected and stored using optimal conditions for glucagon analysis as described previously [8].

2.2. Measurement of Glucagon. We used four immune-based assays for measurement of glucagon: (A) an in-house C-terminal RIA (codename 4305) [6, 8, 10]; (B) Mercodia sandwich ELISA (spectrophotometry) (cat# 10-1271-01, Uppsala, Sweden); (C) sandwich ELISA from MSD (chemiluminescence) (cat# K151HCC-1, MD 21201, USA); and (D) sandwich ELISA from Cis-Bio (homogeneous time-resolved fluorescence) (cat# 62GLCPEK, Codolet, France). Assays were carried out as per protocol according to the manufacturers' instructions. Samples were kept cold (ice-bath) at all times, and all samples were measured simultaneously in a single run to eliminate interassay variance.

2.3. Statistics. To analyze changes in glucagon levels over time, a one-way ANOVA for repeated measurements followed by a Bonferroni post hoc analysis was performed for each of the four assays. To compare the ability of the assays to detect changes in glucagon levels, we created a generalized regression model (ANCOVA) with glucagon as dependent variable and time (minutes) and method (assay) as independent variables. Net area under the curve (delta changes from time zero to 160 minutes relative to the individual baselines) (nAUC) was calculated using the trapezoidal rule and differences were tested using a two-sided test. A power calculation was made based on the following assumptions: normality of data distribution, homoscedasticity, one-sample t-test, quantification limits and coefficient of variations *provided by the manufacturers*, an alpha value of 0.05, and a sample size of five. The calculation showed that the power to detect significant changes (of 5%) in glucagon levels ranged from 79% to 84% across the four assays. $P < 0.05$ was considered significant. Calculations were made using GraphPad Prism version 6.04 for Windows, GraphPad Software, La Jolla, California, USA, http://www.graphpad.com/, and STAT14, Boston, MA, USA. For illustrations we used the Adobe CS6 software suite (California, USA).

3. Results

The recoveries of synthetic glucagon in pooled human plasma ($N = 4$) were 95 ± 11% (assay A), 104 ± 5% (assay B), 75 ± 15% (assay C), and 67 ± 21% (assay D). Glucagon levels dropped significantly compared to baseline (time = 0 min) in both saline and atropine treated groups ($P < 0.01$) when samples were measured using assay A (Figure 1(a)) and assay B (Figure 1(b)) but not with assay C (Figure 1(c), $P = 0.31$) and assay D (Figure 1(d), $P = 0.24$). Assay A was significantly different ($P < 0.05$) from assays C and D but not assay B ($P = 0.43$). Assay B was significantly different from assays C and D ($P < 0.05$) whereas there were no differences between assays C and D ($P = 0.27$). nAUCs during infusion of saline and atropine, respectively, for assay A and assay B were significantly different ($P < 0.001$), indicating further suppression of glucagon secretion with atropine addition. For assays C and D, nAUCs were significantly different between atropine ($P < 0.01$) and saline, indicating that atropine weakly suppressed glucagon levels compared to the clamp alone, where nAUCs did not show significance compared to baseline (zero) by one-side t-test ($P = 0.11$ and $P = 0.17$).

4. Discussion

Immune-based detection methods utilize the extreme binding energy of antibodies which may have equilibrium constants reaching values of 10^{12} L/mol, providing these methods with a potential to measure very low concentrations. However, the use of antibodies relies on their specificity and the antigen-antibody reaction may also may be sensitive to the so-called matrix effects, that is, interference from components in plasma including a variety of high-abundant plasma molecules or proteins (e.g., albumin and immunoglobulins), leading to unspecific interference in antibody-antigen interaction [11].

Assay D uses the homogeneous time-resolved fluorescence technology which combines fluorescence resonance energy transfer technology (FRET) with time-resolved measurement (TR) [12]. HRTF is mainly used in (*in vitro*) primary

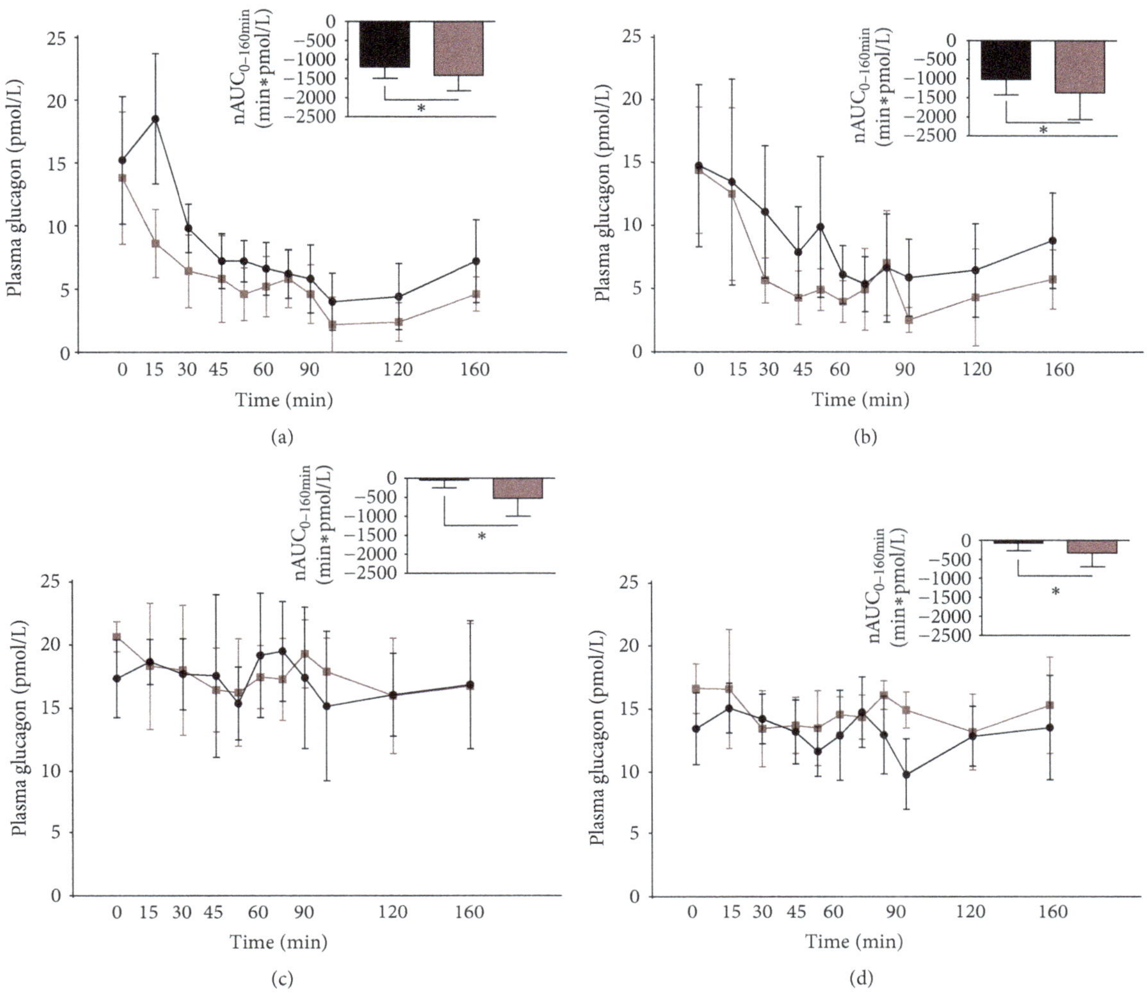

FIGURE 1: Plasma glucagon levels of five healthy participants during a 6 mmol/L glucose clamp with simultaneous infusion of either saline (black) or atropine (red). (a) depicts assay A, a radioimmunoassay; (b) depicts assay B, a spectrophotometrically based ELISA; (c) depicts assay C, a chemiluminescence based ELISA; and (d) depicts assay D, a homogeneous time-resolved fluorescence based ELISA. Net area under the curve (nAUC) is depicted separately at upper right quadrant on (a), (b), (c), and (d). * represents a significant two-sided t-test comparing saline nAUC to atropine nAUC. Data illustrated as mean ± standard deviation.

and secondary screening phases of drug development. However, its usefulness in highly sensitive immunoassays required for detection of 1 pmol/L differences in glucagon levels may be questioned. In contrast, assay C applies an electrochemiluminescence approach: when excited by electrical stimulation, labeled molecules emit light, which then is detected by cameras. The most generic ELISA used in our study is assay B, involving spectrophotometry detection; a chromogenic substrate is added to sample wells, which is then cleaved by an enzyme, for example, horseradish peroxidase, coupled to the detection antibody. Assay A is a radioimmunoassay utilizing competition between radioactively labeled antigen and unlabeled antigen (peptide standard or sample with unknown concentration) for binding to a limited number of specific antibody binding sites. Although it is the most simple, with regard to technology, the data clearly shows that assays A and B perform significantly better than assays C and D. However, a requirement for such a performance is the application of antibodies with sufficient binding energy (and specificity), which is often the crucial step in assay development.

In this study, we highlight the crucial importance of choosing the "right" immune-based method when analyzing endogenous glucagon. We have exemplified the challenge by demonstrating that changes in measured glucagon levels depend on the assay used (Figure 1); where assays A and B clearly register the attenuation of glucagon levels during a glucose clamp, assays C and D did not. The basal levels measured were comparable, around 15 pmol/L (although assay C showed slightly higher levels, around 20 pmol/L). This may reflect a specificity problem in assay C; for example, this assay could be cross-reacting with glucagon-like molecules (oxyntomodulin, glicentin, or glucagon-like peptide-1 [7, 11]) although not stated by the manufacturers. Otherwise, the difference between the assays, although not formally tested here, most likely reflects differences in sensitivity and therefore ability to detect dynamic changes in the very low picomolar range. In a previous study [6], a sensitivity analysis was carried out for assays A and B (where assay A was more sensitive), and, in another study of other commercially available assays [7], sensitivity was clearly insufficient to allow analysis in this concentration range. In addition, we recently demonstrated that measured glucagon levels in subjects with renal dysfunction may erroneously appear elevated, probably due to cross-reactions with N-terminal elongated inactive isoforms of the glucagon molecule (1–61) when analyzed with conventional single antibody C-terminal radioimmunoassays [6]. Importantly for interpretation of clinical studies, the potential instability of glucagon during inappropriate sample preparation and storage, such as multiple freeze-thaw cycles or storing plasma samples at room temperature for more than 1 hour, should also be considered [8].

Novel mass-spectrometry based detection (e.g., selected reaction monitoring (SRM)) of low-abundant peptides as glucagon [13] may in the future facilitate validation of immune-based detection methods. Unfortunately, current mass-spectrometry based methods still depend on 2D-gel extraction techniques or bead-coupled antibodies [14] both of which have questionable recoveries and specificity. However, in the future mass-spectrometry based detection methods may involve label-free (be it chemical or antibody based) purification steps as recently demonstrated [15] and may therefore provide accurate validation.

In conclusion, levels of glucagon are increasingly being used as outcome measures in clinical trials and the reliability of the glucagon assays employed is therefore critical for appropriate interpretation of the data.

Conflict of Interests

Cis-Bio provided assay kits without imposing restrictions on the study design or interpretation of results. Otherwise the authors have no dualities of interest to declare.

Authors' Contribution

Nicolai J. Wewer Albrechtsen, Simon Veedfald, Astrid Plamboeck, Carolyn F. Deacon, Filip K. Knop, Tina Vilsboll, Bolette Hartmann, and Jens J. Holst provided substantial contribution to the concept and design; Nicolai J. Wewer Albrechtsen, Simon Veedfald, and Jens J. Holst substantially contributed to analysis and interpretation of data; Nicolai J. Wewer Albrechtsen, Simon Veedfald, and Jens J. Holst drafted the paper; Astrid Plamboeck, Carolyn F. Deacon, Bolette Hartmann, Tina Vilsboll, and Filip K. Knop revised the paper critically for important intellectual content. All authors have provided final approval of the version to be published. Jens J. Holst is responsible for the integrity of the work as a whole. Nicolai J. Wewer Albrechtsen and Simon Veedfald contributed equally to the study and are co-first authors.

Acknowledgments

The authors acknowledge support from NNF Center for Basic Metabolic Research, University of Copenhagen, NNF Application no. 13563 (Novo Nordisk Foundation, Denmark), The Danish Council for Independent Research (DFF, 1333-00206A), Augustinus Foundation 14-0962, European Molecular Biology Organisation, and the European Foundation for the Study of Diabetes.

References

[1] P. E. Cryer, "Mechanisms of hypoglycemia-associated autonomic failure in diabetes," *The New England Journal of Medicine*, vol. 369, no. 4, pp. 362–372, 2013.

[2] J. E. Campbell and D. J. Drucker, "Islet α cells and glucagon—critical regulators of energy homeostasis," *Nature Reviews Endocrinology*, vol. 11, no. 6, pp. 329–338, 2015.

[3] F. K. Knop, T. Vilsbøll, S. Madsbad, J. J. Holst, and T. Krarup, "Inappropriate suppression of glucagon during OGTT but not during isoglycaemic i.v. glucose infusion contributes to the reduced incretin effect in type 2 diabetes mellitus," *Diabetologia*, vol. 50, no. 4, pp. 797–805, 2007.

[4] P. Raskin and R. H. Unger, "Hyperglucagonemia and its suppression," *The New England Journal of Medicine*, vol. 299, no. 9, pp. 433–436, 1978.

[5] P. Shah, A. Vella, A. Basu, R. Basu, W. F. Schwenk, and R. A. Rizza, "Lack of suppression of glucagon contributes to postprandial hyperglycemia in subjects with type 2 diabetes mellitus," *The Journal of Clinical Endocrinology & Metabolism*, vol. 85, no. 11, pp. 4053–4059, 2000.

[6] N. J. Wewer Albrechtsen, B. Hartmann, S. Veedfald et al., "Hyperglucagonaemia analysed by glucagon sandwich ELISA: nonspecific interference or truly elevated levels?" *Diabetologia*, vol. 57, no. 9, pp. 1919–1926, 2014.

[7] M. J. Bak, N. W. Albrechtsen, J. Pedersen et al., "Specificity and sensitivity of commercially available assays for glucagon and oxyntomodulin measurement in humans," *European Journal of Endocrinology*, vol. 170, no. 4, pp. 529–538, 2014.

[8] N. J. Wewer Albrechtsen, M. J. Bak, B. Hartmann et al., "Stability of glucagon-like peptide 1 and glucagon in human plasma," *Endocrine Connections*, vol. 4, no. 1, pp. 50–57, 2015.

[9] A. Plamboeck, S. Veedfald, C. F. Deacon et al., "The role of efferent cholinergic transmission for the insulinotropic and glucagonostatic effects of GLP-1," *American Journal of Physiology—Regulatory, Integrative and Comparative Physiology*, vol. 309, no. 5, pp. R544–R551, 2015.

[10] J. J. Holst, "Evidence that glicentin contains the entire sequence of glucagon," *The Biochemical Journal*, vol. 187, no. 2, pp. 337–343, 1980.

[11] R. E. Kuhre, N. J. W. Albrechtsen, B. Hartmann, C. F. Deacon, and J. J. Holst, "Measurement of the incretin hormones: glucagon-like peptide-1 and glucose-dependent insulinotropic peptide," *Journal of Diabetes and Its Complications*, vol. 29, no. 3, pp. 445–450, 2015.

[12] F. Degorce, A. Card, S. Soh, E. Trinquet, G. P. Knapik, and B. Xie, "HTRF: a technology tailored for drug discovery—a review of theoretical aspects and recent applications," *Current Chemical Genomics*, vol. 3, no. 1, pp. 22–32, 2009.

[13] J. W. Howard, R. G. Kay, T. Tan et al., "Development of a high-throughput UHPLC–MS/MS (SRM) method for the

quantitation of endogenous glucagon from human plasma," *Bioanalysis*, vol. 6, no. 24, pp. 3295–3309, 2014.

[14] A. Y. H. Lee, D. L. Chappell, M. J. Bak et al., "Multiplexed quantification of proglucagon-derived peptides by immunoaffinity enrichment and tandem mass spectrometry after a meal tolerance test," *Clinical Chemistry*, 2015.

[15] N. J. Wewer Albrechtsen, D. Hornburg, S. Torang, R. E. Kuhre, C. F. Deacon, F. Meissner et al., "A novel immune-based approach for measurement of the anorectic gut hormone oxyntomodulin: changes after gastric bypass surgery," *Diabetes*, 2015.

14

The Actions of Lyophilized Apple Peel on the Electrical Activity and Organization of the Ventricular Syncytium of the Hearts of Diabetic Rats

Elideth Martínez-Ladrón de Guevara,[1] Nury Pérez-Hernández,[2] Miguel Ángel Villalobos-López,[3] David Guillermo Pérez-Ishiwara,[2] Juan Santiago Salas-Benito,[2] Alejandro Martínez Martínez,[1] and Vicente Hernández-García[1]

[1] *Institute of Biomedical Sciences, Autonomous University of Ciudad Juárez, 32310 Ciudad Juárez, CHIH, Mexico*
[2] *National School of Medicine and Homeopathy, National Polytechnic Institute, 07320 Mexico City, DF, Mexico*
[3] *Centre for Research in Applied Biotechnology, National Polytechnic Institute, 90700 Tepetitla, TLAX, Mexico*

Correspondence should be addressed to Vicente Hernández-García; vicherna@uacj.mx

Academic Editor: Hiroshi Okamoto

This study was designed to examine the effects of lyophilized red delicious apple peel (RDP) on the action potentials (APs) and the input resistance-threshold current relationship. The experiments were performed on isolated papillary heart muscles from healthy male rats, healthy male rats treated with RDP, diabetic male rats, and diabetic male rats treated with RDP. The preparation was superfused with oxygenated Tyrode's solution at 37°C. The stimulation and the recording of the APs, the input resistance, and the threshold current were made using conventional electrophysiological methods. The RDP presented no significant effect in normal rats. Equivalent doses in diabetic rats reduced the APD and ARP. The relationship between input resistance and threshold current established an inverse correlation. The results indicate the following: (1) The functional structure of the cardiac ventricular syncytium in healthy rats is heterogeneous, in terms of input resistance and threshold current. Diabetes further accentuates the heterogeneity. (2) As a consequence, conduction block occurs and increases the possibility of reentrant arrhythmias. (3) These modifications in the ventricular syncytium, coupled with the increase in the ARP, are the adequate substrate so that, with diabetes, the heart becomes more arrhythmogenic. (4) RDP decreases the APD, the ARP, and most syncytium irregularity caused by diabetes.

1. Introduction

The cultivation of the apple (*Malus domestica*) for human consumption dates back centuries, and apples are now estimated to be the third most commonly consumed fruit, after bananas and citrus [1]. Epidemiological studies have related the ingestion of one apple or more a day to the prevention of pulmonary and colon cancers [2], cardiovascular disease, type 2 diabetes, pulmonary disorders, and Alzheimer's disease [3]. Some apple components have even been found to have beneficial effects with regard to cognitive loss with ageing, osteoporosis, gastrointestinal protection, and the maintenance of body weight [4]. The protective effects are attributed to phytochemical compounds such as triterpenes and polyphenols due to their antioxidant properties. Furthermore, the apple contains large amounts of free polyphenols [5]. However, the composition of phytochemicals depends on factors including the variety, cultivation conditions, harvesting, soil, and climate, in addition to the type of fruit tissue that is considered (peel, pulp, and seed). The peel contains the greatest amount of polyphenols because it is the main physical, chemical, and biological protection of the fruit from the external environment [1].

The relationship between oxidative stress with diabetes and its micro- and macrovascular complications has been known for years, but the mechanisms involved have only relatively recently begun to be understood. Interestingly, the redox state and diabetic cardiomyopathy that involves both mechanical and electrical cardiac dysfunction [6] are closely related [7] and are responsible for an increased vulnerability to developing heart arrhythmias and sudden death. Nonetheless, to date, there has been only one study, which indicates that red delicious apple peel (RDP) has direct actions on the heart's electrical activity with diabetic cardiomyopathy [8]. Within this context, the objectives of this study are (1) to evaluate and compare the action of the 50 mg/kg dose of RDP on the duration of cardiac action potentials (APs) at 30, 50, and 90% in normal and diabetic rats and (2) to analyse the functional organization of the ventricular syncytium through the input resistance versus threshold current curve of the hearts of control rats, control rats with RDP, diabetic rats, and diabetic rats with RDP administered daily for 90 days. The results obtained indicate that (1) RDP induced a significant decrease in action potential duration (APD) and absolute refractory period (ARP); (2) the cardiac syncytium in healthy animals and in those with diabetes is heterogeneous, in terms of input resistance and intracellular thresholds. However, in animals with diabetes, this irregularity is more accentuated; and (3) RDP administered orally to diabetic rats attenuates the irregularities of the relationship between input resistance and threshold current.

2. Methods

2.1. Apple Peel. The production of apple varieties in Mexico is mainly concentrated on the Golden Delicious and Red Delicious varieties [9]. Only red apple varieties contain anthocyanins; these flavonoids are responsible for the red and blue tones occurring in various fruits, such as grapes, berries, and figs. For this reason we decided to use the Red Delicious variety, which also has the highest concentration of free polyphenols [10–12].

Red Delicious apples, harvested in 2011, were purchased in the market of Ciudad Juarez, CHIH. To obtain the apple peels, a manual peeler was employed once the fruit was washed. The peels were immediately stored at −80°C. The lyophilization was performed using a 6-litre Labconco FreeZone lyophilizer. Once the peels were lyophilized, they were pulverized to obtain a fine powder that was vacuum-packed in plastic bags, shielded in black plastic bags, and stored at −20°C until being utilized. Thus, the biological activity of the polyphenols was preserved.

The proximate analysis of the RDP was performed according to the official methodology outlined by the *Association of Official Analytical Chemists* (AOAC) [13]. The total nitrogen was determined by the Kjeldahl technique, and the crude protein was calculated by multiplying the total nitrogen by 6.25. The crude fat was quantified by the Soxhlet technique. The carbohydrates were quantified by means of the difference of the other components. The fibre was quantified after their acid and alkaline digestion.

Phenol extraction was performed using 20 g of RDP dissolved in 125 mL of 80% methanol. The total phenolic content was determined with the modified Folin-Ciocalteu colorimetric method [14]. The measurement was compared to a standard curve of gallic acid, and the results were expressed in units of mg of gallic acid equivalent (GAE) per 100 g dry weight.

The determination and quantification of the isomers of chlorogenic acid and epicatechin were performed in the laboratories of the *Silliker* Company at *Mérieux NutriSciences* in Grand Prairie, TX, USA.

2.2. Animal Model. The male Wistar rats that were used were acquired from *Rismart* and *Research Global Solutions* in Mexico City. The rats were maintained at a constant temperature of 25°C with a LD 12 : 12 cycle. Both food and water were always offered *ad libitum*. The treatment period was equivalent to 90 days, and 36 rats were utilized. They were divided into four groups: control ($n = 10$), control with RDP treatment ($n = 4$), type 1 diabetes ($n = 11$), and type 1 diabetes with RDP treatment ($n = 11$).

2.2.1. Groups with Apple Peel. The groups treated with RDP received a daily dose of 150 mg/kg. The concentrate was dissolved in distilled water in small volumes and administered orally with a tuberculin syringe. The dose was equated to the daily consumption of the peels of three apples/day ingested by an adult man weighing 70 kg.

2.2.2. Induction of Diabetes Mellitus. The induction of diabetes mellitus type 1 was accomplished using a single intraperitoneal administration of 45 mg/kg of streptozotocin (STZ, *Sigma Chemical Company*) dissolved in a citrate buffer at pH 4.8. To decrease the mortality due to the hypoglycaemia generated by the STZ, 60 mM of sugar water was provided *ad libitum* for one week. The glycaemia of the blood was determined at eight days after STZ injection using a commercial blood glucose metre (*OneTouch Ultra 2*). For this study, only those rats with glycaemia values above 150 mg/dL were used. All experiments were performed according to the guidelines established by the Ethics Committee for Experimental Animals of the Autonomous University of Ciudad Juárez.

2.2.3. Electrophysiological Experiments. Prior to experimentation, the rats were anesthetized with sodium pentobarbital at 50 mg/kg and 0.2 units of heparin/mL. Once an animal was anesthetized, its abdomen was opened; from this area, cardiac puncture was performed, and a 4 mL blood sample was obtained. Then, proceeding to the isolation of the heart, it was placed in an isolated tissue chamber and continuously perfused with oxygenated Tyrode's solution at 37°C. Under these conditions and by dissection of the left ventricle, the left ventricular papillary muscles were isolated. The preparation thus obtained was stimulated through external bipolar silver electrodes coated with insulating material, except for the tip, at a basic cycle of 500 milliseconds. The stimuli were rectangular pulses of one millisecond in duration and an intensity 1.5 times the threshold, obtained from a Digitimer model D4030 pulse generator and passed through a Digitimer model DS2 stimulus isolation unit. When the propagation of premature responses (extrasystoles) was explored, the preparation was stimulated regularly at a basic cycle of 500 milliseconds and, after applying eight basic stimuli, a test stimulus was introduced through the same pair of stimulation electrodes at different time intervals. The intracellular action potentials were obtained using glass microelectrodes filled with 3 M KCl solution and with a tip resistance of between 10 and 20 megaohms. The signal obtained by the microelectrodes was passed through high input impedance amplifiers, WPI model 750, and an HV Electrometer model 400E. The recording of the APs was performed on the screen of a Tektronix model TDS3034B oscilloscope. The records were stored on a Dell model GX520 computer for further quantitative analysis.

2.2.4. Biochemical Analyses. The quantifications of glucose and glycosylated haemoglobin (HbA_{1c}) were determined at 90 days by spectrometry in the Servalab Clinical Laboratory (Puebla, Mexico). To determine the glucose concentration, a Glucose PAP kit (ELITech Clinical Systems) was used in a Vitros DT60 Chemistry System, whereas the HbA_{1c} was performed with a LabonaCheck A_{1c} kit in an HbA_{1c} Analyser. The evaluation of the plasma insulin levels was performed by chemiluminescence in the Italo Gaya Laboratory (Puebla, Mexico).

2.3. Statistical Analysis. The data were analysed with GraphPad Prism version 4.00 for Windows (GraphPad Software, La Jolla, California, USA). The numerical results are expressed as mean values ± SEM (standard error of the mean). The differences observed between the control and the treated groups were assessed using unpaired two-tailed Student's t-test. Values were considered statistically significant at $p < 0.05$.

TABLE 1: Analysis of the composition of the lyophilized apple peel (RD).

Component	%
Moisture	81.5
Ash	1.45
Crude protein	0.02
Crude fat	0.35
Carbohydrates	15
Crude fibre	1.59

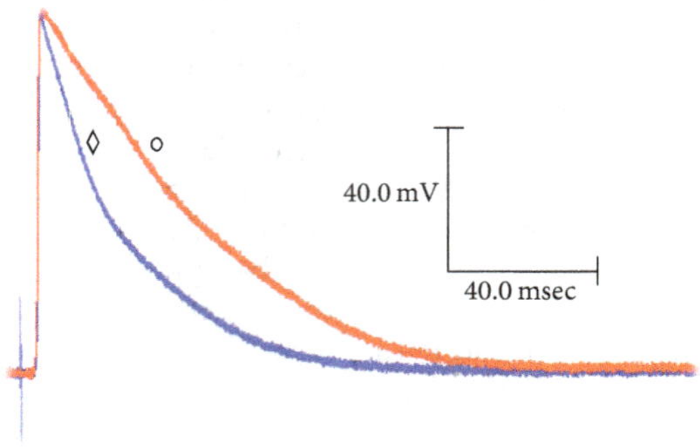

FIGURE 1: Changes in the action potential with diabetes. Representative action potentials obtained from a cell of the papillary muscle of the left ventricle of the heart of control rats and diabetic rats at a basic cycle of 500 milliseconds.

3. Results

3.1. Analysis of the Apple Peel. Table 1 shows the principal components and their values in % of RDP. The polyphenol content was 1,100 μg GAE/100 g dry weight. Specifically, the isomers of chlorogenic acid and epicatechin were present at a concentration of 0.1148 and 2.35 mg/g dry weight, respectively. The determination of the total polyphenols by means of the Folin-Ciocalteu method depends on the extraction of the polyphenols and the units used to report them; thus, it is difficult to compare the results. However, the levels of chlorogenic acid and epicatechin in the peels are in line with those published by other authors [2]. Both chlorogenic acid and epicatechin are the most abundant polyphenols in the apple [4].

3.2. Criteria for Considering Diabetogenesis in Wistar Rats. Table 2 presents variables relating to the body weight and biochemical blood parameters of the rats 90 days after diabetes mellitus was induced.

3.3. Action Potentials

3.3.1. Characteristics of the Action Potentials (APs) of the Hearts of the Control Rats and the Diabetic Rats. Figure 1 shows the overlapping mean APs, recorded in the isolated papillary muscles of hearts from the control rats (blue diamond) and the diabetic rats (red circle), evoked by a basic 500-millisecond cycle.

Figure 2 shows the result of averaging the APs of the diabetic rats and the diabetic rats treated for 90 days with 150 mg/kg of RDP.

Figure 3 summarizes the APD at 30, 50, and 90% and the ARP of the control rats, the diabetic rats, and the diabetic rats treated with RDP.

3.4. Modifications Occurring in the Ventricular Syncytium Muscle with Diabetes

3.4.1. Determination of the Input Resistance and Intracellular Thresholds in the Papillary Muscles of Control Rats and Diabetic Rats Using the Method [14]. Concisely, (1) the papillary heart muscles of the rat present a syncytial geometric organization and (2) to evaluate the possible potential changes of this syncytial organization, it is necessary to quantify the parameters of the input resistance and the threshold current (necessary to evoke a propagated AP).

To quantify the input resistance and the threshold current, two microelectrodes penetrating the same cell were used. The microelectrodes were cemented or glued, aligned under a microscope, and separated between their tips at a distance of approximately 10 μm. The microelectrodes were mounted in a double micromanipulator (Narishige MD-4)

TABLE 2: Body weight and biochemical parameters of the rats after 90 days of treatment.

	Weight (g)	Glucose (mg/dL)	Insulin (μUI/mL)	HbA_{1C} (%)
Control ($n = 11$)	501.00 ± 13.22	196.50 ± 10.33	0.3455 ± 0.01575	4.282 ± 0.3009
D ($n = 11$)	363.20 ± 29.80*	487.10 ± 23.98*	0.1545 ± 0.03123*	6.009 ± 0.1984*
D + RDP ($n = 8$)	366.40 ± 10.67*	511.50 ± 58.35*	0.1500 ± 0.03727*	6.000 ± 0.1753*

Mean ± SEM; $^{*}p < 0.05$, control versus diabetes.

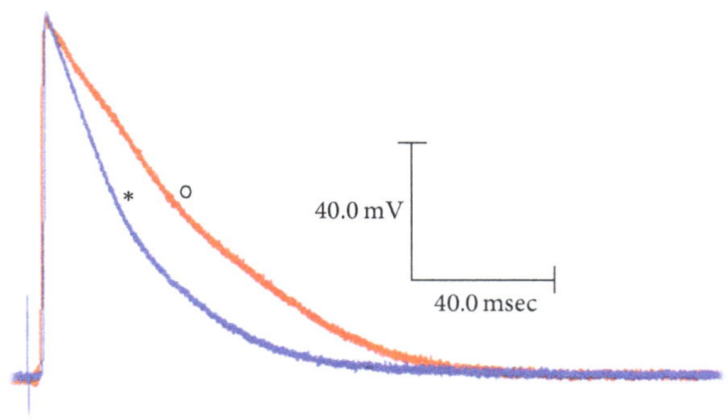

FIGURE 2: Action of the apple peel on the action potentials of diabetic rats. Typical transmembrane potentials obtained in the papillary muscles of the heart of diabetic rats and diabetic rats with apple peel at a basic cycle of 500 milliseconds.

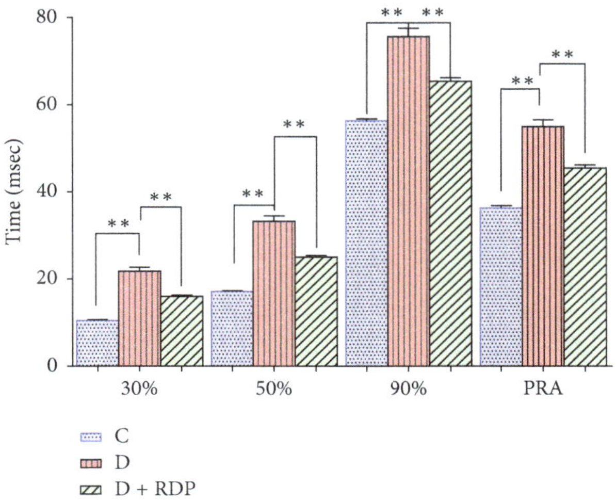

FIGURE 3: Mean values ± SEM of the quantified parameters of the action potentials recorded in the papillary muscles of the hearts of control rats ($n = 225$), diabetic rats ($n = 110$), and diabetic rats receiving apple peel for 90 days ($n = 169$) at a basic cycle of 500 milliseconds. The symbols (∗∗) indicate that the differences between the different groups are significant ($p < 0.05$).

with independent vertical movement. With this system, it was possible to impale the two microelectrodes in the same cell or in two adjacent cells connected by their *nexus*. Under these strict conditions, depolarizing or hyperpolarizing current pulses were injected through one microelectrode, and, with the other, the changes in the transmembrane potential were recorded.

Figure 4 shows the steps that were followed to quantify the input resistance and the intracellular thresholds in the papillary muscles of the control rats. The top trace in Figure 4(a) shows the injection of three constant current hyperpolarizing pulses, in late diastole, with a duration of 7.0 milliseconds and intensities of 35, 68, and 100 nanoamperes, and their corresponding variations in the membrane potential of 5, 10, and 16 millivolts (lower trace). By plotting the change in membrane potential with respect to the injected current, a straight line is obtained, with a slope that is the value of the input resistance. In Figure 4(b), the current polarity is inverted, and a pulse of depolarizing current is injected. The pulse duration is 7.0 milliseconds, and its intensity is gradually increased until it can evoke an action potential. In this case, the intracellular threshold is 805.5 nanoamperes. Figure 4(c) shows the simultaneity and the same configuration of the depolarization phase of the action potentials recorded in the same cell by both of the microelectrodes. Finally, in Figure 4(d), the zero potential of both action potentials recorded in the same cell is obtained. Therefore, it is important to note that the value of the input resistance of the cell will be valid provided that the requirements shown in Figures 4(c) and 4(d) are met.

Using this procedure, sufficient data on the input resistance and threshold current were obtained in the control rats to show that their product (ohms × amperes = volts) equals a mean value of 30 mV. In other words, the experimental results are fitted to the theoretical curve of an equilateral hyperbola in the form $Y = K/X$, where K is a constant with a value equalling 30 mV; and the XY product (resistance × current) is the drop in potential that corresponds to the value of the constant, K, with units in volts. These experimental relationships are shown in Figure 5, with a function, F, and $p < 0.05$. In this graph, the experimental values of the input resistance ranged between 24 and 171.4 KΩ, and the minimum current threshold necessary to initiate propagated responses ranged from 175 to 1,220 nanoamperes.

Because the preparation of the papillary muscle of the rat heart maintains its force of contraction, the duration of the impalement of the microelectrodes is brief. Determining the threshold is achieved by small amplitude steps of increasing current until initiating an AP; consequently, our threshold values lacked absolute precision. Therefore, if the input resistance and threshold current are adequately related, with the equation of an equilateral hyperbola with constant value, $K = 30$ mV, then we can quantify the intracellular thresholds

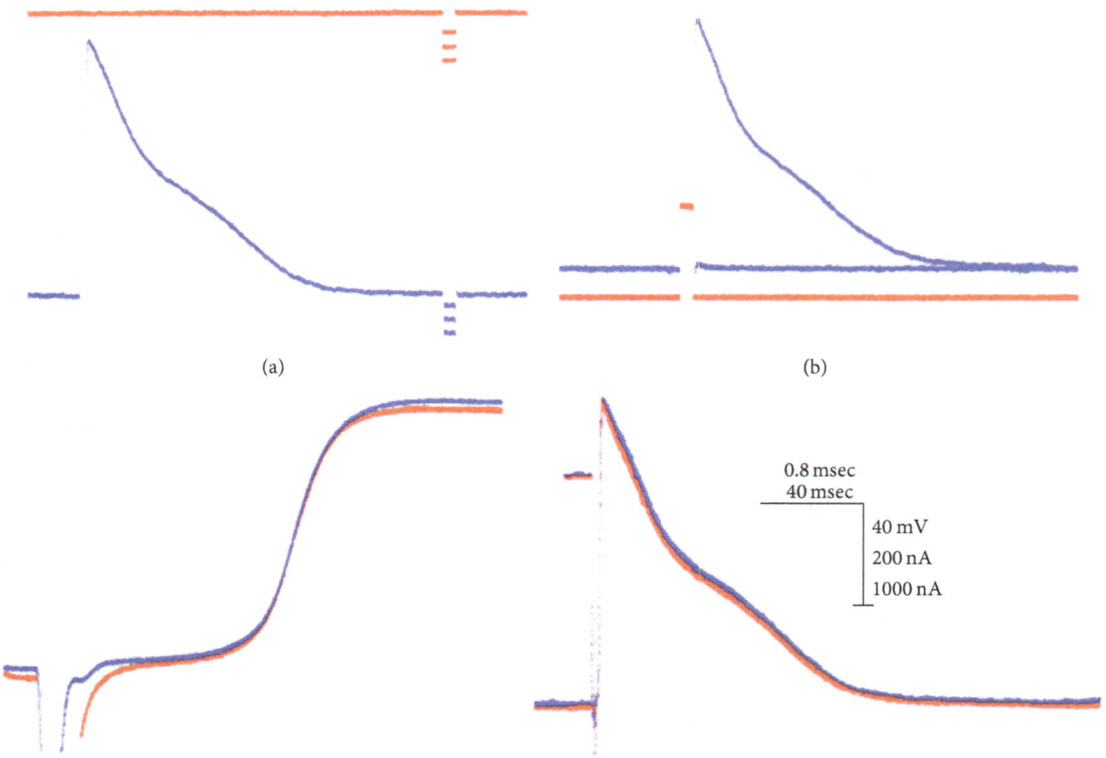

(a) (b)

(c) (d)

Figure 4: Procedure for determining the input resistance. Steps followed to quantify the input resistance and the intracellular thresholds in the papillary muscles of the hearts of the control rats: (a) injection of the pulse current in late diastole to evaluate the input resistance; (b) determination of the intracellular threshold; (c) simultaneity and shape of the depolarization phase of the action potentials; (d) zero potential of both records obtained from the same cell.

more precisely and explore more of the cells in the papillary muscles, impaling two independent microelectrodes at different sites in the preparation. Thus, we can inject the current in smaller steps through one electrode up to the threshold and record the propagated AP through the other. Under these conditions, the input resistance values can be calculated with the equation of the equilateral hyperbola: $Y = K/X$.

3.4.2. Relationship between Input Resistance and Threshold Current in the Hearts of the Control Rats and the Control Rats with Treatment. To make the electrode impalement technique more efficient, obtain a greater amount of experimental data, and have more precise current threshold values, the microelectrode recording the APs remains fixed somewhere in the biological preparation, and the other microelectrode is impaled into many other sites of the papillary muscle for the determination of their thresholds. These data are now used to calculate their corresponding input resistance.

Figure 6 shows the relationships between the papillary muscles of the control rats and the papillary muscles of the control rats treated with 150 mg/kg of RDP over a 90-day period. The values for the input resistance found in the control rats are between 24 and 316.5 KΩ, and their corresponding threshold currents range from 94 to 1,232 nanoamperes. Similar input resistance and threshold current values were observed in both groups.

3.4.3. Relationships between Input Resistances and Threshold Currents in the Control Rats and the Diabetic Rats. Figure 7 shows the changes between the input resistance and threshold current values due to the diabetogenic effects. Wide variations in input resistances, ranging from 24 to 814.1 KΩ, in threshold currents, ranging from 36 to 1,232 nanoamperes, and the resting membrane potential of -77.50 ± 0.3554 mV ($n = 109$) were found in the papillary muscles of the diabetic rats, while in the control rats the variations in input resistance range from 24 to 316.5 KΩ and corresponding threshold current ranges from 1,232 to 94 nanoamps with a resting membrane potential of -76.62 ± 0.5664 mV ($n = 252$). Observe the displacement towards higher input resistance values and low thresholds in the hearts of the diabetic rats.

3.4.4. The Input Resistance-Threshold Current Relationship in the Diabetic Rats and the Diabetic Rats with RDP Treatment. Figure 8 shows the effects of RDP on the input resistance-threshold current values obtained in the papillary muscles of the diabetic rats and the diabetic rats treated with RDP. The results clearly indicate a reduction in diabetogenic effects due to the administration of the RDP, based on the values of the input resistance and threshold current.

3.4.5. Propagation of Premature Responses and Reentrant Activity in the Diabetic Rats. The modifications in the input

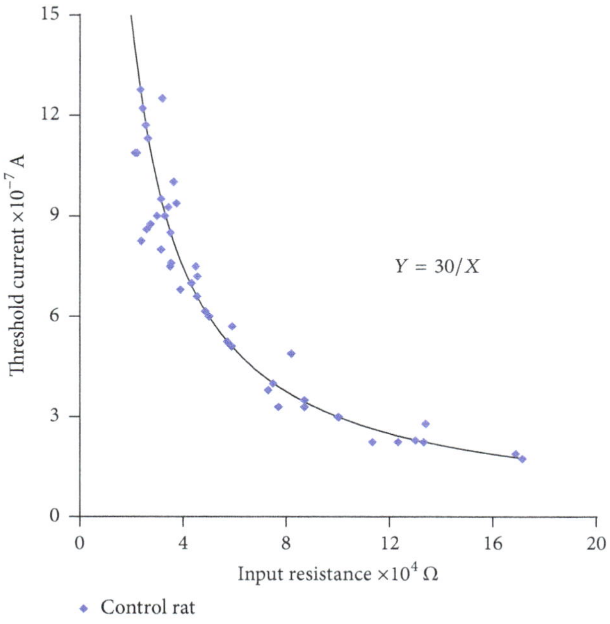

FIGURE 5: Fit relationship of the experimental input resistance-current threshold values (blue) with respect to the theoretical curve (black). Values obtained in the cells of the papillary muscle of the heart of the control rats. The continuous curve corresponds to an equilateral hyperbola defined by the equation $Y = K/X$, where $K = 30$ mV. For each input resistance value, there is a corresponding threshold current value adequately conforming to the theoretical curve, which is established by the statistical analysis of $R^2 = 0.92$ and $p < 0.05$.

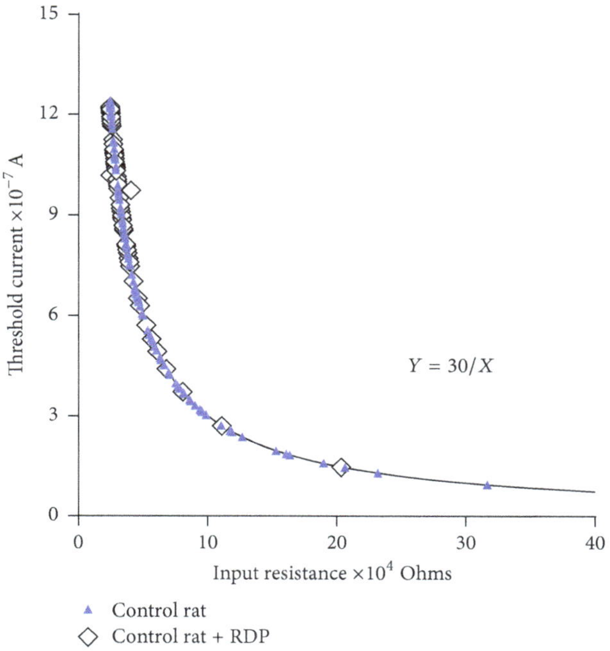

FIGURE 6: Input resistance-current threshold relationship in control rats and control rats with RDP treatment (150 mg/kg). The values of the input resistance were calculated using the equation of the equilateral hyperbola, $Y = K/X$, where Y is the threshold current quantified experimentally and $K = 30$ mV is the constant value. Filled symbols: control rats; unfilled symbols: control rats + RDP.

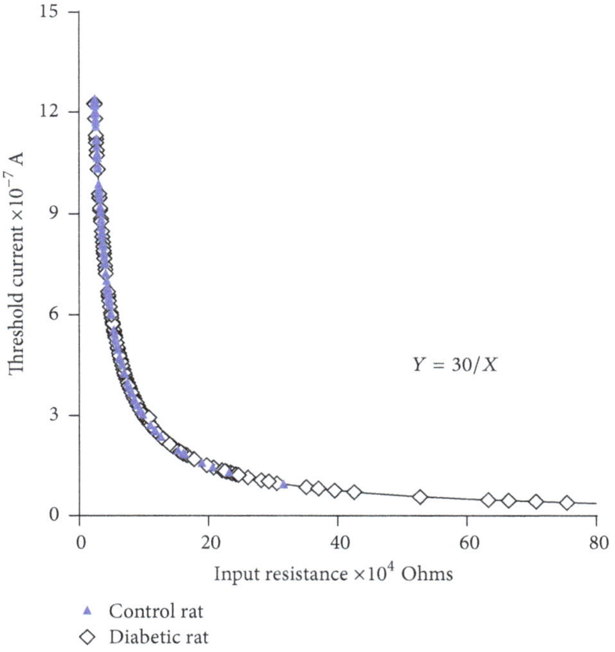

FIGURE 7: Input resistance versus threshold current relationship in the control rats and diabetic rats. The relationship obtained in the papillary muscle of the heart of the control rats and the rats with diabetes. The continuous line corresponds to the theoretical equilateral hyperbola, $Y = 30/X$. Filled symbols: control rats; unfilled symbols: diabetic rats.

resistance and the intracellular threshold found in the papillary muscles of the rats with diabetes can cause the propagation of APs that may become critical; under these conditions, reentrant bioelectrical activity may arise which initiates ventricular fibrillations and sudden death.

Figure 9 shows the response evoked by the application of an early extrasystole in the papillary muscle of diabetic rats. The upper trace corresponds to the APs recorded in the area proximal to the site of the external stimulation electrodes; the lower trace corresponds to the APs recorded in a site distal to the stimulation electrodes. The first response corresponds to the last of a series of eight APs evoked by basic stimuli. The second response corresponds to the activity generated by a test stimulus applied 40 milliseconds after the last basic stimulus. It is observed that the AP evoked by the test pulse is followed by two APs (asterisks) that were not initiated by stimulation, which demonstrates the hypersensitivity of the ventricular syncytium of diabetic rats to generate reentrant action potential activity.

Another example of reentrant activity is shown in Figure 10. This result provides additional evidence that when a test pulse is applied early, the evoked response is followed by multiple reentrant activity. In this case, the last two reentrant action potentials are conducted in a retrograde direction.

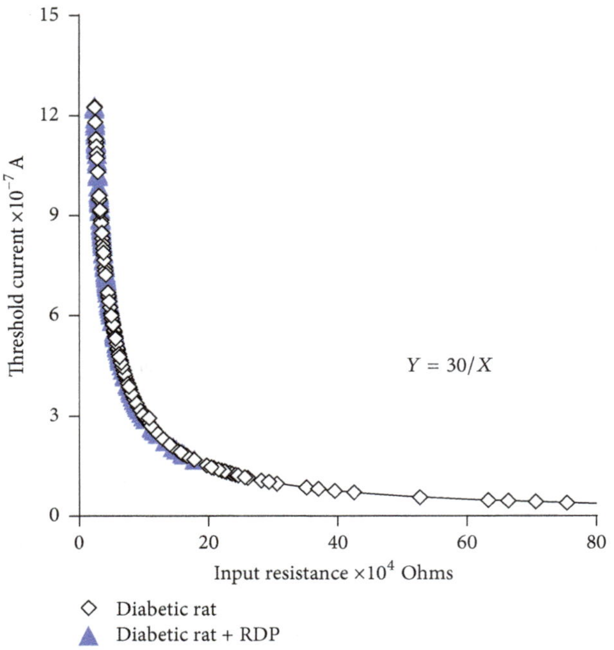

FIGURE 8: Changes in the input resistance-current threshold relationships in diabetic rats and diabetic rats treated with RDP; 150 mg/kg for 90 days. Filled symbols: diabetic rats; unfilled symbols: diabetic + RDP.

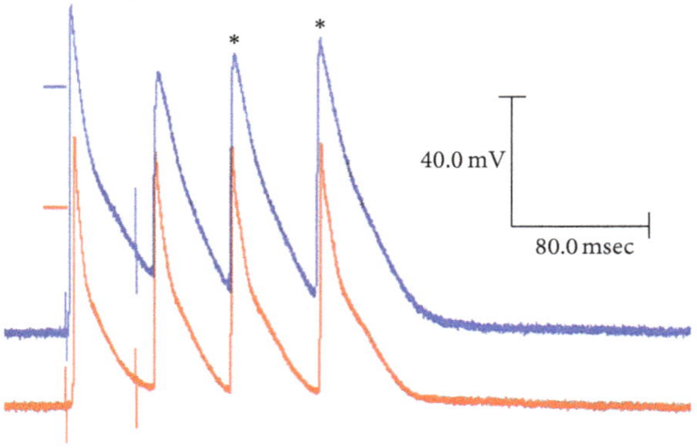

FIGURE 9: Reentrant activity initiated by the application of an early extrasystole. The traces shown correspond to action potentials recorded in the papillary muscles of diabetic rats, in the area proximal (upper trace) and the area distal (lower trace) to the stimulation site, at a basic cycle of 500 milliseconds. Observe that, after the implementation of the extrasystole, two responses (asterisks) not evoked by stimulation appear, corresponding to a type of reentrant activity.

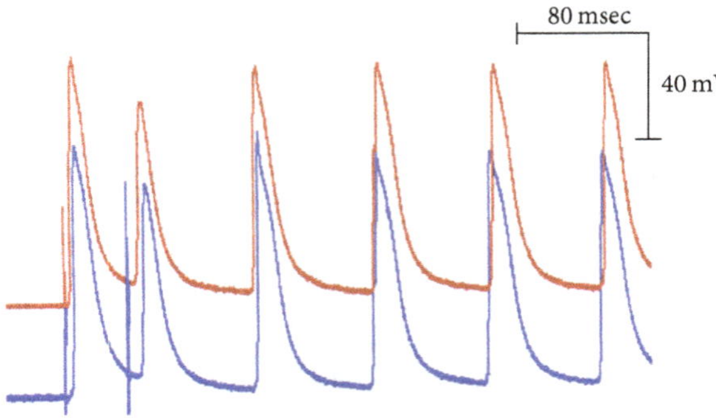

FIGURE 10: Change of direction in the propagation of the wavefront. Observe that the first three responses (basic, test, and first reentrant) are propagated from the stimulation site towards the rest of the preparation, whereas the last three following reentrant responses propagate in the opposite direction.

4. Discussion

This study was designed with the purpose of obtaining solid experimental evidence of the effects of RDP on diabetic cardiomyopathy. A well-established model of diabetes induced by streptozotocin in the rat was used for this purpose [15, 16]. The effects of RDP were quantified with the electrophysiological parameters of the papillary muscle of the hearts of male Wistar rats. The electrophysiological properties studied included (1) the duration of the ARP and APs at 30, 50, and 90% of their repolarization and (2) the organization of the ventricular syncytium muscle in terms of the input resistance-current threshold relationship in control rats, control rats treated with RDP, diabetic rats, and diabetic rats treated with RDP.

It is important and necessary to clarify that we are unable to provide an adequate explanation of or the mechanisms that are involved in the actions and effects of the RDP for the following reasons: (1) This is the first study in which the action of RDP is assessed. (2) All of the biologically active components of RDP are not known. (3) Their concentrations and pharmacokinetic and pharmacodynamic properties prevent us from formulating an explanation. Considering the foregoing and with the aforementioned reservations, we interpret the actions of RDP on the hearts of diabetic rats.

4.1. Action Potentials. The results obtained clearly show that the duration of the action potentials increases in the papillary heart muscles of the diabetic rats compared to the control rats (Figures 1 and 3) [16–20]. Additionally, the increase in the duration of the action potential is more pronounced at 30% than at 90%. There are several ionic currents that intervene spatially and temporally in the repolarization of the action potential in the ventricular myocardium of the rat. The early phase of ventricular repolarization is performed by the activation of two potassium currents ($I_K{}^+$), the transient outward current (I_{to}) and the delayed rectifier current (I_K) [21], whereas the late phase of repolarization is due to the activation of the Na^+/Ca^{2+} exchanger current, which is responsible for the final elongation of the repolarization of the action potential [22]. Furthermore, the increase observed in the early phase of the repolarization of the action potentials in the diabetic rats is due to the decrease in the potassium currents, I_{to} and I_K [16, 18, 20], whereas the increase in $APD_{90\%}$ is attributed to the increase in the Na^+/Ca^{2+} exchanger current, causing an overload of Ca^{2+} in the ventricular myocytes [23–25].

Figures 2 and 3 show that the supplementation of apple peels to the diabetic rats for 90 days after having induced diabetes significantly decreased the duration of the action potentials and the ARP. Results similar to those shown in this study have been obtained by other authors [26]. It has been reported that the polyphenols contained in apple extract decrease the duration of the action potential in the ventricular myocytes of the mouse heart with dilated cardiomyopathy. Such a decrease in the APD is the result of an increased K^+ current (I_{K1}), induced by the polyphenols extract. The results obtained in the papillary muscles of diabetic rats with treatment can be explained if we assume that the RDP has the same types of polyphenols and is at concentrations similar to those found in the apple extracts tested [25]. Consequently, the RDP could cause an increase in the transient outward K^+ current ($I_{k_{to}}$), given that it is the principal K^+ current affected in the ventricular myocytes of the hearts of diabetic rats [16, 20]. Indeed, it is necessary to measure this current in the ventricular myocytes of the diabetic rats to provide a more sustainable affirmation.

4.2. Organization of the Ventricular Syncytium of the Rat Heart. Our study was conducted in the isolated papillary muscles of the left ventricle of the rat heart. Before considering the interpretation of the results, in which the organization of the ventricular functional syncytium was analysed, we must consider the following factors:

(1) The first work in which the organization of the ventricular functional syncytium was analysed [27] was developed in the right anterior papillary muscle of the dog heart. This preparation has been used extensively in studies of heart electrophysiology. The morphologies of the intracellular action potentials revealed the existence of three functionally distinct areas in the right anterior papillary muscle of the dog heart [28]. The proximal and middle thirds are composed of muscle tissue and specialized conduction tissue. The distal third contains only ventricular muscle. The same authors designated the end portion of the conduction tissue as terminal Purkinje fibres. The terminal Purkinje fibres establish low-resistance electrical contact with the ventricular muscle fibres and give rise to the Purkinje-muscle junctions. In this manner, the preparation of the papillary muscle of the dog provides a syncytium composed of different cellular elements that can be easily identified.

(2) Nonetheless, the rat is an experimental model widely used in cardiac electrophysiology studies. To date, there is no interest in performing the classification made in the anterior papillary muscle of the dog in the papillary muscle of the left ventricle of the rat [28]. With that condition, it is assumed that there is a similar functional structure in their proximal and middle thirds (composed of specialized conduction fibres and ordinary ventricular muscle cells). This asseveration is supported by the similarity of the input resistance values evaluated in the proximal and middle thirds (high resistance values and low thresholds). Low resistance values and high thresholds are found in the distal third, which indicates that the distal third may possibly be composed exclusively of muscle tissue. Thus, the homology is considered applicable in all mammals.

4.2.1. The Input Resistance-Threshold Current Relationship in the Papillary Muscles of the Control Rats. The knowledge of the structural organization of the ventricular syncytium is made possible through the study of its active and passive functional properties. The foregoing involves first determining the characteristics of the generation and propagation of its APs. In making these determinations, understanding its behaviour as a functional syncytium is favoured, in addition to the importance that it represents for the structural geometry of the organization of the cardiac ventricular syncytium. It also helps to explain, under normal conditions, the proper propagation of the APs, even when there is a low margin of safety for the propagation [29].

It was observed that the experimental data on the input resistance-threshold current obtained in the cardiac syncytial system of the rat fit an equilateral hyperbola (Figures 5, 6, 7, and 8) and that the values of the input resistance and intracellular thresholds change, with relatively broad ranges.

These results show the following characteristics of the mammalian ventricular functional syncytium [27]:

(1) The input resistance and threshold current are inversely related.

(2) The functional organization of the ventricular syncytium in the left papillary muscle of the rat heart is irregular in terms of the values of the input resistance and the current threshold for initiating an action potential. However, they maintain the same constant value; $K = 30$ mV.

(3) In terms of the threshold current, the cellular excitability is different in each of the explored sites of the papillary muscle preparation.

Therefore, in relatively small areas, the extension of the abundance of low resistance junctions can be an important parameter that can determine and explain the hyperbolic nature of the relationship between the input resistance and the current threshold [27]. With this experimental evidence, it is possible to explain the results obtained. We conclude that the papillary heart muscles from the control rats constitute an irregular syncytium and that the principal cause for this lack of homogeneity is the possible nonuniformity of the spatial distribution of the *nexus* (Figures 5 and 6). Similarly, the experimental data indicate that the smaller the value of the input resistance, the higher the threshold current. The only way we can explain this fact is by assuming that the density of the *nexus* varies from one small area to the next. The small areas that we refer to would be the amount of cells needed to permit the formation of the wavefront [30], and, under these circumstances, every initiation of a wavefront will have a different threshold and, consequently, will present a different *nexus* density. The results shown in Figures 5 and 6 indicate the lack of homogeneity in the ventricular syncytium of the hearts of the control rats.

4.2.2. The Input Resistance-Threshold Current Relationship in the Papillary Muscles of the Diabetic Rats. The irregularity of the ventricular syncytium of the hearts of healthy rats does not imply ventricular electrophysiological abnormalities. However, under pathological conditions such as diabetes (Figure 7), the heterogeneity of the cardiac syncytium is accentuated in these new conditions and increases the probability of the development of lethal arrhythmias. The greater heterogeneity found in the heart of the diabetic rats includes areas of tissue in the papillary muscle with higher input resistance values and lower intracellular thresholds, which implies the existence of areas of tissue with less *nexus* density in the papillary muscle. This phenomenon, observed with high input resistance values and low threshold current values, is firmly supported by studies in diabetic rats in which the decreases in the expression of connexin 43 were found, in addition to the redistribution of their *nexus* [31, 32].

4.2.3. Reentrant Activity in the Ventricular Syncytium of the Diabetic Rats. The accentuated changes in the values of the input resistance and the intracellular thresholds found in the papillary muscles of the diabetic rats become critical to the propagation of the APs. Under these conditions, a wavefront originating from a low-resistance area (high threshold) to high-resistance area (low threshold) propagates easily. However, the opposite case, in which an area of high resistance (low threshold) comes into contact with an area of low resistance (high threshold), faces greater difficulty in propagation because the depolarizing current provided by the wavefront is insufficient for reaching the threshold. Consequently, blocking of the propagation occurs at the site of low resistance, and reentrant activity is facilitated [33]. Figures 9 and 10 clearly show that this phenomenon occurs.

With regard to the results obtained in the papillary muscles of the diabetic rats, it follows that the phenomena exhibited in the propagation of premature responses are the result of discontinuous propagation. Under these conditions, two factors that can cause conduction block in the ventricular syncytium are added: (1) the small efficacy of the premature action potentials, as physiological stimulus, and (2) the irregularity in the input resistance and the intracellular threshold for initiating propagated action potentials (cellular excitability). It is well known that the propagation of the AP in areas of tissue whose excitability is found to be reduced (low input resistance) is performed through electronic potentials [30] and that the magnitude and temporal development of such potentials depend on the organizational geometry of the syncytium.

This study presents two important findings: (1) simultaneous modifications in the input resistance-intracellular threshold in the hearts of diabetic rats and (2) the alterations in the propagation of premature responses. These phenomena allow us to provide an adequate explanation of the arrhythmogenic phenomenon shown by the heart in pathological situations such as diabetes; furthermore, they produce a partial understanding with respect to the high vulnerability of the heart in presenting ventricular fibrillation and sudden death.

4.2.4. Action of the RDP on the Input Resistance-Threshold Current Relationship in the Papillary Muscles of the Hearts of the Control Rats and the Diabetic Rats. Under normal conditions, the daily ingestion of at least one apple is sufficient to decrease the incidence of cardiovascular disease and/or diabetic cardiomyopathy. The dose of RDP provided to the healthy rats for 90 days maintained the heterogeneity of the ventricular syncytium observed in the papillary muscles of the healthy rats (Figure 6). However, the oral supplementation of RDP to the diabetic rats attenuated the increase in the input resistance and the decrease in the threshold current (Figure 8). We noted above (Figure 7) that the increase in the heterogeneity of the ventricular syncytium in the diabetic rats occurs due to a decrease in the density of the *nexus*, which causes an increase in the input resistance values and a decrease in the intracellular thresholds. These changes are supported by the decreased expression of connexin 43, and, therefore, the spatial redistribution of the *nexus* occurs [31, 32]. In the papillary muscles of the diabetic rats with RDP, lower input resistance values and higher current thresholds were found. These magnitudes were similar to those obtained in the control rats. The latter indicates that, in the papillary muscles of the diabetic rats with RDP, there are areas of tissue with a greater density of *nexus*. This observed phenomenon can be explained if we consider that the alterations that occur in the diabetic rats may also occur in dilated cardiomyopathy in the mouse. In this model of dilated cardiomyopathy [26], it was reported that oral supplementation of the mice with an extract of polyphenols contained in the apple increased the expression of connexin 43; consequently, there was an increase in the density and interconnection of the *nexus* in the cardiac myocytes.

Finally, the decrease in the amplitudes of the heterogeneities of the ventricular syncytium and the decrease in the absolute refractory period are two factors that favour the disappearance of the critical propagation of action potentials. Therefore, the heart becomes less vulnerable to arrhythmias. We conclude that apple peel has protective effects on diabetic cardiomyopathy.

5. Conclusions

(1) The ventricular syncytium of the control rats is heterogeneous.

(2) In diabetic cardiomyopathy, the organization of the ventricular syncytium muscle proceeds with functional modifications that are evaluated in terms of input resistance and threshold current.

(3) The propagation of premature responses is associated with conduction blocks.

(4) The hearts of rats with induced diabetes are more vulnerable to reentrant arrhythmias.

(5) The apple peel achieves its protective action by reducing the ARP and attenuating the modifications that the ventricular syncytium suffers during diabetes.

Abbreviations

APD: Action potential duration
GAE: Gallic acid equivalents
STZ: Streptozotocin
AP: Action potential
ARP: Absolute refractory period
RDP: Red Delicious apple peel.

Conflict of Interests

The authors declare that there is no conflict of interests regarding the publication of this paper.

Acknowledgment

The authors would like to express their gratitude to the *Consejo Nacional de Ciencia y Tecnología* (CONACyT, Mexico) (National Council of Science and Technology) for the economic scholarship awarded (no. 60485).

References

[1] T. K. McGhie, S. Hudault, R. C. M. Lunken, and J. T. Christeller, "Apple peels, from seven cultivars, have lipase-inhibitory activity and contain numerous ursenoic acids as identified by LC-ESI-QTOF-HRMS," *Journal of Agricultural and Food Chemistry*, vol. 60, no. 1, pp. 482–491, 2012.

[2] A. Francini and L. Sebastiani, "Phenolic compounds in apple (Malus x domestica Borkh.): compounds characterization and stability during postharvest and after processing," *Antioxidants*, vol. 2, no. 3, pp. 181–193, 2013.

[3] D. A. Hyson, "A comprehensive review of apples and apple components and their relationship to human health," *Advances in Nutrition*, vol. 2, no. 5, pp. 408–420, 2011.

[4] C. M. Andre, J. M. Greenwood, E. G. Walker et al., "Anti-inflammatory procyanidins and triterpenes in 109 apple varieties," *Journal of Agricultural and Food Chemistry*, vol. 60, no. 42, pp. 10546–10554, 2012.

[5] J. Bizjak, M. Mikulic-Petkovsek, F. Stampar, and R. Veberic, "Changes in primary metabolites and polyphenols in the peel of 'braeburn' apples (*Malus domestica* Borkh.) during advanced maturation," *Journal of Agricultural and Food Chemistry*, vol. 61, no. 43, pp. 10283–10292, 2013.

[6] A. Nygren, M. L. Olson, K. Y. Chen, T. Emmett, G. Kargacin, and Y. Shimoni, "Propagation of the cardiac impulse in the diabetic rat heart: reduced conduction reserve," *Journal of Physiology*, vol. 580, no. 2, pp. 543–560, 2007.

[7] N. T. Aggarwal and J. C. Makielski, "Redox control of cardiac excitability," *Antioxidants and Redox Signaling*, vol. 18, no. 4, pp. 432–468, 2013.

[8] E. Martinez-Ladron de Guevara, N. Pérez-Hernández, M. A. Villalobos-López, F. Félix Durán, and V. Hernández García, "Actions of the apple peel on electrical activity of the heart of rats with type 1 diabetes," in *Proceedings of the 1st PanAmerican Congress of Physiological Sciences*, abstract 04-36, p. 83, Foz do Iguaçu, Brazil, 2014.

[9] Secretariat of Finance and Public Credit, "Panorama of the apple," April 2014, http://www.financierarural.gob.mx/informacionsectorrural/Panoramas/Panorama%20Manzana%20(abr%202014).pdf.

[10] U. Imeh and S. Khokhar, "Distribution of conjugated and free phenols in fruits: antioxidant activity and cultivar variations," *Journal of Agricultural and Food Chemistry*, vol. 50, no. 22, pp. 6301–6306, 2002.

[11] R. Tsao, R. Yang, J. C. Young, and H. Zhu, "Polyphenolic profiles in eight apple cultivars using high-performance liquid chromatography (HPLC)," *Journal of Agricultural and Food Chemistry*, vol. 51, no. 21, pp. 6347–6353, 2003.

[12] K. Wolfe, X. Wu, and R. H. Liu, "Antioxidant activity of apple peels," *Journal of Agricultural and Food Chemistry*, vol. 51, no. 3, pp. 609–614, 2003.

[13] Association Official Analytical Chemists (AOAC), *Official Methods of Analysis*, AOAC, Washington, DC, USA, 16th edition, 1995.

[14] V. L. Singleton and J. A. Rossi Jr., "Colorimetry of total phenolics with phosphomolybdic-phosphotungstic acid reagents," *American Journal of Enology and Viticulture*, vol. 16, no. 3, pp. 144–158, 1965.

[15] F. S. Fein, L. B. Kornstein, J. E. Strobeck, J. M. Capasso, and E. H. Sonnenblick, "Altered myocardial mechanics in diabetic rats," *Circulation Research*, vol. 47, no. 6, pp. 922–933, 1980.

[16] Y. Shimoni, L. Firek, D. Severson, and W. Giles, "Short-term diabetes alters K^+ currents in rat ventricular myocytes," *Circulation Research*, vol. 74, no. 4, pp. 620–628, 1994.

[17] F. S. Fein, R. S. Aronson, C. Nordin, B. Miller-Green, and E. H. Sonnenblick, "Altered myocardial response to ouabain in diabetic rats: mechanics and electrophysiology," *Journal of Molecular and Cellular Cardiology*, vol. 15, no. 11, pp. 769–784, 1983.

[18] J. Magyar, Z. Rusznák, P. Szentesi, G. Szûcs, and L. Kovács, "Action potentials and potassium currents in rat ventricular muscle during experimental diabetes," *Journal of Molecular and Cellular Cardiology*, vol. 24, no. 8, pp. 841–853, 1992.

[19] P. Jourdon and D. Feuvray, "Calcium and potassium currents in ventricular myocytes isolated from diabetic rats," *The Journal of Physiology*, vol. 470, no. 1, pp. 411–429, 1993.

[20] Y. Shimoni, D. Severson, and W. Giles, "Thyroid status and diabetes modulate regional differences in potassium currents in rat ventricle," *The Journal of Physiology*, vol. 488, no. 3, pp. 673–688, 1995.

[21] M. Apkon and J. M. Nerbonne, "Characterization of two distinct depolarization-activated K^+ currents in isolated adult rat ventricular myocytes," *Journal of General Physiology*, vol. 97, no. 5, pp. 973–1011, 1991.

[22] M. R. Mitchell, T. Powell, D. A. Terrar, and V. W. Twist, "The effects of ryanodine, EGTA and low-sodium on action potentials in rat and guinea-pig ventricular myocytes: evidence for two inward currents during the plateau," *British Journal of Pharmacology*, vol. 81, no. 3, pp. 543–550, 1984.

[23] J. R. Lopez, T. Banyasz, T. Kavacs, F. A. Sreter, and G. Szücs, "Defective myoplasmatic Ca^{2+} homeostasis in vetricular muscle in diabetic cardiomyopathic rats," *Biophysical Journal*, vol. 53, article 161a, 1988, (abstract).

[24] S. Nobe, M. Aomine, M. Arita, S. Ito, and R. Takaki, "Chronic diabetes mellitus prolongs action potential duration of rat ventricular muscles: circumstantial evidence for impaired Ca^{2+} channel," *Cardiovascular Research*, vol. 24, no. 5, pp. 381–389, 1990.

[25] D. Lagadic-Gossmann, K. J. Buckler, K. Le Prigent, and D. Feuvray, "Altered Ca^{2+} handling in ventricular myocytes isolated from diabetic rats," *The American Journal of Physiology—Heart*

and Circulatory Physiology, vol. 270, no. 5, pp. H1529–H1537, 1996.

[26] T. Sunagawa, T. Shimizu, A. Matsumoto et al., "Cardiac electrophysiological alterations in heart/muscle-specific manganese-superoxide dismutase-deficient mice: prevention by a dietary antioxidant polyphenol," *BioMed Research International*, vol. 2014, Article ID 704291, 12 pages, 2014.

[27] C. Mendez and V. Hernandez, "Inverse relation between input resistance and threshold current in canine cardiac syncytium," *Journal of Cardiovascular Electrophysiology*, vol. 12, no. 3, pp. 337–342, 2001.

[28] K. Matsuda, A. Kamillama, and T. Hoshi, "Configuration of the transmembrane potential of the Purkinje-muscle fiber junction and its analysis," in *Electrophysiology and Ultrastructure of the Heart*, pp. 177–187, Grune & Stratton, New York, NY, USA, 1967.

[29] C. Mendez, W. J. Mueller, and X. Urguiaga, "Propagation of impulses across the Purkinje fiber-muscle junctions in the dog heart," *Circulation Research*, vol. 26, no. 2, pp. 135–150, 1970.

[30] C. Mendez and G. K. Moe, "Some characteristics of transmembrane potentials of AV nodal cells during propagation of premature beats," *Circulation Research*, vol. 19, no. 6, pp. 933–1010, 1966.

[31] H. Lin, K. Ogawa, I. Imanaga, and N. Tribulova, "Remodeling of connexin 43 in the diabetic rat heart," *Molecular and Cellular Biochemistry*, vol. 290, no. 1-2, pp. 69–78, 2006.

[32] L. Okruhlicova, N. Tribulova, M. Mišejkova et al., "Gap junction remodelling is involved in the susceptibility of diabetic rats to hypokalemia-induced ventricular fibrillation," *Acta Histochemica*, vol. 104, no. 4, pp. 387–391, 2002.

[33] B. I. Sasyniuk and C. Mendez, "A mechanism for reentry in canine ventricular tissue," *Circulation Research*, vol. 28, pp. 3–15, 1971.

15

Puerarin Improves Diabetic Aorta Injury by Inhibiting NADPH Oxidase-Derived Oxidative Stress in STZ-Induced Diabetic Rats

Wenping Li,[1,2] Wenwen Zhao,[3] Qin Wu,[1] Yuanfu Lu,[1] Jingshan Shi,[1] and Xiuping Chen[3]

[1] *Key Lab for Pharmacology of Ministry of Education, Department of Pharmacology, Zunyi Medical College, Zunyi 563003, China*
[2] *Chengdu Chronic Diseases Hospital, Chengdu 610083, China*
[3] *State Key Laboratory of Quality Research in Chinese Medicine, Institute of Chinese Medical Sciences, University of Macau, Macau*

Correspondence should be addressed to Jingshan Shi; shijs@zmc.edu.cn and Xiuping Chen; xpchen@umac.mo

Academic Editor: Hiroshi Okamoto

Objective. Puerarin is a natural flavonoid isolated from the TCM lobed kudzuvine root. This study investigated the effect and mechanisms of puerarin on diabetic aorta in rats. *Methods.* Streptozotocin- (STZ-) induced diabetic rats were administered with puerarin for 3 weeks. Levels of serum insulin (INS), PGE2, endothelin (ET), glycated hemoglobin (GHb), H_2O_2, and nitric oxide (NO) in rats were measured by ELISA and colorimetric assay kits. The aortas were stained with H&E. Moreover, the mRNA expression of ICAM-1, LOX-1, NADPH oxidase 2 (NOX2), and NOX4 and the protein expression of ICAM-1, LOX-1, NF-κB p65, E-selectin, NOX2, and NOX4 in aorta tissues were measured by real-time PCR and Western blot, respectively. The localization of ICAM-1, NF-κB p65, NOX2, and NOX4 in the aorta tissues was also determined through immunohistochemistry. *Results.* Puerarin treatment exerted no effect on fasting blood glucose levels but significantly reduced the serum levels of INS, GHb, PGE2, ET, H_2O_2, and NO. In addition, puerarin improved the pathological alterations and inhibited the expression of ICAM-1, LOX-1, NOX2, and NOX4 at both mRNA and protein levels. Puerarin also significantly reduced the number of cells showing positive staining for ICAM-1, NOX2, NOX4, and NF-κB p65. *Conclusion.* Puerarin demonstrated protective effect on the STZ-induced diabetic rat aorta. The protective mechanisms may include regulation of NF-κB and inhibition of NOX2 and NOX4 followed by inhibition of cell adhesion molecule expression.

1. Introduction

Diabetes, a chronic disease characterized by hyperglycemia, has become a major health crisis worldwide. The global prevalence of diabetes in 382 million people in 2013 is estimated to rise to 592 million by 2035 [1]. Diabetes leads to an array of chronic microvascular (retinopathy, nephropathy, and neuropathy) and macrovascular (atherosclerosis, ischemic heart disease, stroke, and peripheral vascular disease) complications. These chronic complications are the major causes of the reduced quality of life among diabetics, increased burden to the health care system, and increased diabetes-related mortality [2]. Although the microvascular complications are directly related to the severity and duration of hyperglycemia, the macrovascular complications are the primary causes of mortality, with myocardial infarction and stroke accounting for 80% of all deaths among T2DM patients [3]. Therefore, inhibiting and alleviating the macrovascular complications have become a major challenge in diabetes treatment.

The vascular functions are tightly regulated by a series of vasoactive agents such as nitric oxide (NO), PGE2, and endothelin (ET) [4]. Furthermore, the adhesion molecules such as intercellular adhesion molecule-1 (ICAM-1) and lectin-like oxidized low-density lipoprotein receptor-1 (LOX-1) play important roles in endothelial dysfunction and vascular injury [5]. In addition, the NADPH oxidase (NOX family), one of the main sources of reactive oxygen species (ROS) in vascular, and NF-κB, the key transcription factor in regulating adhesion molecular expression, play important roles in diabetic vascular complications [6, 7].

Puerarin is a natural, flavonoid-rich component of the Chinese herb lobed kudzuvine root. Previous findings showed that puerarin contains multiple bioactive compounds and has been widely used to treat cardiovascular and cerebrovascular diseases, osteonecrosis, Parkinson's disease, Alzheimer's disease, endometriosis, osteoporosis, liver injury, inflammation, and cancer [8, 9]. Studies also showed that puerarin improves diabetic complications by reducing blood glucose [10] and enhancing glucose uptake [11], thereby preventing retinopathy [12], improving insulin resistance (IR) [13], protecting the pancreatic beta cells [14], improving cardiac function [15], and inhibiting oxidative stress [16], among others. However, its effect on diabetic macrovascular complications remains unclear. In the current research, the effect of puerarin on macrovascular complications was investigated in streptozotocin- (STZ-) induced diabetic rats.

2. Methods

2.1. Reagents. Puerarin injection was purchased from Hunan WZT Pharmaceutical Co., Ltd. (China). The STZ was obtained from Sigma (USA). The primers for ICAM-1, LOX-1, NADPH oxidase 2 (NOX2), NOX4, and β-actin were purchased from Generay, Inc. (Shanghai, China). The primary antibodies for ICAM-1, LOX-1, and NF-κB p65 were purchased from Proteintech Group, Inc. (Wuhan, China), Abcam (USA), and Boster (Wuhan, China), respectively, whereas those for NOX2, NOX4, and E-selectin were purchased from Santa Cruz Biotechnology.

2.2. Animals. Male Sprague Dawley rats (250–280 g) were purchased from the Experimental Animal Center of Daping Hospital. This study was approved by the Animal Ethics Committee of Zunyi Medical College. All rats were maintained on a 12 h alternating light/dark cycle at $22 \pm 2^{\circ}$C and 55%–60% humidity. Diabetes was induced by intraperitoneal (i.p.) injection of freshly prepared STZ in citrate buffer (dissolved in 0.1 mmol/L citrate buffer, pH 4.2–4.5) at a dosage of 60 mg/kg/day for 3 consecutive days. Eight nondiabetic control rats received an equal volume of citric buffer only. Rats with blood glucose levels of ≥16.7 mmol/L after 72 h administration of STZ were considered diabetic. These diabetic rats (24 rats) were randomly divided into 3 groups (8 each) and were administered with or without puerarin (18 and 45 mg/kg/day i.p.) for 3 weeks. Body weight and blood glucose levels were measured twice a week.

2.3. Determination of Fasting Blood Glucose (FBG). FBG was determined twice a week by using ONETOUCH Ultra Glucometer (Johnson & Johnson, USA) in accordance with the manufacturer's instructions.

2.4. Determination of Serum Insulin (INS), Glycated Hemoglobin (GHb), PGE2, ET, H_2O_2, and NO Levels. Serum levels of INS, GHb, PGE2, ET, H_2O_2, and NO were determined using commercial ELISA kits (R&D, USA) in accordance with the manufacturer's instructions.

2.5. H&E Staining. Aorta specimens were fixed in 4% neutral formaldehyde solution. After dehydration with graded alcohol solutions and xylene, the specimens were embedded in paraffin. The specimens were then cut into 5 μm thick cross sections and stained with H&E by conventional method.

2.6. RT-PCR. Total RNA was extracted from the aorta specimens with Trizol (Invitrogen) for cDNA synthesis by using a reverse transcription reaction kit (TaKaRa). Table 1 shows the primers for ICAM-1, LOX-1, NOX2, NOX4, and β-actin.

2.7. Western Blot. Total proteins were extracted from the aorta, and the protein contents were determined using a BCA Protein Assay Kit (Generay). Proteins (50 μg) were subjected to 8%–10% SDS-PAGE and then transferred onto PVDF membranes. After blocking with 5% nonfat milk in TBST at room temperature for 1 h, the membranes were washed thrice with TBST and then incubated overnight with specific primary antibodies (1 : 500–1 : 1000) at 4°C. After washing with 5% nonfat milk/TBST, the membranes were incubated with horseradish peroxidase-conjugated secondary antibodies at room temperature for 2 h. Protein-antibody complexes were detected by ECL Advanced Western Blot Detection Kit.

2.8. Immunohistochemistry. After the consecutive steps of deparaffinization, deactivation of endogenous peroxidase with 3% H_2O_2, and antigen blocking with 5% BSA-PBS, the sections were incubated with ICAM-1, NF-κB, NOX2, and NOX4 antibodies (1 : 50 dilution) at 37°C for 2 h. After rinsing thrice with PBS, the sections were incubated with secondary antibody (Gene Tech, Shanghai, China) for 30 min at 37°C and then stained using DAB chromogen kit (Beijing Zhongshan Golden Bridge Biotechnology Co., Ltd.).

2.9. Statistical Analysis. Data were expressed as means ± SD of at least three separate experiments. Statistical analysis was performed using SPSS 16.0, and differences between groups were analyzed by one-way ANOVA. A value of $p < 0.05$ was considered statistically significant.

3. Results

3.1. Effect of Puerarin on Body Weight and FBG. The average body weight of the control group increased significantly, whereas that of the model group decreased considerably. Puerarin treatment exerted no effect on body weight (Figure 1(a)). Moreover, the mean FBG of the control group was 5.1 mmol/L, which increased to 20.8 mmol/L after STZ injection approximately fourfold. Compared with the model group, the FBG levels of the high-dosage treatment group decreased, but this disparity was not statistically significant (Figure 1(b)).

3.2. Effect of Puerarin on Serum INS and GHb. Compared with the control group, the serum levels of INS and GHb in the diabetic rats increased significantly. Low-dose puerarin exerted no effect on either INS or GHb, whereas high-dose puerarin significantly reduced both INS and GHb levels (Figures 1(c) and 1(d)).

TABLE 1: Primers for RT-PCR.

Gene	Forward primer (5′-3′)	Reverse primer (5′-3′)
NOX4	CAGTCAAACAGATGGATACAGA	ATAGAACTGGGTCCACAGCAGA
ICAM-1	GCTCAGGTATCCATCCATCCC	AGTTCGTCTTTCATCCAGTTAGTCT
LOX-1	TAACTGGGAAAAAAGTCGGGAGAAT	AATGGGAAGTTGCTTGTAAGACGAA
NOX2	TGAATCTCAGGCCAATCACTTT	ATGGTCTTGAACTCGTTATCCC
β-actin	CTGAACCCTAAGGCCAACCG	GACCGAGGCATACAGGGACAA

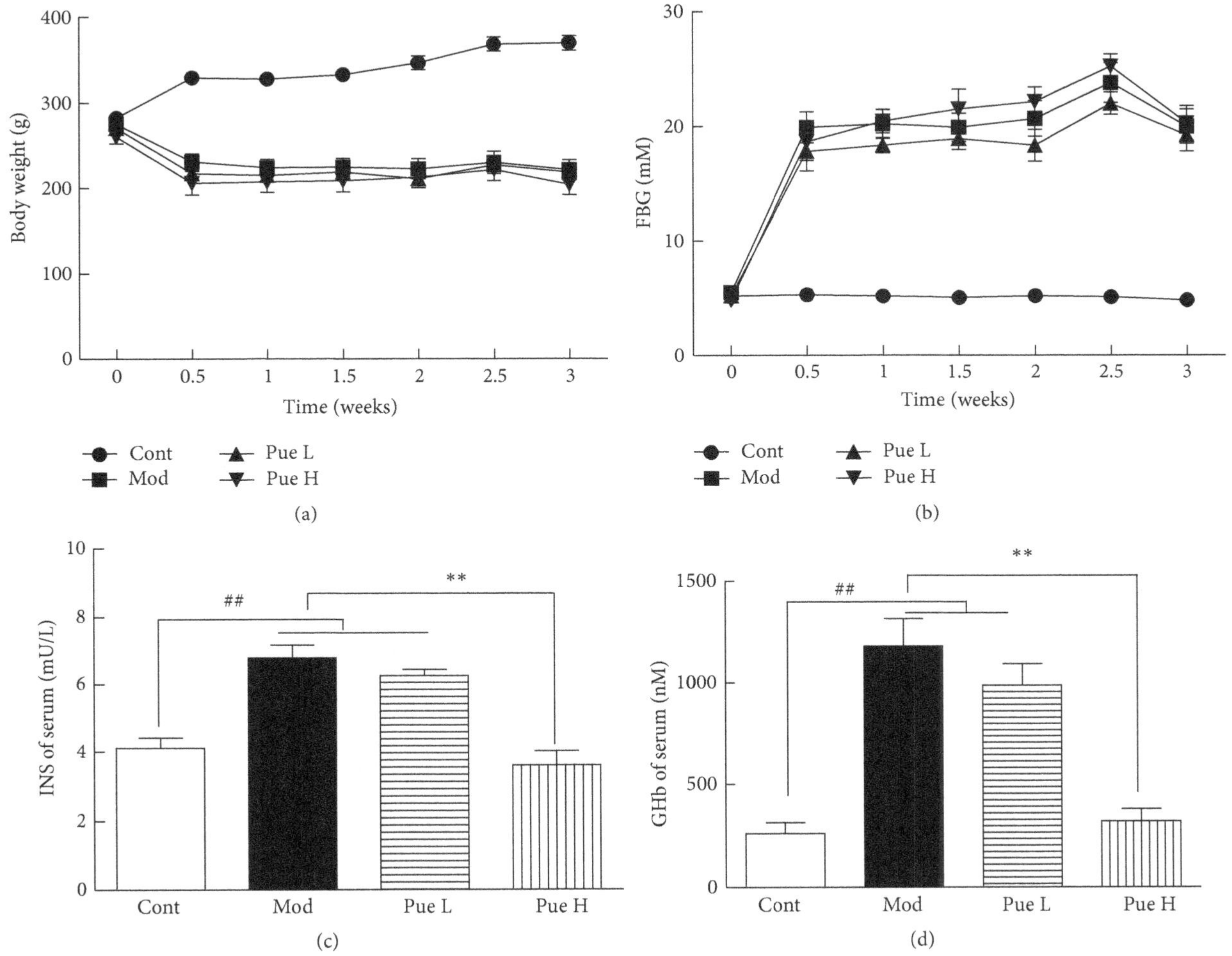

FIGURE 1: Effect of puerarin on body weight (a), FBG (b), serum INS (c), and GHb in STZ-induced diabetic rats. $^{##}p < 0.01$ versus Cont; $^{**}p < 0.01$ versus Mod. Cont, control group; Mod, diabetic model group; Pue L, low dosage of puerarin; Pue H, high dosage of puerarin.

3.3. Effects of Puerarin on Serum PGE2, ET, H_2O_2, and NO. Compared with the control group, the serum levels of PGE2, ET, H_2O_2, and NO in diabetic rats significantly increased. These parameters were not affected by low-dose puerarin but significantly reduced by high-dose puerarin (Figure 2).

3.4. Effect of Puerarin on Aorta Alterations. H&E staining showed that the structure of each layer of the aorta was normal, and the smooth muscle cells were neatly arranged in rows. No damage or injury was observed in the control group, whereas the aortic wall was thickened and the adventitial fibrosis increased in the diabetic group. Furthermore, ruptured smooth muscles and increased nucleus were observed. These alterations were improved by both dosages of puerarin treatment, especially the high-dosage treatment (Figure 3).

3.5. Effect of Puerarin on mRNA Expression of ICAM-1, LOX-1, NOX2, and NOX4. Compared with the control group, the mRNA expression of ICAM-1, LOX-1, NOX2, and NOX4 increased significantly in diabetic rats. The mRNA expression levels of these genes were inhibited by puerarin in a dose-dependent manner (Figure 4).

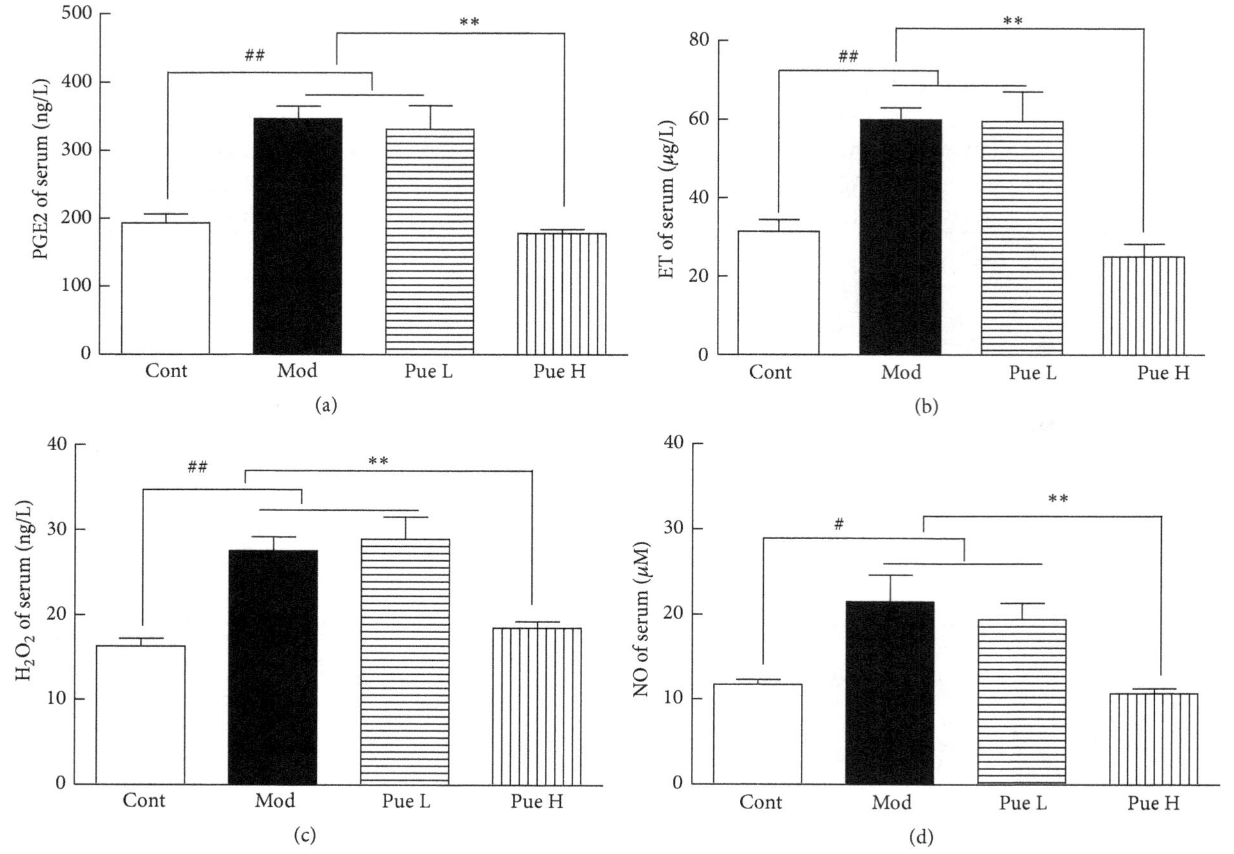

FIGURE 2: Effect of puerarin on serum PGE2 (a), ET (b), H_2O_2(c), and NO (d) in STZ-induced diabetic rats. $^{\#\#}p < 0.01$ versus Cont; $^{**}p < 0.01$ versus Mod. Cont, control group; Mod, diabetic model group; Pue L, low dosage of puerarin; Pue H, high dosage of puerarin.

3.6. Effect of Puerarin on Protein Expression of ICAM-1, LOX-1, NOX2, NOX4, E-Selectin, and NF-κB p65. Compared with the control group, the protein expression levels of ICAM-1, LOX-1, and E-selectin (Figure 5), as well as those of NOX2, NOX4, and NF-κB p65 (Figure 6), increased significantly in diabetic rats and were inhibited by puerarin.

3.7. Effect of Puerarin on Localization of ICAM-1, NF-κB p65, NOX2, and NOX4. ICAM-1, NOX2, NOX4, and NF-κB p65 were lowly expressed in the endothelial and smooth muscle cells of the control group. By contrast, their expression increased significantly, especially in the smooth muscle cells of the aorta of diabetic rats, as indicated by the conspicuous brown granules. Puerarin treatment significantly reduced the amount of brown granules, suggesting the reduced expression of these proteins (Figure 7). Furthermore, high dosage of puerarin can almost completely inhibit the expression of ICAM-1 and NOX2.

4. Discussion

Diabetes, regardless of its clinical categories, is a metabolic disease characterized by high blood glucose level over a prolonged period. The diabetic vascular complications, the main cause of diabetic death, are closely connected with the sustained increase of glucose. In this study, we established a diabetic model with dramatic increase of glucose level, increase of serum INS, and decrease of body weight. Though these characteristics are not identical to classical type 1 or type 2 diabetic rat models, the increased glucose level was useful for the exploration of vascular protective agents.

Puerarin has been approved by the SFDA of China as an adjuvant treatment of coronary heart disease, myocardial infarction, and cerebrovascular disease. The present study investigated the effect of puerarin on the aorta of diabetic rats. STZ injection significantly induced hyperglycemia, increased INS, and reduced body weight, suggesting the development of diabetes. Puerarin exerted no effect on FBG of the STZ-induced diabetic rats, and this finding is consistent with previous report [17]. However, She et al. [16] showed that puerarin treatment reduced blood glucose levels and increased body weight. This disparity may be ascribed to the difference in dosage. Our dosage is less than half of that used by She et al. [16]. Moreover, blood GHb level plays a pivotal role in monitoring the long-term glycemic status of diabetes mellitus patients [18]. In the current study, although puerarin exerted no effect on FBG, puerarin reduced GHb, and this finding is consistent with previous observation on puerarin-treated diabetic patients [19]. Previous research also showed

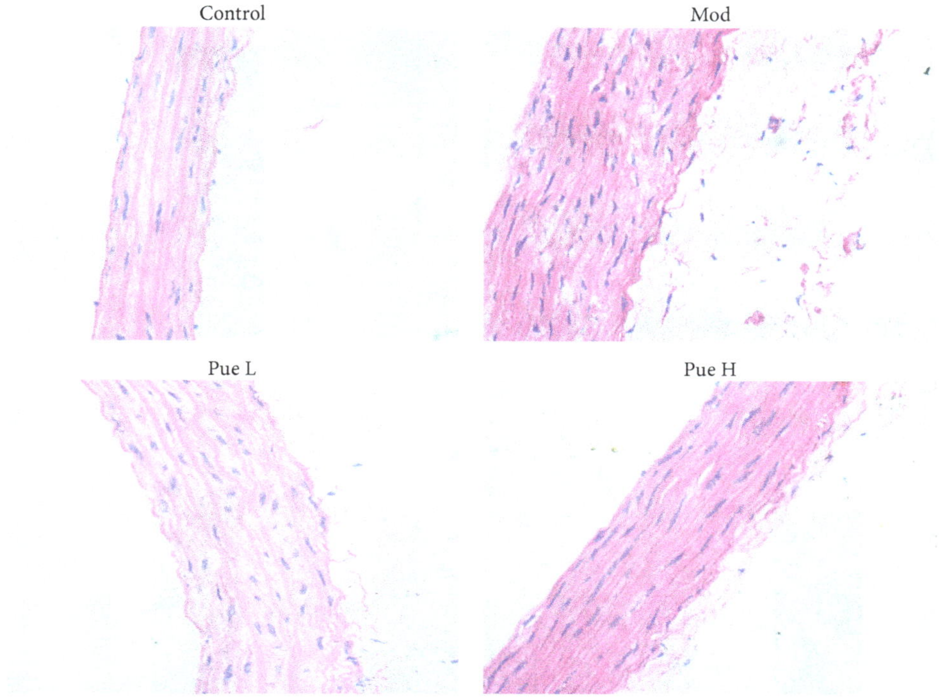

FIGURE 3: Effect of puerarin on morphological alterations in STZ-induced diabetic rats. H&E staining, 200x. Pue L, low dosage of puerarin; Pue H, high dosage of puerarin.

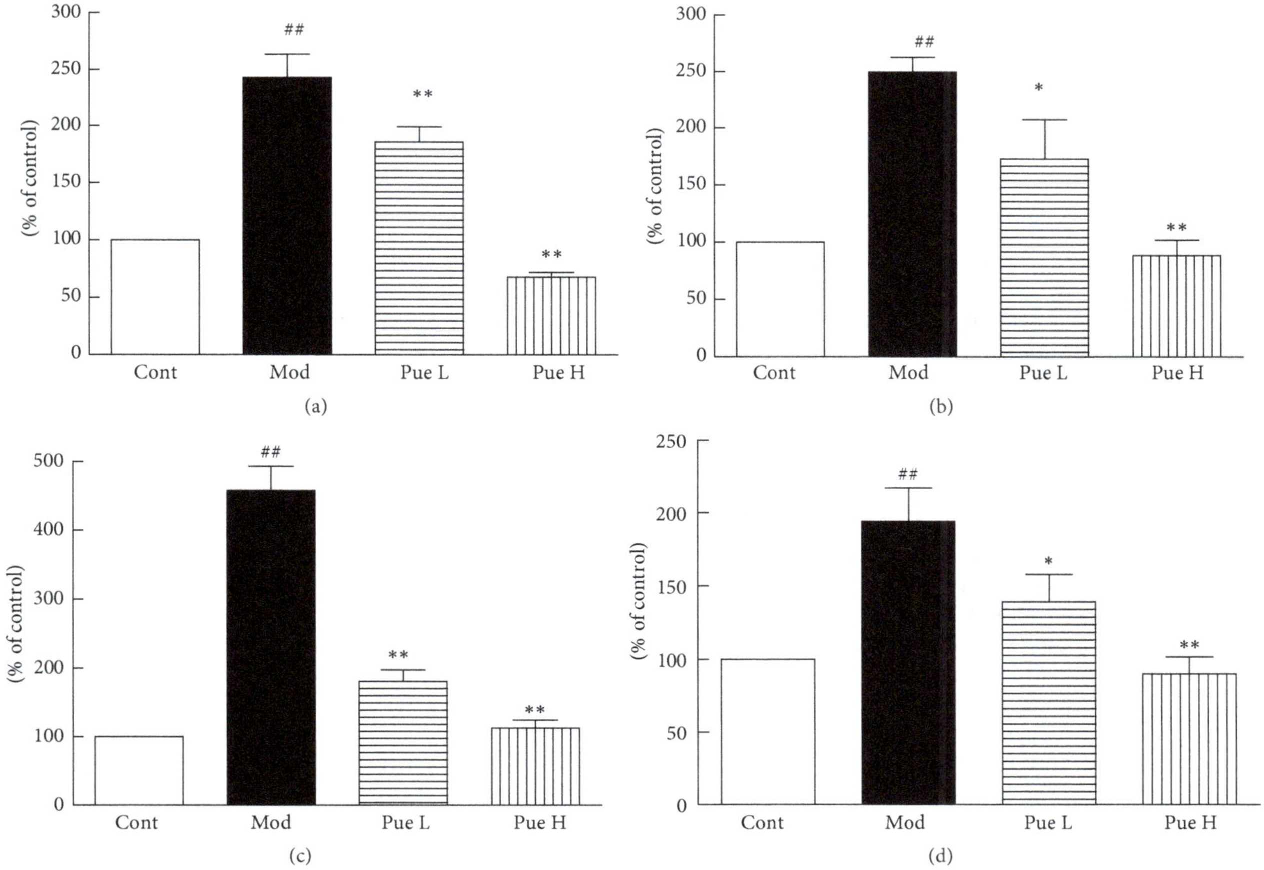

FIGURE 4: Effect of puerarin on mRNA expression of ICAM-1 (a), LOX-1 (b), NOX2 (c), and NOX4 (d) in the aorta of STZ-induced diabetic rats. $^{\#\#}p < 0.01$ versus Cont; $^{*}p < 0.05$ and $^{**}p < 0.01$ versus Mod. Cont, control group; Mod, diabetic model group; Pue L, low dosage of puerarin; Pue H, high dosage of puerarin.

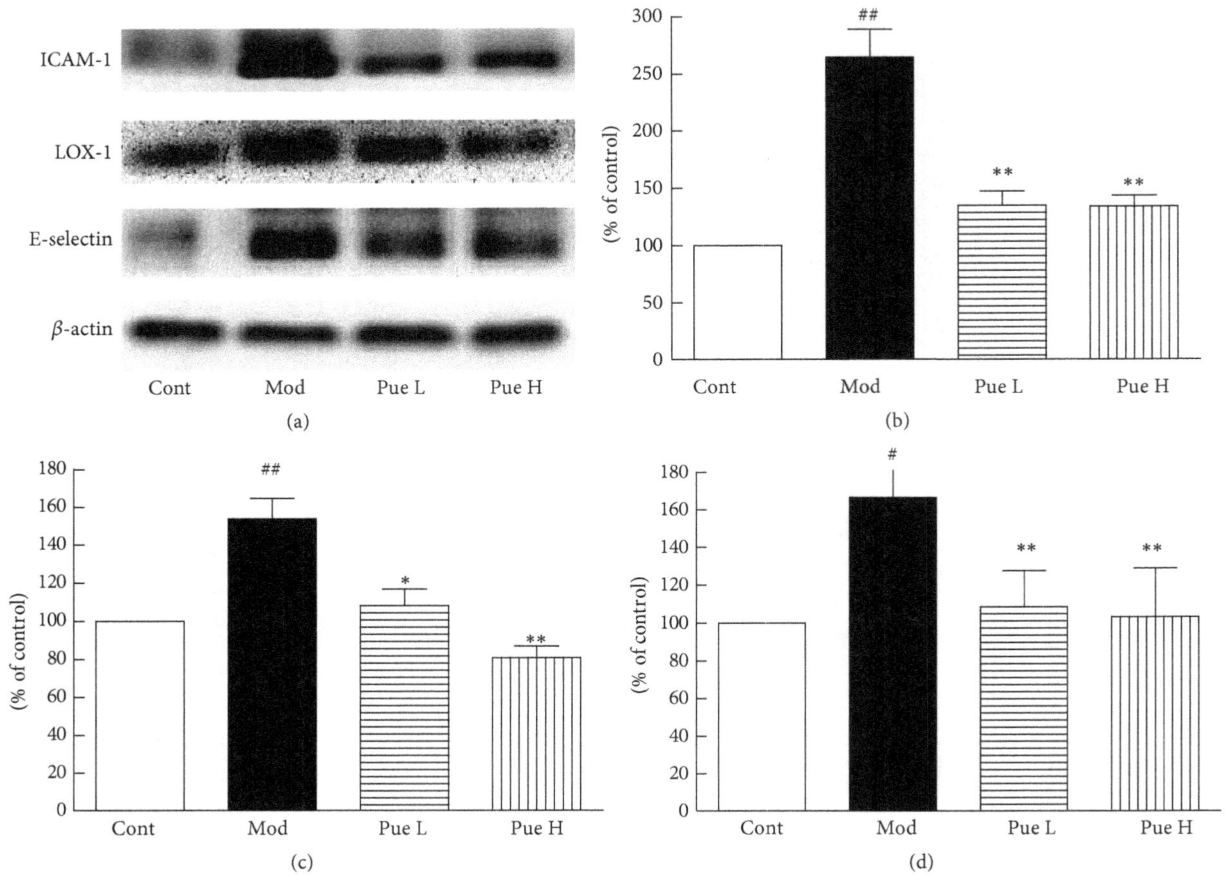

FIGURE 5: Effect of puerarin on protein expression of ICAM-1, LOX-1, and E-selectin (a) in the aorta of STZ-induced diabetic rats; statistical results for ICAM-1 (b), LOX-1 (c), and E-selectin (d). $^{\#}p < 0.05$ and $^{\#\#}p < 0.01$ versus Cont; $^{*}p < 0.05$ and $^{**}p < 0.01$ versus Mod. Cont, control group; Mod, diabetic model group; Pue L, low dosage of puerarin; Pue H, high dosage of puerarin.

that puerarin reversed the reduced INS in STZ-induced diabetic mice [20]. By contrast, we found that puerarin reversed the increased INS in STZ-induced diabetic rats. This effect of puerarin may be associated with its influence on IR [13]. The contraction and relaxation of vessels are strictly and precisely controlled by vasoactive substances, such as angiotensin II, ET, PGEs, and NO. Consistent with previous reports [21, 22], serum NO and H_2O_2 concentrations were significantly increased in diabetic rats. Although physiological levels of NO and H_2O_2 positively regulate the vascular function and homeostasis, nitrosative and oxidative stresses caused by excessive generation of them result in alterations of vascular reactivity and lead to vascular toxicity [23]. Increased PGE2 and ET secretions in diabetic vascular bed [24] and placenta [25] were also observed. These changes reflected diabetic vascular dysfunction, which was partly reversed by puerarin, suggesting that puerarin affects diabetic vascular nitrosative and oxidative stresses, and restored vascular tension. Furthermore, pathological alterations were detected in diabetic aorta. The thickened media were mainly caused by the proliferation of vascular smooth muscles, possibly resulting from increased amount of glucose [26]. These observations are consistent with the recent findings in which puerarin attenuates calcification of vascular smooth muscle cells (VSMCs) [27] and attenuates high-glucose- and diabetes-induced VSMC proliferation [28].

The vascular adhesion molecules ICAM-1, LOX-1, and E-selectin serve as biomarkers of vascular inflammation. Enhanced expression of these molecules was observed in high-glucose-treated endothelial cells [29, 30]. In the present study, both the expression of ICAM-1 and LOX-1 at mRNA and protein levels and the protein expression of E-selectin increased in diabetic aorta. Moreover, immunohistochemistry results showed that increased ICAM-1 was observed not only in endothelial cells but also in VSMCs. Puerarin inhibited the expression of these adhesion molecules, suggesting its inhibitory effect on vascular inflammation.

Oxidative stress plays a key role in diabetic complications in the kidney, heart, eye, or vasculature [31]. NOX is a major source of reactive oxygen species (ROS) and is a critical mediator of redox signaling in diabetes [32]. The NOX family comprises seven members, including NOX1–5, DUOX1, and DUOX2. NOX2 and NOX4 are widely expressed in vascular endothelial cells and VSMCs [32, 33]. We found herein a low expression of both NOX2 and NOX4 at mRNA and protein levels in the aorta. Immunohistochemistry results

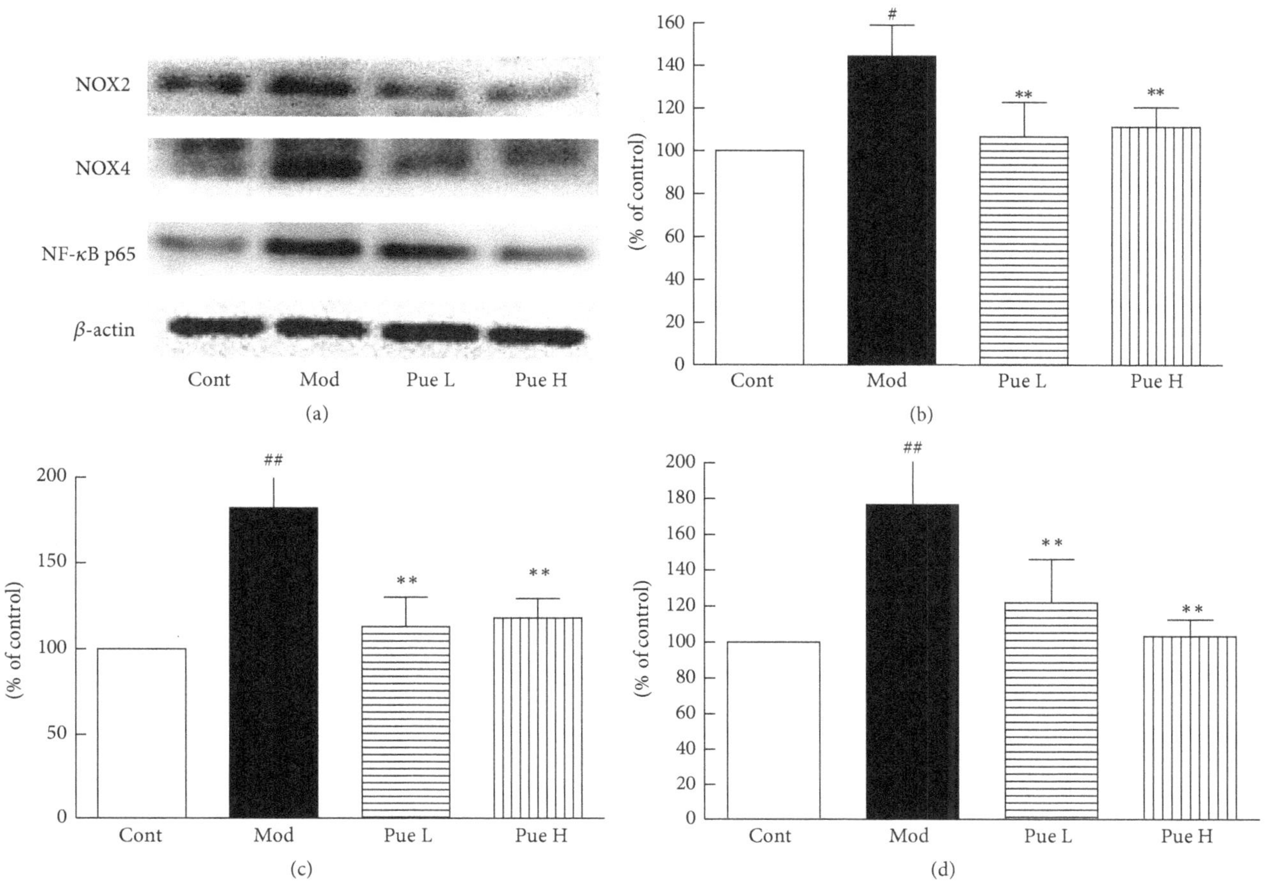

FIGURE 6: Effect of puerarin on protein expression of NOX2, NOX4, and NF-κB p65 (a) in the aorta of STZ-induced diabetic rats; statistical results for NOX2 (b), NOX4 (c), and NF-κB p65 (d). $^{\#}p < 0.05$ and $^{\#\#}p < 0.01$ versus Cont; $^{*}p < 0.05$ and $^{**}p < 0.01$ versus Mod. Cont, control group; Mod, diabetic model group; Pue L, low dosage of puerarin; Pue H, high dosage of puerarin.

also showed that both endothelial cells and VSMCs expressed NOX2 and NOX4. In addition, their expression was significantly increased in STZ-induced diabetic rats, especially in their VSMCs. These results suggested that NOX was activated in diabetic aorta. Furthermore, superoxide anion and H_2O_2 are the main products of NOX2 and NOX4, respectively, and the increased serum H_2O_2 concentration is possibly caused by NOX4 activation. Previous studies showed that puerarin inhibits high-glucose-induced VSMC proliferation by interfering with PKCβ2/Rac1-dependent ROS [28]; moreover, puerarin inhibits retinal pericyte apoptosis induced by the end products of advanced glycation *in vitro* and *in vivo* by inhibiting NOX-related oxidative stress [34]. The inhibitory effect of puerarin on NOX2 and NOX4 expression in diabetic aorta suggested that the beneficial effect of puerarin is attributed to its inhibitory effect on NOX.

ROS is a key upstream activator of the NF-κB pathway [35], which consequently regulates the expression of LOX-1, ICAM-1, and E-selectin [36–39]. The NF-κB pathway was activated as evidenced by the increased protein expression of NF-κB p65 in the diabetic aorta. Furthermore, the expression of NF-κB p65 was colocalized with those of NOX2, NOX4, and ICAM-1, suggesting the potential role of NF-κB. The inhibitory effect of puerarin on NF-κB is possibly caused by the inhibitory effect of puerarin on NOX2 and NOX4, as well as its antioxidant activities [9].

In summary, this study showed that puerarin protected the diabetic aorta by inhibiting oxidative stress and adhesion molecule expression. This finding proves that puerarin can improve the macrovascular complications of diabetes.

Conflict of Interests

The authors declare no conflict of interests related to the present work.

Acknowledgments

This study was supported by the Science and Technology Development Fund, Macau (FDCT) (021/2012/A1), and the National Natural Science Foundation of China (no. 81160048).

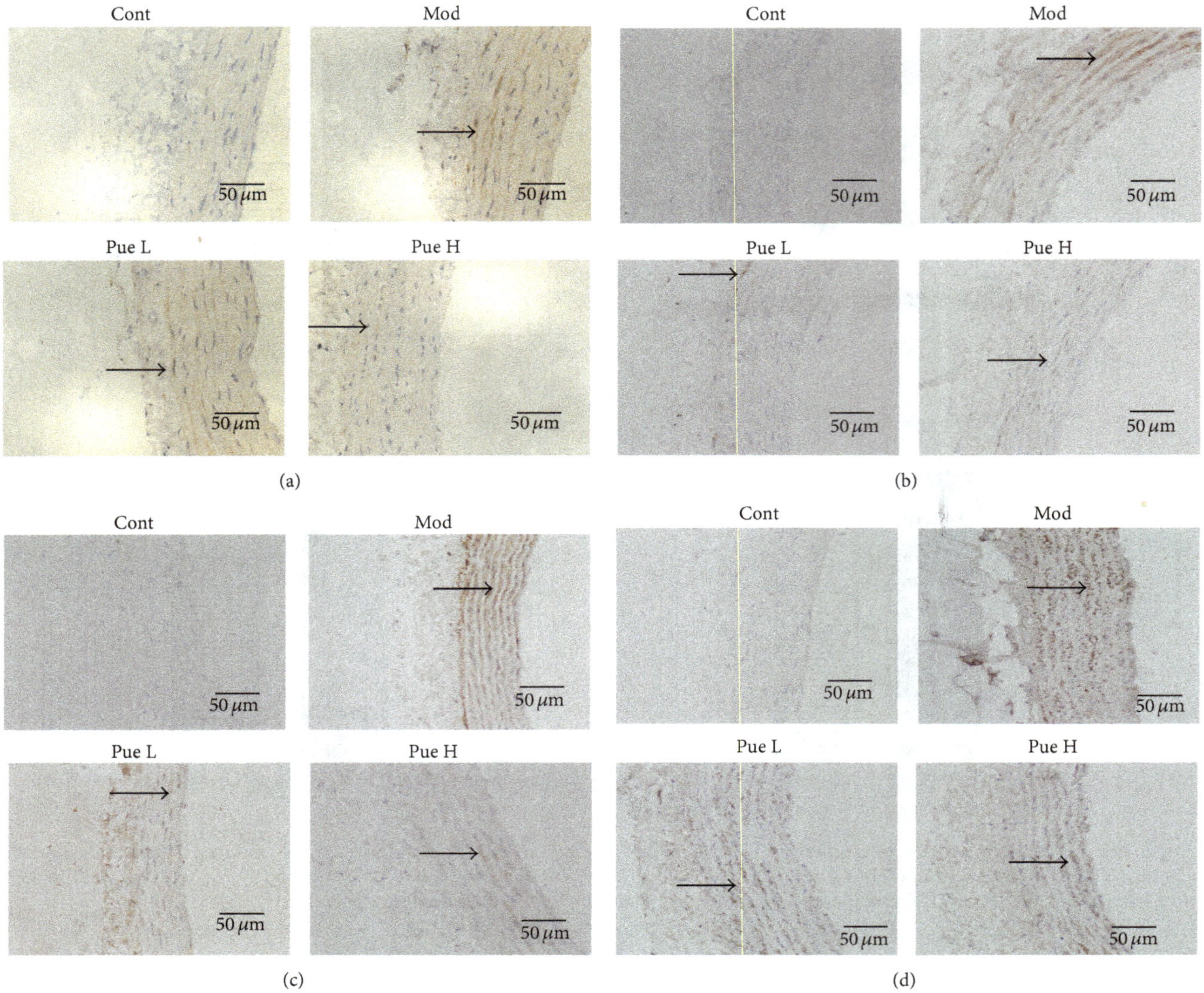

FIGURE 7: Effect of puerarin on localization of ICAM-1 (a), NOX2 (b), NOX4 (c), and NF-κB p65 (d) proteins in the aorta as revealed by immunohistochemistry. Arrows, intensive expression.

References

[1] N. G. Forouhi and N. J. Wareham, "Epidemiology of diabetes," *Medicine*, vol. 42, no. 12, pp. 698–702, 2014.

[2] Z. Liu, C. Fu, W. Wang, and B. Xu, "Prevalence of chronic complications of type 2 diabetes mellitus in outpatients—a cross-sectional hospital based survey in urban China," *Health and Quality of Life Outcomes*, vol. 8, article 62, 2010.

[3] E. Ferrannini and R. A. DeFronzo, "Impact of glucose-lowering drugs on cardiovascular disease in type 2 diabetes," *European Heart Journal*, vol. 36, no. 34, pp. 2288–2296, 2015.

[4] J. Xu and M.-H. Zou, "Molecular insights and therapeutic targets for diabetic endothelial dysfunction," *Circulation*, vol. 120, no. 13, pp. 1266–1286, 2009.

[5] T. Kita, N. Kume, M. Minami et al., "Role of oxidized LDL in atherosclerosis," *Annals of the New York Academy of Sciences*, vol. 947, pp. 199–206, 2001.

[6] A. Manea, "NADPH oxidase-derived reactive oxygen species: involvement in vascular physiology and pathology," *Cell and Tissue Research*, vol. 342, no. 3, pp. 325–339, 2010.

[7] L. Xiao, Y. Liu, and N. Wang, "New paradigms in inflammatory signaling in vascular endothelial cells," *The American Journal of Physiology—Heart and Circulatory Physiology*, vol. 306, no. 3, pp. H317–H325, 2014.

[8] S.-Y. Wei, Y. Chen, and X.-Y. Xu, "Progress on the pharmacological research of puerarin: a review," *Chinese Journal of Natural Medicines*, vol. 12, no. 6, pp. 407–414, 2014.

[9] Y.-X. Zhou, H. Zhang, and C. Peng, "Puerarin: a review of pharmacological effects," *Phytotherapy Research*, vol. 28, no. 7, pp. 961–975, 2014.

[10] F.-L. Hsu, I.-M. Liu, D.-H. Kuo, W.-C. Chen, H.-C. Su, and J.-T. Cheng, "Antihyperglycemic effect of puerarin in streptozotocin-induced diabetic rats," *Journal of Natural Products*, vol. 66, no. 6, pp. 788–792, 2003.

[11] E. Kato and J. Kawabata, "Glucose uptake enhancing activity of puerarin and the role of C-glucoside suggested from activity of related compounds," *Bioorganic and Medicinal Chemistry Letters*, vol. 20, no. 15, pp. 4333–4336, 2010.

[12] Y. Teng, H. Cui, M. Yang et al., "Protective effect of puerarin on diabetic retinopathy in rats," *Molecular Biology Reports*, vol. 36, no. 5, pp. 1129–1133, 2009.

[13] W. Zhang, C.-Q. Liu, P.-W. Wang et al., "Puerarin improves insulin resistance and modulates adipokine expression in rats fed a high-fat diet," *European Journal of Pharmacology*, vol. 649, no. 1–3, pp. 398–402, 2010.

[14] Z. Li, Z. Shangguan, Y. Liu et al., "Puerarin protects pancreatic β-cell survival via PI3K/Akt signaling pathway," *Journal of Molecular Endocrinology*, vol. 53, no. 1, pp. 71–79, 2014.

[15] W. Cheng, P. Wu, Y. Du et al., "Puerarin improves cardiac function through regulation of energy metabolism in Streptozotocin-Nicotinamide induced diabetic mice after myocardial infarction," *Biochemical and Biophysical Research Communications*, vol. 463, no. 4, pp. 1108–1114, 2015.

[16] S. She, W. Liu, T. Li, and Y. Hong, "Effects of puerarin in STZ-induced diabetic rats by oxidative stress and the TGF-β1/Smad2 pathway," *Food and Function*, vol. 5, no. 5, pp. 944–950, 2014.

[17] Y. Zhong, X. Zhang, X. Cai, K. Wang, Y. Chen, and Y. Deng, "Puerarin attenuated early diabetic kidney injury through down-regulation of matrix metalloproteinase 9 in streptozotocin-induced diabetic rats," *PLoS ONE*, vol. 9, no. 1, Article ID e85690, 2014.

[18] F. Braga, A. Dolci, A. Mosca, and M. Panteghini, "Biological variability of glycated hemoglobin," *Clinica Chimica Acta*, vol. 411, no. 21-22, pp. 1606–1610, 2010.

[19] N. Li, "The influence of puerarin on glycated hemoglobin, MDA, and SOD in diabetic patients," *Guangxi Medical Journal*, vol. 19, p. 3, 1997.

[20] K. Wu, T. Liang, X. Duan, L. Xu, K. Zhang, and R. Li, "Anti-diabetic effects of puerarin, isolated from *Pueraria lobata* (Willd.), on streptozotocin-diabetogenic mice through promoting insulin expression and ameliorating metabolic function," *Food and Chemical Toxicology*, vol. 60, pp. 341–347, 2013.

[21] S.-J. Yang, W. Je Lee, E.-A. Kim et al., "Effects of *N*-adamantyl-4-methylthiazol-2-amine on hyperglycemia, hyperlipidemia and oxidative stress in streptozotocin-induced diabetic rats," *European Journal of Pharmacology*, vol. 736, pp. 26–34, 2014.

[22] N. Giribabu, K. E. Kumar, S. S. Rekha et al., "*Chlorophytum borivilianum* (Safed Musli) root extract prevents impairment in characteristics and elevation of oxidative stress in sperm of streptozotocin-induced adult male diabetic Wistar rats," *BMC Complementary and Alternative Medicine*, vol. 14, article 291, 2014.

[23] C. Szabo, "Role of nitrosative stress in the pathogenesis of diabetic vascular dysfunction," *British Journal of Pharmacology*, vol. 156, no. 5, pp. 713–727, 2009.

[24] K. Fujii, M. Soma, Y.-S. Huang, M. S. Manku, and D. F. Horrobin, "Increased release of prostaglandins from the mesenteric vascular bed of diabetic animals: the effects of glucose and insulin," *Prostaglandins, Leukotrienes and Medicine*, vol. 24, no. 2-3, pp. 151–161, 1986.

[25] E. Capobianco, A. Jawerbaum, V. White, C. Pustovrh, D. Sinner, and E. T. Gonzalez, "Elevated levels of endothelin-1 and prostaglandin E_2 and their effect on nitric oxide generation in placental tissue from neonatal streptozotocin-induced diabetic rats," *Prostaglandins Leukotrienes and Essential Fatty Acids*, vol. 68, no. 3, pp. 225–231, 2003.

[26] W.-Y. Wu, H. Yan, X.-B. Wang et al., "Sodium tanshinone IIA silate inhibits high glucose-induced vascular smooth muscle cell proliferation and migration through activation of amp-activated protein kinase," *PLoS ONE*, vol. 9, no. 4, Article ID e94957, 2014.

[27] Q. Lu, D.-X. Xiang, H.-Y. Yuan, Y. Xiao, L.-Q. Yuan, and H.-B. Li, "Puerarin attenuates calcification of vascular smooth muscle cells," *American Journal of Chinese Medicine*, vol. 42, no. 2, pp. 337–347, 2014.

[28] L.-H. Zhu, L. Wang, D. Wang et al., "Puerarin attenuates high-glucose-and diabetes-induced vascular smooth muscle cell proliferation by blocking PKCβ2/Rac1-dependent signaling," *Free Radical Biology and Medicine*, vol. 48, no. 4, pp. 471–482, 2010.

[29] M. Zhu, J. Chen, H. Jiang, and C. Miao, "Propofol protects against high glucose-induced endothelial adhesion molecules expression in human umbilical vein endothelial cells," *Cardiovascular Diabetology*, vol. 12, no. 1, article 13, 2013.

[30] L. Li, T. Sawamura, and G. Renier, "Glucose enhances endothelial LOX-1 expression: role for LOX-1 in glucose-induced human monocyte adhesion to endothelium," *Diabetes*, vol. 52, no. 7, pp. 1843–1850, 2003.

[31] J. M. Forbes and M. E. Cooper, "Mechanisms of diabetic complications," *Physiological Reviews*, vol. 93, no. 1, pp. 137–188, 2013.

[32] Y. Gorin and K. Block, "Nox as a target for diabetic complications," *Clinical Science*, vol. 125, no. 8, pp. 361–382, 2013.

[33] A. Schramm, P. Matusik, G. Osmenda, and T. J. Guzik, "Targeting NADPH oxidases in vascular pharmacology," *Vascular Pharmacology*, vol. 56, no. 5-6, pp. 216–231, 2012.

[34] J. Kim, K. M. Kim, C.-S. Kim et al., "Puerarin inhibits the retinal pericyte apoptosis induced by advanced glycation end products in vitro and in vivo by inhibiting NADPH oxidase-related oxidative stress," *Free Radical Biology and Medicine*, vol. 53, no. 2, pp. 357–365, 2012.

[35] M. Buelna-Chontal and C. Zazueta, "Redox activation of Nrf2 & NF-κB: a double end sword?" *Cellular Signalling*, vol. 25, no. 12, pp. 2548–2557, 2013.

[36] L. Cominacini, A. Fratta Pasini, U. Garbin et al., "Oxidized low density lipoprotein (ox-LDL) binding to ox-LDL receptor-1 in endothelial cells induces the activation of NF-κB through an increased production of intracellular reactive oxygen species," *The Journal of Biological Chemistry*, vol. 275, no. 17, pp. 12633–12638, 2000.

[37] Y. Sun and X. Chen, "Ox-LDL-induced LOX-1 expression in vascular smooth muscle cells: role of reactive oxygen species," *Fundamental and Clinical Pharmacology*, vol. 25, no. 5, pp. 572–579, 2011.

[38] R. B. Ning, J. Zhu, D. J. Chai et al., "RXR agonists inhibit high glucose-induced upregulation of inflammation by suppressing activation of the NADPH oxidase-nuclear factor-κB pathway in human endothelial cells," *Genetics and Molecular Research*, vol. 12, no. 4, pp. 6692–6707, 2013.

[39] G.-F. Wang, S.-Y. Wu, W. Xu et al., "Geniposide inhibits high glucose-induced cell adhesion through the NF-kappaB signaling pathway in human umbilical vein endothelial cells," *Acta Pharmacologica Sinica*, vol. 31, no. 8, pp. 953–962, 2010.

16

Effects of the New Aldose Reductase Inhibitor Benzofuroxane Derivative BF-5m on High Glucose Induced Prolongation of Cardiac QT Interval and Increase of Coronary Perfusion Pressure

C. Di Filippo,[1] B. Ferraro,[1] R. Maisto,[1] M. C. Trotta,[1] N. Di Carluccio,[1] S. Sartini,[2] C. La Motta,[2] F. Ferraraccio,[3] F. Rossi,[1] and M. D'Amico[1]

[1]*Department of Experimental Medicine, Section of Pharmacology "L. Donatelli", Second University of Naples, 80138 Naples, Italy*
[2]*Department of Pharmacy, University of Pisa, 56126 Pisa, Italy*
[3]*Department of Clinical, Public and Preventive Medicine, Second University of Naples, 80138 Naples, Italy*

Correspondence should be addressed to C. Di Filippo; clara.difilippo@unina2.it

Academic Editor: Shi Fang Yan

This study investigated the effects of the new aldose reductase inhibitor benzofuroxane derivative 5(6)-(benzo[*d*]thiazol-2-ylmethoxy)benzofuroxane (BF-5m) on the prolongation of cardiac QT interval and increase of coronary perfusion pressure (CPP) in isolated, high glucose (33.3 mM D-glucose) perfused rat hearts. BF-5m was dissolved in the Krebs solution at a final concentration of 0.01 μM, 0.05 μM, and 0.1 μM. 33.3 mM D-glucose caused a prolongation of the QT interval and increase of CPP up to values of 190 ± 12 ms and 110 ± 8 mmHg with respect to the values of hearts perfused with standard Krebs solution (11.1 mM D-glucose). The QT prolongation was reduced by 10%, 32%, and 41%, respectively, for the concentration of BF-5m 0.01 μM, 0.05 μM, and 0.1 μM. Similarly, the CPP was reduced by 20% for BF-5m 0.05 μM and by 32% for BF-5m 0.1 μM. BF-5m also increased the expression levels of sirtuin 1, MnSOD, eNOS, and FOXO-1, into the heart. The beneficial actions of BF-5m were partly abolished by the pretreatment of the rats with the inhibitor of the sirtuin 1 activity EX527 (10 mg/kg/day/7 days i.p.) prior to perfusion of the hearts with high glucose + BF-5m (0.1 μM). Therefore, BF-5m supplies cardioprotection from the high glucose induced QT prolongation and increase of CPP.

1. Introduction

Hyperglycemia during the diabetes has detrimental effects on various organs including eye, kidney, central nervous system, and heart [1]. Hyperglycemia favors the insurgence of coronary artery disease, peripheral arterial diseases, cardiomyopathy, angina, and myocardial infarction [1]. Among these, the most dangerous consequence of the hyperglycemia is the prolongation of the cardiac QT interval, which leads diabetic patients to sudden death [2]. Long cardiac QT interval is partly sensitive to antioxidant drugs acting on the nitric oxide bioavailability, glycosylated products, accumulation of reactive oxygen species, and impairment of ionic pumps in models of isolated high glucose perfused heart [3, 4]. Increased interest, therefore, has gained the discovery of new drugs that may modulate pathways involved in glucose metabolism and hyperglycemia-induced modifications, in order to produce cardiovascular protection. In this context, one pathway that could be targeted is the aldose reductase (ALR2), because it contributes to the deleterious actions of hyperglycemia onto the cardiovascular system by inducing oxidative damage into the heart following diabetes [5–9].

Recently, Sartini et al. [10] discovered a series of new benzofuroxane derivatives which inhibits the aldose reductase (ALR2). These compounds spontaneously release NO, possess a hydroxyl radical scavenging activity, and account for multieffective agents for the treatment of cardiovascular diabetic complications. For this, the first aim of the study was to investigate the effects of the BF-5m, on the prolongation of cardiac QT interval and increase of the CPP induced by perfusion with high glucose of isolated rat heart.

In addition, since the action of ALR2 on glucose metabolism is linked to depletion into the cells of the cofactor NAD+ [11] and SIRT1 is a NAD1-dependent protein deacetylase which belongs to a class of proteins that lead to improved energy consumption, limitation of oxidative stress, and reduced DNA damage [12, 13], the second aim of the study was to investigate whether there is an involvement of the sirtuin 1 (SIRT1) in the cardiac effects of BF-5m. SIRT1 is one of the better characterized sirtuins with multiple protective actions in many pathological conditions, through involvement of several molecular pathways, deacetylation of mediators of oxidative stress, inflammation, apoptosis, and transcription factors, and plays an important role in the regulation of glucose consumption by regulating insulin expression in vivo [14, 15]. SIRT1 also has strong antioxidant action [16].

2. Material and Methods

2.1. Drug. BF-5m, 5(6)-(benzo[*d*]thiazol-2-ylmethoxy)benzofuroxane, was synthesized at the Department of Pharmacy of the University of Pisa, Italy, following a previously reported procedure [10]. Briefly, alkylation of the commercially available 4-amino-3-nitrophenol with chloroacetonitrile, in the presence of anhydrous potassium carbonate, provided the 2-(4-amino-3-nitrophenoxy)acetonitrile which, through reaction with o-aminothiophenol, gave the key intermediate 4-[(benzo[*d*]thiazol-2-yl)methoxy]-2-nitrobenzenamine. Treatment with sodium nitrite in concentrated hydrochloric acid and then with sodium azide in water gave the corresponding azido-derivative, which cyclized to the target inhibitor, 5(6)-(benzo[*d*]thiazol-2-ylmethoxy)benzofuroxane, when heated under reflux in acetic acid.

2.2. Isolated Heart Preparation. Male Sprague-Dawley rats (3-4 months old, with a weight of 210 ± 20 g) were anaesthetised with urethane (1.2 mg/kg i.p.) and heparinized (sodium heparin, 250 IU, i.p. 10 min before heart removal). Subsequently, the hearts were quickly excised and placed in ice-cold Krebs solution (composition in mmol/L: 11.1 D(+)-glucose; 1.4 $CaCl_2$; 118.5 NaCl; 25.0 $NaHCO_3$; 1.2 $MgSO_4$; 1.2 NaH_2PO_4; 4.0 KCl). Then, the hearts were connected to a Langendorff apparatus via the aorta and retrogradely perfused at 37°C under constant flow (9-10 mL/min) with the Krebs solution bubbled with 95% O_2-5% CO_2 and composed as described above.

A total of 82 hearts were used. Of these, 12 were excluded having a sinus rate of <210 beats per minute or a coronary perfusion pressure (CPP) <60 mmHg between 5 and 15 min after beginning of the perfusion; hearts not in sinus rhythm during the study were also excluded. The remaining 70 hearts having a sinus rate of >210 beats per minute or CPP > 60 mmHg, between 5 and 15 min after beginning, were used in the study and divided into the following experimental groups (n = 10 rats for each group): (i) control: hearts perfused for 2 hours with a Krebs solution containing D-glucose at 11.1 mM [4, 5]; (ii) high glu: hearts perfused for 2 hours with Krebs solution containing D-glucose at 33.3 mM [4, 5]; (iii) high glu + DMSO: hearts perfused with Krebs solution containing 1% DMSO + D-glucose at 33.3 mM; (iv) high glu + BF-5m: hearts perfused for 2 hours with Krebs solution containing D-glucose at 33.3 mM + BF-5m (0.01 μM in 1% DMSO); (v) high glu + BF-5m: hearts perfused for 2 hours with Krebs solution containing D-glucose at 33.3 mM + BF-5m (0.05 μM, in 1% DMSO); (vi) high glu + BF-5m: hearts perfused for two hours with Krebs solution containing D-glucose at 33.3 mM + BF-5m (0.1 μM, in 1% DMSO). Moreover, in order to assess the role of SIRT1 in the BF-5m cardiac effects additional studies were done on 10 hearts excised from rats pretreated for 7 days (10 mg/kg/day i.p.) [17] with EX527 and perfused with a Krebs solution with high glucose + BF-5m 0.1 μM. In these the QT interval, CPP values, and biochemical parameters mentioned below were monitored.

2.3. QT Interval and CPP Measurements. QT interval, for each heart, was recorded by a unipolar ECG with a stainless steel wire electrode in the apex of left ventricular muscle mass, with a second electrode connected to the aorta. This electrode arrangement gave clear P waves and ventricular complexes. An ECG (chart speed 50 mm/s) was recorded for 4 min every 10 min for 2 h. The ECG was analysed and heart rate (RR interval) and the width of the ventricular complex (QT) at 100% repolarization (QT100) were measured. The CPP in the aortic line was monitored using a Statham Spectramed pressure transducer connected to a chart recorder (Grass, 79E, Quincy, MA, USA). Temperature was maintained constant by means of a heated (37°C) water jacket. On establishing a stable value (20–30 min following cannulation) CPP was calculated according to Di Filippo et al. [4]. Briefly, CPP value was expressed either as the mean of each 10-min value throughout the entire experiment or as the mean of the steady-state increment above baseline when an increase of CPP was evident during an experiment. All experimental procedures were approved by Animal Care Ethical Committee of the Naples University in accordance with Italian (Decree 116/92) and European Community (E.C. L358/1 18/12/86) guidelines on the use and protection of laboratory animals.

2.4. Hematoxylin and Eosin Staining. At the end of the perfusion period the hearts were cut into two halves and one was immediately frozen in liquid nitrogen and stored at −80°C. The hematoxylin and eosin staining was conducted according to Marfella et al. [18] protocol and 200x magnification pictures were taken.

2.5. Western Blot Analysis and SIRT1 Activity Assay. Western blotting analysis was performed from the homogenized frozen biopsy according to Di Filippo et al. [19]. We used (i) primary anti-SIRT1 antibody (1 : 1000, Abcam, Cambridge, UK), (ii) specific monoclonal antibody directed against FOXO-1 (1:500, Millipore, California, USA), (iii) anti-MnSOD primary antibody (1 : 800, Millipore, California, USA), (iv) anti-β-actin monoclonal antibody (1 : 1000, Sigma-Aldrich), and (v) anti-eNOS sc-654 (1 : 500, Santa Cruz Biotech, USA) with an enhanced chemiluminescence detection reagent (ECL), quantified by densitometry using a BioRad ChemiDoc MP Imaging system. The following secondary antibodies were used: goat anti-mouse (1:1000, Santa Cruz Biotech, USA) and goat anti-rabbit (1:1000, Santa Cruz Biotech, USA). The deacetylase activity of SIRT1 was measured by means of a commercial fluorometric kit (Abcam, Cambridge, UK) and normalized by protein content.

2.6. Sorbitol Assay in Heart Samples. A procedure early described in literature [20] with slight modifications was used to assess the sorbitol levels in the heart homogenates by fluorimetry. Briefly, one mL of the supernatants was incubated for 5 min at 37°C in presence of 50 μmol glycine buffer, 2 μmol magnesium chloride, and 0.2 μmol nicotinamide adenine dinucleotide (NAD) and reaction initiated by the addition of 0.6 U of sorbitol dehydrogenase. A standard curve was constructed with sorbitol from 0.4 to 10 μg/mL; the fluorescence from NADH formation was measured at 450 nm and expressed as sorbitol μg/mL.

2.7. RNA Isolation and Quantification. Total RNA was extracted from the heart tissue (~50 mg) using the Rneasy Plus Mini Kit (Qiagen) according the manufacturer's protocol from Animal Cells. Then RNA was quantified using NanoDrop 2000c Spectrophotometer (Thermo Scientific, Waltham, MA, USA) according to Rossi et al. [21].

2.8. RNA Retrotranscription and Real Time PCR Reaction. cDNA synthesis was obtained using SuperScript III Reverse Transcriptase Kit (Invitrogen, USA) starting from 1.5 μg of total RNA. In the subsequent q-PCR reaction performed with Power SYBR Green PCR Master Mix (Applied Biosystems, UK), SIRT1 mRNA has been quantified and normalized using β-actin as housekeeping gene in CFX96 Real Time System (BioRad) cycler (BioRad Laboratories, Inc.). Primers sequences were as follows: 5′-TGTTTCCTGTGGGATACCTGA-3′ (sense) and 5′-TGAAGAATGGTCTTGGGTCTTT-3′ (antisense) for SIRT1 and 5′-CGAGTACAACCTTCTTGCAG-3′ (sense) and 5′-TTCTGACCCATACCCACCAT-3′ (antisense) for β-actin. Relative quantification of gene expression was normalized to beta-actin using the $2^{-\Delta\Delta Ct}$ method [19, 21].

2.9. Statistical Analysis. Data are expressed as means ± standard error of the mean (s.e.m.). Student's t-test (when only two groups were compared) or one-way ANOVA followed by Dunnett's test (more than two experimental groups) was used. $P < 0.05$ was considered statistically significant.

3. Results

Figure 1 shows representative pictures of the heart structure derangement caused by perfusion of the hearts with the a Krebs solution containing high glucose concentration (D-glucose, 33.3 mM) with respect to the hearts perfused with a Krebs solution containing normal glucose concentration (D-glucose, 11.1 M), in presence or absence of the first active dose of the compound BF-5m (e.g., 0.05 μM). There was clear evidence of a damaged structure with no or few signs of well tissue organization (e.g., bands, Z line) following high glucose perfusion. In contrast, a discrete preservation of the heart structure was seen in rat hearts perfused with high glucose + BF-5m with an almost intact structure of the tissue. This cardiac preservation disappeared when the rats were pretreated with the SIRT1 activity inhibitor EX527 (10 mg/kg/day/7 days i.p.) and then perfused with high glucose + BF-5m 0.1 μM (Figure 1).

3.1. BF-5m Decreased QT Interval and CPP in Rats Hearts Perfused with the High Glucose Concentration. 11.1 mM glucose (control) exhibited a QT interval of 112 ± 5 ms and a CPP of 70 ± 3 mmHg. These values were increased up to 190 ± 12 ms ($P < 0.01$ versus control) for QT and up to 110 ± 8 mmHg ($P < 0.01$ versus control) for CPP in the heart perfused with glucose 33.3 mM. The addition of BF-5m (0.01 μM; 0.05 μM; 0.1 μM) to Krebs solution containing a high glucose concentration diminished the QT interval of 10%, 32%, and 41% with calculated values of 170 ± 14 ms, 130 ± 12 ms, and 113 ± 20 ms, respectively. Similarly, the CPP was reduced by 3% (107±12 mmHg), 20% (88±5 mmHg), and 32% by BF-5m (Figure 2). Pretreatment (7 days) of the rats with EX527 prior to the perfusion of the hearts with high glu + BF-5m 0.1 μM decreased the BF-5m cardioprotection by reporting the QT interval at 174 ± 11 ms ($P < 0.01$) and CCP at 102 ± 7 mmHg ($P < 0.01$ versus high glu + BF-5m 0.1 μM) (Figure 2).

3.2. Effects of BF-5m on SIRT1 Levels and Activity in Rats Hearts Perfused with the High Glucose Concentration. Figure 3 showed that SIRT1 gene and protein expression significantly decreased in rat hearts perfused for two hours with Krebs solution containing a high glucose concentration ($P < 0.01$ versus control). Addition of BF-5m at 0.01, 0.05, and 0.1 μM to the Krebs solution plus glucose at 33.3 mM significantly increased the cardiac SIRT1 gene expression (e.g., +65%, +160%, and +227%) and protein levels (e.g., +50%, +105%, and +160%; Figure 3). SIRT1 deacetylase activity was significantly increased in heart homogenates from high glu + BF-5m with respect to the activity measured in hearts from high glu. The SIRT1 deacetylase activity was 450 ± 32 RFU/μg of protein in high glu perfused hearts; 492 ± 48 RFU/μg of protein in high glu + BF-5m 0.01 μM; 726 ± 64 RFU/μg of protein in high glu + BF-5m 0.51 μM; 1149 ± 86 RFU/μg of protein in high glu + BF-5m 0.1 μM.

EX527 pretreatment (10 mg/kg/day/7 days i.p.) did not affect SIRT1 gene and protein expression levels but diminished (−57%) the BF-5m cardioprotection (Figures 1 and 2).

3.3. Effects of BF-5m on MnSOD, eNOS Expression, and Tissue Sorbitol Content. As shown in Figures 4(a)–4(c), the perfusion of the hearts with high glu + BF-5m (0.01 μM; 0.05 μM; 0.1 μM) increased the levels of MnSOD and eNOS compared to the hearts perfused with the high glucose only. In contrast, the effects of 0.1 μM BF-5m on MnSOD and eNOS were decreased by the EX527 pretreatment (Figures 4(a)–4(c)). The tissue sorbitol content as marker of the aldose reductase activity was increased in heart perfused with high glu with respect to the content of vehicle. This increase was not

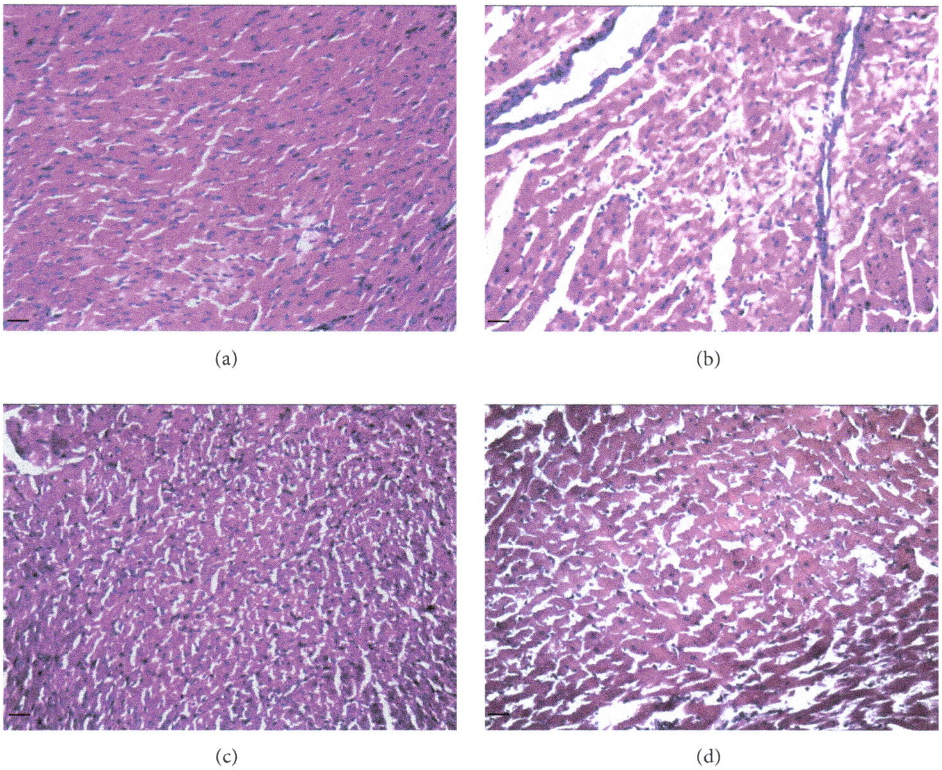

FIGURE 1: Representative pictures from hematoxylin and eosin staining of cardiac tissue. Rat hearts were perfused with Krebs solution containing (a) D-glucose 11.1 mM (control); (b) glucose 33.3 mM (high glu); (c) high glu + BF-5m (0.1 μM); (d) high glu + BF-5m (0.1 μM) + EX527 (10 mg/kg/day i.p.). 200x magnification; scale bar = 100 μm.

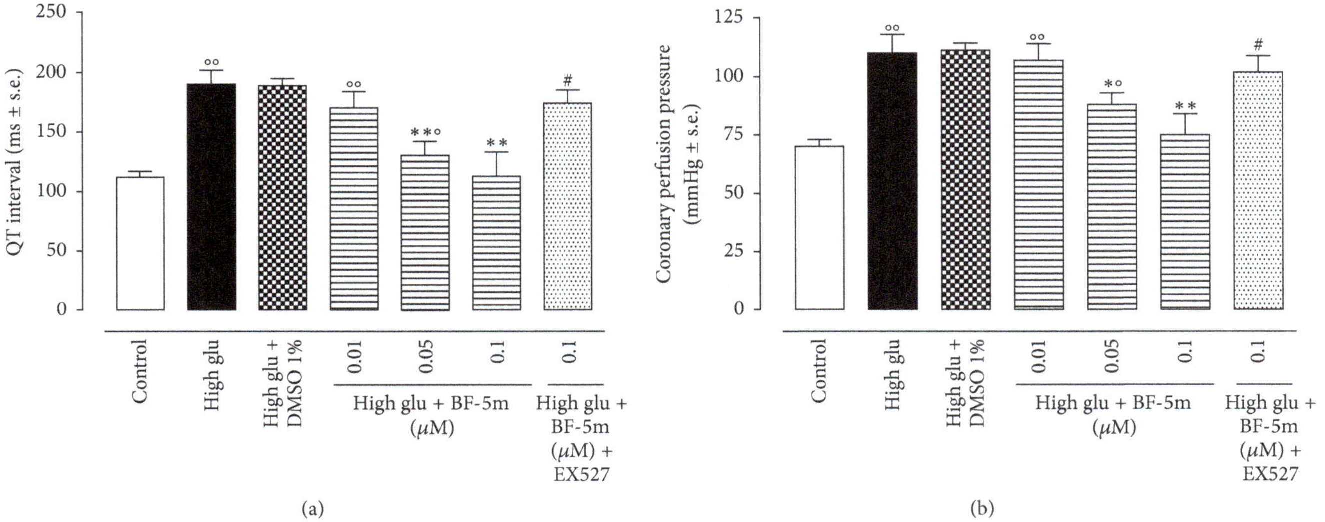

FIGURE 2: (a) Cardiac QT interval in hearts of Sprague-Dawley rats perfused for two hours in a Langendorff apparatus with Krebs solution containing D-glucose 11.1 mM (control); glucose 11.1 mM + DMSO 1% (vehicle); glucose 33.3 mM (high glu); high glu + BF-5m (0.01, 0.05, and 0.1 μM); high glu + BF-5m (0.1 μM) + EX527 (10 mg/kg/day i.p.). (b) Coronary perfusion pressure (CPP) recorded on a Power Lab system following exposure of perfused hearts to the same treatments as in panel (a). Values are expressed as the mean of 10 observations ± s.e.m. Significant differences *versus* control are reported as $^{\circ}P < 0.05$ and $^{\circ\circ}P < 0.01$; significant differences *versus* high glu are reported as $^{*}P < 0.05$ and $^{**}P < 0.01$; significant differences *versus* high glu + BF-5m 0.1 μM are reported as $^{\#}P < 0.01$.

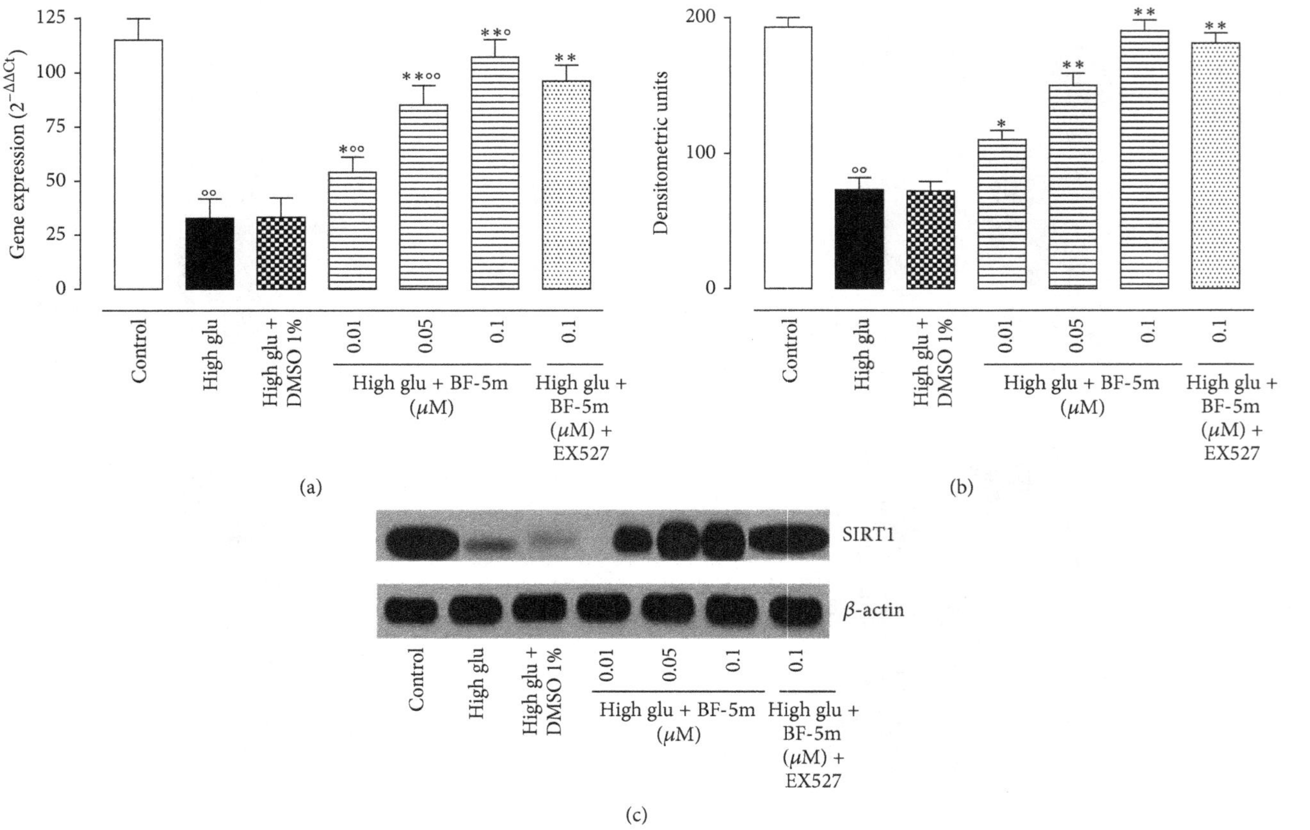

Figure 3: (a) SIRT1 in perfused hearts following treatment with D-glucose 11.1 mM (control); glucose 11.1 mM + DMSO 1% (vehicle); glucose 33.3 mM (high glu); high glu + BF-5m (0.01, 0.05, and 0.1 μM); high glu + BF-5m (0.1 μM) + EX527 (10 mg/kg/day i.p.). Total RNA was extracted from the hearts and reverse transcribed into cDNA using superscript reverse transcriptase system. The expression of SIRT1 was quantified by qPCR using commercially available rat primers. Results are expressed as arbitrary units based on calculation of $2^{-\Delta\Delta Ct}$ method. $^{\circ}P < 0.01$ *versus* control; $^{*}P < 0.05$ and $^{**}P < 0.01$ *versus* high glu. (b) Addition of BF-5m (0.01, 0.05, and 0.1 μM) to the high glucose Krebs solution dose-dependently increased the expression of SIRT1. Results are derived from western blotting (panel (c) representative) and expressed as densitometric units (mean ± s.e.m. of $n = 10$ observations for each group). Significant differences *versus* control are reported as $^{\circ}P < 0.05$ and $^{\circ\circ}P < 0.01$; significant differences *versus* high glu are reported as $^{*}P < 0.05$ and $^{**}P < 0.01$; significant differences *versus* high glu + BF-5m 0.1 μM are reported as $^{\circ}P < 0.01$.

observed after the treatment of the rats with the BF-5m at all the concentration used (Figure 4(d)).

3.4. Effect of BF-5m on FOXO-1. BF-5m modified the levels of cardiac FOXO-1 (Forkhead transcription factor 1), which is a direct target of SIRT1. Western blotting analysis showed lower expression of this protein in hearts perfused with high glucose solution. This was reported towards the control values by high glu + BF-5m (Figure 5). The inhibitor of SIRT1 activity EX527 also inhibited the restoring of FOXO-1 levels operated by the BF-5m (Figure 5).

4. Discussion

Here we show that inhibition of the endogenous enzyme aldose reductase (ALR2) activity by the newly synthetized benzofuroxane derivative 5(6)-(benzo[*d*]thiazol-2-ylmethoxy)benzofuroxane (BF-5m) results in cardioprotection from the electrical instability and increased vasomotor tone caused by high levels of glucose into the heart. This cardioprotection is characterized by reduction of the long cardiac QT interval and the decrease of the coronary perfusion pressure (CPP). The ALR2 is a critical enzyme when there is a high glucose condition into cells and tissues since this by catalyzing the reduction of glucose to sorbitol [22] favors accumulation of this polyol into the cell cytoplasm of organs and tissues and determines local generation of reactive oxygen species and damage [22]. Over the years many compounds have shown potent inhibitory effects against the enzyme aldose reductase (ALR2) including, for example, epalrestat, fidarestat, lidorestat, and sorbinil [22–24]. However, some of these were withdrawn from clinical trials because they showed undesirable effects such as skin reactions or liver toxicity [25]. Numerous efforts have been made, therefore, to identify molecules that could effectively block the activity of ALR2, limit the negative effects from prolonged exposure to high glucose, and possibly have few or no side effects. Among these, Sartini et al. [10] proposed a novel class of nonhydantoin noncarboxylic acid

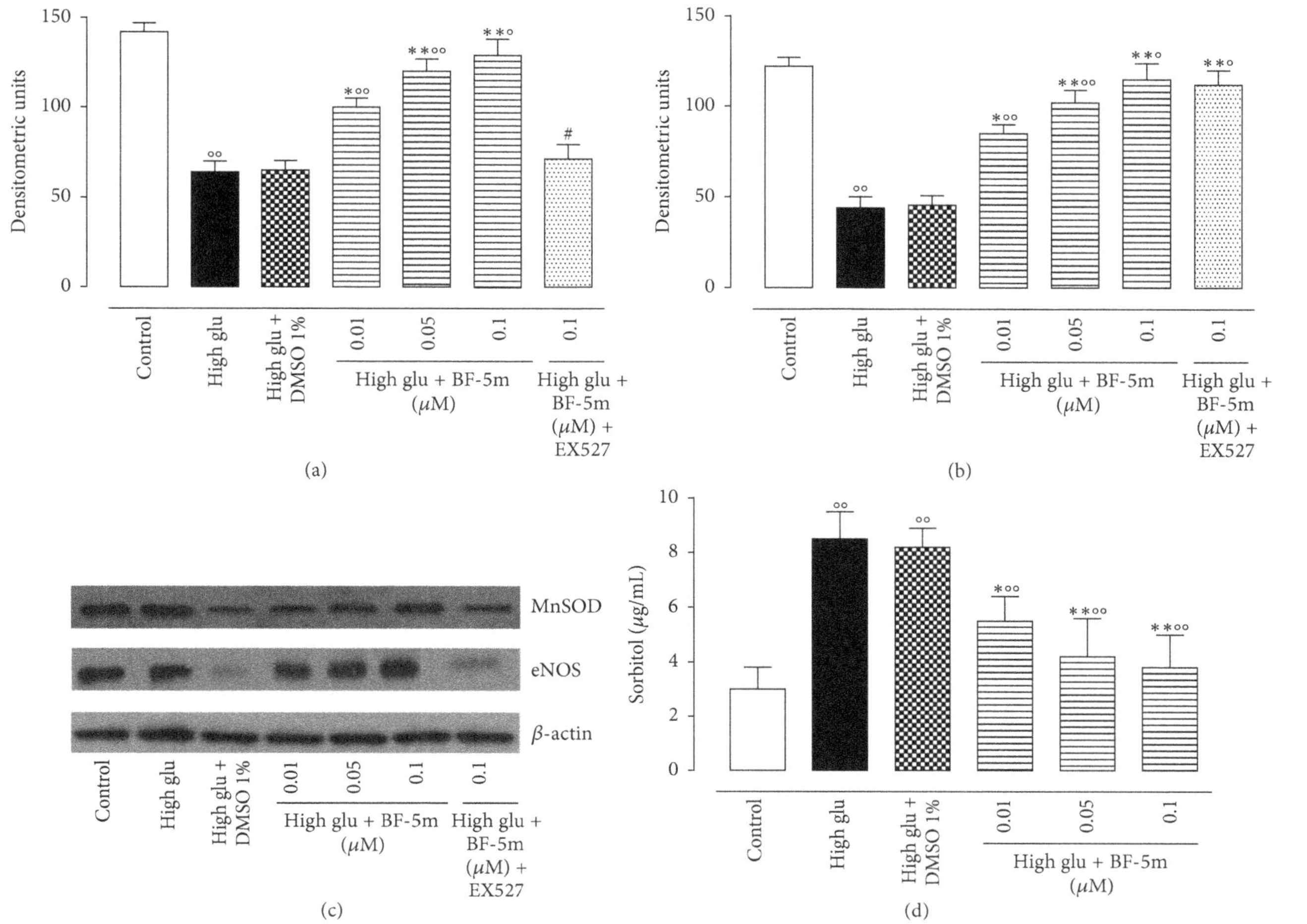

FIGURE 4: (a) MnSOD expression in hearts perfused with glucose 11.1 mM (control); glucose 11.1 mM + DMSO 1% (vehicle); glucose 33.3 mM (high glu); high glu + BF-5m (0.01, 0.05, and 0.1 μM); high glu + BF-5m (0.1 μM) + EX527 (10 mg/kg/day i.p.). (b) eNOS expression levels in hearts perfused as in panel (a). Results are derived from western blotting (panel (c) representative) and expressed as densitometric units; (d) tissue sorbitol content (μg/mL). Mean $\pm$ s.e.m. of $n = 10$ observations for each group. Significant differences *versus* control are reported as $^{\circ}P < 0.05$ and $^{\circ\circ}P < 0.01$; significant differences *versus* high glu are reported as $^{*}P < 0.05$ and $^{**}P < 0.01$; significant differences *versus* high glu + BF-5m 0.1 μM are reported as $^{\#}P < 0.01$.

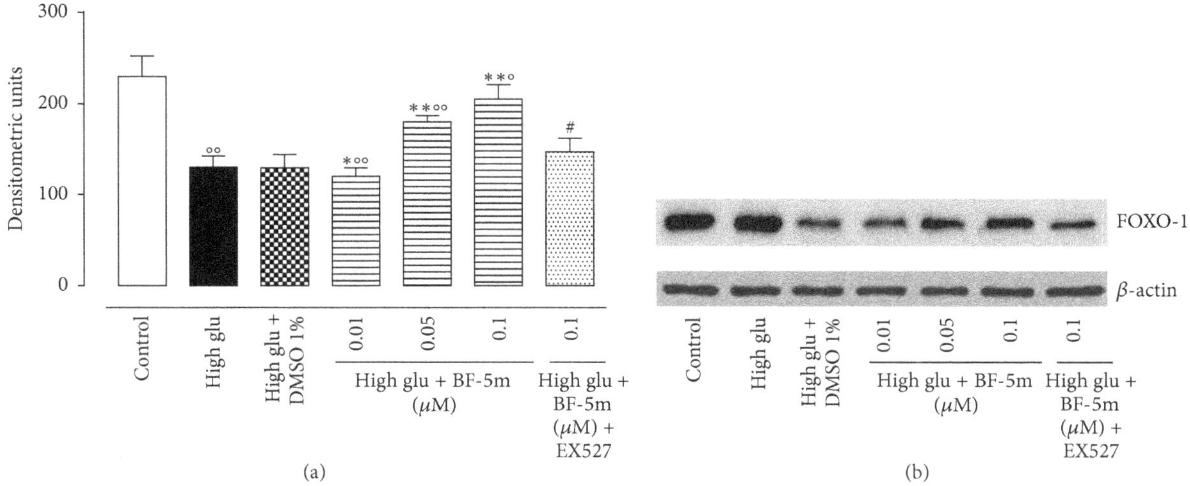

FIGURE 5: (a) Expression of FOXO-1 in hearts perfused with glucose 11.1 mM (control); glucose 11.1 mM + DMSO 1% (vehicle); glucose 33.3 mM (high glu); high glu + BF-5m (0.01, 0.05, and 0.1 μM); high glu + BF-5m (0.1 μM) + EX527 (10 mg/kg/day i.p.). Results are derived from western blotting (panel (b) representative) and expressed as densitometric units and represented the mean $\pm$ s.e.m. of $n = 10$ observations for each group. Significant differences *versus* control are reported as $^{\circ}P < 0.05$ and $^{\circ\circ}P < 0.01$; significant differences *versus* high glu are reported as $^{*}P < 0.05$ and $^{**}P < 0.01$; significant differences *versus* high glu + BF-5m 0.1 μM are reported as $^{\#}P < 0.01$.

inhibitors, featuring the benzofuroxane core [22, 26] as new scaffold interacting with the so-called ALR2 anion site. Merging submicromolar ALR2 inhibitory activities with significant ROS scavenging properties, these compounds have been identified as the ideal therapeutic treatment for the high glucose-related pathologies [10] as could be the alterations of cardiac electrical stability. Effectively, BF-5m reduced the prolongation of cardiac QT interval, sensitive marker of electrical instability, in our setting.

BF-5m also promotes increase of the expression and activity of endogenous antioxidant pathways and free radical scavengers such as SIRT1 and MnSOD, its downstream target [27], into the heart following exposure to a high glucose stimulus. Indeed, the high glucose to the heart caused decrease of the protein SIRT1 into the tissue, an effect that was reverted by the BF-5m. SIRT1 is NAD1-dependent protein deacetylase which belongs to a class of proteins that lead to improved energy consumption, limitation of oxidative stress, and reduced DNA damage [12, 13]. SIRT1, through involvement of several molecular pathways and deacetylation of mediators of oxidative stress, inflammation, apoptosis, and transcription factors, possesses multiple protective actions in many pathological conditions. SIRT1 also plays an important role in the regulation of insulin expression by glucose concentration [14, 15]. So, back to our game, BF-5m was able to reduce the structural and functional cardiac derangement caused by high glucose into the myocardium through the modulation of SIRT1 activity. This result is also confirmed by the reduction in the expression of the Forkhead transcription factor 1 (FOXO-1), the direct downstream product of SIRT1 activity into tissues. FOXO-1 is a transcription factor that is regulated by SIRT1 through its deacetylase activity [28, 29] and it regulates gluconeogenesis, glycogenolysis, and adipogenesis [30]. From the clinical point of view, upregulated FOXO-1 raises a state of insulin resistance and diabetes, due to a loss of insulin sensitivity, and the consequent hyperglycemia or high glucose accelerates cellular damage [31]. In our case, a condition of diminished activity of FOXO-1 caused by high glucose may be one of the actors accounting for an altered homeostasis at cardiac levels which may have led to reduced perfusion of heart and finally electrical instability.

5. Conclusions

These results suggest that the new aldose reductase inhibitor benzofuroxane derivative BF-5m supplies cardioprotection from the high glucose induced QT prolongation and increase of CPP. The mechanism of action involves the increase of SIRT1 protein and activity into the heart tissue, together with the modulation of the expression and activity of its downstream mediators MnSOD and FOXO-1.

Conflict of Interests

The authors declare that there is no conflict of interests regarding the publication of this paper.

References

[1] D. M. Nathan, "Diabetes: advances in diagnosis and treatment," *The Journal of the American Medical Association*, vol. 314, no. 10, pp. 1052–1062, 2015.

[2] R. Marfella, F. Nappo, L. De Angelis, M. Siniscalchi, F. Rossi, and D. Giugliano, "The effect of acute hyperglycaemia on QTc duration in healthy man," *Diabetologia*, vol. 43, no. 5, pp. 571–575, 2000.

[3] A. Ceriello, L. Quagliaro, M. D'Amico et al., "Acute hyperglycemia induces nitrotyrosine formation and apoptosis in perfused heart from rat," *Diabetes*, vol. 51, no. 4, pp. 1076–1082, 2002.

[4] C. Di Filippo, M. D'Amico, R. Marfella, L. Berrino, D. Giugliano, and F. Rossi, "Endothelin-1 receptor antagonists reduce cardiac electrical instability induced by high glucose in rats," *Naunyn-Schmiedeberg's Archives of Pharmacology*, vol. 366, no. 3, pp. 193–197, 2002.

[5] N.-H. Son, R. Ananthakrishnan, S. Yu et al., "Cardiomyocyte aldose reductase causes heart failure and impairs recovery from ischemia," *PLoS ONE*, vol. 7, no. 9, Article ID e46549, 2012.

[6] M. Abdillahi, R. Ananthakrishnan, S. Vedantham et al., "Aldose reductase modulates cardiac glycogen synthase kinase-3β phosphorylation during ischemia-reperfusion," *American Journal of Physiology—Heart and Circulatory Physiology*, vol. 303, no. 3, pp. H297–H308, 2012.

[7] Q. Li, Y. C. Hwang, R. Ananthakrishnan, P. J. Oates, D. Guberski, and R. Ravichandran, "Polyol pathway and modulation of ischemia-reperfusion injury in Type 2 diabetic BBZ rat hearts," *Cardiovascular Diabetology*, vol. 7, article 33, 2008.

[8] R. K. Vikramadithyan, Y. Hu, H.-L. Noh et al., "Human aldose reductase expression accelerates diabetic atherosclerosis in transgenic mice," *Journal of Clinical Investigation*, vol. 115, no. 9, pp. 2434–2443, 2005.

[9] M. Kaneko, L. Bucciarelli, Y. C. Hwang et al., "Aldose reductase and AGE-RAGE pathways: key players in myocardial ischemic injury," *Annals of the New York Academy of Sciences*, vol. 1043, pp. 702–709, 2005.

[10] S. Sartini, S. Cosconati, L. Marinelli et al., "Benzofuroxane derivatives as multi-effective agents for the treatment of cardiovascular diabetic complications. Synthesis, functional evaluation, and molecular modeling studies," *Journal of Medicinal Chemistry*, vol. 55, no. 23, pp. 10523–10531, 2012.

[11] A. Y. W. Lee and S. S. M. Chung, "Contributions of polyol pathway to oxidative stress in diabetic cataract," *The FASEB Journal*, vol. 13, no. 1, pp. 23–30, 1999.

[12] T. Finkel, C.-X. Deng, and R. Mostoslavsky, "Recent progress in the biology and physiology of sirtuins," *Nature*, vol. 460, no. 7255, pp. 587–591, 2009.

[13] S. Imai and J. Yoshino, "The importance of NAMPT/NAD/SIRT1 in the systemic regulation of metabolism and ageing," *Diabetes, Obesity and Metabolism*, vol. 15, no. 3, pp. 26–33, 2013.

[14] S. K. Chakrabarti, J. Francis, S. M. Ziesmann, J. C. Garmey, and R. G. Mirmira, "Covalent histone modifications underlie the developmental regulation of insulin gene transcription in pancreatic beta cells," *The Journal of Biological Chemistry*, vol. 278, no. 26, pp. 23617–23623, 2003.

[15] A. L. Mosley and S. Özcan, "Glucose regulates insulin gene transcription by hyperacetylation of histone H4," *The Journal of Biological Chemistry*, vol. 278, no. 22, pp. 19660–19666, 2003.

[16] Y. Hu, N. Zhang, Q. Fan et al., "Protective efficacy of carnosic acid against hydrogen peroxide induced oxidative injury in HepG2 cells through the SIRT1 pathway," *Canadian Journal of Physiology and Pharmacology*, vol. 93, no. 8, pp. 625–631, 2015.

[17] J. M. Solomon, R. Pasupuleti, L. Xu et al., "Inhibition of SIRT1 catalytic activity increases p53 acetylation but does not alter cell survival following DNA damage," *Molecular and Cellular Biology*, vol. 26, no. 1, pp. 28–38, 2006.

[18] R. Marfella, C. Di Filippo, M. Portoghese et al., "Myocardial lipid accumulation in patients with pressure-overloaded heart and metabolic syndrome," *Journal of Lipid Research*, vol. 50, no. 11, pp. 2314–2323, 2009.

[19] C. Di Filippo, M. V. Zippo, R. Maisto et al., "inhibition of ocular aldose reductase by a new benzofuroxane derivative ameliorates rat endotoxic uveitis," *Mediators of Inflammation*, vol. 2014, Article ID 857958, 9 pages, 2014.

[20] G. B. Reddy, A. Satyanarayana, N. Balakrishna et al., "Erythrocyte aldose reductase activity and sorbitol levels in diabetic retinopathy," *Molecular Vision*, vol. 14, pp. 593–601, 2008.

[21] S. Rossi, C. Di Filippo, C. Gesualdo et al., "Protection from endotoxic uveitis by intravitreal resolvin D1: involvement of lymphocytes, miRNAs, ubiquitin-proteasome, and M1/M2 macrophages," *Mediators of Inflammation*, vol. 2015, Article ID 149381, 12 pages, 2015.

[22] C. Veeresham, A. Rama Rao, and K. Asres, "Aldose reductase inhibitors of plant origin," *Phytotherapy Research*, vol. 28, no. 3, pp. 317–333, 2014.

[23] H. Cerecetto and W. Porcal, "Pharmacological properties of furoxans and benzofuroxans: recent developments," *Mini-Reviews in Medicinal Chemistry*, vol. 5, no. 1, pp. 57–67, 2005.

[24] S. Zhang, X. Chen, S. Parveen et al., "Effect of C7 modifications on benzothiadiazine-1,1-dioxide derivatives on their inhibitory activity and selectivity toward aldose reductase," *ChemMedChem*, vol. 8, no. 4, pp. 603–613, 2013.

[25] W. Sun, P. J. Oates, J. B. Coutcher, C. Gerhardinger, and M. Lorenzi, "A selective aldose reductase inhibitor of a new structural class prevents or reverses early retinal abnormalities in experimental diabetic retinopathy," *Diabetes*, vol. 55, no. 10, pp. 2757–2762, 2006.

[26] S. Cosconati, L. Marinelli, C. La Motta et al., "Pursuing aldose reductase inhibitors through in situ cross-docking and similarity-based virtual screening," *Journal of Medicinal Chemistry*, vol. 52, no. 18, pp. 5578–5581, 2009.

[27] A. I. Malik and K. B. Storey, "Transcriptional regulation of antioxidant enzymes by FoxO1 under dehydration stress," *Gene*, vol. 485, no. 2, pp. 114–119, 2011.

[28] A. Brunet, L. B. Sweeney, J. F. Sturgill et al., "Stress-dependent regulation of FOXO transcription factors by the SIRT1 deacetylase," *Science*, vol. 303, no. 5666, pp. 2011–2015, 2004.

[29] M. C. Motta, N. Divecha, M. Lemieux et al., "Mammalian SIRT1 represses forkhead transcription factors," *Cell*, vol. 116, no. 4, pp. 551–563, 2004.

[30] J. Nakae, T. Kitamura, Y. Kitamura, W. H. Biggs III, K. C. Arden, and D. Accili, "The forkhead transcription factor Foxo1 regulates adipocyte differentiation," *Developmental Cell*, vol. 4, no. 1, pp. 119–129, 2003.

[31] R. Mortuza, S. Chen, B. Feng, S. Sen, and S. Chakrabarti, "High glucose induced alteration of SIRTs in endothelial cells causes rapid aging in a p300 and FOXO regulated pathway," *PLoS ONE*, vol. 8, no. 1, Article ID e54514, 2013.

17

Effect of Ranirestat on Sensory and Motor Nerve Function in Japanese Patients with Diabetic Polyneuropathy: A Randomized Double-Blind Placebo-Controlled Study

Jo Satoh,[1] Nobuo Kohara,[2] Kenji Sekiguchi,[3] and Yasuyuki Yamaguchi[4]

[1]*NTT-EAST Tohoku Hospital, 2-29-1 Yamato-machi, Wakabayashi-ku, Sendai, Miyagi 984-8560, Japan*
[2]*Department of Neurology, Kobe City Medical Center General Hospital, 4-6 Minatojima-Nakamachi, Chuo-ku, Kobe, Hyogo 650-0046, Japan*
[3]*Division of Neurology, Kobe University Graduate School of Medicine, 7-5-2 Kusunoki-cho, Chuo-ku, Kobe, Hyogo 650-0017, Japan*
[4]*Sumitomo Dainippon Pharma, Co., Ltd., 6-8 Doshomachi 2-chome, Chuo-ku, Osaka 541-0045, Japan*

Correspondence should be addressed to Jo Satoh; josatoh@nifty.com

Academic Editor: Rodica Pop-Busui

We conducted a 26-week oral-administration study of ranirestat (an aldose reductase inhibitor) at a once-daily dose of 20 mg to evaluate its efficacy and safety in Japanese patients with diabetic polyneuropathy (DPN). The primary endpoint was summed change in sensory nerve conduction velocity (NCV) for the bilateral sural and proximal median sensory nerves. The sensory NCV was significantly ($P = 0.006$) improved by ranirestat. On clinical symptoms evaluated with the use of modified Toronto Clinical Neuropathy Score (mTCNS), obvious efficacy was not found in total score. However, improvement in the sensory test domain of the mTCNS was significant ($P = 0.037$) in a subgroup of patients diagnosed with neuropathy according to the TCNS severity classification. No clinically significant effects on safety parameters including hepatic and renal functions were observed. Our results indicate that ranirestat is effective on DPN (Japic CTI-121994).

1. Introduction

Diabetic polyneuropathy (DPN) is one of the most frequent diabetic complications. Its onset and progression cause deterioration of sensory, motor, and autonomic nerve functions, markedly reducing patients' quality of life (QOL). The onset mechanism is complex and remains to be clarified. Activation of the polyol pathway may be responsible for DPN. The polyol pathway is a side pathway metabolizing excess (or unused) glucose to sorbitol. It is thus suggested that intracellular sorbitol production (which is increased by accelerated metabolism in the hyperglycemic condition) may trigger the development and progression of DPN [1].

Aldose reductase (AR) is a rate-limiting enzyme that controls the polyol pathway. AR inhibitors (ARIs), expected to ameliorate DPN, have been extensively developed. A promising ARI zenarestat not only reduced sorbitol production and improved nerve conduction velocity (NCV), but also significantly increased myelinated nerve fiber density in the sural nerve via reducing the sorbitol concentration by 80% or more. These findings imply the usefulness of ARIs in the treatment of DPN [2].

Ranirestat is an ARI synthesized by Sumitomo-Dainippon Pharma Co., Ltd. It has already been demonstrated that ranirestat orally administered for 12 weeks significantly inhibited accumulation of sorbitol within the sural nerve: a dosage of 20 mg/day reduced accumulation by 83.5%. Furthermore, the 12-week treatment improved sensory NCV (the change from baseline reached 1 m/s). Even after an additional 48-week treatment, the improved sensory NCV was long maintained and associated with ameliorated peroneal motor NCV [3, 4]. On the basis of these results, we carried out the present clinical trial to explore the effectiveness and safety of ranirestat in Japanese DPN patients.

2. Materials and Methods

2.1. Study Design. This study was a multicenter (20 sites in Japan), double-blind, randomized, placebo-controlled study in which patients with DPN were assigned to either ranirestat 20 mg/day or placebo administered after breakfast as a once-daily dose for 26 weeks. The 20 mg/day dose was selected because it was associated with an 83.5% inhibition of sorbitol accumulation in the 12-week biopsy study [3]. The following procedures were performed at entry for each patient: medical history, physical examinations, nerve conduction studies (NCS), and both the Toronto Clinical Neuropathy Score (TCNS) and modified TCNS (mTCNS) [5–7]. Clinical laboratory tests were performed at every visit. An ECG was examined every month and at last visit. Adverse events were recorded. At weeks 12 and 26, NCS, TCNS, and mTCNS were repeated.

The primary end point was the summed change in sensory NCV from baseline of the bilateral sural and proximal median sensory nerves. Secondary end points were the changes for individual NCVs, amplitudes, minimum F-wave latencies (MFWL), TCNS, and mTCNS.

2.2. Patients. We enrolled patients who met the following entry criteria: age 20–70 years, either sex, type 1 or 2 diabetes for at least 6 months, glycemic control stable for at least 6 weeks before entry, and HbA1c (≥7.4% but ≤11.5%) [8, 9]. DPN was diagnosed when two of the following four modified San Antonio criteria were present: (1) symptoms of DPN, (2) signs of DPN, (3) abnormal results of NCS with at least two abnormal nerves (meeting this criterion was mandatory), and (4) abnormal vibration perception threshold (<10 seconds using a 128 Hz tuning fork). The requirement for both sural nerves potential amplitude responses of at least 1.0 μV insured the presence of viable nerve fibers to allow accurate measurements and avoided inclusion of patients with severe neuropathy who would not be expected to respond. Since a sural nerve generally shows symmetrical responses, the difference in sural nerve potential amplitude and conduction velocity between the right and left legs should be limited (amplitude <6.0 μV, NCV <7.0 m/s). Patients with nondiabetic neuropathy were excluded, as well as those with any clinically significant abnormal clinical laboratory parameter or any abnormal liver function test.

The institutional review boards at each center reviewed and approved the study protocol. All patients provided written informed consent at screening. The study was performed in accordance with the guidelines expressed in the Declaration of Helsinki.

2.3. Electrophysiological Measurements. A training meeting was held with investigators to review the protocol and procedures. Testing was standardized for measurement of temperature, side of testing, stimulation protocol, averaging of sensory potentials, and measurement of latencies and amplitudes.

Standardized techniques with temperature controlled and distal distances fixed were used for NCS. The minimum temperature was maintained at 31°C in the forearm and 30°C in the lower calf. If limb temperature was lower than specified, the limbs tested were warmed in a heating water bath before starting the test. It was recommended to warm cold legs in hot water at approximately 40°C for at least 20 min before performing the test. Unilateral NCSs were performed on the nondominant median motor, dominant tibial motor, and nondominant median sensory nerves. Bilateral NCSs were performed on the sural sensory nerves. Sensory NCSs were performed antidromically. All stimulation and recording were performed using surface electrodes. The fixed distal surface electrode distances for motor NCS were 60 mm for the median nerve and 80 mm for the tibial nerve. Corresponding distances for sensory NCS were 20 mm proximal to the distal wrist crease for the median nerve and 140 mm for the sural nerve. Measurements of distances, response latencies, and amplitudes were performed in a standard fashion using onset latencies and baseline-to-peak amplitudes. Measurements from the initial positive peak to negative peak were made for sensory responses. F-waves were generated for all motor nerves with 16 supramaximal stimuli per nerve, and the minimal reproducible latency of at least three responses was measured. The examiners had access to the previous temperatures, distances, and results through this trial. Results of the screening NCS for each patient were reviewed and the eligibility of each patient was decided by the Nerve Conduction Study Assessment Committee before randomization. This central supervision ensured consistency of study procedures and high quality of data under blinding [10].

2.4. Clinical Measurements. Symptoms and signs were assessed with the mTCNS and TCNS. TCNS is a validated and reliable way to assess clinical findings in DPN [5]. The TCNS has been modified to better capture sensory test results reflecting early dysfunction in DPN, also to improve the sensitivity and specificity of the original TCNS [6, 7]. The mTCNS includes a symptom domain and a sensory test domain. In the symptom domain, the course of development of "Pain, Numbness, Tingling, Weakness, and Ataxia in Foot and Upper limb" is separated into 4 stages: 0 = absent, 1 = present but not interfering with the sense of well-being or activities of daily living, 2 = present and interfering with the sense of well-being but not with activities of daily living, and 3 = present and interfering with both the sense of well-being and activities of daily living. In the sensory test domain, "Pinprick, Temperature, Light Touch, Vibration, and Position Sense" were assessed as 0 = normal, 1 = reduced at the toes only, 2 = reduced to a level above the toes, but only up to the ankles, and 3 = reduced to a level above the ankles and/or absent at the toes. The mTCNS scale varies from 0 (no signs or no symptoms of DPN) to 33 (all symptoms and signs of DPN present with a maximum score of 18 symptom points and 15 sensory test points).

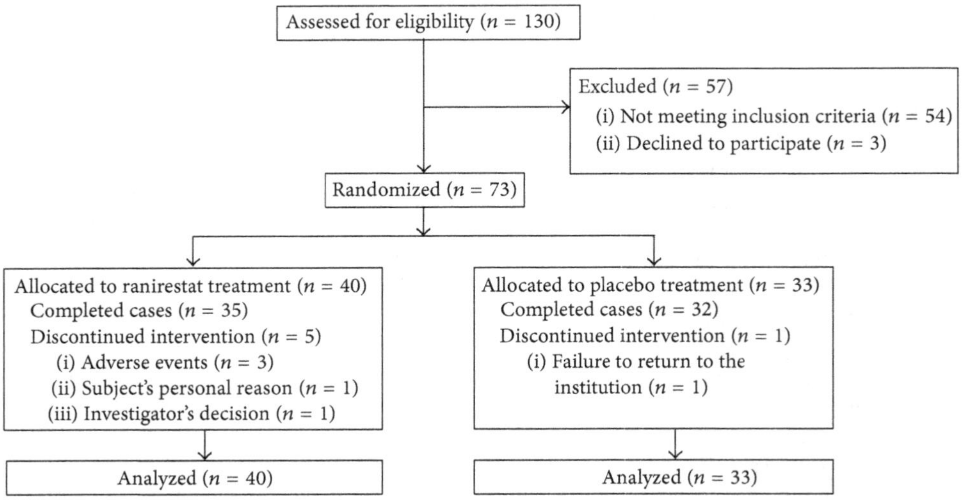

FIGURE 1: Study flow diagram.

2.5. Statistical Analyses. The full analysis set was used in the efficacy analysis and included all randomized patients but excluded those receiving no investigational drug and those with no efficacy data (Figure 1). Changes from baseline to the last observation in efficacy variables were compared between the treatment groups. The last observation was recorded at week 26. When no data were available at week 26, the last observation carried forward (LOCF) approach was used.

The data were compared between groups by analysis of covariance using group as a factor and baseline values as a covariate. The changes were determined by group at each visit for which summary statistics were calculated and plotted against visit. Within-group differences were tested using the paired Student t-test by group and visit. For binary data, the number and percentage were determined by group and visit and compared between the groups using the Fisher exact test. For ordinal data, the number and percentage were determined by group and visit and compared between the groups using the Mantel test.

3. Results

3.1. Demographic Profiles of the Patients. We screened 130 patients and excluded 57 patients for not meeting the inclusion criteria or meeting the exclusion criteria at screening (n = 54) and for withdrawing their consent prior to randomization (n = 3). Seventy-three patients were randomized to either ranirestat or placebo (40 : 33), and all 73 received an investigational drug (Figure 1). The baseline characteristics for these 73 patients are summarized in Table 1. Some differences in HbA1c between the ranirestat and placebo groups were observed at baseline.

3.2. Electrophysiological Measurements. Because the magnitude of change in the individual NCV varied, the sensory NCVs were summed to comprehensively evaluate each sensory nerve's function. The summed sensory NCV (primary endpoint) was the sum of the NCV in the bilateral sural sensory nerves and proximal median sensory nerves. Distal median sensory NCV was not included in the summed sensory NCV in order to avoid the possible influence of carpal tunnel syndrome. The baseline characteristics are summarized in Table 2.

For the summed sensory NCV, the change from baseline to the last observation was 7.28 ± 1.27 m/s (least squares mean [LSM] $\pm$ SE) in the ranirestat group and 1.92 ± 1.39 m/s in the placebo group (Table 3). Analysis of covariance of the changes in the summed sensory NCV at the last observation using drug group as a factor and the summed sensory NCV at baseline as a covariate detected a significant improvement in the ranirestat group compared with the placebo group ($P = 0.006$).

In order to investigate how the imbalance of baseline HbA1c between the two groups influences the results, analysis of covariance (ANCOVA) was conducted to assess change in summed sensory NCV from the baseline to the last observation, controlling for HbA1c by adding baseline HbA1c as a covariate, in reference to the ICH E9 guideline. The changes in summed sensory NCV were 7.54 ± 1.29 m/s in the ranirestat group and 1.60 ± 1.42 m/s in the placebo group, indicating significant difference between the two groups ($P = 0.003$). There was no significant effect of baseline HbA1c because the changes before and after adding the covariate of baseline HbA1c were similar.

Table 3 also shows that the improvement of NCV from baseline to the last observation in the individual nerves was consistently significant in the ranirestat group ($P <$ 0.001–0.030) for all except the median motor NCV. The change in the placebo group did not achieve significance. The between-group differences in proximal median sensory NCV were significant ($P = 0.019$). There was a tendency of significant between-group difference in median motor NCV ($P = 0.051$).

The change in the amplitude of each nerve is shown in Table 4. Analysis of covariance of the change at the last

TABLE 1: Summary of baseline characteristics.

	Ranirestat (n = 40)	Placebo (n = 33)	P values
Male sex	23 (57.5)	24 (72.7)	0.176
Age (years)	58.9 ± 8.7	58.2 ± 7.5	0.708
BMI (kg/m^2)	24.63 ± 2.97	25.34 ± 4.12	0.396
Type of diabetes			
Type I	3 (7.5)	4 (12.1)	0.505
Type II	37 (92.5)	29 (87.9)	
Diabetes duration (years)	15.7 ± 7.3	15.2 ± 7.4	0.751
Neuropathy duration (years)	5.1 ± 3.8	4.9 ± 3.1	0.846
HbA1c (%)	7.67 ± 0.70	8.05 ± 0.93	0.046

Data are n (%) for sex and type of diabetes and means ± SD for other parameters. P values for sex and type of diabetes were obtained from χ^2 tests. P values for other parameters were obtained from Student t-tests.

TABLE 2: Summary of the baseline nerve conduction study and mTCNS.

	Ranirestat (n = 40)	Placebo (n = 33)	P values
Nerve conduction velocity (m/s)			
Summed sensory NCV	146.37 ± 13.47	146.13 ± 12.75	0.940
Right sural sensory NCV	44.15 ± 4.88	45.11 ± 5.05	0.420
Left sural sensory NCV	43.81 ± 5.85	44.71 ± 4.96	0.491
Proximal median sensory NCV	57.96 ± 5.58	56.08 ± 4.68	0.132
Distal median sensory NCV	46.13 ± 8.76	44.35 ± 9.90	0.419
Median motor NCV	51.45 ± 4.30	50.47 ± 3.53	0.299
Tibial motor NCV	39.79 ± 4.44	39.76 ± 3.71	0.975
F-wave latency (ms)			
Median motor MFWL	27.29 ± 2.95	28.88 ± 2.00	0.010
Tibial motor MFWL	50.98 ± 5.28	52.55 ± 4.21	0.180
mTCNS (pt)			
Total score	7.6 ± 5.8	7.3 ± 4.4	0.806
Symptom domain	3.0 ± 2.7	3.1 ± 2.6	0.917
Sensory domain	4.6 ± 3.7	4.2 ± 3.0	0.647

Data are mean ± SD. P values for other parameters were obtained from Student t-tests.
mTCNS total score is the sum of symptom domain and sensory domain scores. The symptom domain score is the sum of individual symptom scores, and the sensory domain score is the sum of individual sensory scores.

TABLE 3: Changes from baseline in the summed sensory NCV and individual NCV.

		Ranirestat (n = 40)	Placebo (n = 33)	P values
Sensory NCV (m/s)				
Summed sensory	Baseline	146.37 ± 13.47	146.13 ± 12.75	0.006
	Change	7.28 ± 9.56	1.92 ± 7.46	
Right sural sensory	Baseline	44.15 ± 4.88	45.11 ± 5.05	0.088
	Change	2.84 ± 4.17	0.77 ± 4.60	
Left sural sensory	Baseline	43.81 ± 5.85	44.71 ± 4.96	0.183
	Change	2.91 ± 4.61	1.30 ± 4.22	
Proximal median sensory	Baseline	57.96 ± 5.58	56.08 ± 4.68	0.019
	Change	1.40 ± 3.91	−0.28 ± 4.01	
Distal median sensory	Baseline	46.13 ± 8.76	44.35 ± 9.90	0.153
	Change	1.97 ± 4.46	0.73 ± 3.51	
Motor NCV (m/s)				
Median motor	Baseline	51.45 ± 4.30	50.47 ± 3.53	0.051
	Change	0.95 ± 3.30	−0.11 ± 2.73	
Tibial motor	Baseline	39.79 ± 4.44	39.76 ± 3.71	0.152
	Change	1.18 ± 2.63	0.35 ± 2.36	

Data shown are mean ± SD change from baseline to last observation carried forward. P values were obtained from an ANCOVA model with change from baseline to the last observation and the baseline value as a covariate.

Table 4: Changes from baseline in the individual nerve amplitudes.

		Ranirestat (n = 40)	Placebo (n = 33)	P values
Sensory nerve amplitude (μV)				
Right sural nerve	Baseline	4.26 ± 2.15	4.15 ± 2.91	0.442
	Change	0.15 ± 2.41	0.18 ± 1.02	
Left sural nerve	Baseline	4.48 ± 2.53	4.67 ± 3.48	0.332
	Change	−0.01 ± 2.71	−0.57 ± 1.67	
Proximal median sensory	Baseline	7.83 ± 4.67	6.53 ± 3.99	0.208
	Change	0.66 ± 3.02	−0.05 ± 2.83	
Distal median sensory	Baseline	15.70 ± 9.24	12.20 ± 7.87	0.465
	Change	0.18 ± 4.33	−0.23 ± 3.24	
Motor nerve amplitude (mV)				
Proximal median motor	Baseline	6.99 ± 2.91	7.22 ± 2.53	0.026
	Change	0.39 ± 1.53	−0.41 ± 1.40	
Distal median motor	Baseline	7.36 ± 3.01	7.74 ± 2.60	0.019
	Change	0.41 ± 1.46	−0.44 ± 1.43	
Proximal tibial motor	Baseline	6.03 ± 3.32	5.35 ± 2.55	0.477
	Change	−0.23 ± 1.60	0.12 ± 1.77	
Distal tibial motor	Baseline	8.57 ± 4.45	8.23 ± 3.49	0.821
	Change	−0.30 ± 2.33	−0.35 ± 2.41	

Data shown are mean ± SD change from baseline to last observation carried forward. P values were obtained from an ANCOVA model with change from baseline to the last observation and the baseline value as a covariate.

observation detected a significant difference for the proximal (P = 0.026) and distal (P = 0.019) median motor nerves between the ranirestat group and the placebo group.

MFWL was measured for each motor nerve. The change in MFWL did not show prolongation for the ranirestat group. The improvement in the tibial motor MFWL was significant (50.12 ± 4.69 msec versus 50.98 ± 5.28 msec, P = 0.007). However, analysis of covariance for each nerve detected no significant improvement for the ranirestat group compared to the placebo group.

3.3. Clinical Measurements. Figure 2 shows our mTCNS findings. The total score improved at 12 weeks in the two groups, and no between-group difference was observed in the change from baseline at the final evaluation. By domain, similar time-course changes were seen in the symptom domain in the two groups, while ranirestat change tended to increase at the final evaluation in the sensory test domain. An additional analysis in a subgroup of patients with mild to severe neuropathy according to the TCNS severity classification revealed significant improvements in the sensory test domain in the ranirestat group (P = 0.037), although there was no between-group difference in total score change at the final evaluation.

3.4. Safety. Ranirestat 20 mg/day was well tolerated for 26 weeks. The prevalence of adverse events was similar in both groups: 33 of 40 patients (82.5%) in the ranirestat group and 29 of 33 (87.9%) in the placebo group. In the ranirestat group, 3 serious adverse events (appendicitis perforated, peritonitis, and spinal compression fracture) were noted, but all were judged by the investigator to be unrelated to ranirestat (Table 5). No clinically significant changes were observed for the other safety parameters.

Table 5: Summary of adverse event.

	Ranirestat (n = 40)	Placebo (n = 33)
Adverse event	33 (82.5)	29 (87.9)
Serious adverse event	3 (7.5)	0 (0.0)
Adverse drug reaction	11 (27.5)	11 (33.3)

Data are n (%).

4. Discussion

This clinical trial has demonstrated that oral administration of ranirestat at 20 mg/day for 26 weeks, as compared with placebo, significantly improved the primary endpoint of summed sensory NCV: summed sensory NCVs in the ranirestat group increased after 12-week treatment and were significantly higher than that in the placebo group at the final evaluation (P = 0.006). In a proof-of-concept study conducted in North America, 12-week treatment with ranirestat 20 mg/day reduced the sorbitol concentration in the sural nerve by more than 80% and ameliorated sensory nerve NCV [3]. These study results were reproduced in the present study carried out in Japanese patients with DPN. Blood glucose control is critical for the treatment of DPN, as indicated by the results of a large-scale clinical trial [11]. The blood glucose control status may affect the results of our study. Since an imbalance in HbA1c was found at baseline in the present study, we investigated whether the blood glucose control status at baseline affected the study results.

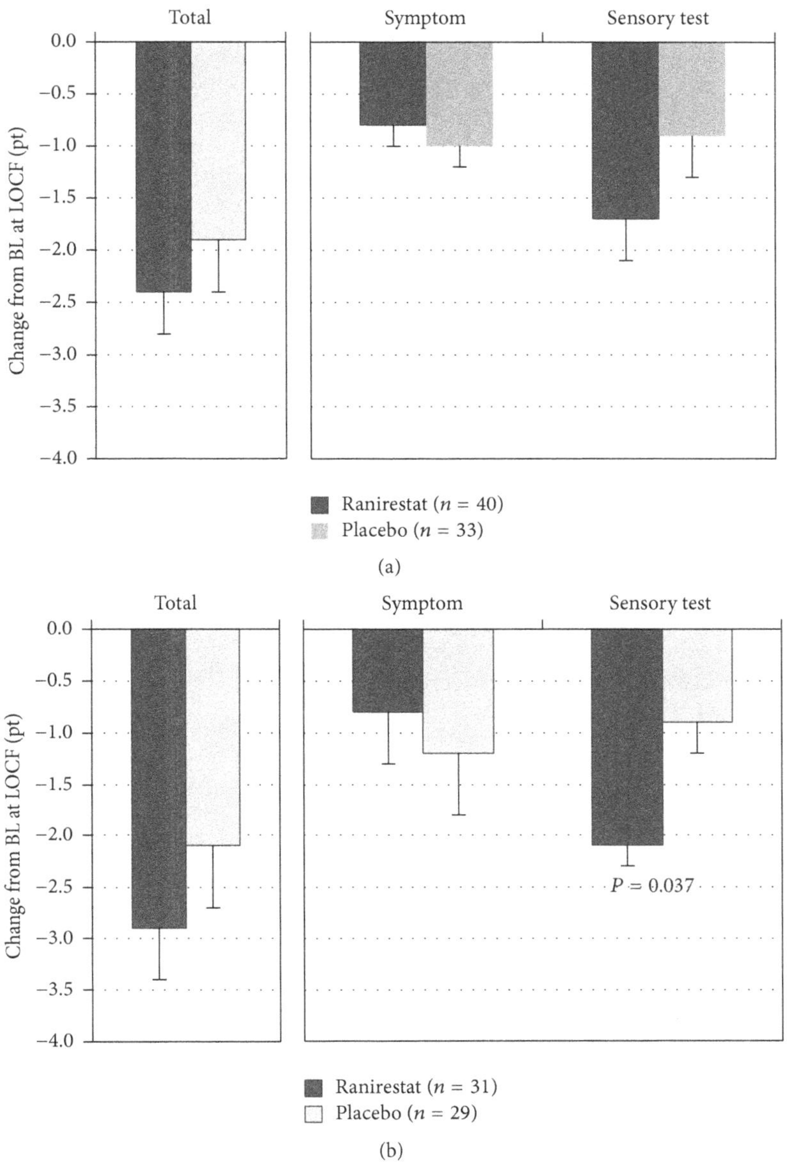

FIGURE 2: Changes from baseline in the mTCNS. (a) Full analysis set. Data shown are LS mean ± SE change from baseline (BL) at LOCF in the mTCNS. (b) Subgroup of patients with mild to severe neuropathy diagnosed according to the TCNS severity classification at BL. Data shown are LS mean ± SE change from BL at LOCF in the mTCNS. P values were obtained from an ANCOVA model with change from baseline to the last observation and the baseline value as a covariate.

Using baseline HbA1c as another covariate on the basis of the ICH E9 guideline, we performed an additional analysis of summed sensory NCV and found the significance of differences between the ranirestat and placebo groups had remained unchanged ($P = 0.0034$): the robustness of our results was thereby confirmed.

We did additional analyses. The changes from baseline to last observation in HbA1c were +0.26% in the ranirestat group versus +0.07% in the placebo group; there were no significant changes from baseline in the two groups. Furthermore, we performed a subgroup analysis of summed sensory NCV, via dividing participants into "well-controlled" (improved or unchanged HbA1c [ΔHbA1c $\leq$ 0%]) and "poorly controlled" (deteriorated HbA1c [ΔHbA1c > 0%]). The change from baseline in summed sensory NCV was 9.4 m/s for ranirestat ($n = 23$) versus 4.1 m/s for placebo ($n = 12$) in "well-controlled" participants and 3.8 m/s for ranirestat ($n = 14$) versus 0.5 m/s for placebo ($n = 19$) in "poorly controlled" participants. In either subgroup, ranirestat produced greater changes, indicating that difference in blood glucose control during the study period had no effect on the results or conclusions in this study. Thus, we consider that baseline HbA1c imbalance has no relevant effect on study conclusions. Nevertheless, as the present study is a small-scale trial with limited subgroup analysis, a further study involving a larger number of participants is desired for a valid conclusion.

DPN is a systemic neuropathy that damages both the sensory and motor nerves as well as both the upper and lower limbs. Its fundamental treatment is strict control of blood glucose. The landmark Diabetes Control and Complication Trial followed up patients receiving intensive treatment and those receiving conventional treatment for 5 years and reported that NCV at 5 years was lower by more than 1 m/s in the conventional treatment group than the intensive treatment group. In the present study, we examined and evaluated a sensory nerve and a motor nerve in both the upper and lower limbs. NCV increased from the baseline value in all ranirestat-treated nerves. Compared with placebo, ranirestat significantly increased proximal-median sensory NCV ($P = 0.019$). These findings imply that the effect of ranirestat is not limited to a particular nerve but extends to all peripheral nerves. In this study, NCV of each nerve tested was higher by 0.83 to 2.17 m/s in the ranirestat group than in the placebo group, indicating that ranirestat and strict control of blood glucose play equally potent roles in maintaining nerve function. A clinical trial using median motor NCV (MMNCV) as a parameter for long-term treatment with epalrestat (the only ARI in clinical use) reported that epalrestat significantly reduced MMNCV deterioration by 0.78 m/s at one year, by 1.21 m/s at 2 years, and by 1.60 m/s at 3 years as compared with the control [12]. In this study, the difference in MMNCV between the ranirestat and placebo groups was 1.06 m/s ($P = 0.051$). In regard to NCV, these findings indicate that ranirestat can be expected to exert an effect as potent as the existing therapeutic epalrestat.

In parallel to the present trial, a phase III clinical trial of ranirestat was carried out in North America. Bril et al. reported that summed motor NCV was significantly improved by ranirestat, but summed sensory NCV was not [13]. On the other hand, in our study, summed sensory NCV was significantly improved, whereas motor NCV was not significantly changed, although there was a tendency of significant between-group difference in median motor NCV ($P = 0.051$). It is difficult to clearly elucidate the reason for the different results between two trials. However, there may be a couple of possibilities. The cohort size was different between their and our trial. The number of participants in their trial was more than three times as large as ours. It may be one of reasons that summed motor NCV was significantly improved in their trial [13].

As for summed sensory NCV, measurement of sensory NCV using surface electrodes is affected by a variety of conditions such as skin temperature and measurement site condition, because the amplitude of sensory nerve action potential (measured in microvolts) is markedly lower than that of compound muscle action potential (measured in millivolts). To overcome these difficulties, measurement in NCS was performed more precisely by standardization of measuring methods, use of common procedures, and intensive evaluation in the core laboratory to increase data reproducibility in the phase III trial and our trial. However, a large difference in demographic characteristics of patients such as BMI might partially affect condition of measurement sites such as subcutaneous tissue; BMI (mean ± SD) was 25.0 ± 3.5 in our study versus 33.1 ± 6.8 in the North America study [13].

DPN is a nerve-degenerative disease that progresses slowly and is characterized by a variety of clinical manifestations including subjective symptoms (such as spontaneous pain; positive symptoms) and sensory deterioration (negative symptoms) associated with progression of nerve destruction. In this study, these various clinical symptoms were evaluated with the use of an mTCNS (with symptom domain dedicated to positive symptoms and sensory test domain dedicated to negative symptoms). Both the original mTCNS and Japanese version are recognized as valid and reliable evaluation tools [6, 7]. In this study, the total score of mTCNS improved at 12 weeks in both groups and no between-group difference in change from baseline was found at the final evaluation: no obvious effect of ranirestat was observed on clinical symptoms. Since the mTCNS used in this study is based on the TCNS, all patients were divided into two subgroups, based on TCNS severity. One subgroup of patients with TCNS total score ≤5 (9 in the ranirestat group and 4 in the placebo group) was excluded in order to perform an additional analysis. In the other subgroup of patients with TCNS total score ≥6, ranirestat elicited significant improvement in the sensory test domain, as compared with placebo ($P = 0.037$). As sensory test results have been reported to well correlate with risk of foot ulcers [14], improvement in negative signs is important for preventing foot ulcers and avoiding limb amputation, which are targets of DPN treatment. The subgroup analysis in this trial indicated the effectiveness of ranirestat on sensory signs. Nevertheless, the efficacy of ranirestat on clinical symptoms remains to be elucidated, probably because this trial was limited by short treatment duration and presence of a placebo effect. Evaluation using mTCNS in the phase III trial of ranirestat in North America also demonstrated that mTCNS scores were improved in the all groups including placebo at 12 weeks and no efficacy of ranirestat was detected at 52 weeks [13]. Placebo effects were also noted in the recent phase II/III studies of ranirestat with 2-year treatment duration (in Asia, Europe, North America, and Russia) and resulted in a failure to demonstrate significant efficacy on clinical symptoms [15]. For evaluation of clinical symptoms of DPN, different scales have been used in different clinical trials. Placebo effects have been observed in multiple trials, perhaps not only in trials using the mTCNS [16, 17]. In our and other studies, blood glucose was relatively well controlled and maintained, which might be attributable to lack of deterioration in the placebo group. Because DPN is slowly progressive, it may be necessary to design a study with longer duration of more than 2 years [18] and with a more sensitive tool for assessing or detecting clinical symptoms.

Regarding the adverse events in this study, there was no particular difference between the two groups; adverse effects on hepatic and/or renal function associated with use of other drugs were also undetectable. These findings assure the safety of the 26-week treatment with ranirestat at a daily dose of 20 mg.

5. Conclusions

As compared with placebo, ranirestat administered to Japanese DPN patients at a once-daily dose of 20 mg for 26 weeks significantly improved summed sensory NCV. A subgroup analysis revealed that treatment with ranirestat led to significant improvement in clinical signs (i.e., increased the sensory test domain score of the mTCNS). There was no particular safety problem. These findings indicate the effectiveness of ranirestat on DPN. However, this study aiming at proof-of-concept was limited by its short-term treatment duration and small number of patients. Further studies are needed to establish the efficacy of ranirestat in the treatment of DPN.

Conflict of Interests

Jo Satoh, Nobuo Kohara, and Kenji Sekiguchi have received consultation fees from Dainippon Sumitomo Pharma. Yasuyuki Yamaguchi is an employee of Dainippon Sumitomo Pharma.

Acknowledgments

This work was supported by Sumitomo Dinippon Pharma, Co., Ltd. Nobuo Kohara and Kenji Sekiguchi have served as the evaluation committee of nerve conduction study. List of principal investigators is as follows: Katsuyuki Yanagisawa (Sapporo City General Hospital), Masatomo Sekiguchi (JA Sapporo-Kosei General Hospital), Kazushi Misawa (Manda Memorial Hospital), Yoshihito Kaneko (Iwate Medical University Hospital), Masaei Kakizaki (Tohoku Kosei-Nenkin Hospital), Hiroaki Seino (Ota Nishinouchi Hospital, Ota General Hospital), Sane Ishikawa (Omiya Medical Center, Jichi Medical University Hospital), Michio Hayashi (Kanto Medical Center, NTT East), Yasuhisa Kato (Nagoya Medical Center), Tsuyoshi Tanaka (Mie Central Medical Center), Shigeo Kono (Kyoto Medical Center), Ryohei Todo (Osaka Medical Center), Kazuyuki Hida (Okayama Medical Center), Kenji Takahashi (Kurashiki Central Hospital), Michihiro Matsuki (Kawasaki Medical University Hospital), Ryo Nagase (Tsuyama Central Hospital), Atsuo Yamada (Kure Medical Center), Kazufumi Ishida (Hiroshima General Hospital), Hideaki Jinnouchi (Jinnouchi Hospital), and Kiichiro Higashi (Kumamoto Medical Center).

References

[1] S. Yagihashi, H. Mizukami, and K. Sugimoto, "Mechanism of diabetic neuropathy: where are we now and where to go?" *Journal of Diabetes Investigation*, vol. 2, no. 1, pp. 18–32, 2011.

[2] D. A. Greene, J. C. Arezzo, and M. B. Brown, "Effect of aldose reductase inhibition on nerve conduction and morphometry in diabetic neuropathy," *Neurology*, vol. 53, no. 3, pp. 580–591, 1999.

[3] V. Bril, R. A. Buchanan, and The AS-3201 Study Group, "Aldose reductase inhibition by AS-3201 in sural nerve from patients with diabetic sensorimotor polyneuropathy," *Diabetes Care*, vol. 27, no. 10, pp. 2369–2375, 2004.

[4] V. Bril and R. A. Buchanan, "Long-term effects of ranirestat (AS-3201) on peripheral nerve function in patients with diabetic sensorimotor polyneuropathy," *Diabetes Care*, vol. 29, no. 1, pp. 68–72, 2006.

[5] V. Bril and B. A. Perkins, "Validation of the Toronto Clinical Scoring System for diabetic polyneuropathy," *Diabetes Care*, vol. 25, no. 11, pp. 2048–2052, 2002.

[6] V. Bril, S. Tomioka, R. A. Buchanan, B. A. Perkins, and The mTCNS Study Group, "Reliability and validity of the modified Toronto Clinical Neuropathy Score in diabetic sensorimotor polyneuropathy," *Diabetic Medicine*, vol. 26, no. 3, pp. 240–246, 2009.

[7] J. Satoh, N. Kohara, and C. Hamada, "Assessment of the reliability of a Japanese version of the modified toronto clinical neuropathy score in Japanese patients with diabetic sensorimotor polyneuropathy," *Journal of the Japan Diabetes Society*, vol. 56, no. 12, pp. 932–937, 2013.

[8] A. Kashiwagi, M. Kasuga, E. Araki et al., "International clinical harmonization of glycated hemoglobin in Japan: from Japan Diabetes Society to National Glycohemoglobin Standardization Program values," *Diabetology International*, vol. 3, no. 1, pp. 8–10, 2012.

[9] A. Kashiwagi, M. Kasuga, E. Araki et al., "International clinical harmonization of glycated hemoglobin in Japan: from Japan Diabetes Society to National Glycohemoglobin Standardization Program values," *Journal of Diabetes Investigation*, vol. 3, no. 1, pp. 39–40, 2012.

[10] V. Bril, R. Ellison, M. Ngo et al., "Electrophysiological monitoring in clinical trials," *Muscle and Nerve*, vol. 21, no. 11, pp. 1368–1373, 1998.

[11] Diabetes Control and Complications Trial Research Group, "Effect of intensive diabetes treatment on nerve conduction in the Diabetes Control and Complications Trial," *Annals of Neurology*, vol. 38, no. 6, pp. 869–880, 1995.

[12] N. Hotta, Y. Akanuma, R. Kawamori et al., "Long-term clinical effects of epalrestat, an aldose reductase inhibitor, on diabetic peripheral neuropathy: the 3-year, multicenter, comparative aldose reductase inhibitor-diabetes complications trial," *Diabetes Care*, vol. 29, no. 7, pp. 1538–1544, 2006.

[13] V. Bril, T. Hirose, S. Tomioka, and R. Buchanan, "Ranirestat for the management of diabetic sensorimotor polyneuropathy," *Diabetes Care*, vol. 32, no. 7, pp. 1256–1260, 2009.

[14] C. A. Abbott, A. L. Carrington, H. Ashe et al., "The North-West Diabetes Foot Care Study: incidence of, and risk factors for, new diabetic foot ulceration in a community-based patient cohort," *Diabetic Medicine*, vol. 19, no. 5, pp. 377–384, 2002.

[15] M. Polydefkis, J. Arezzo, M. Nash et al., "Safety and efficacy of ranirestat in patients with mild-to-moderate diabetic sensorimotor polyneuropathy," *Journal of the Peripheral Nervous System*, vol. 20, no. 4, pp. 363–371, 2015.

[16] A. I. Vinik, V. Bril, P. Kempler et al., "Treatment of symptomatic diabetic peripheral neuropathy with the protein kinase C β-inhibitor ruboxistaurin mesylate during a 1-year, randomized, placebo-controlled, double-blind clinical trial," *Clinical Therapeutics*, vol. 27, no. 8, pp. 1164–1180, 2005.

[17] D. Ziegler, A. Ametov, A. Barinov et al., "Oral treatment with α-lipoic acid improves symptomatic diabetic polyneuropathy," *Diabetes Care*, vol. 29, no. 11, pp. 2365–2370, 2006.

[18] C. Laudadio and A. A. F. Sima, "Progression rates of diabetic neuropathy in placebo patients in an 18-month clinical trial," *Journal of Diabetes and Its Complications*, vol. 12, no. 3, pp. 121–127, 1988.

18

The Four-Herb Chinese Medicine Formula Tuo-Li-Xiao-Du-San Accelerates Cutaneous Wound Healing in Streptozotocin-Induced Diabetic Rats through Reducing Inflammation and Increasing Angiogenesis

Xiao-na Zhang, Ze-jun Ma, Ying Wang, Yu-zhu Li, Bei Sun, Xin Guo, Cong-qing Pan, and Li-ming Chen

2011 Collaborative Innovation Center of Tianjin for Medical Epigenetics, Key Laboratory of Hormone and Development of Ministry of Health, Metabolic Disease Hospital and Tianjin Institute of Endocrinology, Tianjin Medical University, Tianjin 300070, China

Correspondence should be addressed to Cong-qing Pan; cq.pan@163.com and Li-ming Chen; chenliming3266@163.com

Academic Editor: Didac Mauricio

Impaired wound healing in diabetic patients is a serious complication that often leads to amputation or even death with limited effective treatments. Tuo-Li-Xiao-Du-San (TLXDS), a traditional Chinese medicine formula for refractory wounds, has been prescribed for nearly 400 years in China and shows good efficacy in promoting healing. In this study, we explored the effect of TLXDS on healing of diabetic wounds and investigated underlying mechanisms. Four weeks after intravenous injection of streptozotocin, two full-thickness excisional wounds were created with a 10 mm diameter sterile biopsy punch on the back of rats. The ethanol extract of TLXDS was given once daily by oral gavage. Wound area, histological change, inflammation, angiogenesis, and collagen synthesis were evaluated. TLXDS treatment significantly accelerated healing of diabetic rats and improved the healing quality. These effects were associated with reduced neutrophil infiltration and macrophage accumulation, enhanced angiogenesis, and increased collagen deposition. This study shows that TLXDS improves diabetes-impaired wound healing.

1. Introduction

Nonhealing wound is a hallmark of diabetes and the leading cause of nontraumatic lower extremity amputation. The lifetime risk of a person with diabetes developing a chronic foot ulcer could be as high as 25% [1]. However, the treatments for it are limited and the cost is high [2]. Therefore, developing effective and economical therapies for correcting impaired healing of diabetic wounds is an urgent clinical demand. Diabetes impairs wound healing through magnifying the inflammatory response, inhibiting angiogenesis, and decreasing extracellular matrix (ECM) deposition [3]. The ideal treatment relies on correcting the multiple deficits simultaneously through highly integrated therapeutic approaches. Traditional Chinese medicine (TCM) is characterized by the use of herbal formulas that are usually grouped by two or more medicinal herbs, which can effectively produce synergetic effects to be greater than the sum of the individual effects and reduce side effects, providing novel therapeutic strategies for diabetic ulcer. Studies showed that combining TCM with conventional treatments in diabetic wound management received better clinical outcome [4].

Tuo-Li-Xiao-Du-San (TLXDS) is a refined Chinese medicine formula consisting of four herbs: Danggui (*Radix Angelica sinensis*), Huangqi (*Radix Astragali*), Baizhi (*Angelica dahurica*), and Zaojiaoci (*thorns of Gleditsia sinensis*), in the ratio of 5 : 5 : 4 : 4 (15 g for the former two and 12 g for the latter two). It is derived from "orthodox manual of surgery" ("Wai Ke Zheng Zong" in Chinese) formulated by a famous TCM physician Shigong Chen in 1617 AD and has been used for the treatment of various refractory wounds, including pressure ulcer, venous leg ulcer, abscesses, and carbuncle. In Chinese medicine theory, TLXDS includes the therapeutic method of "TUO" represented by *Radix Angelica sinensis* and *Radix Astragali* and the therapeutic method of "TOU" represented by *Angelica dahurica* and thorns of *Gleditsia sinensis*. Therapeutic method of "TUO" means raising "Qi" (vital energy) and nourishing "Blood" (body circulation), while therapeutic method of "TOU" refers to cleansing wound environment and eliminating toxins. For the pharmacological action of each single herb in TLXDS, *Radix Astragali* is used as "Qi" invigorator [5] and *Angelica sinensis* is prescribed as blood circulation activator [6]; *Angelica dahurica* is classified as a sweat-inducing drug able to counter harmful external influences on the skin, such as cold, heat, dampness, and dryness [7]; the thorns of *Gleditsia sinensis* have been used for the treatment of inflammatory diseases including swelling, suppuration, carbuncle, and skin diseases [8]. Hundreds of years of practice has proven the wound healing effect of TLXDS on various refractory wounds [9], and the pharmacological actions of herbs in TLXDS suggest it might be a potential remedy for diabetic wound. However, the effect of TLXDS on healing of diabetic wounds has not been explored before. The purpose of this study is to evaluate the efficacy of TLXDS on diabetic wound by using an excisional cutaneous wound model of streptozotocin-induced diabetic rats and also to clarify its active mechanism by immunohistochemical, qRT-PCR, and western blot analyses.

2. Materials and Methods

2.1. Preparation of Tuo-Li-Xiao-Du-San Ethanol Extract. Tuo-Li-Xiao-Du-San is comprised of four herbs, *Astragalus membranaceus*, *Angelica sinensis*, *Angelica dahurica*, and thorns of *Gleditsia sinensis*, in the ratio of 5 : 5 : 4 : 4 (15 g for the former two and 12 g for the latter two). The herbs were obtained from and authenticated by TASLY Pharmaceutical Group Co. Ltd. (Tianjin, China). The 70% ethanol extract of mixture of four herbs was prepared by the department of Pharmaceutical Sciences, Tianjin University of Traditional Chinese Medicine (Tianjin, China) using standardized procedure [10, 11]. Briefly, the crude herbs were powered and then extracted by 70% ethanol for three times. Gather the extracts and filter to remove the solid fragment. The solvents were removed by freeze-drying. The condensate was stored at −20°C. The extracts are freshly prepared by dissolving in sterile water to an appropriate concentration as herb solution for the later experiment.

2.2. Animals. Sprague-Dawley male rats ($n = 120$, 10 weeks old, SPF) weighing 290 ± 10 g were purchased from Beijing HFK Bioscience Co., Ltd. (Beijing, China). Rats were housed under pathogen-free conditions at the Chinese Academy of medical Sciences & Peking Union Medical College Institute of Biomedical Engineering Animal SPF facility (Tianjin, China). Rats were maintained at controlled temperature (22–25°C) and relative humidity (50%–60%) on a 12 h light-dark cycle and fed a commercial pellet diet with food and water available *ad libitum*. This study was approved by Experimental Animal Ethical Committee of Tianjin Medical University, and all procedures with animals complied with rules of the Guide for the Care and Use of Laboratory Animals of the National Institutes of Health as well as the guidelines of the Animal Welfare Act.

2.3. Induction of Diabetes. After overnight fasting, diabetes was induced by a single intravenous injection of STZ (Sigma-Aldrich, St. Louis, MO, USA) at a dose of 50 mg/kg body weight in 0.1 mol/L citrate-phosphate buffer, pH 4.5. Control rats were injected with citrate buffer alone. Blood glucose concentration was monitored using an Accu-Chek Aviva glucometer (Roche Diagnostics GmbH, Germany) from tail vein blood. Animals with random blood glucose levels ≥16.7 mmol/L for three consecutive tests were considered diabetic.

2.4. Wound Model and TLXDS Treatment. Wound-healing model of rats was induced as described before [12]. Four weeks after STZ injection, control and diabetic rats were anesthetized by intraperitoneal injection of sodium pentobarbital (30 mg/kg body weight). The dorsal hair of rats was shaved and two 10 mm diameter full thickness wounds were created with a sterile biopsy punch. Diabetic rats were randomly allotted to diabetic treated with TLXDS (DM + TLXDS group, $n = 36$) and diabetic without drug treatment (DM group, $n = 36$), while nondiabetic rats were placed in the normal control group (NC group, $n = 10$). Rats of these three groups were randomly allocated to four experimental end points (i.e., days 5, 8, 11, and 14, 7–10 animals for each end point). Rats in TLXDS group received TLXDS ethanol extract 1.1 mL/0.2 kg body weight once daily by oral gavage starting from day 0 to each end point, and rats in NC and DM group received 1.1 mL/0.2 kg body weight water once daily by oral gavage. The dose of each herb used in rats was 1.5 g/kg body weight for *Angelica sinensis* and *Astragalus membranaceus*, 1.2 g/kg body weight for *Angelica dahurica* and *Gleditsia sinensis* thorns, which was calculated according to the dose used in patients (0.25 g/kg and 0.2 g/kg, resp.). At each experimental end point, the animals were killed simultaneously by euthanasia.

2.5. Macroscopic Analysis. The ulcers were photographed every other day with a digital camera. The percentage of completely closed ulcers was calculated with the NIH Image J analyzer by tracing the wound margin and calculating pixel area. Wound closure was calculated as Percentage Closed = [(Area on Day 0 − Open Area on Final Day)/Area on Day 0] × 100.

2.6. Immunohistochemistry. The wounds, together with unwounded skin margins, were excised, fixed with 10% formaldehyde, and embedded with paraffin. The sections (4 μm thick) were then deparaffinized and rehydrated. Antigen retrieval was performed at 95°C by microwave in 0.01 mol/L sodium citrate buffer (pH 6.0). Endogenous peroxidase activity was quenched by exposing to 3% H_2O_2. After blocking with 5% BSA in PBS, the sections were incubated with anti-CD68 (1 : 100, Thermo Fisher Scientific), anti-MPO (1 : 100, Thermo Fisher Scientific), anti-CD31 (1 : 200, Santa Cruz Biotechnology), anti-desmin (1 : 100, Thermo Fisher Scientific), and anti-collagen I (1 : 100, Thermo Fisher Scientific), respectively, followed by incubating with the corresponding HRP-conjugated secondary antibodies. The antigen-antibody complex was visualized with a Diaminobenzidine (DAB) kit. For evaluation of staining, the overview of the positive-signal density was scored semiquantitatively as 1 (absent), 2 (low), 3 (medium), 4 (strong), and 5 (very strong). The median of scores from three observers, who were blinded to the treatment, was used for comparisons.

2.7. Collagen Estimation (Hydroxyproline Content). Wound tissues were analyzed for hydroxyproline content, which is basic constituent of collagen. The collagen composed of amino acid (hydroxyproline) is the major component of extracellular tissue, which gives strength and support. Breakdown of collagen liberates free hydroxyproline and its peptides. Measurement of hydroxyproline hence can be used as a biochemical marker for tissue collagen and an index for collagen turnover. Hydroxyproline content was analyzed using a hydroxyproline assay kit (Sigma-Aldrich, St. Louis, MO, USA) according to the manufacturer's instructions. Dilute 10 μL of the 1 mg/mL hydroxyproline standard solution with 90 μL of water to prepare a 0.1 mg/mL standard solution. Add 0, 2, 4, 6, 8, and 10 μL of the 0.1 mg/mL hydroxyproline standard solution into a 96-well plate, generating 0 (blank), 0.2, 0.4, 0.6, 0.8, and 1.0 μg/well standards. Homogenize 10 mg tissue in 100 μL of water and transfer it to a 2.0 mL polypropylene tube. Add 100 μL of concentrated hydrochloric acid (HCl, ~12 M), cap tightly and hydrolyze at 120°C for 3 hours. Transfer 10–50 μL of supernatant to a 96 well plate. Place plates in a 60°C oven to dry samples. Add 100 μL of the Chloramine T/Oxidation Buffer Mixture to each sample and standard well. Incubate at room temperature for 5 minutes. Add 100 μL of the Diluted DMAB Reagent to each sample and standard well and incubate for 90 minutes at 60°C. Measure the absorbance at 560 nm (A560). The concentration of the sample was calculated as

$$\begin{aligned} &\text{Concentration of the sample} \\ &\quad = \frac{\text{OD of the sample}}{\text{OD of standard}} \\ &\quad \times \text{Concentration of standard}. \end{aligned} \tag{1}$$

2.8. Real-Time Quantitative PCR. Total RNA from rat ulcer was extracted using Trizol (Invitrogen, Grand Island, NY). RNA purity and integrity were assessed by spectrophotometric analysis. A total of 3 μg of RNA was reverse-transcribed using a RevertAid kit (Thermo Fisher Scientific, Waltham, MA). Reverse transcription polymerase chain reaction (RT-PCR) was performed using the CFX96 real-time PCR system (Bio-Rad, USA) with the SYBR Green PCR Kit (Takara, Otsu, Japan) for rat VEGF-A, PDGF-BB, IL-1β, and TNF-α. Primer sequences are as follows: for VEGF-A 5′ TCA AAC CTC ACC AAA GCC 3′ and 5′ GGT GAG AGG TCT AGT TCC 3′; for PDGF-BB 5′ CGC CTG CTG CAC AGA GAC 3′ and 5′ CCG CGA GAT CTG GAA CAC 3′; for IL-1β 5′ AGA AGA AGA TGG AAA AGC 3′ and 5′ CGA CCA TTG CTG TTT CCT 3′; for TNF-α 5′ TCC CAG GTT CTC TTC AAG G 3′ and 5′ GTA CAT GGG CTC ATA CCA G 3′; for GAPDH 5′ TAC CCA CGG CAA GTT CAA CG 3′ and 5′ CAC CAG CAT CAC CCC ATT TG 3′. GAPDH was defined as the reference gene. Data were analyzed with $2^{-\Delta\Delta CT}$ method.

2.9. Western Blot Analysis. Protein contents of VEGF-A, PDGF-BB, IL-1β, and TNF-α in ulcer tissue homogenates were evaluated by western blot. In brief, the protein concentrations of homogenates were determined using a BCA protein assay (Pierce Biotechnology, Rockford, IL, USA). Equivalent amount of protein samples (30 μg) was separated on an SDS polyacrylamide gel and transferred onto a polyvinylidene difluoride membrane (Millipore). After blocking in TBS containing 5% nonfat milk for 2 h at room temperature, the membranes were incubated overnight with 1:1,000 diluted anti-VEGF-A (Abcam), 1:2000 diluted anti-PDGF-BB (Abcam), 1:200 diluted anti-IL-1β (Santa Cruz Biotechnology), 1:500 diluted anti-TNF-α (Abcam), and 1:8000 diluted anti-β-actin (Tianjin Sungene Biotech Co., Ltd.), respectively. Binding of the primary antibody was detected using a HRP-conjugated secondary antibody (Tianjin Sungene Biotech Co., Ltd.). Positive bands were visualized using an ECL kit (Bio-Rad) and then captured on X-ray film. Housekeeping protein β-actin was used as a loading control. The density of each band was quantified using Quantity One software (Bio-Rad Laboratory) and normalized to their respective control.

2.10. Statistical Analysis. Data are presented as means ± SEM. Statistical analysis were performed using SPSS 16.0 software. One-way analysis of variance (ANOVA) test was used to determine statistical significance. $P < 0.05$ was considered to indicate a statistically significant difference.

3. Results

3.1. Diabetes Induction and Blood Glucose Level. During the 4-week diabetes induction period, 90% (72/80) of the STZ-injected rats became consistently hyperglycemic and were included in this study. During the treatment period, blood glucose levels of rats in DM group and DM + TLXDS group were significantly higher than those of rats in NC group ($P < 0.05$), and no significant difference was observed between DM group and DM + TLXDS group ($P > 0.05$), indicating that TLXDS had no effects on blood glucose (Figure 1).

3.2. Administration of TLXDS Accelerated Wound Healing. As shown in Figure 2, by the end of observation (14 days after wounding), nondiabetic wounds completely healed, while most of the diabetic wounds remained open with a low average closure rate of 61.6%. TLXDS began to significantly improve diabetic wound closure 4 days after wounding (24% versus 14%, $P < 0.05$), and by the end of observation, TLXDS increased the healing rate of diabetic wound by 25.2% (86.8% versus 61.6%, $P < 0.01$).

3.3. Administration of TLXDS Reduced Inflammatory Cells Infiltration and Stimulated Inflammation Resolution. Uncontrolled inflammation is a major characteristic of diabetic wounds. We assessed histological changes by HE staining on day 5 (Figure 3(a)) and populations of neutrophil and macrophage at the wound site by determining the constitutively expressed molecular markers MPO (for neutrophils) and CD68 (for macrophages) on day 14

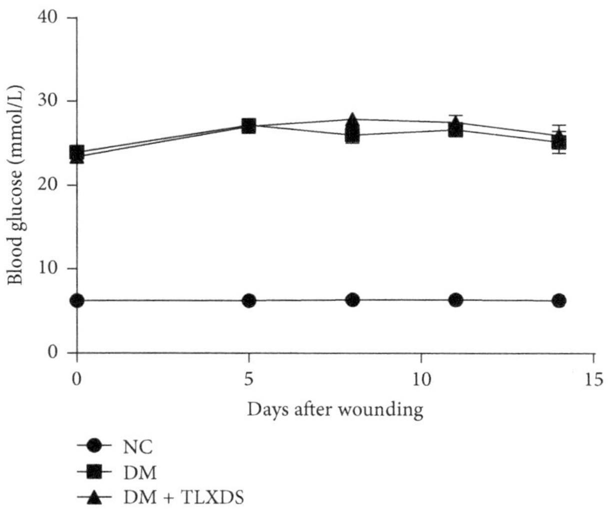

FIGURE 1: Blood glucose levels monitored during the treatment period. During the study period, the level of blood glucose was significantly higher in both DM and TLXDS-treated rats compared with the NC rats ($P < 0.05$). No significant difference between DM and TLXDS-treated groups was seen ($P > 0.05$). On day 0, $n = 40$ for NC, $n = 36$ for DM and DM + TLXDS; on day 5, $n = 39$ for NC, $n = 34$ for DM, and $n = 35$ for DM + TLXDS; on day 8, $n = 29$ for NC, $n = 23$ for DM, and $n = 26$ for DM + TLXDS; on day 11, $n = 19$ for NC, $n = 15$ for DM, and $n = 16$ for DM + TLXDS; on day 14, $n = 9$ for NC, $n = 7$ for DM, and $n = 8$ for DM + TLXDS.

(Figures 3(b), 3(c), and 3(d)). The infiltration of inflammatory cells and concomitant tissue necrosis in diabetic wounds was much stronger compared with nondiabetic wounds on day 5 (Figure 3(a)). Moreover, the inflammation resolution of untreated diabetic rats was significantly delayed, which was characterized by increased and prolonged neutrophils and macrophages influx on day 14 (Figure 3(b)). Administration of TLXDS led to a marked decline in inflammatory cells infiltration and tissue necrosis on days 5 and an accelerated resolution of neutrophils and macrophages on day 14 ($P < 0.05$).

3.4. Administration of TLXDS Augmented Neovascularization and Increased Granulation Tissue Deposition. Neovascularization is an essential event in the development of granulation tissue. We evaluated the growth and maturation of blood vessels by immunostaining of endothelial cell marker CD31 and pericyte marker desmin, respectively (Figure 4). The vessel density of untreated diabetic wounds was significantly decreased compared with nondiabetic wounds ($P < 0.05$), and the pericyte coverage of new vessels was discrete and incomplete. TLXDS treatment significantly enhanced neovascularization of diabetic wounds, demonstrated by increased CD31 staining. Besides, the pericyte recruitment was restored by TLXDS administration, suggesting that new vessels in TLXDS treated wounds were more mature, stable, and functional.

Meanwhile, Masson's trichrome staining and immunohistochemistry of type I collagen showed that the deposition of ECM in diabetic wounds on day 14 after wounding was significantly impaired compared with nondiabetic wounds, which was restored by the administration of TLXDS (Figure 5). Consistently, the hydroxyproline content in diabetic wounds was decreased significantly compared with nondiabetic wounds on day 14 (5.42 ± 0.29 versus 12.03 ± 0.24 μg/mg tissue, $P < 0.05$). Administration of TLXDS increased hydroxyproline content in diabetic ulcers on day 14 (7.38 ± 0.22 versus 5.42 ± 0.29 μg/mg tissue, $P < 0.05$).

3.5. Administration of TLXDS Increased Expression of Angiogenic Factors and Reduced Inflammatory Cytokine Expression. Impaired angiogenic factors production accounts for the compromised neovascularization of diabetic wounds. Therefore, we performed real-time PCR and western blotting to investigate whether TLXDS increased neovascularization through increasing angiogenic factors expression. As expected, VEGF-A and PDGF-BB levels of diabetic wounds failed to rise on day 5 after wounding to initiate the angiogenic response as compared with nondiabetic wounds (Figures 6(a), 6(c), 6(d), 6(g), and 6(h)). TLXDS increased VEGF-A and PDGF-BB expression on day 5 after wounding when active angiogenesis was undergoing ($P < 0.05$).

TLXDS stimulated inflammation resolution in diabetic wounds. Therefore, we examined the effect of TLXDS on inflammatory cytokines expression on both gene and protein levels. On day 11 after wounding, expression of inflammatory cytokines, such as IL-1β and TNF-α, was significantly higher in diabetic wounds than in nondiabetic wounds ($P < 0.05$), and TLXDS markedly reduced these inflammatory cytokine expression (Figures 6(b), 6(e), 6(f), 6(i), and 6(j)).

4. Discussion

Impaired wound healing is a serious complication in diabetes, leading to prolonged hospitalization and even amputation. However, there are limited effective and safe treatments. In this study, we demonstrated that a traditional Chinese medicine formula for refractory ulcers, named Tuo-Li-Xiao-Du-San (TLXDS), significantly improved wound healing of STZ-induced diabetic rats through reducing inflammation, increasing angiogenesis and collagen deposition.

Wounds go through three sequential and coordinate phases, inflammation, tissue formation, and tissue remodeling, to restore morphological and functional integrity [13]. Diabetes impairs wound healing through magnifying the inflammatory response, inhibiting angiogenesis, and decreasing ECM deposition [3]. Inflammation is the first and indispensable response after acute skin injury, usually subsiding in less than 5 days after wounding [14]. However, metabolic defects, such as hyperglycemia and oxidative stress, induce excessive proinflammatory cytokines (IL-1β, TNF-α, etc.) production [15, 16], sustaining a prolonged influx of neutrophils and macrophages [14, 17, 18]. As shown in the present study (Figure 3), diabetic wounds were still stuck in large amount inflammatory cells infiltration and apparent tissue necrosis on day 5 after wounding, while nondiabetic wounds already moved forward to the proliferative stage of

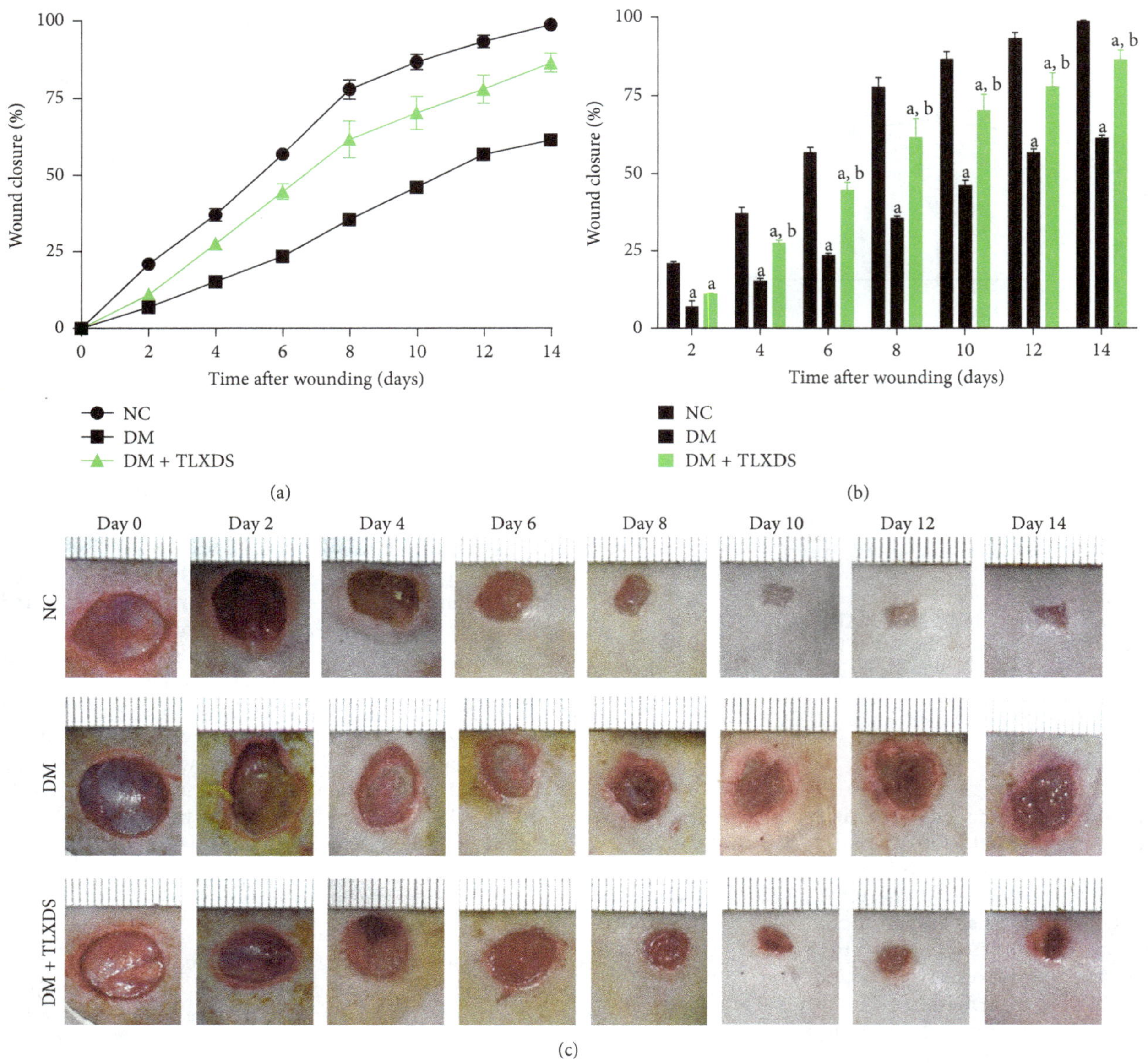

FIGURE 2: TLXDS treatment accelerated wound healing in diabetic rats. Percentage of wound closure (mean ± SEM) of 10 mm punch biopsies was monitored every other day until day 14 (a, b). Healing of diabetic wounds was significantly delayed compared with nondiabetic wounds at all observation time points ($P < 0.05$). TLXDS began to significantly improve wound closure on day 4 ($P < 0.05$). At the end of observation (14 days), 86.8% of the wounding area healed in DM + TLXDS group, while the closure rate in DM group was only 61.6%. (c) Typical photographs of wound healing for each group. $^{a}P < 0.05$, compared with NC group, and $^{b}P < 0.05$, compared with DM group. $n = 7$ for each group at each monitored time point.

healing. Moreover, by 14 days after wounding, neutrophils and macrophages were still abundant in diabetic wounds. Persisting inflammatory cells create a protease (neutrophil elastase, MMPs, and gelatinase) rich hostile microenvironment [19], resulting in extracellular matrix and growth factors degradation [20, 21]. Therefore, diabetic wounds are entrapped in a self-sustaining cycle of chronic inflammation and never get mature enough to move forward to the next stage of healing. The present study showed that administration of TLXDS significantly accelerated inflammation resolution by decreasing the expression of inflammatory cytokines, such as IL-1β and TNF-α, and thereby reducing the neutrophils and macrophages abundance in diabetic wounds. Reducing inflammation by TLXDS treatment might provide a favorable microenvironment for other repair cells to play their roles in healing the wounds.

In response to hypoxia after injury, endothelial cells and pericytes are recruited by angiogenic factors from existing vessels and proliferate to form new and functional blood vessels which provide the essential oxygen and blood supply for regenerating new tissues, a process known as neovascularization [22, 23]. Inadequate neovascularization

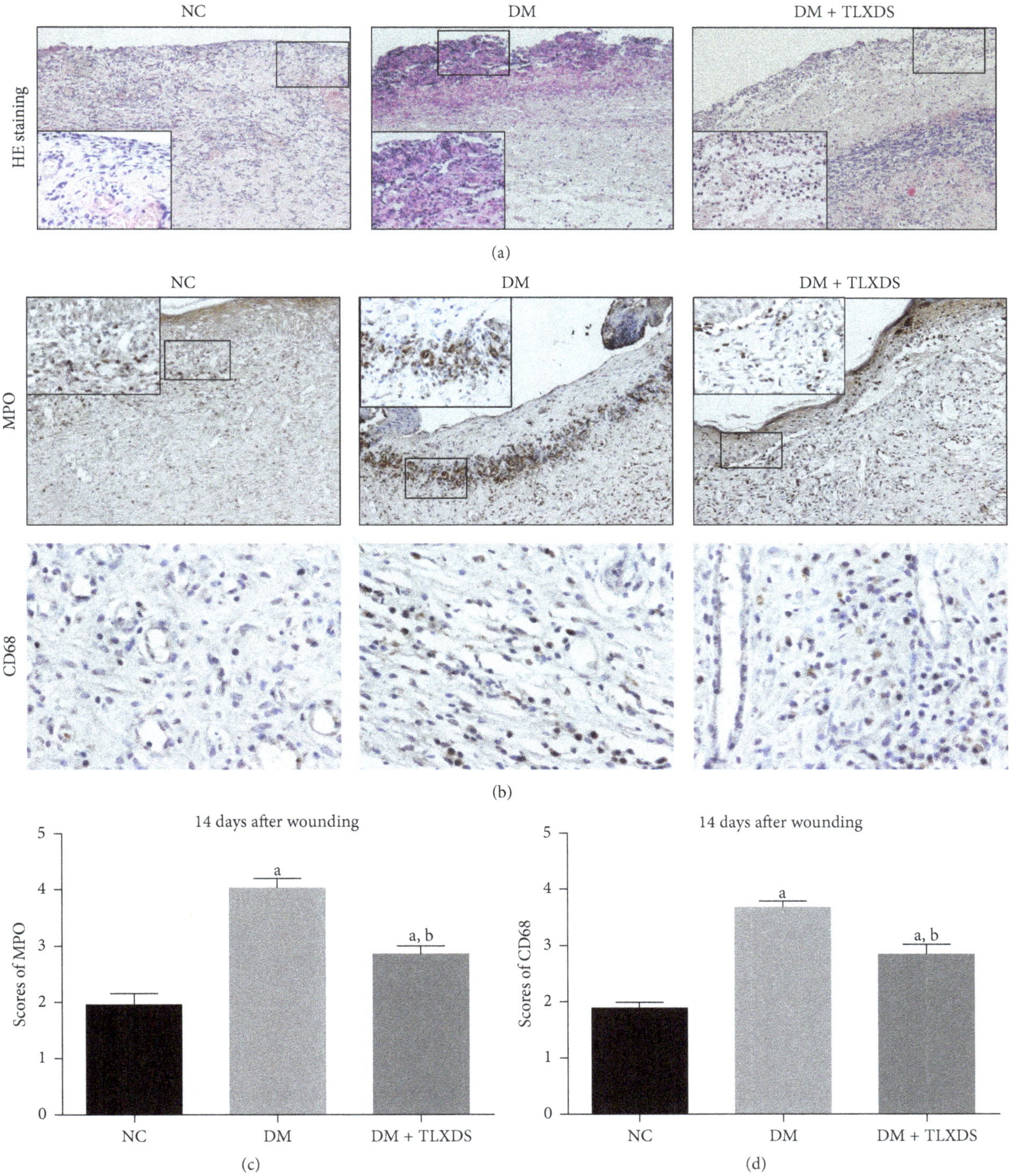

FIGURE 3: Effects of TLXDS treatment on inflammatory cells infiltration and inflammation resolution assessed by hematoxylin and eosin-(H&E-) stained histology on day 5 (a) and immunohistochemistry of MPO and CD68 on day 14 (b). Original magnification ×100 and insert magnification ×400. (c) and (d) Scores of MPO and CD68 staining. $n = 7$ for each group. Data are represented as means ± SEM. $^{a}P < 0.05$, compared with NC group, and $^{b}P < 0.05$, compared with DM group.

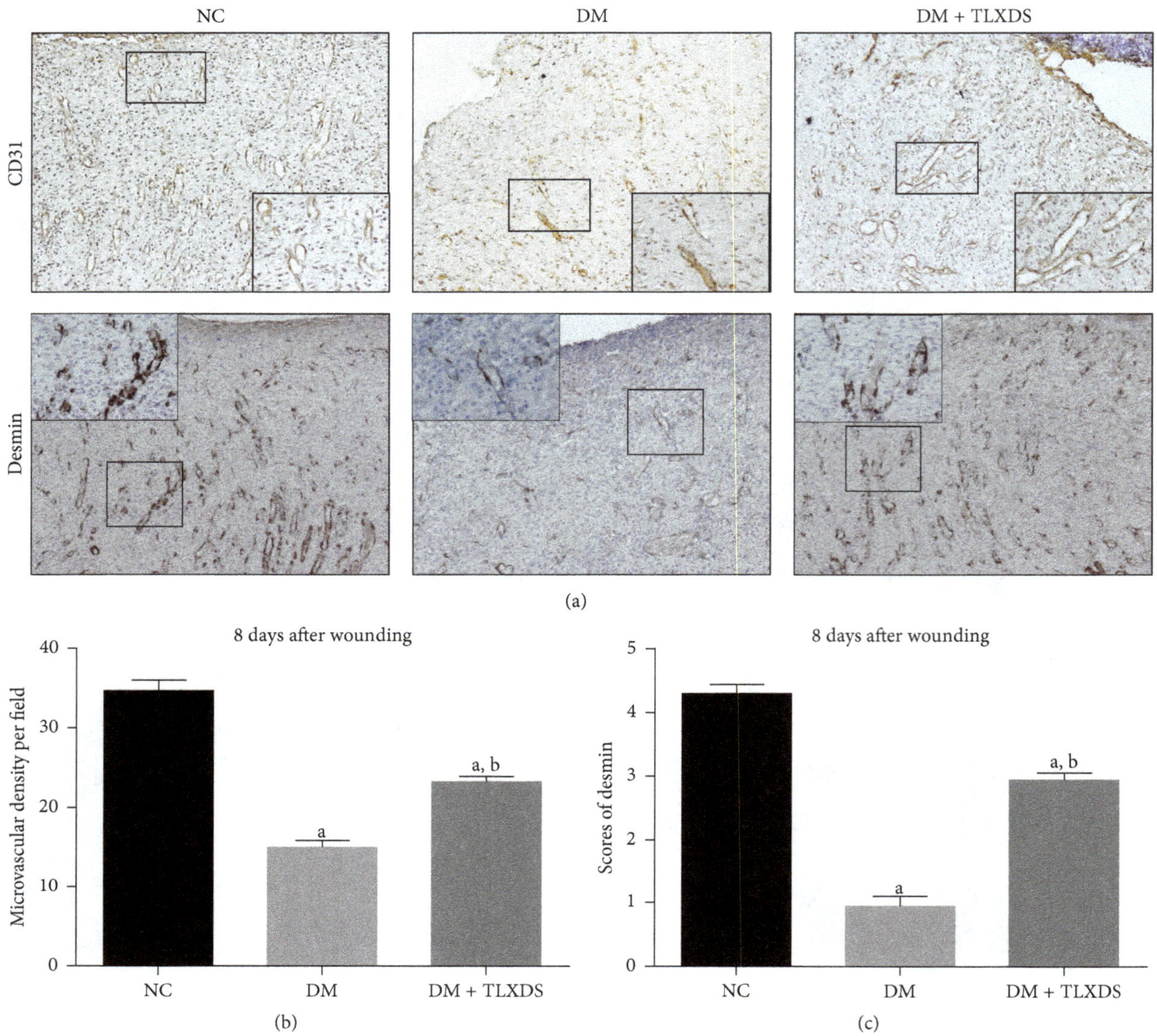

FIGURE 4: Effects of TLXDS treatment on angiogenesis assessed by the endothelial cell marker CD31 and pericyte marker desmin immunohistochemistry, respectively. (a) Representative CD31 and desmin-staining sections of NC group, DM group, and DM + TLXDS group on day 8 after wounding, respectively. Original magnification ×100 and inset magnification ×400. (b) Five "hot spots" in each specimen in which the CD31 antibody signal was the most intense were chosen and captured. The number of blood vessels was then counted by two investigators who were blinded to the treatment of the rats using the "manual tagging" feature in Image Pro-Plus software package. (c) Graphic visualization of scores of desmin staining on day 8. $n = 7$ for each group. Data are presented as means ± SEM. $^{a}P < 0.05$, compared with NC group; $^{b}P < 0.05$, compared with DM group.

is a cardinal feature of nonhealing diabetic wounds. The mechanisms underlying this impairment are studied a lot and now researchers widely accept that inadequate production of angiogenic growth factors, such as VEGF and PDGF, is a fundamental cause [24–26]. In this study, we observed that TLXDS restores diabetes-impaired neovascularization by increasing recruitment of both endothelial cells and pericytes. The mechanisms of TLXDS's effects in boosting angiogenesis of diabetic wounds might be related, at least in part, to the correction of reduced production of angiogenic growth factors, such as VEGF-A and PDGF-BB, which is demonstrated in this study.

Furthermore, Masson's trichrome staining and collagen type I immunohistochemistry demonstrated that TLXDS treatment increased collagen production of diabetic wounds significantly, which is important for functional recovery and healing quality [27]. This effect is probably secondary to the combined action of reduced inflammation and increased angiogenesis, since the degradation of ECM was decreased and the synthesis was fueled.

Compound formulae, usually called "FuFang" in Chinese, are combinations of TCM prescribed for treating various diseases in China. The therapeutic potencies of herbs are found additive, or even synergistic, when used

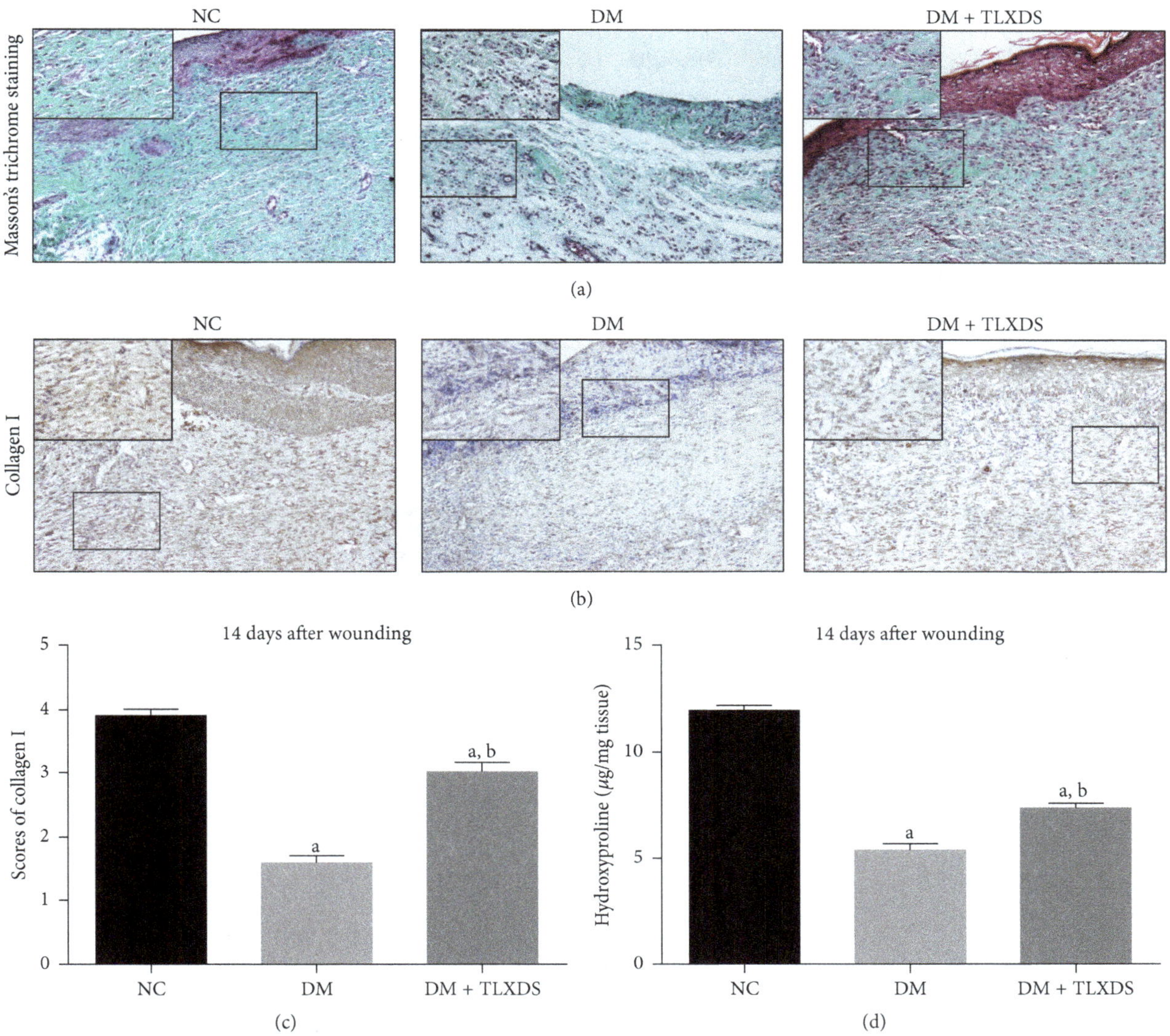

FIGURE 5: Effect of TLXDS treatment on extracellular matrix deposition evaluated by Masson's trichrome staining and collagen type I immunohistochemistry. Representative Masson's trichrome staining (a) and collagen type I staining sections (b) of NC, DM, and DM + TLXDS groups on day 14 after wounding. (c) Graphic visualization of scores of collagen type I staining on day 14. (d) Hydroxyproline content in the granulation tissue of each group on day 14. $n = 7$ for each group. Data are presented as means ± SEM. $^{a}P < 0.05$, compared with NC group, and $^{b}P < 0.05$, compared with DM group.

as combination. This is a great advantage for compound formulae in TCM. In Chinese medicine theory, TLXDS includes the therapeutic method of "TUO" which means raising "Qi" (vital energy) and nourishing "Blood" (body circulation) and the therapeutic method "TOU" which means cleansing wound environment and eliminating toxins. Recent researches show constituents of "TOU method," *Angelica dahurica* and thorns of *Gleditsia sinensis*, exhibit antibacterial and anti-inflammatory activities [28, 29]; the constituents of "TUO method," *Astragalus membranaceus* and *Angelica sinensis*, promote angiogenesis and the expression of angiogenic growth factors [30, 31]. Oftentimes, hundreds or even thousands of years of clinical practice has optimized formulae in TCM. The present study showed that TLXDS improves diabetic wounding healing as indicated in the ancient Chinese medicine theory and modern researching literature. There is great possibility that combining "TOU method" and "TUO method" can produce complementary and synergistic effects. It is of great interest in the future for us to reveal whether pleiotropic effects on diabetic wound healing of TLXDS in diabetic rats are attributed to the synergistic action between TUO method and TOU method. Furthermore, to clarify the active ingredients in TLXDS is of great practical significance as well.

It is noticeable that ulcer healing in diabetic ulcer and diabetic foot is complicated with many chronic problems, including long-term uncontrolled hyperglycemia, peripheral vascular disease, neuropathies, excessive pressure to the wound sites, and infection secondary to compromised immunity [2]. One pathogenic abnormality can lead to

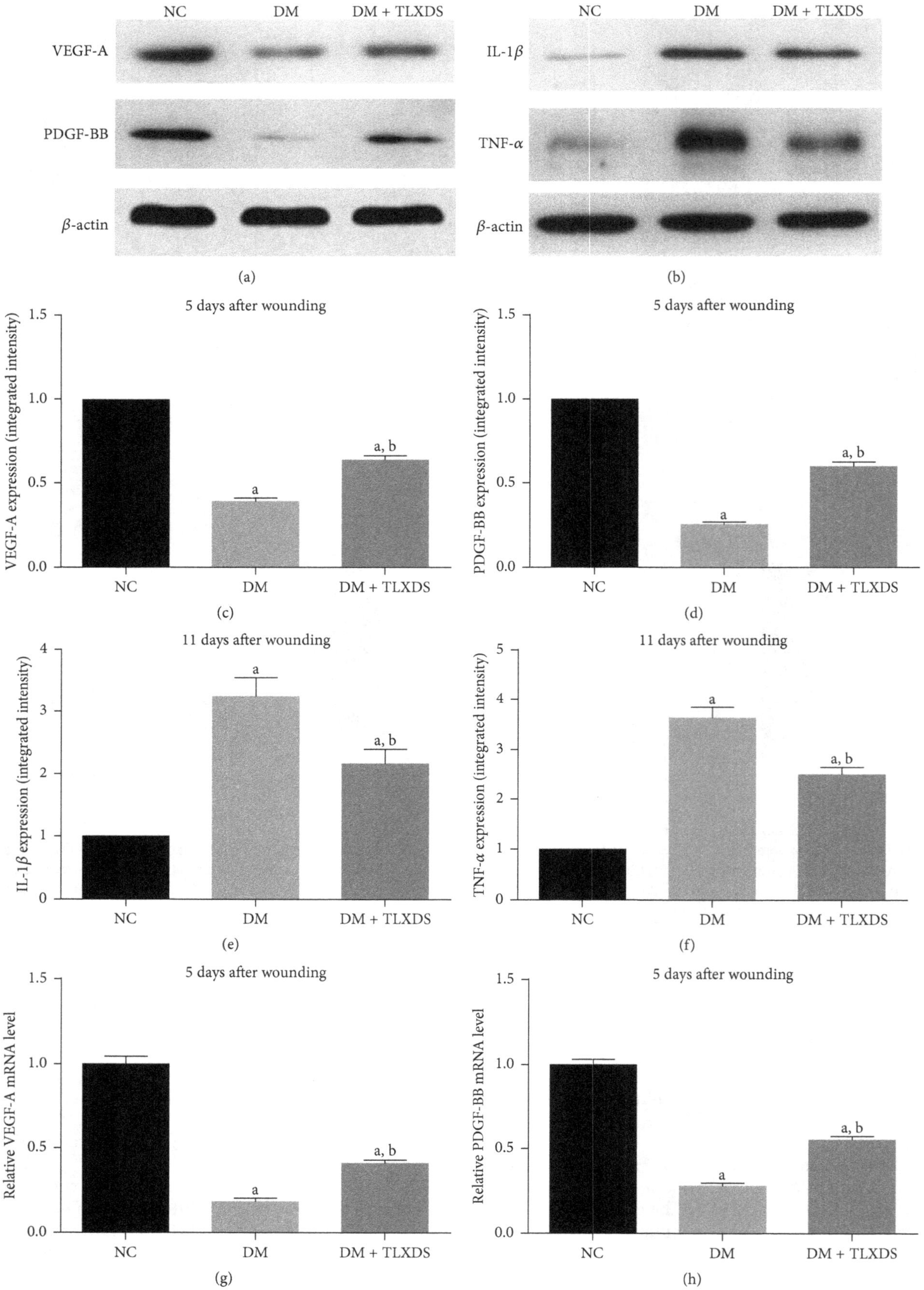

Figure 6: Continued.

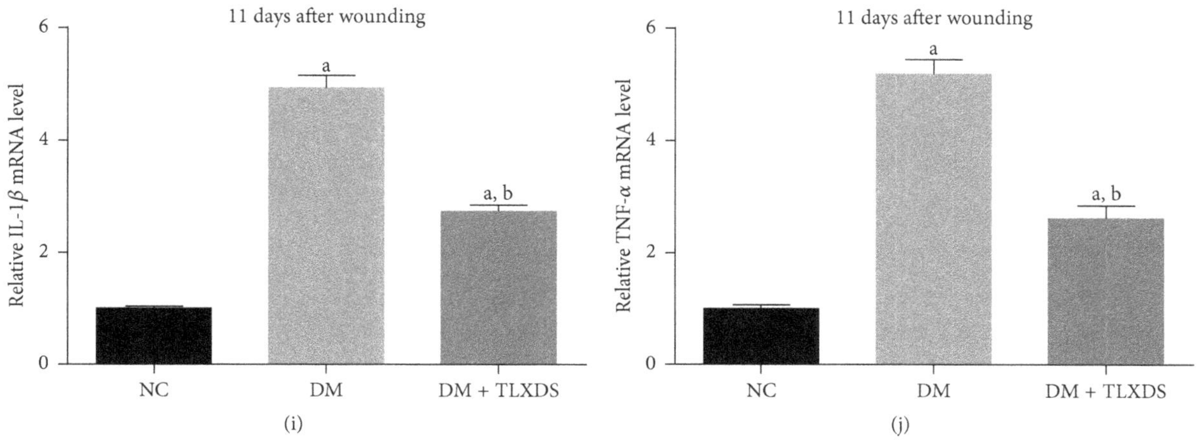

FIGURE 6: Effect of TLXDS treatment on the vascular endothelial growth factor-A (VEGF-A), platelet-derived growth factor BB (PDGF-BB), interleukin-1β (IL-1-β), and tumor necrosis factor-α (TNF-α) expressions assessed by western blot and real-time PCR analysis. Representative immunoblots of VEGF and PDGF-BB on day 5 after wounding ((a), $n = 9$ for each group), IL-1-β and TNF-α on day 11 after wounding ((b), $n = 7$ for each group). Quantifications of the bands (c–f). Quantification of VEGF-A, PDGF-BB, IL-1-β, and TNF-α mRNA expression (g–j). Data are presented as means ± SEM. $^aP < 0.05$, compared with NC group, and $^bP < 0.05$, compared with DM group.

another, developing vicious cycles of pathogenicity in the diabetic chronic ulcers. Considering the heterogeneity and complexity of human diabetic foot, no single animal model is capable of fully recapitulating each clinical scenario [32]. In the present study, we employed a widely used STZ-induced diabetic animal wound model [33, 34] to simulate the hyperglycemic state of diabetics and its impairment on wound healing. The results showed that TLXDS treatment is able to correct the abnormal healing process induced by hyperglycemia through reducing inflammation, increasing angiogenesis, and collagen deposition. Whether TLXDS could improve other abnormalities leading to diabetic foot, such as vascular disease and neuropathies, will be a constructive investigative direction in our further research work by using appropriate animal or cell models. And whether these findings can be extrapolated to the situation encountered in diabetic foot in patients still needs further investigation in clinical trials.

In summary, this study showed that TLXDS, a traditional Chinese medicine formula for refractory ulcers, has a positive effect on diabetes-impaired wounds. The improved wound healing is associated with reduced inflammation, increased angiogenesis, and collagen deposition after TLXDS treatment. The oral administration of traditional Chinese herbal medicine could provide an alternative and effective approach for diabetic foot ulcer therapy.

Conflict of Interests

All authors declare that there is no conflict of interests regarding the publication of this paper.

Authors' Contribution

Xiao-na Zhang, Ze-jun Ma, Cong-qing Pan, and Li-ming Chen designed the study; Xiao-na Zhang, Ze-jun Ma, Ying Wang, Yu-zhu Li, Bei Sun, and Xin Guo performed the research; Xiao-na Zhang and Ze-jun Ma wrote the paper. Xiao-na Zhang and Ze-jun Ma contributed equally to this study.

Acknowledgment

This work was supported by the National Natural Science Foundation of China (nos. 81273916 and 81373846).

References

[1] N. Singh, D. G. Armstrong, and B. A. Lipsky, "Preventing foot ulcers in patients with diabetes," *Journal of the American Medical Association*, vol. 293, no. 2, pp. 217–228, 2005.

[2] P. R. Cavanagh, B. A. Lipsky, A. W. Bradbury, and G. Botek, "Treatment for diabetic foot ulcers," *The Lancet*, vol. 366, no. 9498, pp. 1725–1735, 2005.

[3] V. Falanga, "Wound healing and its impairment in the diabetic foot," *The Lancet*, vol. 366, no. 9498, pp. 1736–1743, 2005.

[4] M. Chen, H. Zheng, L.-P. Yin, and C.-G. Xie, "Is oral administration of Chinese herbal medicine effective and safe as an adjunctive therapy for managing diabetic foot ulcers? A systematic review and meta-analysis," *Journal of Alternative and Complementary Medicine*, vol. 16, no. 8, pp. 889–898, 2010.

[5] X. Q. Ma, Q. Shi, J. A. Duan, T. T. X. Dong, and K. W. K. Tsim, "Chemical analysis of Radix Astragali (Huangqi) in China: a comparison with its adulterants and seasonal variations," *Journal of Agricultural and Food Chemistry*, vol. 50, no. 17, pp. 4861–4866, 2002.

[6] Y.-C. Wu and C.-L. Hsieh, "Pharmacological effects of *Radix Angelica Sinensis* (*Danggui*) on cerebral infarction," *Chinese Medicine*, vol. 6, article 32, 2011.

[7] A. Chevallier, *Encyclopedia of Medicinal Plants*, Dorling Kindersley Limited, London, UK, 2001.

[8] D. K. Ahn, *Illustrated Book of Korean Medicinal Herbs*, Kyohak Publishing, 2003.

[9] H. Fuming, "Commentary on researching progresses of TUO-Li-Xiao-Du-San," *Chinese Archives Of Traditional Chinese Medicine*, vol. 26, no. 3, pp. 598–599, 2008.

[10] S. Ling, L. Nheu, A. Dai, Z. Guo, and P. Komesaroff, "Effects of four medicinal herbs on human vascular endothelial cells in culture," *International Journal of Cardiology*, vol. 128, no. 3, pp. 350–358, 2008.

[11] J.-S. Sun, G.-C. Dong, C.-Y. Lin et al., "The effect of Gu-Sui-Bu (Drynaria fortunei J. Sm) immobilized modified calcium hydrogenphosphate on bone cell activities," *Biomaterials*, vol. 24, no. 5, pp. 873–882, 2003.

[12] C.-C. E. Lan, C.-S. Wu, S.-M. Huang, I.-H. Wu, and G.-S. Chen, "High-glucose environment enhanced oxidative stress and increased interleukin-8 secretion from keratinocytes," *Diabetes*, vol. 62, no. 7, pp. 2530–2538, 2013.

[13] P. Martin, "Wound healing—aiming for perfect skin regeneration," *Science*, vol. 276, no. 5309, pp. 75–81, 1997.

[14] S. A. Eming, T. Krieg, and J. M. Davidson, "Inflammation in wound repair: molecular and cellular mechanisms," *Journal of Investigative Dermatology*, vol. 127, no. 3, pp. 514–525, 2007.

[15] M. R. Dasu, S. Devaraj, and I. Jialal, "High glucose induces IL-1β expression in human monocytes: mechanistic insights," *American Journal of Physiology—Endocrinology and Metabolism*, vol. 293, no. 1, pp. E337–E346, 2007.

[16] M. F. Siqueira, J. Li, L. Chehab et al., "Impaired wound healing in mouse models of diabetes is mediated by TNF-α dysregulation and associated with enhanced activation of forkhead box O1 (FOXO1)," *Diabetologia*, vol. 53, no. 2, pp. 378–388, 2010.

[17] R. E. Mirza, M. M. Fang, W. J. Ennis, and T. J. Kohl, "Blocking interleukin-1β induces a healing-associated wound macrophage phenotype and improves healing in type 2 diabetes," *Diabetes*, vol. 62, no. 7, pp. 2579–2587, 2013.

[18] C. Wetzler, H. Kampfer, B. Stallmeyer, J. Pfeilschifter, and S. Frank, "Large and sustained induction of chemokines during impaired wound healing in the genetically diabetic mouse: prolonged persistence of neutrophils and macrophages during the late phase of repair," *Journal of Investigative Dermatology*, vol. 115, no. 2, pp. 245–253, 2000.

[19] S. J. Wall, D. Bevan, D. W. Thomas, K. G. Harding, D. R. Edwards, and G. Murphy, "Differential expression of matrix metalloproteinases during impaired wound healing of the diabetes mouse," *Journal of Investigative Dermatology*, vol. 119, no. 1, pp. 91–98, 2002.

[20] A. N. Moor, D. J. Vachon, and L. J. Gould, "Proteolytic activity in wound fluids and tissues derived from chronic venous leg ulcers," *Wound Repair and Regeneration*, vol. 17, no. 6, pp. 832–839, 2009.

[21] S. Herrick, G. Ashcroft, G. Ireland, M. Horan, C. McCollum, and M. Ferguson, "Up-regulation of elastase in acute wounds of healthy aged humans and chronic venous leg ulcers are associated with matrix degradation," *Laboratory Investigation*, vol. 77, no. 3, pp. 281–288, 1997.

[22] A. Hoeben, B. Landuyt, M. S. Highley, H. Wildiers, A. T. Van Oosterom, and E. A. De Bruijn, "Vascular endothelial growth factor and angiogenesis," *Pharmacological Reviews*, vol. 56, no. 4, pp. 549–580, 2004.

[23] P. Carmeliet, "Angiogenesis in life, disease and medicine," *Nature*, vol. 438, no. 7070, pp. 932–936, 2005.

[24] H.-D. Beer, M. T. Longaker, and S. Werner, "Reduced expression of PDGF and PDGF receptors during impaired wound healing," *Journal of Investigative Dermatology*, vol. 109, no. 2, pp. 132–138, 1997.

[25] S. Frank, G. Hübner, G. Breier, M. T. Longaker, D. G. Greenhalgh, and S. Werner, "Regulation of vascular endothelial growth factor expression in cultured keratinocytes. Implications for normal and impaired wound healing," *The Journal of Biological Chemistry*, vol. 270, no. 21, pp. 12607–12613, 1995.

[26] A. Rivard, M. Silver, D. Chen et al., "Rescue of diabetes-related impairment of angiogenesis by intramuscular gene therapy with adeno-VEGF," *The American Journal of Pathology*, vol. 154, no. 2, pp. 355–363, 1999.

[27] J. E. Glim, M. van Egmond, F. B. Niessen, V. Everts, and R. H. J. Beelen, "Detrimental dermal wound healing: what can we learn from the oral mucosa?" *Wound Repair and Regeneration*, vol. 21, no. 5, pp. 648–660, 2013.

[28] D. Lechner, M. Stavri, M. Oluwatuyi, R. Pereda-Miranda, and S. Gibbons, "The anti-staphylococcal activity of *Angelica dahurica* (Bai Zhi)," *Phytochemistry*, vol. 65, no. 3, pp. 331–335, 2004.

[29] H. H. Ha, S. Y. Park, W. S. Ko, and Y. Kim, "*Gleditsia sinensis* thorns inhibit the production of NO through NF-κB suppression in LPS-stimulated macrophages," *Journal of Ethnopharmacology*, vol. 118, no. 3, pp. 429–434, 2008.

[30] J. C.-W. Tam, C.-H. Ko, K.-M. Lau et al., "A Chinese 2-herb formula (NF3) promotes hindlimb ischemia-induced neovascularization and wound healing of diabetic rats," *Journal of Diabetes and its Complications*, vol. 28, no. 4, pp. 436–447, 2014.

[31] H.-W. Lam, H.-C. Lin, S.-C. Lao et al., "The angiogenic effects of *Angelica sinensis* extract on HUVEC in vitro and zebrafish in vivo," *Journal of Cellular Biochemistry*, vol. 103, no. 1, pp. 195–211, 2008.

[32] R. Nunan, K. G. Harding, and P. Martin, "Clinical challenges of chronic wounds: searching for an optimal animal model to recapitulate their complexity," *Disease Models and Mechanisms*, vol. 7, no. 11, pp. 1205–1213, 2014.

[33] C.-C. E. Lan, C.-S. Wu, S.-M. Huang, I.-H. Wu, and G.-S. Chen, "High-glucose environment enhanced oxidative stress and increased interleukin-8 secretion from keratinocytes: new insights into impaired diabetic wound healing," *Diabetes*, vol. 62, no. 7, pp. 2530–2538, 2013.

[34] M. Tong, B. Tuk, P. Shang et al., "Diabetes-impaired wound healing is improved by matrix therapy with heparan sulfate glycosaminoglycan mimetic OTR4120 in rats," *Diabetes*, vol. 61, no. 10, pp. 2633–2641, 2012.

19

Genetic Analysis and Follow-Up of 25 Neonatal Diabetes Mellitus Patients in China

Bingyan Cao,[1] Chunxiu Gong,[1] Di Wu,[1] Chaoxia Lu,[2] Fang Liu,[2] Xiaojing Liu,[3] Yingxian Zhang,[3] Yi Gu,[1] Zhan Qi,[4] Xiaoqiao Li,[1] Min Liu,[1] Wenjing Li,[1] Chang Su,[1] Xuejun Liang,[1] and Mei Feng[5]

[1]*Department of Pediatric Endocrinology and Genetic Metabolism, Beijing Children's Hospital, Capital Medical University, Beijing 100045, China*
[2]*Institute of Basic Medical Sciences, Peking Union Medical College, Beijing 100730, China*
[3]*Department of Endocrinology and Genetic Metabolism, Zhengzhou Children's Hospital, Zhengzhou 450053, China*
[4]*Department of Pediatrics, Beijing Children's Hospital, Capital Medical University, Beijing 100045, China*
[5]*Department of Endocrinology, Shanxi Children's Hospital, Taiyuan 030013, China*

Correspondence should be addressed to Chunxiu Gong; chunxiugong@163.com

Academic Editor: Adam Kretowski

Aims. To study the clinical features, genetic etiology, and the correlation between phenotype and genotype of neonatal diabetes mellitus (NDM) in Chinese patients. *Methods.* We reviewed the medical records of 25 NDM patients along with their follow-up details. Molecular genetic analysis was performed. We compared the HbA1c levels between PNDM group and infantile-onset T1DM patients. *Results.* Of 25 NDM patients, 18 (72.0%) were PNDM and 7 (28.0%) were TNDM. Among 18 PNDM cases, 6 (33.3%) had known KATP channel mutations (KATP-PNDM). There were six non-KATP mutations, five novel mutations, including *INS*, *EIF2AK3* ($n = 2$), *GLIS3*, and *SLC19A2*, one known *EIF2AK3* mutation. There are two *ABCC8* mutations in TNDM cases and one paternal UPD6q24. Five of the six KATP-PNDM patients were tried for glyburide transition, and 3 were successfully switched to glyburide. Mean HbA1c of PNDM was not significantly different from infantile onset T1DM (7.2% versus 7.4%, $P = 0.41$). *Conclusion.* PNDM accounted for 72% of NDM patients. About one-third of PNDM and TNDM patients had KATP mutations. The genetic etiology could be determined in 50% of PNDM and 43% of TNDM cases. PNDM patients achieved good glycemic control with insulin or glyburide therapy. The etiology of NDM suggests polygenic inheritance.

1. Introduction

Neonatal diabetes mellitus (NDM) occurs within the first six months of life. Depending on clinical outcomes, it is classified into Transient Neonatal Diabetes Mellitus (TNDM) and Permanent Neonatal Diabetes Mellitus (PNDM) [1]. TNDM, which accounts for 50% to 60% of NDM, goes into remission after treatment for an average period of 12 weeks. PNDM, on the other hand, is a lifelong disease without remission. TNDM is usually diagnosed within one month after birth with a median age at diagnosis of 6 days. It is characterized by intrauterine growth retardation (IUGR), less frequent diabetic ketoacidosis, requirement of low initial dose of insulin for treatment, and early remission. About 50% of TNDM patients, however, may have relapse in adulthood and require lifelong insulin maintenance therapy [2]. The clinical features of TNDM and PNDM overlap, and the typing is based on clinical remission on follow-up. PNDM should be considered if insulin requirement persists for up to 18 months [3].

More than 20 pathogenic genes have been identified in PNDM, of which the most common are *KCNJ11* and *ABCC8* encoding the Kir6.2 and SUR1 subunits of KATP channel accounting for 40% to 60% [4, 5]. Mutations in *KCNJ11* and *ABCC8* lead to persistence of KATP channel in the open state inducing membrane hyperpolarization and impaired insulin secretion. The *INS* gene mutation is the secondary cause. Other infrequent mutations include *GCK*, *PDX1*,

EIF2AK3, *PTF1A*, *IPF1*, *GLIS3*, *RFX6*, *SLC2A2*, *SLC19A2*, *FOXP3*, *GATA6*, *MNX1*, *NEUROD1*, and *HNF1B* [6]. TNDM is caused by defects associated with overexpression of paternally expressed genes in the imprinted region of chromosome 6q24 in 70% cases. Three reported defects include (1) paternal uniparental disomy of chromosome 6 (UPD6); (2) paternally inherited duplication of 6q24 (duplication); and (3) maternal hypomethylation at 6q24 [7]. About 26% of the patients contain mutations in *KCNJ11*, *ABCC8*, *INS*, or *HNF1B*. The genetic etiology remains currently unknown in 40% of NDM cases [8].

In vitro and clinical studies suggest that treatment with oral sulfonylurea can close KATP channel and improve glycemic control and neuropsychological development [9, 10]. Only patients with mutations identified in the *KCNJ11* or *ABCC8* genes benefit from sulfonylureas. However, 10% of patients with *KCNJ11* and 15% *ABCC8* mutations fail to achieve glycemic control when insulin therapy is switched to oral sulfonylureas. Therefore, molecular diagnosis is vital not only in accurate typing but also for better prognostication [5].

We summarized the clinical features, molecular typing, treatment, and 1- to 13-year follow-up of 25 cases of NDM in order to better understand the clinical treatment and prognosis.

2. Subjects and Methods

2.1. Patients. The present study included 25 patients diagnosed with NDM including 18 PNDM and 7 TNDM from Beijing Children's Hospital, Zhengzhou Children's Hospital, and Shanxi Children's Hospital, from 2001 to 2013. Diagnostic criteria for NDM [11] were as follows: (1) age at onset <6 months; (2) hyperglycemia sustained for ≥2 weeks; (3) insulin dependence; and (4) exclusion of hyperglycemia caused by stress and infection and drug therapies.

The symptoms at onset and laboratory reports were obtained from medical records. The family history of diabetes mellitus, especially glucose metabolism in parents, was recorded for every patient. Clinical follow-up started with diagnosis at 3- to 6-month intervals, subsequently. Height and weight were measured using normal growth chart of Chinese children. The self-reported frequency of severe hypoglycemia was recorded, and HbA1c was measured at every visit. All the data between years 2012 and 2013 were analyzed.

Patients aged below 18 months, showing normal blood glucose (fasting glucose < 5.6 mmol/L, postprandial glucose < 7.8 mmol/L) and HbA1c (<6.0%) without the need for insulin or oral hypoglycemic treatment, were defined as TNDM. Patients aged more than 18 months and requiring insulin or oral hypoglycemic agents to maintain normal glucose were defined as PNDM [3].

This study was approved by the Ethics Committee of Beijing Children's Hospital of Capital Medical University and all parents have signed the informed consent.

2.2. Sample Collection and DNA Extraction. Upon NDM diagnosis, 2 mL of blood samples was collected in ethylenediaminetetraacetic acid (EDTA) tubes from 25 patients and stored at −20°C. DNA was extracted from peripheral blood leukocytes using kits (QIAGEN, Valencia, CA).

2.3. Gene Mutation Analysis. Samples were tested for *KCNJ11* and *ABCC8* mutations using Sanger sequencing annually, usually within 1 year after diagnosis. Sanger sequencing of the *EIF2AK3* was undertaken in one patient because of the presence of typical features of *Wolcott-Rallison syndrome*. The negative PNDM cases were screened using Ion Torrent platform as described previously [12]. Genes associated with NDM include *KCNJ11*, *ABCC8*, *INS*, *GCK*, *PDX1*, *EIF2AK3*, *PTF1A*, *IPF1*, *GLIS3*, *RFX6*, *SLC2A2*, *SLC19A2*, *FOXP3*, *GATA6*, *MNX1*, *NEUROD1*, and *HNF1B*. Subsequently, Sanger sequencing was used to validate the screened mutations and in parents for inherited or *de novo* mutations. Confirmed mutations were then searched in the human gene mutation database (HGMD), dbSNP138, thousand genomes, and recent reviews. For all mutations, software Polyphen-2 was used to predict the pathogenicity (http://genetics.bwh.harvard.edu/pph2/).

Microarray comparative genomic hybridization was performed in 5 TNDM patients, in whom *ABCC8* and *KCNJ11* mutations were excluded. We used 4 μL–10 μL of patient DNA for the assay, DNA amplification, tagging, and hybridization according to the manufacturer's protocol. The array slides were scanned on an iScan Reader (Illumina). Data analysis was performed using GenomeStudio version 2010.1, KaryoStudio version 1.2 (Illumina, standard settings), and Nexus Copy Number 5.0 (BioDiscovery, El Segundo, CA, USA). The positive case was subjected to haplotype analysis using highly polymorphic short tandem repeat (STR) markers that span both arms of chromosome 6 [13].

We recalled KATP-PNDM patients to switch from insulin injection to oral glyburide, usually within 18 months of diagnosis. The transfer was carried out using a protocol that was similar to that described previously [8]. Glyburide was started at a dose of 0.1 mg per kilogram twice daily and was increased daily by 0.2 mg per kilogram. The dose of glyburide was increased until insulin independence was achieved or the dose was at least 0.8 mg per kilogram per day. The change to sulfonylureas was considered to be successful if a patient was able to stop insulin treatment completely at any dose of glyburide and was deemed to be unsuccessful if insulin was still required with a dose of glyburide at least 0.8 mg per kilogram per day. All trials were performed during hospitalization.

Type 1 diabetic patients with age of onset between 6 months and 2 years were matched one-to-one with those of PNDM (15 patients with recorded HbA1c). T1DM patients hospitalized during the same period as PNDM group with positive autoimmune antibody (ICA, GAD, or IAA) and comparable age, sex, duration of illness, and time of sample/data collection were selected as the control group. The HbA1c between the two groups was compared. The HbA1c of the PNDM group was tested at least 6 months after glyburide treatment.

2.4. Statistical Analysis. Statistical analysis was performed using chi-square test and Student's t-test using SPSS 19.0

TABLE 1: Clinical characteristics of NDM patients.

	NDM	PNDM	TNDM
Cases	25	18	7
Male (female)	14 (11)	11 (7)	3 (4)[#]
Birth weight (kg, mean ± SD)	2.6 ± 0.5	2.7 ± 0.5	2.4 ± 0.6[#]
Age at diagnosis (Days, mean ± SD)	74.4 ± 41.4	81.3 ± 42.7	56.7 ± 34.6[#]
DK/DKA (%)	68.0%	77.8%	42.9%[#]
Symptoms (cases)		Infection (6) Decreased responsiveness (5) Polydipsia, polyuria (2) Urine sticky (4) Seizures (2)	Infection (4) Polydipsia, polyuria (1) Seizures (2)
Physical development on follow-up (cases)		Physical and mental retardation (4), others are normal	Intellectual and physical development is normal
Genetic testing (cases)		*KCNJ11* (5) *ABCC8* (1) *INS* (1) *EIF2AK3* (3) *SLC19A2* (1) *GLIS3* (1)	*ABCC8* (2) Paternal uniparental disomy of 6q24 (1)
Therapy (cases)		Glyburide (3) Insulin (15)	Remission in 2 weeks to 1 year after insulin therapy (6)
Average HbA1c at the last follow-up (cases had recorded results)		7.2% (15)	5.5% (5)

[#]No significant differences compared with PNDM ($P > 0.05$).

(SPSS Inc., Chicago, IL, USA) software. Continuous data were analyzed using Student's t-test, and categorical data was analyzed using chi-square test.

3. Results

3.1. Baseline Characteristics of Patients. Table 1 shows the baseline characteristics of 25 NDM patients. Based on follow-up, 18 cases were typed as PNDM (72.0%) and 7 cases as TNDM (28.0%). No statistical differences were found between the two types with age of onset, birth weight, and DK/DKA prevalence ($P > 0.05$) (see Table 1). The clinical features of PNDM and TNDM are summarized in Table 2. All patients were treated with insulin initially. All patients were born to nonconsanguineous parents.

3.2. Genetic Analysis. In PNDM cases, twelve mutations were identified. Direct sequencing identified the most frequent mutations involving KATP channel ($n = 6$) including *KCNJ11* ($n = 5$) and *ABCC8* mutation ($n = 1$), all of which were identified earlier. The non-KATP mutations ($n = 6$) including *INS*, *EIF2AK3* ($n = 3$), *GLIS3*, and *SLC19A2* were identified and five were confirmed as novel mutations. In the TNDM, we found 2 cases harbouring *ABCC8* mutation and 1 case with UPD6. The mutations are summarized in Table 2.

3.3. Follow-Up of NDM Cases

3.3.1. PNDM. All patients were treated with insulin initially. Following stable glucose control with insulin, transition from insulin to oral sulfonylureas was attempted in five of six KATP-PNDM cases. Finally, three cases (60%) were successfully placed on glyburide; one switched back to insulin as there was no response to glyburide; one stopped oral glyburide because of serious gastrointestinal reactions; and in another case glyburide was not tried because of loss of follow-up. The mean HbA1c of PNDM during the last visit was 7.2 ± 0.8%, which was similar to that of the infant-onset T1DM group (Table 3).

Except in 4 PNDM cases, the height and development were found to be normal on follow-up. The patients who presented with convulsion at the onset showed no further convulsions.

Among patients with positive mutations, case 1 carrying *KCNJ11*p.R201H mutation had congenital cataract. Glyburide therapy was also stopped in case 1 due to gastrointestinal reactions and it was switched back to regular insulin treatment with good glycemic control. Case 2 with *KCNJ11*p.R201H mutation and case 3 with *KCNJ11*p.G53S mutation achieved good blood glucose levels with no hypoglycemia with glyburide treatment. Case 5 bearing *KCNJ11*p.E229K mutation was lost to follow-up 1 year after

Table 2: Clinical profile and gene analysis of NDM.

Subtype	Number	Gender	Term or preterm	HbA1c at diagnosis (%)	Age at last visit (yr)	HbA1c (%) at last visit	Height (cm) (percentile)	Weight (kg) (percentile)	Mutant gene	Inherited from Father	Inherited from Mother	*De novo* mutation	Specific clinical features	Mutation	Zygosity	Insulin/glyburide therapy (age at transfer)
P	1	M	Term	13.7	4.1	6.1%	107.0 (P75)	17.0 (P50)	*KCNJ11*			p.R201H	Congenital cataract	c.602G>A; p.R201H	HET	Insulin/interruption because of side effects (1 yr)
P	2	F	Term	4.0	2.0	6.0%	88.0 (P50–75)	12.5 (P50–75)	*KCNJ11*			p.R201H		c.602G>A; p.R201H	HET	Glyburide response (0.7 mg/kg/d) (3 months)
P	3	M	Term	9.6	1.5	6.5%	81.0 (P25)	11.0 (P10–P25)	*KCNJ11*			p.G53S		c.157C>T; p.G53S	HET	Glyburide response (0.4 mg/kg/d) (7 months)
P	4	M	Term	8.1	2.5	7.5%	85.0 (P3)	11.0 (P3)	*KCNJ11*			p.V59M	iDEND	c.175G>A; p.V59M	HET	Glyburide response (4 months)
P	5	M	Term						*KCNJ11*		p.E229K			c.685G>A; p.E229K	HET	Insulin/no transition because of lost to follow-up
P	6	F	Term	9.6	5.1	8.0%	105.0 (P10)	15.0 (P3–10)	*ABCC8*		p.R825W			c.2473C>T; p.R825W	HET	Insulin/no response (4 months)
P	7	F	Term	9.8	1.5	7.0%	83.0 (P50–75)	11.5 (P25–50)	*INS*					c.293C>A; p.S98I	HET	Insulin
P	8	F	Term	14.2	1.5				*GLIS3*	No sample	No sample		Died of liver and kidney failure at 1.5 years of age	c.2570T>A; p.F857Y	HET	Insulin
P	9	M	Term	10.4	5.0	7.9%	110.0 (P25–P50)	17.5 (P10–P25)	*SLC19A2*	No sample	No sample		Moderate normocytic anemia	c.1213A>G; p.T405A	HET	Insulin
P	10	M	Term	9.5	13.9	7.0%	140.0 (<P3)	30.0 (<P3)	*EIF2AK3*	p.C532STOP			WRS	c.1798A>T; p.C532STOP	HET	Insulin
P	11	F	Term	11.2	1.5	7.5%	74.3 (<P3)	8.0 (<P3)	*EIF2AK3*	p.leu182leufsX19	p.Arg588Ter		WRS	c.1762C>T, p.Arg588Ter; c.544delC, p.leu182leufsX19	HET	Insulin
P	12	F	Term	9.8	4.5	7.5%	106.0 (P50)	15.0 (P10)								Insulin (0.8 IU/kg/d)
P	13	M	Term	15.8	2.0	7.9%	89.5 (P50–P75)	13.0 (P50)								Insulin (based on glucose, injection once every other day)
P	14	M	Term	4.38	0.6		62.0 (<P3)	4.0 (<P3)					Died of DKA at 7 months of age Intellectual and physical retardation			Insulin
P	15	M	Term	5.2	6.0	8.2%	115.0 (P25)	18.5 (P10–P25)								Insulin
P	16	M	Term		5.0	7.4%	113.0 (P75)	20 (P50–75)								Insulin
P	17	M	Term	5.9	3.0	7.3%	98.0 (P50–75)	17.0 (P90)								Insulin
P	18	F	Term		4.0	7.6%	105.0 (P75)	16.0 (P50)								Insulin

TABLE 2: Continued.

Subtype	Number	Gender	Term or preterm	HbA1c at diagnosis (%)	Age at last visit (yr)	HbA1c (%) at last visit	Height (cm) (percentile)	Weight (kg) (percentile)	Mutant gene	Inherited from Father	Inherited from Mother	*De novo* mutation	Specific clinical features	Mutation	Zygosity	Insulin/glyburide therapy (age at transfer)
T	19	F	Term	7.1	1.8				*ABCC8*		p.G296R			c.886G>A; p.G296R	HET	
T	20	M	Term	10.2	1.8	5.6%	83.6 (P25–50)	11.2 (P25–50)	*ABCC8*		p.D212E			c.636G>T; p.D212E	HET	
T	21	F	Term	9.6	5.8	5.7%	110.5 (P25–50)	20.0 (P50)	UPD6							
T	22	F	Term	7.4	4.8	5.6%	110.0 (P50)	19.0 (P75)								
T	23	M	Term		5.5	5.6%	112.5 (P25–50)	18.0 (P10–25)								
T	24	M	Term	9.9	3.7	5.2%	102.3 (P75)	16.5 (P50–75)								
T	25	F	Term		4.0											

Table 3: Comparison of HbA1c between PNDM and infantile onset T1DM groups.

	PNDM	T1DM	P value
N	15	15	
M (F)	10 (5)	10 (5)	1.00
Onset of age (years)	0.2 ± 0.1	1.3 ± 0.5	0.00
Age at follow-up (years)	4.0 ± 2.9	4.4 ± 2.1	0.70
Duration of illness (years)	3.8 ± 2.9	3.1 ± 1.9	0.44
HbA1c at follow-up (%)	7.2 ± 0.8	7.4 ± 0.9	0.41

diagnosis, while he showed good response to initial insulin therapy but failed to undergo glyburide therapy later. Case 6 carrying the *ABCC8* p.R825W mutation failed to respond to glyburide (0.4 mg/kg/d), and the insulin dose was not reduced. During follow-up, insulin therapy once or twice daily was administered to the child depending on the blood glucose level. Case 7 carrying *INS* mutation achieved good glucose control with insulin therapy. All these patients exhibited normal physical and mental development.

PNDM was associated with special syndromes. Case 4 (*KCNJ11*p.V59M) had intellectual and physical retardation without epilepsy and hence was diagnosed as iDEND syndrome. This patient was given intermittent glyburide therapy (following parental request) but died of DKA at 2 years of age in local hospital. Case 8 (*GLIS3* p.F857Y) had liver dysfunction but improved by following supportive therapy. This patient died of liver and kidney failure at 1.5 years of age. Case 9 (*SLC19A2* p.T405A) presented with moderate anemia (hemoglobin, 70 g/L), which improved with oral iron therapy. Case 10 (*EIF2AK3* p.C532STOP) was accompanied with intellectual and physical retardation, short stature, multiple skeletal dysplasia, and hypothyroidism, diagnosed as *Wolcott-Rallison syndrome*. Case 11 who manifested physical retardation and skeletal dysplasia showed compound heterozygous mutations in *EIF2AK3*.

There were three deaths (Cases 4, 8, and 14). Case 14 died of DKA at 7 months of age, several days after diagnosis. The patient also showed weight loss and mental and physical retardation with negative results on genetic screening.

3.3.2. TNDM. Remission among TNDM cases in our cohort was ascertained from 2 weeks to 1 year after diagnosis. None of these patients showed any congenital abnormalities such as macroglossia, umbilical hernia, dysmorphic facial features, hematopoietic dysfunction or abnormal hearing, and heart, liver, or kidney function. The development and height were normal. None of them had acanthosis nigricans. The oldest patient was 5 years old, with no recurrence of diabetes. No specific features were observed in patient carrying *ABCC8* mutations and UPD6 compared with the other TNDM cases carrying negative genetic results.

4. Discussion

The NDM patients generally presented with infection or decreased responsiveness at the onset, without the typical symptoms such as polyuria, polydipsia, polyphagia, and weight loss. In the present study, approximately 30% were TNDM patients, which is similar to the previous reports [4]. There were no differences between PNDM and TNDM patients in age of onset, birth-weight, and prevalence of DKA, making it difficult to clinically distinguish between the two types. Therefore, the typing was based on clinical remission during follow-up. The remission of TNDM cases was from 2 weeks to 1 year. The oldest child on follow-up was 5 years old with no recurrence of diabetes. Of the patients carrying *KCNJ11* and *ABCC8* mutations, there was developmental delay in one patient diagnosed as iDEND, including one with congenital cataract. Busiah et al. [14] found that patients with mutations in KATP channel subunit genes presented with developmental coordination disorders including visual-spatial dyspraxia and attention deficits but not developmental delay or epilepsy. Therefore, adults with a history of neonatal diabetes mellitus should be tested for neuropsychological dysfunction and developmental defects.

We identified six mutations in KATP channel that were previously reported and six non-KATP mutations in PNDM cases, five of which were not identified until now, and found two KATP mutations in TNDM cases. Three cases were placed on glyburide therapy and 15 cases were on insulin therapy, with good glycemic control in most cases.

In this study, we evaluated the gene mutations and clinical manifestations of PNDM cases. We identified two cases of p.R201H mutations, which were the most common *KCNJ11* mutations without neurological abnormalities. These mutations have been confirmed at CpG dinucleotide, resulting in decreased sensitivity of KATP channels to ATP. Glucose stimulation reduces insulin secretion, whereas sulfonylureas stimulate the secretion, explaining the rationale of glyburide therapy. Of the two cases, one was responsive to glyburide and the other presented with severe gastrointestinal reactions and parental worries about side effects and therefore discontinued despite recommendations to the contrary.

The second mutation of *KCNJ11* revealed in the present study was p.V59M. Generally, patients with this mutation cause a triad of developmental delay, epilepsy, and neonatal diabetes (DEND syndrome), or without epilepsy (intermediate DEND (iDEND) syndrome). The neurological symptoms are attributable to the presence of Kir6.2 in nerve and brain tissue. One case with iDEND in the present study responded favorably to oral glyburide therapy. Glyburide not only controls blood glucose levels, but also ameliorates the neurological symptoms. However, this patient died of DKA attributed to glyburide therapy cessation.

The third mutation was *KCNJ11*p.G53S, located between Kir6.2 and SUR1. The patient with this mutation in the present study was successfully switched from insulin to glyburide, leading to HbA1c level of 6.5%.

The fourth mutation was *KCNJ11*p.E229K, which induces NDM without neurological manifestations but was lost to follow-up. As reported, p.E229 and p.G53 mutations cause both PNDM and TNDM [15, 16]. In our study, they were classified as PNDM. The patient with *KCNJ11*p.G53S underwent low dose glyburide (0.4 mg/kg/d), consistent with previous reports [17].

Another case we identified with *ABCC8* p.R825W mutation was not responsive to glyburide transition. The mean effective dosage of glyburide is 0.5~0.6 mg/kg/d for SUR1 mutations [17]. The glyburide dosage of 0.4 mg/kg/d was not effective. The insulin dosage was not reduced during glyburide therapy. The patient manifested nausea and poor appetite. The parents stopped glyburide due to the side effects. At follow-up, the patient was on insulin therapy and refused to be treated with glyburide. Physicians must be cautious before using sulfonylureas as they are not licensed in children and may have side effects. The glyburide transition can only be tried as an inpatient procedure to avoid diabetic ketoacidosis in those young children who may be unresponsive to glyburide and need careful monitoring [18]. Parents who carried the same *KCNJ11* or *ABCC8* mutations showed no neonatal diabetes mellitus symptoms or past history of abnormal glucose metabolism. The phenomenon suggests that KATP mutations have variable clinical phenotypes, with the symptoms varying from TNDM or PNDM. The mild and transient manifestations during neonatal period were missed, with possible risk of relapse in the future. The glucose metabolism of parents carrying the same mutations as their children needs to be monitored.

The success rate of glyburide transition among cases with KATP mutations of 60.0% in the present study is lower than that reported from other countries. One reason for the low success rate could be the side effects of glyburide such as nausea and vomiting that affected its clinical application in infants in the present study. Diarrhea is the common reported side effects of glyburide but has not been seen in our patients. The failed transitions due to side effects were not reported in other studies, suggesting that Chinese children respond differently to glyburide compared with other ethnic groups. The small sample size may be another reason for such a response. We also found a novel *INS* mutation causing simple diabetes.

Other NDM mutations were associated with specific manifestations. Case 1 manifesting mental and physical retardation, hypothyroidism, and multiple epiphyseal dysplasia was diagnosed with WRS, as reported by Sang et al. [19]. Sanger sequencing yielded a sole heterozygous mutation in this patient, which was inherited from father. This nonsense mutation resulted in a truncated protein of 532 amino acid residues. The loss of kinase in the catalytic domain resulted in a complete loss of function. WRS is an autosomal recessive disorder. Therefore, we should also ascertain other genes causing PNDM. The Italian PNDM patient had heterozygous mutations in both *KCNJ11* and *GCK* genes [20], suggesting that NDM may be a polygenic disease. However, no NGS was performed. We decided to monitor the father for diabetic symptoms. Case 18 was also diagnosed as WRS carrying compound heterozygous mutations of *EIF2AK3*, inherited from father and mother, respectively, with one mutation reported and another deletion mutation resulting in a truncated protein. NDM patients with *GLIS3* gene mutation may also manifest congenital hypothyroidism, glaucoma, liver fibrosis, and polycystic kidney disease. The patient with *GLIS3* mutation showed hepatic dysfunction without liver fibrosis and polycystic kidney disease at onset but eventually died of liver and kidney failure 1 year later in a local hospital. The thyroid function was normal in this patient on follow-up. *GLIS3* mutations have been reported to be autosomal recessive resulting in a variable clinical phenotype. Only one heterozygous mutation was found in this patient. Polyphen analysis further indicated a possible causative mutation. Another genetic variant was needed for further study.

SLC19A2 gene mutations causing NDM lead to the development of diabetes, deafness and megaloblastic anemia. This syndrome can be ameliorated by thiamine, so it is called thiamine-responsive megaloblastic anaemia (TRMA) [21]. Our patient with *SLC19A2* mutation exhibited moderate normocytic anemia with no hearing abnormalities at diagnosis. Only one heterozygous mutation was detected by NGS. Polyphen analysis indicated possible causative mutations but not SNP. Another mutation in a non-coding region or a large deletion may be found by Sanger sequencing of the whole gene or with multiplex ligation probe amplification technology (MLPA), respectively.

The genetic etiology of NDM suggests polygenic inheritance. The classification of TNDM and PNDM should be reconsidered. A diagnosis of diabetes in parents who carried the mutations cannot be excluded. We need additional and longer follow-up of cases to establish a TNDM diagnosis or PNDM remission.

Diarrhea is one of the manifestations of IPEX (immune dysregulation, polyendocrinopathy, enteropathy, and X-linked syndrome), which is caused by *FOXP3* mutation. IPEX may also present with autoimmune thyroid disease, exfoliative dermatitis, and sepsis caused by immune dysregulation [22]. Identification of a *FOXP3* mutation suggests possible prenatal testing. Case 14 presenting with diarrhea and fever was negative for *FOXP3* mutations using NGS.

The mutations in KATP channel accounted for 33.3% of PNDM, including 27.8% in *KCNJ11* mutations and 5.6% in *ABCC8* mutations, similar to the reported data. *INS* gene mutation accounted for 5.6%. We diagnosed two cases of WRS (11.2% of all PNDM cases), which is now recognized as the most frequent cause of PNDM in consanguineous children [23, 24]. In addition, rare gene mutations (*GLIS3*, *SLC19A2*, etc.) also were associated with specific clinical manifestations. Therefore, in view of the high mutation rate of *KCNJ11* in PNDM and high correlation between genotype and phenotype, we suggest screening for *KCNJ11* mutations first in NDM cases, followed by *ABCC8* screen and genes associated with specific complications. It is difficult to distinguish TNDM from PNDM initially during the illness. NGS has been used worldwide to detect mutations in PNDM or TNDM.

PNDM children on insulin and glyburide therapy were found to have good glycemic control (mean HbA1c 7.2%) during follow-up, which is similar to infantile onset T1DM group. It was probably associated with younger age at onset, need for a lower insulin dose, and better residual pancreatic β cell function. The onset age of PNDM and T1DM is usually different, although the duration of illness is comparable, which is the most important factor affecting the HbA1c level.

TNDM is associated with chromosome 6q24 imprinting abnormalities in 70% of cases. The syndrome is associated with giant tongue, umbilical hernia, facial deformity, kidney abnormalities, congenital heart disease, hypothyroidism, and intrauterine growth retardation (>95%). Array-CGH could be used to detect UPD6 and duplication simultaneously, so it may be a cost-effective genetic analysis method for TNDM cases. In our study, all the TNDM cases did not exhibit the specific manifestations mentioned above. Recurrence of TNDM resulting from *KCNJ11*, *ABCC8*, and 6q24 mutations might respond to treatment with sulfonylurea [3, 25]. It should be noted that the pathophysiological mechanism of 6q24 mutations is not clear and thus the most appropriate treatment remains unclear.

In the present study, PNDM accounted for 72%; the onset symptoms are not typical. Seizure may be seen initially in NDM cases making it remain misdiagnosed. About one-third of PNDM and TNDM patients had KATP mutations. Only one TNDM case had paternal uniparental disomy of chromosome 6q24. The genetic etiology could not be determined in 50% of PNDM and 57% of TNDM cases. However, no maternal hypomethylation at Chr6q24 was detected, which may have affected the mutational analysis of the TNDM cohort. Glyburide was effective in most KATP-PNDM patients. Most NDM patients achieved good glycemic control (HbA1c < 7.5%) and there was no significant difference when compared to infantile onset T1DM.

Conflict of Interests

The authors declare no conflict of interests.

Acknowledgments

A portion of this work was supported by the Open Research Project of Shanghai Key Laboratory of Diabetes Mellitus (SHKLD-KF-1304). The authors thank the patients and their relatives for providing the study samples. They also thank the referring hospitals and clinicians.

References

[1] E. L. Edghill and A. T. Hattersley, "Genetic disorders of the pancreatic beta cell and diabetes (permanent neonatal diabetes and maturity-onset diabetes of the young)," in *Pancreatic Beta Cell in Health and Disease*, S. Seino and G. I. Bell, Eds., pp. 389–420, Springer, Tokyo, Japan, 2008.

[2] I. K. Temple, R. J. Gardner, D. J. G. Mackay, J. C. K. Barber, D. O. Robinson, and J. P. H. Shield, "Transient neonatal diabetes: widening the understanding of the etiopathogenesis of diabetes," *Diabetes*, vol. 49, no. 8, pp. 1359–1366, 2000.

[3] D. J. G. Mackay and I. K. Temple, "Transient neonatal diabetes mellitus type 1," *American Journal of Medical Genetics Part C: Seminars in Medical Genetics*, vol. 154, no. 3, pp. 335–342, 2010.

[4] A. P. Babenko, M. Polak, H. Cavé et al., "Activating mutations in the ABCC8 gene in neonatal diabetes mellitus," *The New England Journal of Medicine*, vol. 355, no. 5, pp. 456–466, 2006.

[5] A. L. Gloyn, E. R. Pearson, J. F. Antcliff et al., "Activating mutations in the gene encoding the ATP-sensitive potassium-channel subunit Kir6.2 and permanent neonatal diabetes," *The New England Journal of Medicine*, vol. 350, no. 18, pp. 1838–1849, 2004.

[6] M. Vaxillaire, A. Bonnefond, and P. Froguel, "The lessons of early-onset monogenic diabetes for the understanding of diabetes pathogenesis," *Best Practice & Research: Clinical Endocrinology & Metabolism*, vol. 26, no. 2, pp. 171–187, 2012.

[7] L. E. Docherty, S. Kabwama, A. Lehmann et al., "Clinical presentation of 6q24 transient neonatal diabetes mellitus (6q24 TNDM) and genotype-phenotype correlation in an international cohort of patients," *Diabetologia*, vol. 56, no. 4, pp. 758–762, 2013.

[8] E. L. Edghill, S. E. Flanagan, A.-M. Patch et al., "Insulin mutation screening in 1,044 patients with diabetes: mutations in the INS gene are a common cause of neonatal diabetes but a rare cause of diabetes diagnosed in childhood or adulthood," *Diabetes*, vol. 57, no. 4, pp. 1034–1042, 2008.

[9] E. R. Pearson, I. Flechtner, P. R. Njølstad et al., "Switching from insulin to oral sulfonylureas in patients with diabetes due to Kir6.2 mutations," *The New England Journal of Medicine*, vol. 355, no. 5, pp. 467–477, 2006.

[10] G. Tonini, C. Bizzarri, R. Bonfanti et al., "Sulfonylurea treatment outweighs insulin therapy in short-term metabolic control of patients with permanent neonatal diabetes mellitus due to activating mutations of the *KCNJ11* (*KIR6.2*) gene," *Diabetologia*, vol. 49, no. 9, pp. 2210–2213, 2006.

[11] International Diabetes Federation, *Global IDF/ISPAD Guideline for Diabetes in Childhood and Adolescents*, International Diabetes Federation, 2011.

[12] C. Gong, S. Huang, C. Su et al., "Congenital hyperinsulinism in Chinese patients: 5-yr treatment outcome of 95 clinical cases with genetic analysis of 55 cases," *Pediatric Diabetes*, 2015.

[13] I. Salahshourifar, A. S. Halim, W. A. W. Sulaiman, and B. A. Zilfalil, "Maternal uniparental heterodisomy of chromosome 6 in a boy with an isolated cleft lip and palate," *American Journal of Medical Genetics Part A*, vol. 152, no. 7, pp. 1818–1821, 2010.

[14] K. Busiah, S. Drunat, L. Vaivre-Douret et al., "Neuropsychological dysfunction and developmental defects associated with genetic changes in infants with neonatal diabetes mellitus: a prospective cohort study," *The Lancet Diabetes & Endocrinology*, vol. 1, no. 3, pp. 199–207, 2013.

[15] T. Klupa, J. Skupien, B. Mirkiewicz-Sieradzka et al., "Efficacy and safety of sulfonylurea use in permanent neonatal diabetes due to KCNJ11 gene mutations: 34-month median follow-up," *Diabetes Technology & Therapeutics*, vol. 12, no. 5, pp. 387–391, 2010.

[16] S. E. Flanagan, A.-M. Patch, D. J. G. Mackay et al., "Mutations in ATP-sensitive K^+ channel genes cause transient neonatal diabetes and permanent diabetes in childhood or adulthood," *Diabetes*, vol. 56, no. 7, pp. 1930–1937, 2007.

[17] M. Rafiq, S. E. Flanagan, A. M. Patch, B. M. Shields, S. Ellard, and A. T. Hattersley, "Effective treatment with oral sulfonylureas in patients with diabetes due to sulfonylurea receptor 1 (SUR1) mutations. Neonatal Diabetes International Collaborative Group," *Diabetes Care*, vol. 31, no. 2, pp. 204–209, 2008.

[18] D. Carmody, C. D. Bell, J. L. Hwang et al., "Sulfonylurea treatment before genetic testing in neonatal diabetes: pros and cons," *Journal of Clinical Endocrinology and Metabolism*, vol. 99, no. 12, pp. E2709–E2714, 2014.

[19] Y. Sang, M. Liu, W. Yang, J. Yan, Chengzhu, and G. Ni, "A novel EIF2AK3 mutation leading to Wolcott-Rallison syndrome

in a Chinese child," *Journal of Pediatric Endocrinology & Metabolism*, vol. 24, no. 3-4, pp. 181–184, 2011.

[20] O. Massa, D. Iafusco, E. D'Amato, A. L. Gloyn, A. T. Hattersley, and B. Pasquino, "KCNJ11 activating mutations in Italian patients with permanent neonatal diabetes. Early onset diabetes study group of the Italian Society of Pediatric Endocrinology and Diabetology," *Human Mutation*, vol. 25, pp. 22–27, 2005.

[21] V. Labay, T. Raz, D. Baron et al., "Mutations in SLC19A2 cause thiamine-responsive megaloblastic anaemia associated with diabetes mellitus and deafness," *Nature Genetics*, vol. 22, no. 3, pp. 300–304, 1999.

[22] R. S. Wildin, S. Smyk-Pearson, and A. H. Filipovich, "Clinical and molecular features of the immunodysregulation, polyendocrinopathy, enteropathy, X linked (IPEX) syndrome," *Journal of Medical Genetics*, vol. 39, no. 8, pp. 537–545, 2002.

[23] H. Demirbilek, V. B. Arya, M. N. Ozbek et al., "Clinical characteristics and molecular genetic analysis of 22 patients with neonatal diabetes from the South-Eastern region of Turkey: predominance of non-KATP channel mutations," *European Journal of Endocrinology*, vol. 172, no. 6, pp. 697–705, 2015.

[24] S. Jahnavi, V. Poovazhagi, S. Kanthimathi, V. Gayathri, V. Mohan, and V. Radha, "EIF2AK3 mutations in South Indian children with permanent neonatal diabetes mellitus associated with Wolcott-Rallison syndrome," *Pediatric Diabetes*, vol. 15, no. 4, pp. 313–318, 2014.

[25] P. Proks, C. Girard, S. Haider et al., "A gating mutation at the internal mouth of the Kir6.2 pore is associated with DEND syndrome," *EMBO Reports*, vol. 6, no. 5, pp. 470–475, 2005.

20

The Stricter the Better? The Relationship between Targeted HbA_{1c} Values and Metabolic Control of Pediatric Type 1 Diabetes Mellitus

Marcin Braun,[1] Bartlomiej Tomasik,[1] Ewa Wrona,[1] Wojciech Fendler,[1] Przemyslawa Jarosz-Chobot,[2] Agnieszka Szadkowska,[1] Agnieszka Zmysłowska,[1] Jayne Wilson,[3] and Wojciech Mlynarski[1]

[1] *Department of Pediatrics, Oncology, Hematology and Diabetology, Medical University of Lodz, Sporna 36/50, 91-738 Lodz, Poland*
[2] *Department of Pediatrics, Endocrinology and Diabetology, Medical University of Silesia, Medykow 16, 40-752 Katowice, Poland*
[3] *Cancer Research UK Clinical Trials Unit, School of Cancer Sciences, University of Birmingham, Vincent Drive, Edgbaston, Birmingham B15 2TT, UK*

Correspondence should be addressed to Wojciech Mlynarski; wojciech.mlynarski@umed.lodz.pl

Academic Editor: Francisco J. Ruperez

Introduction. It remains unclear how HbA_{1c} recommendations influence metabolic control of paediatric patients with type 1 diabetes mellitus. To evaluate this we compared reported HbA_{1c} with guideline thresholds. *Materials and Methods.* We searched systematically MEDLINE and EMBASE for studies reporting on HbA_{1c} in children with T1DM and grouped them according to targeted HbA_{1c} obtained from regional guidelines. We assessed the discrepancies in the metabolic control between these groups by comparing mean HbA_{1c} extracted from each study and the differences between actual and targeted HbA_{1c}. *Results.* We included 105 from 1365 searched studies. The median (IQR) HbA_{1c} for the study population was 8.30% (8.00%–8.70%) and was lower in "6.5%" than in "7.5%" as targeted HbA_{1c} level (8.20% (7.85%–8.57%) versus 8.40% (8.20%–8.80%); $p = 0.028$). Median difference between actual and targeted HbA_{1c} was 1.20% (0.80%–1.70%) and was higher in "6.5%" than in "7.5%" (1.70% (1.30%–2.07%) versus 0.90% (0.70%–1.30%), resp.; $p < 0.001$). *Conclusions.* Our study indicates that the 7.5% threshold results in HbA_{1c} levels being closer to the therapeutic goal, but the actual values are still higher than those observed in the "6.5%" group. A meta-analysis of raw data from national registries or a prospective study comparing both approaches is warranted as the next step to examine this subject further.

1. Introduction

Despite the crucial role of HbA_{1c} in the management of diabetes, substantial differences among diabetic associations regarding targeted levels of this parameter are still present. The stricter approach is represented by the European Society of Cardiology (ESC) and recommends 6.5% (48 mmol/mol) of HbA_{1c} [1], whilst the International Society for Pediatric and Adolescent Diabetes (ISPAD), International Diabetes Federation (IDF), and American Diabetes Association (ADA) advocate 7.5% (58 mmol/mol) as the valid target of HbA_{1c} [2, 3].

The Hvidøre Study Group on Childhood Diabetes observed significant differences in average HbA_{1c} levels among 21 large pediatric diabetes centres from 17 countries in Europe, Japan, and North America [4]. The authors of this study suggested that there might be several reasons for these discrepancies. One possible explanation might be bound to guideline values of desirable HbA_{1c} level that differ depending on the diabetic association.

Both the Diabetes Control and Complications Trial (DCCT) and the Epidemiology of Diabetes Interventions and Complications Study (EDIC) have shown that early intensive therapy of patients with type 1 diabetes results in better metabolic control [5, 6]. The differences in metabolic control between conventional therapy and functional intensive insulin treatment cohorts were directly correlated with strikingly different treatment outcomes (e.g., any cardiovascular disease event was reduced by 42% in the intensive metabolic control arm). Taking into consideration the results of DCCT and EDIC studies, if the difference among targeted HbA_{1c} levels of 1% was related to a different metabolic control, this would have an impact on long-term complications of diabetes mellitus. Recent cohort studies have shown that metabolic control of patients with T1DM has significantly improved during the last decade and better metabolic control resulted in superior outcome which supports aforementioned observations [7, 8].

In view of the controversy of the role of HbA_{1c} guidelines and the fact that, in majority of cases, they are set arbitrarily, we have conducted this study to examine the influence of HbA_{1c} targets on metabolic control of type 1 diabetes in pediatric population [9].

2. Materials and Methods

2.1. Guideline Identification. The data on guideline HbA_{1c} values in each country or region at the time of the study were obtained from official websites of national/regional diabetic associations. In case of lack of information consultants were contacted by phone or e-mail.

2.2. Reported HbA_{1c} Levels: Data Sources and Searches. Publications which reported HbA_{1c} levels were sought using systematic review techniques. A systematic search was undertaken using terms for pediatric/children/juvenile diabetes mellitus type 1, glycated haemoglobin A_{1c}, and insulin-based therapy in the following databases: OVID MEDLINE, EMBASE, Cochrane Database of Systematic Reviews (CDSR), National Institute for Health and Clinical Excellence (NICE) database, Scottish Intercollegiate Guidelines (SIGN) database, Database of Reviews of Effects (DARE), and Health Technology Assessment (HTA/NHS EED). The searches were conducted between 1st January 2008 and 26th August 2013, with no language restrictions. We searched for studies with T1DM pediatric patients (≤18 years) being treated for at least 1 year. The patients had to have at least one HbA_{1c} level measurement taken after December 2007. In cases of interventional studies, we utilized the HbA_{1c} levels recorded prior to the planned intervention. We excluded studies with less than 50 participants. The study design and search strategy are available in the Supporting Information, available online at http://dx.doi.org/10.1155/2016/5490258.

2.3. Study Selection. Two reviewers independently assessed searched papers for eligibility: firstly by screening titles and abstracts and secondly by examining full-text papers of studies included after screening. The same strategy was used for both data bits' extraction. All disagreements were resolved by the discussion between reviewers.

In order to reduce bias caused by overlapping studies we contacted corresponding authors of papers, which we found to be based on common national diabetic registries or which had at least one common author or when the research was done in the same institution. When we detected that the results of several papers overlapped each other and we could not obtain separated data, we chose the study with the largest sample.

2.4. Data Extraction. Data were extracted onto a predefined form. HbA_{1c} levels representing populations of each study were calculated by combining the mean values for all investigated groups. If applicable, all values were transformed and presented as percentage of the total haemoglobin level by using standard HbA_{1c} units' converter [10]. HbA_{1c} measurements had to be performed using high-performance liquid chromatography meeting the DCCT standard. For interventional studies HbA_{1c} values were extracted before implementation of preplanned intervention.

2.5. Data Synthesis and Statistical Analysis. Subgroup analyses were undertaken according to the following: gross domestic product (GDP; high-income country is defined to have a GDP above US$12,746 in 2013) [11], number of patients in each study, age, duration of type 1 diabetes mellitus, prevalence of acute complications (hypoglycaemia and ketoacidosis), and type of therapy (continuous subcutaneous insulin infusion and multiple daily injection). If studies were conducted across multiple countries we checked whether guideline values were homogenous among them and allocated to appropriate groups. If targeted values were different in individual studies and we could not extract separate data for each country we excluded such studies from the quantitative analyses. In order to compare compliance, the difference between actual and targeted guideline HbA_{1c} value was calculated for each study (ΔHbA_{1c}).

Nominal variables were given as numbers with appropriate percentage whereas continuous variables were given as medians with interquartile ranges (IQR). For pairwise comparisons of continuous variables, the Mann-Whitney U (MWU) test was used. For multigroup comparisons Kruskal-Wallis one-way analysis of variance with additional post hoc tests within subgroups was used. Correlations were assessed using Spearman's rank correlation coefficient. Multivariate analyses were made using linear regression (GLM) weighted by the logarithm of number of participants in included studies. The multivariate model was fitted including all the variables that had reached statistical significance in the univariate analyses. Meta-analysis for comparison of adherence to guideline values was conducted using differences between mean and guideline HbA_{1c} levels. I^2 values to assess the heterogeneity between studies were calculated and results above 50% were considered as being of high heterogeneity. Statistical significance was set at $p \leq 0.05$; 95% confidence intervals were calculated. Statistical analysis was performed with usage of STATISTICA 10.0 software (StatSoft, Tulsa, OK, USA).

3. Results

3.1. Studies' Selection. The systematic searches for published HbA_{1c} levels yielded 1365 records. Eight hundred thirty of them were excluded after screening by title and abstract and further 77 were excluded due to duplication. Three hundred and fifty-three papers were excluded after full-text paper analysis. One hundred five studies were included for the final analyses, involving 91393 patients. In 25 studies only the abstract was available. The flowchart for the study selection

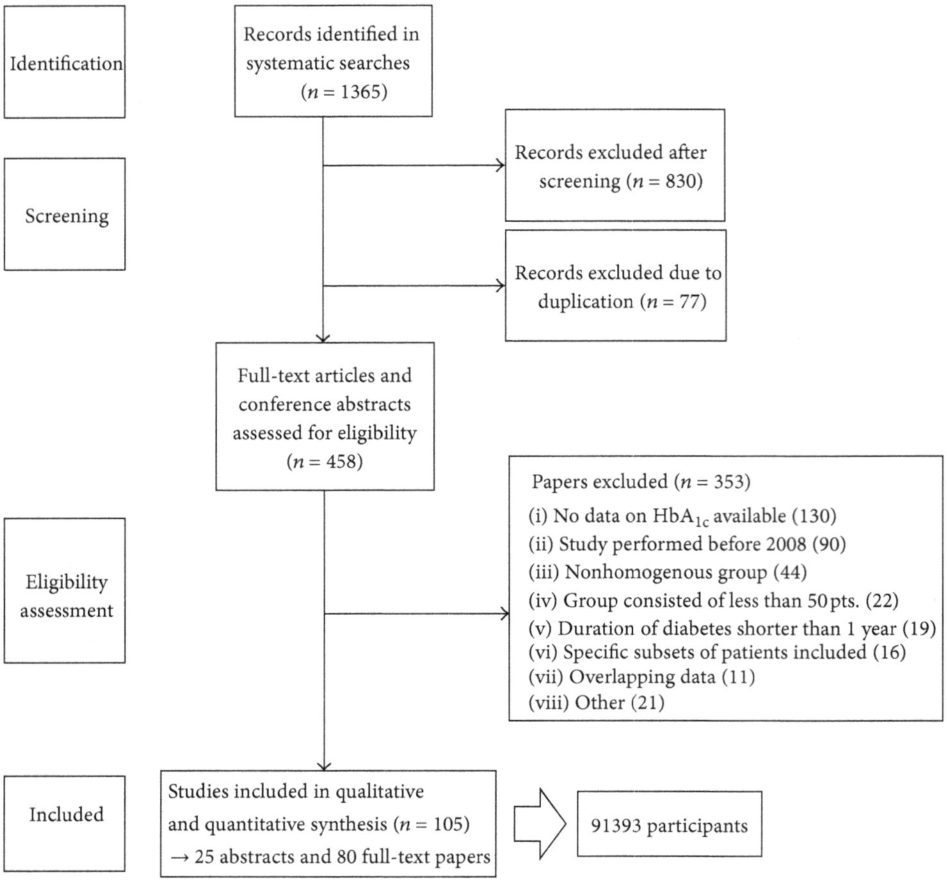

FIGURE 1: Flowchart for studies' selection process.

process with detailed reasons for exclusion is presented in Figure 1.

3.2. Studies' Characteristics and Allocation of Countries and Regions regarding Guideline Values. Of the 105 studies yielding HbA_{1c} level data 47 (44.76%) were cross-sectional, 40 (38.10%) were cohort, 9 (8.57%) were case-series or case-control, and 9 (8.57%) were interventional (including 5 randomized clinical trials). The eligible studies came from 18 countries (at least one country from Africa, Asia, Australia, Europe, South America, and North America). Forty-three (40.95%) studies were from European Union (21 of them (48.84%) were represented by 3 countries—UK (9 studies), Poland (6 studies), and Germany (6 studies)), whilst 39 (37.14%) were from the USA. Fifty-five (52.38%) studies were allocated to the group of "7.5% (58 mmol/mol)" as guideline HbA_{1c} value; 42 (40.00%) were allocated to the group of "6.5% (48 mmol/mol)." The guideline values from remaining studies (7.62%) were not homogenous and thus we excluded them from further analyses (the complete data for comparisons among all three study groups are available in Supporting Information). Ninety-five (90.48%) studies were conducted in high-income countries. The smallest study enrolled 50 patients [12], whilst the biggest one included 42881 individuals (cross-sectional study from Germany, Austria, and Switzerland) [13]. The median number of enrolled patients was 146 (IQR: 90–368). Median age within the studies was 12.79 (IQR: 11.60–13.77) years and median duration of diabetes was 5.20 (IQR: 3.90–6.30) years. In 26 studies (24.76%) patients were treated more frequently with MDI; in 30 (28.57%) of studies CSII was the preferred method of therapy. Only in 5 (4.76%) and in 8 (7.62%) of included studies did acute complications of diabetes mellitus (hypoglycaemia and diabetic ketoacidosis, resp.) occur more frequently in comparison to the prevalence reported in the literature. A detailed table with studies' characteristics and references can be seen in Supporting Information.

3.3. Comparison of HbA_{1c} Levels regarding HbA_{1c} Guideline Values. The median (IQR) HbA_{1c} level in the whole study population was 8.30% (IQR: 8.00%–8.70%) (67 (IQR: 63–72) mmol/mol). Median values for HbA_{1c} in groups regarding guideline values were significantly lower in "6.5" group than in "7.5" group and equalled 8.20% (IQR: 7.85%–8.57%; 66 (IQR: 62–70) mmol/mol) versus 8.40% (IQR: 8.20%–8.80%) (68 (IQR: 66–73) mmol/mol), respectively (MWU—p = 0.028, Figure 2(a); GLM—p = 0.001; beta for "6.5" group = −0.22 (95% CI: −0.34, −0.09)). This difference was significant in linear regression model with studies weighted by logarithm

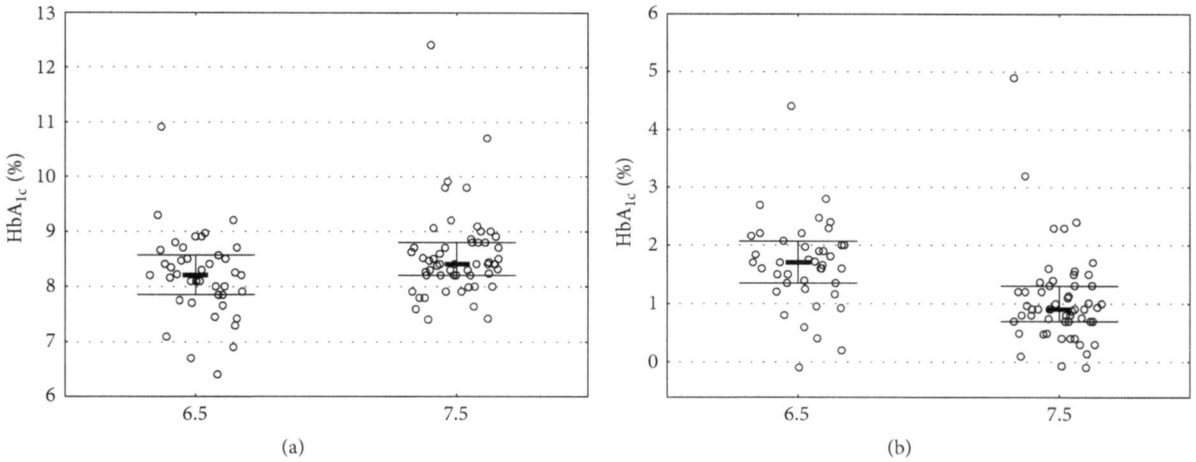

FIGURE 2: (a) Comparison for HbA_{1c} levels between regions of 6.5% and 7.5% as guideline values (MWU test, $p = 0.0162$). (b) Comparison of the difference between HbA_{1c} levels and guideline HbA_{1c} values between regions of 6.5% and 7.5% as guideline values (MWU test, $p < 0.0001$). Bolded line represents median; whiskers represent IQR.

from the number of patients ($p = 0.025$, beta for "6.5" group = −0.16 (95% CI: −0.29, −0.22)).

3.4. Comparison of the Difference between HbA_{1c} Levels and Guideline HbA_{1c} Values. The median ΔHbA_{1c} in the whole study population was 1.20% (IQR: 0.80%–1.70%). Median values for ΔHbA_{1c} in groups regarding guideline values were significantly higher in "6.5" group than in "7.5" group and equalled 1.70% (IQR: 1.30%–2.07%) versus 0.9% (IQR: 0.70%–1.30%) respectively (MWU—$p < 0.001$, Figure 2(b); GLM—$p < 0.001$; beta for "6.5" group = 0.40). The forest plots for meta-analysis of ΔHbA_{1c} are available in the Supporting Information.

3.5. Evaluation of the Effect of Other Variables on HbA_{1c} Level. Study design, publication type, percentage of patients with severe diabetic ketoacidosis or severe hypoglycaemia, type of therapy, GDP per capita, and number of patients did not have a significant impact on HbA_{1c} levels. HbA_{1c} values were significantly lower in countries from Europe (in comparison with the USA). We observed a positive correlation between HbA_{1c} levels and duration of type 1 diabetes and age of patients. All results for discussed comparisons are available in Table 1.

4. Discussion

Taking into consideration the debate regarding the role of HbA_{1c} guidelines and the fact that in majority of cases they are set arbitrarily, we decided to conduct this study to examine the impact of HbA_{1c} targets on metabolic control of type 1 diabetes in pediatric population [14]. Our work suggests that patients treated in centres with lower HbA_{1c} targets have better metabolic control despite being further from reaching their goal than patients from higher target countries. We found that the diabetic populations in countries with 6.5% (48 mmol/mol) as the targeted HbA_{1c} values are represented by actual median levels of HbA_{1c} of 0.2% lower than countries with 7.5% (58 mmol/mol) as targeted levels. Although the adherence was better in the centres with less strict aims of the therapy (median ΔHbA_{1c} 1.70% (1.30%–2.07%) versus 0.90% (0.70%–1.30%), resp.) the final outcome in terms of metabolic control was better in the more strict centres. We found also discrepancies between centres included in our study and this result tends to agree with the main observation of the Hvidøre Study Group [4].

The real reason for discrepancies between guideline levels for HbA_{1c} is likely to be linked to different aims and priorities in the management of diabetes [4, 15]. The teams, which set higher HbA_{1c} goals, are more concerned about risks of intensive therapy, such as hypoglycaemia. Although the previously strong association of low HbA_{1c} with severe hypoglycemia in young individuals with type 1 diabetes has substantially decreased in the last decade [16] this complication is one of the most common fatal acute diabetic complications [17]. Therefore the supporters of less strict metabolic control are willing to make concessions in order to avoid the risk. Higher HbA_{1c} values are also easier to accept and may lead to a better compliance. On the other hand, other teams focus on avoidance of hyperglycaemia, because they are devoted to minimalize the risk of long-term complications from the very first day after the diagnosis of diabetes mellitus. The crucial issue of this approach is to convince patients and their families to put an effort in pursuing stricter metabolic control [15, 18]. Additionally, since recently developed technologies including insulin pumps with low glucose suspend software reduce the risk of hypoglycaemia, the restricted goal is safely achievable [19, 20].

The differences in average HbA_{1c} levels among large diabetic centres have been the area of interest of researchers in pediatric diabetology for years [4, 15, 21–23]. The authors from the Hvidøre Study Group on Childhood Diabetes indicated several reasons, which could lead to discrepancies. The majority of these issues are relatively hard to assess in

TABLE 1: Univariate and multivariate linear model results for HbA_{1c} values regarding HbA_{1c} guideline groups (6.5% and 7.5%) and the other covariates. NA means not applied.

Variable	Groups	Number of studies included in analysis	p value from univariate analysis	p value from multivariate analysis with β parameter (95% CI)	The effect on HbA_{1c} level
HbA_{1c} targeted levels	6.5 (48 mmol/mol) versus 7.5 (58 mmol/mol)	97	0.028	<0.001 $\beta = -0.26$ (−0.40, −0.12)	Lower in "6.5% (48 mmol/mol) countries"
Publication type	Article versus abstract	97	0.967	NA	NA
Hypoglycemia	More versus less frequent	30	0.427	NA	NA
Diabetic ketoacidosis	More versus less frequent	26	0.261	NA	NA
Type of therapy	MDI versus CSII	56	0.249	NA	NA
Study design	Five groups	97	0.356	NA	NA
Location	Europe versus USA	82	0.022	NA	Lower in Europe
GDP per capita ($)	Continuous variable	97	0.127	NA	NA
Number of patients in the study	Continuous variable	97	0.985	NA	NA
Mean age in the study (years)	Continuous variable	93	0.016	0.001 $\beta = 0.29$ (0.12, 0.47)	Positive correlation ($r = 0.25$)
Mean duration of DM in the study (years)	Continuous variable	85	0.037	0.753 $\beta = -0.03$ (−0.20, −0.15)	Positive correlation ($r = 0.23$)

a robust way (e.g., the role of multidisciplinary approach, self-care behaviours, educational models, ethnic or cultural aspects, socioeconomic status, etc.) [24]. Recent findings suggest that the phenomenon of seasonal HbA_{1c} variability in schoolchildren could also affect the results of reported HbA_{1c} results [25]. According to Hvidøre Study Group different guideline values of HbA_{1c} among centres also appear to play a significant role in explaining the differences in metabolic outcomes among pediatric population [15]. The results of our study supports this hypothesis.

Although this is the first study that systematically examines the influence of different guideline HbA_{1c} values on the actual HbA_{1c} levels, it should be stated that our work has several limitations. The problem of overlapping populations in the enrolled studies was particularly hard to eliminate in our review. Although we tried to contact with the authors of the studies, in which such problem might have occurred, the response rate level was lower than 20%. Another issue which affects our study is the fact that more than a half of enrolled studies concerned several countries. Studies from United States of America constituted 37% of all included studies and studies from Poland, Germany, and United Kingdom constituted further 20% when considered together. Additionally it should be mentioned that we included both studies based on national registries (e.g., Germany and Austria or Sweden) and single centre studies. In the major analyses, which we are presenting in this report, we excluded 8 studies due to heterogenous HbA_{1c} guideline values. In our opinion such small number of studies is not representative and analysis of their results would be burdened with high risk of bias. Because we included studies of various designs, from which neither aimed directly to compare groups of different HbA_{1c} guidelines, we found linear regression model weighted by number of participants in each study as most appropriate for our comparisons. We present the results for all comparisons in the Supporting Information. Furthermore, our search was not restricted to studies that contained data on other variables that might have an impact on DMI control. Hence, the results on, for example, acute complications (ketoacidosis and hypoglycemia) were not fully covered in the included papers and our subgroup analysis should be treated with caution. Nevertheless we conducted the analyses on those aspects within representative studies. Only in 5 (4.76%) and in 8 (7.62%) of included studies hypoglycaemia and diabetic ketoacidosis occurred more frequently in comparison to the prevalence reported in the literature. Although this is an ecological study, with its inherent limitations (i.e., cause and effect cannot be proven and confounding factors cannot be eliminated) we attempted to strengthen the data used by employing systematic review techniques to identify and process the published data set that was used for HbA_{1c} levels. By using systematic review techniques for our searches we have attempted to reduce selection and publication biases and by using double data extraction we have reduced possible errors in data collection and analysis. Therefore our study is a robust piece of work for ascertaining the impact of discrepancies between major diabetic associations regarding targeted HbA_{1c} levels in children with type 1 diabetes.

5. Conclusions

Our study shows that the targeted HbA_{1c} level plays an important role in terms of metabolic control in children with type 1 diabetes. The consequences of this observation should be discussed among health care professionals. Target values for HbA_{1c} levels for children and adolescents suffering from type 1 diabetes vary between countries and centres which, in the light of our study, affects metabolic control of the patients and may have an impact on long-term complications in the future. Our study provides a solid basis for rational discussion on the impact of guideline HbA_{1c} values on the metabolic control. According to our findings the "6.5% approach" results in better outcomes, but other factors such as multidisciplinary approach, self-care behaviours, educational models, ethnic or cultural aspects, socioeconomic status, and seasonal variability should be taken into consideration. In our opinion a metaregression of raw data from national registries is warranted as a next step to corroborate our results and finally ascertain the effect of HbA_{1c} guideline values on the metabolic control among children with type 1 diabetes mellitus.

Disclosure

This research received no specific grant from any funding agency in the public, commercial, or not-for-profit sectors.

Conflict of Interests

The authors declare that there is no duality of interest associated with this paper.

Authors' Contribution

Wojciech Mlynarski, Przemyslawa Jarosz-Chobot, Agnieszka Szadkowska, Agnieszka Zmysłowska, and Wojciech Fendler conceived this study. Marcin Braun, Bartlomiej Tomasik, and Ewa Wrona did the searches, selection of studies, data extraction, and statistical analysis. Wojciech Fendler contributed to statistical analysis. Jayne Wilson critically assessed the design and realization of the study. All authors critically reviewed various drafts of the paper, and all authors approved the final version. Wojciech Mlynarski is responsible for the integrity of the work as a whole. Marcin Braun, Bartlomiej Tomasik, and Ewa Wrona contributed equally.

References

[1] ESC Clinical Practice Guidelines, 2013, http://www.escardio.org/Guidelines-&-Education/Clinical-Practice-Guidelines/Diabetes-Pre-Diabetes-and-Cardiovascular-Diseases-developed-with-the-EASD.

[2] Global IDF/ISPAD Guideline for Diabetes in Childhood and Adolescence, 2011, http://www.idf.org/sites/default/files/Diabetes-in-Childhood-and-Adolescence-Guidelines.pdf.

[3] American Diabetes Association, "Standards of medical care in diabetes: children and adolescents," *Diabetes Care*, vol. 38, supplement 1, pp. S70–S76, 2015.

[4] T. Danne, H. B. Mortensen, P. Hougaard et al., "Persistent differences among centers over 3 years in glycemic control and hypoglycemia in a study of 3,805 children and adolescents with type 1 diabetes from the Hvidøre Study Group," *Diabetes Care*, vol. 24, no. 8, pp. 1342–1347, 2001.

[5] The Diabetes Control and Complications Trial Research Group, "The effect of intensive treatment of diabetes on the development and progression of long-term complications in insulin-dependent diabetes mellitus. The Diabetes Control and Complications Trial Research Group," *The New England Journal of Medicine*, vol. 329, pp. 977–986, 1993.

[6] D. M. Nathan, P. A. Cleary, J.-Y. C. Backlund et al., "Intensive diabetes treatment and cardiovascular disease in patients with type 1 diabetes," *The New England Journal of Medicine*, vol. 353, no. 25, pp. 2643–2653, 2005.

[7] K. Dovc, S. S. Telic, L. Lusa et al., "Improved metabolic control in pediatric patients with type 1 diabetes: a nationwide prospective 12-year time trends analysis," *Diabetes Technology and Therapeutics*, vol. 16, no. 1, pp. 33–40, 2014.

[8] D. M. Maahs, J. M. Hermann, S. N. DuBose et al., "Contrasting the clinical care and outcomes of 2,622 children with type 1 diabetes less than 6 years of age in the United States T1D Exchange and German/Austrian DPV registries," *Diabetologia*, vol. 57, no. 8, pp. 1578–1585, 2014.

[9] D. F. Stroup, J. A. Berlin, S. C. Morton et al., "Meta-analysis of observational studies in epidemiology: a proposal for reporting. Meta-analysis of Observational Studies in Epidemiology (MOOSE) group," *Journal of the American Medical Association*, vol. 283, no. 15, pp. 2008–2012, 2000.

[10] NSGP, International Federation of Clinical Chemistry (IFCC) Standardization of HbA1c, 2010, http://www.ngsp.org/docs/IFCCstd.pdf.

[11] Country and Lending Groups, 2015, http://data.worldbank.org/about/country-and-lending-groups#High_income.

[12] Juvenile Diabetes Research Foundation Continuous Glucose Monitoring Study Group, "Effectiveness of continuous glucose monitoring in a clinical care environment: evidence from the Juvenile Diabetes Research Foundation Continuous Glucose Monitoring (JDRF-CGM) trial," *Diabetes Care*, vol. 33, no. 1, pp. 17–22, 2010.

[13] T. R. Rohrer, P. Hennes, A. Thon et al., "Down's syndrome in diabetic patients aged <20 years: an analysis of metabolic status, glycaemic control and autoimmunity in comparison with type 1 diabetes," *Diabetologia*, vol. 53, no. 6, pp. 1070–1075, 2010.

[14] P. Jarosz-Chobot, J. Polańska, M. Myśliwiec et al., "Multicenter cross-sectional analysis of values of glycated haemoglobin (HbA1c) in Polish children and adolescents with long-term type 1 diabetes in Poland: PolPeDiab study group," *Pediatric Endocrinology, Diabetes, and Metabolism*, vol. 18, no. 4, pp. 125–129, 2012.

[15] P. G. F. Swift, T. C. Skinner, C. E. de Beaufort et al., "Target setting in intensive insulin management is associated with metabolic control: the Hvidoere Childhood Diabetes Study Group Centre Differences Study 2005," *Pediatric Diabetes*, vol. 11, no. 4, pp. 271–278, 2010.

[16] B. Karges, J. Rosenbauer, T. Kapellen et al., "Hemoglobin A1c levels and risk of severe hypoglycemia in children and young adults with type 1 diabetes from Germany and Austria: a trend

analysis in a cohort of 37,539 patients between 1995 and 2012," *PLoS Medicine*, vol. 11, no. 10, Article ID e1001742, 2014.

[17] A. Morimoto, Y. Onda, R. Nishimura, H. Sano, K. Utsunomiya, and N. Tajima, "Cause-specific mortality trends in a nationwide population-based cohort of childhood-onset type 1 diabetes in Japan during 35 years of follow-up: the DERI Mortality study," *Diabetologia*, vol. 56, no. 10, pp. 2171–2175, 2013.

[18] M. Boot, L. K. Volkening, D. A. Butler, and L. M. B. Laffel, "The impact of blood glucose and HbA_{1c} goals on glycaemic control in children and adolescents with Type 1 diabetes," *Diabetic Medicine*, vol. 30, no. 3, pp. 333–337, 2013.

[19] T. T. Ly, A. J. M. Brnabic, A. Eggleston et al., "A cost-effectiveness analysis of sensor-augmented insulin pump therapy and automated insulin suspension versus standard pump therapy for hypoglycemic unaware patients with type 1 diabetes," *Value in Health*, vol. 17, no. 5, pp. 561–569, 2014.

[20] M. Stenerson, F. Cameron, D. M. Wilson et al., "The impact of accelerometer and heart rate data on hypoglycemia mitigation in type 1 diabetes," *Journal of Diabetes Science and Technology*, vol. 8, no. 1, pp. 64–69, 2014.

[21] H. B. Mortensen and P. Hougaard, "Comparison of metabolic control in a cross-sectional study of 2,873 children and adolescents with IDDM from 18 countries," *Diabetes Care*, vol. 20, no. 5, pp. 714–720, 1997.

[22] L. Schwartz and D. Drotar, "Defining the nature and impact of goals in children and adolescents with a chronic health condition: a review of research and a theoretical framework," *Journal of Clinical Psychology in Medical Settings*, vol. 13, no. 4, pp. 390–402, 2006.

[23] H. A. Wolpert and B. J. Anderson, "Metabolic control matters: why is the message lost in the translation? The need for realistic goal-setting in diabetes care," *Diabetes Care*, vol. 24, no. 7, pp. 1301–1303, 2001.

[24] F. J. Cameron, T. C. Skinner, C. E. de Beaufort et al., "Are family factors universally related to metabolic outcomes in adolescents with type 1 diabetes?" *Diabetic Medicine*, vol. 25, no. 4, pp. 463–468, 2008.

[25] B. Mianowska, W. Fendler, A. Szadkowska et al., "HbA1c levels in schoolchildren with type 1 diabetes are seasonally variable and dependent on weather conditions," *Diabetologia*, vol. 54, no. 4, pp. 749–756, 2011.

21

Glycaemic Control and Associated Self-Management Behaviours in Diabetic Outpatients: A Hospital Based Observation Study in Lusaka, Zambia

Emmanuel Mwila Musenge,[1] Charles Michelo,[2] Boyd Mudenda,[2] and Alexey Manankov[1]

[1] *Department of Physiological Sciences, School of Medicine, University of Zambia, Ridgeway Campus, P.O. Box 50110, 10101 Lusaka, Zambia*
[2] *Department of Public Health, Section for Epidemiology and Biostatistics, School of Medicine, University of Zambia, Ridgeway Campus, P.O. Box 50110, 10101 Lusaka, Zambia*

Correspondence should be addressed to Emmanuel Mwila Musenge; emmanuel.musenge@unza.zm

Academic Editor: Andrea Tura

Background. The control of *diabetes mellitus* depends on several factors that also include individual lifestyles. We assessed glycaemic control status and self-management behaviours that may influence glycaemic control among diabetic outpatients. *Methods.* This cross-sectional study among 198 consenting randomly selected patients was conducted at the University Teaching Hospital diabetic clinic between September and December 2013 in Lusaka, Zambia. A structured interview schedule was used to collect data on demographic characteristics, self-management behaviours, and laboratory measurements. Binary logistic regression analysis using IBM SPSS for Windows version 20.0 was carried out to predict behaviours that were associated with glycaemic control status. *Results.* The proportion of patients that had good glycaemic control status ($HbA_{1c} \leq 48$ mmol/mol) was 38.7% compared to 61.3% that had poor glycaemic control status ($HbA_{1c} \geq 49$ mmol/mol). Adherence to antidiabetic treatment and fasting plasma glucose predicted glycaemic control status of the patients. However, self-blood glucose monitoring, self-blood glucose monitoring means and exercise did not predict glycaemic control status of the patients. *Conclusion.* We find evidence of poor glycaemic control status among most diabetic patients suggesting that health promotion messages need to take into account both individual and community factors to promote behaviours likely to reduce nonadherence.

1. Introduction

Diabetes mellitus (DM) is a group of metabolic diseases of prolonged hyperglycaemia due to either the pancreas not producing enough insulin, or the cells of the body not responding properly to the insulin produced [1]. It is a major public health problem that is approaching epidemic proportions worldwide [2] and largely associated with lifestyle changes in emerging economies, a double edged sword [3]. The worldwide prevalence of both types 1 and 2 DM among adults was 285 million (6.4%) in 2010 and is predicted to rise to around 439 million (7.8%) by 2030 [4]. Although sub-Saharan Africa has been reported to have an estimated DM adult prevalence of 2.4%, this is probably not just an understatement but the burden is also likely to increase in a few years' time [5].

The progressive nature of the disease requires regular monitoring of glycaemia and, when necessary, intensification of any existing treatment [6]. The most common form of monitoring involves pricking the fingertip to obtain a blood sample, which is tested with a glucometer to determine the patient's blood glucose level. The results from self-glucose monitoring aid the diabetics in decision making on the food, exercise, and use of medications including dose adjustment. This allows diabetics to manage their disease and avoid associated complications of uncontrolled abnormal plasma glucose levels. For type 2 DM, self-management behaviours are an important aspect of management and should be recommended for all diabetic patients. These self-management behaviours include, but are not limited to, adherence and self-blood glucose monitoring (SBGM) as well as exercise and body mass index (BMI) monitoring [7].

One way of monitoring glycaemia reliably is by measuring glycated haemoglobin (HbA_{1c}). Glycated haemoglobin is determined by colorimetry and turbidimetry using the clinical chemistry analyzer. High level of glycated hemoglobin indicates poor control of diabetes and is associated with cardiovascular disease, nephropathy, and retinopathy [8]. Glycated haemoglobin is the primary target of glycaemic control. Measuring HbA_{1c} can be used to reflect average blood glucose levels over the previous 8 to 12 weeks prior to the measurement, thus providing a useful longer-term gauge of glycaemic control [9]. The HbA_{1c} test should be done approximately every 3 months in uncontrolled or at least twice a year in well-controlled diabetic patients.

A number of studies have been conducted among diabetic patients in different parts of the world and most of them aimed to estimate the exact burden and associated factors. In a study by Mahmood and Aamir in Pakistan, over half of the patients had poor diabetic control [10]. Moreira Jr. et al. [11] in Venezuela reported 87% poor glycaemic control status in type 1 and 75% in type 2 diabetic patients. Sobngwi et al. [12] in a six sub-Saharan African countries study revealed that only 29% of the patients had good glycaemic control. The background retinopathy (18%) and cataract (14%) were the most common eye complications while macrovascular disease was rare, and 48% had neuropathy [12]. Erasmus et al. [13] in South Africa reported that 20.1% of patients had good glycaemic control which was associated with obesity. Rwegerera [14] in Tanzania reported 24.2% and 32.9% good glycaemic control using HbA_{1c} and fasting/random blood glucose, respectively.

Satisfaction with current antidiabetic treatment was associated with improved glycaemic control among non-insulin-treated type 2 diabetic patients, but gender and participation in a diabetes education program were not [10, 15]. In addition, adherence to antidiabetic drugs significantly increased with an increase in the number of nondiabetic medications [14]. High cost of medication was significantly associated with antidiabetic treatment nonadherence [14]. Good antidiabetic medication adherence was associated with better glycaemic control, but the results were not statistically significant [11]. Other studies elsewhere revealed poor glycaemic control status in most patients and factors such as treatment satisfaction, gender, treatment adherence, DM knowledge, exercise, and obesity were associated with glycaemic control but multiprofessional care and participation in education programs were not [11, 16, 17]. Most studies did not assess reasons for nonadherence, SBGM, and means as influencers of glycaemic control.

In Zambia, diabetes prevalence is estimated to be at <5% but the associated morbidity and mortality at University Teaching Hospital (UTH) were 7.7% and 20.3%, respectively, in 2010 [18, 19]. The reasons for the increasing morbidity and mortality from DM are unclear although poor or sedentary personal lifestyle could be among the factors contributing to this huge burden. However, there is still scarcity of information on glycaemic control patterns and factors that may be associated with it. The poor glycaemic control among diabetic patients compounded with inadequate self-care in Zambia is such an emerging public health concern needing urgent response.

The health care delivery system in Zambia has a pyramid area based structure, with provision of primary health care (PHC) services in lower health facilities such as health posts (HPs) and health centres (HCs) covering a limited geographical area [18]. The PHC services are supported by the first-, second-, and third-level referral hospitals, through an established referral system. Currently, the hospital referral systems are not working as planned. This is largely due to the insufficient capacities at lower levels, including shortages of health workers, erratic supply of essential drugs and medical supplies, and inequities in the distribution of essential physical infrastructure and equipment to offer services that are appropriate to their level, and also due to the limited scope of services offered by facilities at lower levels [18].

In view of the foregoing, Level two hospitals are forced to operate more as district hospitals, as many patients bypass the HPs and HCs due to the observed capacity challenges. Similarly, Level three (tertiary) hospitals are mainly providing first- and second-level hospital services and this situation amounts to inappropriate use of resources, leading to inefficiencies in service delivery [18]. Thus, rightsizing and strengthening the hospital referral systems would result in reductions in congestion at higher level referral facilities and increase in the efficiency and effectiveness of health service delivery [18].

It is believed that prevention and control strategies need to be multithronged in approach and must encompass both individual and group factors despite the evolving theory of change suggesting that individual factors are very critical and probably more than nonindividual factors [20]. There is evidence of efforts focusing on individual factor such as information, education, and communication on SBGM, exercise, diet, and adherence to antidiabetic treatment. Although these have continued to be emphasised as part of the overall management of DM patients, achieving good glycaemic control has continued to be a challenge and has been considered unattainable among some of the diabetic patients [21].

We aimed to assess the current glycaemic control and self-management behaviours that may affect diabetic control among DM patients attending outpatients diabetic clinic at the UTH in Lusaka, Zambia.

2. Methods

2.1. Design. Data stem from a cross-sectional study, carried out at the UTH diabetic clinic, Lusaka, Zambia. The UTH is the main national referral health centre that treats and reviews patients with various diseases, including DM. The patients attend the diabetic clinic at appointed times as advised by the medical officers for regular monitoring of their disease. All the confirmed diabetic patients on treatment attending outpatients care for at least two years and aged 15 years and above were eligible for the study and newly diagnosed patients that started antidiabetic treatment less than two years were excluded from the study. The patients who agreed to participate in the study provided written informed consent before participating in the study. The study proposal was reviewed and approved by an Independent University of Zambia Biomedical Ethics Committee.

A simple random sampling method was used to accrue eligible consenting patients between September 2013 and December 2013. The sample size and duration of accrual were calculated based on estimated 360 diabetic patients that attend outpatients diabetic clinic and fulfil appointments as well as the proportion of newly referred patients over a four-month period.

Based on Krejcie and Morgan's [22] formula for calculating sample size of a finite population, this gave a calculated sample size of *at least* 186 participants (see sample size calculation below). However, to account for possible exclusions due to refusal to give consent and the need to carry out subgroup analysis, oversampling was ensured to achieve a total of 198 patients who were finally included in the study.

2.2. Sample Size Calculation. We have

$$s = \frac{X^2 NP(1-P)}{d^2(N-1)} + X^2 P(1-P), \quad (1)$$

where s is required sample size. X^2 is the table value of Chi-Square for 1 degree of freedom at the desired confidence level of 0.05 ($1.96^2 = 3.84$) (for 95% CI). N is the population size. P is the population proportion (assumed to be 0.50 since this would provide the maximum sample size). d is the degree of accuracy expressed as a proportion (0.05) (±5% accepted error).

Choose

$$\begin{aligned} X &= 1.96, \\ N &= 360, \\ P &= 0.50, \\ d &= 0.05, \\ s &= \frac{1.96^2 * 360 * 0.5(1-0.5)}{0.05^2(360-1)} + 1.96^2 P(1-0.5), \\ s &= 186. \end{aligned} \quad (2)$$

2.3. Data Collection. General characteristics: a structured interview schedule was used to capture data on demographic characteristics, self-management behaviours, and laboratory results. The interview schedule was developed based on the World Health Organization (WHO) stepwise survey (STEPS) instrument, version three [23]. The same instruments were used on all the patients to ensure reliability and validity. The data on sociodemographic information were collected using a structured interview schedule, and additional data on clinical factors were extracted from medical records and laboratory results of these patients. Thereafter this data was checked for completeness and entered into the EpiData version 3.0.

The weight and height of the patients were measured using a ZT-160 adult weighing mechanical scale model with a height rod (Wuxi Weigher Factory Co., Ltd., Zhejiang, China) whose values were used to compute the BMI based on the formula developed by Lambert Adolphe Jacques Quételet in 1835 [24]. A scientific calculator FX-82ES (CASIO computer company Ltd., Tokyo, Japan) was used to obtain the actual BMI figure by dividing weight in kilograms with height squared in metres which was also verified by the WHO BMI chart [25].

Laboratory measurement (HbA_{1c}): the quantitative determination of HbA_{1c} level in the collected blood from the patients was carried out by the immunoturbidimetry method using the ABX Pentra 400 Automated Clinical Chemistry Analyser (HORIBA ABX SAS, 34184 Montpellier, France), whose technique has been certified by the National Glycohemoglobin Standardisation Program (NGSP) of Australia [26]. The FPG was measured by the enzymatic determination of glucose using the Trinder method using the same analyser [27].

The therapeutic objective of HbA_{1c} has been to obtain values $\leq$ 48 mmol/mol as recommended by the International Diabetes Federation (IDF) and American College of Endocrinology (ACE) and the target for FPG is $\leq$ 6 mmol/L [28].

2.4. Analyses. Statistical analyses were carried out using IBM SPSS Statistics for Windows version 20.0 (IBM Corp., Armonk, NY, USA). The frequencies and descriptive statistics of the variables were calculated. Pearson's Chi-Squared test, Fisher's exact test, and Student's t-test were used to select potential self-management behaviours that may be associated with glycaemic control status. The odds ratio and 95% confidence interval were calculated using multivariate binary logistic regression to identify true potential predictors of glycaemic control while adjusting for confounders. Statistical significance was considered at a P value of less than 0.05.

2.5. Ethics. This study was approved by the University of Zambia Biomedical Research Ethics Committee on reference number 005-07-13. Written informed consent was obtained from all study participants randomly selected which ensured that all eligible persons were given an equal chance to participate or decline. To ensure confidentiality, the interviews were conducted in preselected private spaces within the health facility and participants' identifiers were kept with the hospital in charge as a standard management protocol but they were ultimately delinked from all research documents except through numerical codes. Venipuncture to obtain blood for testing was considered to pose minimal risk and was acceptable to patients as it was considered a standard practice in the disease management. In similar manner, the patients were not given any direct immediate benefits as they were being interviewed within the hospital environment and at the time that they came for routine referral, consultation, monitoring, or review.

3. Results

3.1. Patients' Demographic Characteristics. The demographic characteristics of the patients are shown in Table 1. Of all the

TABLE 1: Demographic characteristics of the patients (n = 198).

Variable	Frequency	Percent
Age		
15–34 years	22	11.1
35–54 years	77	38.9
55 years and above	99	50.0
Total	**198**	**100**
Sex		
Male	79	39.9
Female	119	60.1
Total	**198**	**100**
Education level		
Never/primary	74	37.4
Secondary	92	46.5
College/university	32	16.2
Total	**198**	**100**
*Body mass index (kg/m^2) (n = 190)		
Underweight (≤18.4 kg/m^2)	6	3
Normal (18.5–24.9 kg/m^2)	60	30.3
Overweight (25–29.9 kg/m^2)	70	35.4
Obese (30 or greater kg/m^2)	54	27.3
Total	**190**	**100**

*According to the WHO classification of obesity [29].

patients enrolled for the study (n = 198), median age was 55 years (IQR 45, 62).

3.2. Burden of Diabetes Mellitus. Most (92.9%) of the patients had type 2 DM in contrast to the 7.1% that had type 1 DM. In addition, majority (61.3%) of the patients had poor glycaemic control status and only 38.7% had good glycemic control among those whose data was complete. The mean (SD) FPG of the patients was 9.65 ± 4.96 mmol/L.

3.3. Self-Management Behaviours of the Patients. Most (73.7%) of the patients reported not following the treatment regimen as prescribed (adherence) in contrast to the 52 (26.3%) participants that reported adherence to the type of antidiabetic treatment they were on. Only a few (13.1%) patients reported SBGM at home whereas most (86.1%) of them reported none. Amongst the patients who reported SBGM at home, 13 (6.6%) of the patients reported monitoring glucose control at the public health facility, 2.5% own glucometer, and 4.0% reported glucose monitoring at the private health facility. The majority (59.6%) of the patients were not involved in any type of regular physical exercise.

3.4. Glycaemic Control Status by Characteristics/Self-Management Behaviours. The glycaemic control status of the patients according to the characteristics and self-management behaviours is shown in Table 2. In bivariate analysis, there was an association between glycaemic control status and adherence to treatment and FPG. However, there was no association between age, sex, education, BMI, SBGM, means of SBGM, exercise, and glycaemic control status.

3.5. Predictors of Glycaemic Control Status. The multivariate binary logistic regression model was tested for multicollinearity, Hosmer and Lemeshow test of model fitness for data, and omnibus test of model coefficients and classification accuracy. The dependent variable was glycaemic control status: Good (1) and Poor (0). The results of the multivariate binary logistic regression analysis to predict whether the 9 variable factors, age, sex, education level, BMI, adherence to treatment, SBGM, SBGM means, and exercise, predicted glycaemic control status showed that only adherence to treatment and FPG predicted glycaemic control status of the patients (Table 3). Thus, the patients who do not adhere to antidiabetic treatment and those with mean (SD) FPG, 10.26 ± 5.17 mmol/L, are 68% and 7% less likely to achieve good glycaemic control status (Table 3).

4. Discussion

It is well established that nonadherence rates for chronic disease regimens and for lifestyle changes are generally approximately 50%, and patients with diabetes are particularly prone to regimen adherence problems especially when on multiple treatment regimens including medications, lifestyle, diet, and exercise [30–33]. Consequently, successful management of DM is challenging, yet patients with good self-care behaviours can achieve excellent glycaemic control and avoid frequent diabetic complications.

However, many patients are devoid of optimal self-care behaviours and continue to suffer from complications of the disease. Regular SBGM empowers patients to play a role in the management of diabetes, simultaneously improving their metabolic parameters. Glucometers are frequently used to assess the FPG and the results can prompt and help the patient to adjust the diet (especially carbohydrate intake), exercise, and improve adherence to or modify medication dosage. The consistent use and correct response to the glycaemic results have been shown to improve glycaemic control in type 2 diabetes, consequently preventing or delaying further complications of diabetes [34].

In this study we found evidence of poor glycaemic control which was significantly associated with poor adherence to medication use among diabetic patients that regularly attend medical review at the diabetic clinic. However, poor glycaemic control was not strongly associated with age, sex, education level, SBGM and means of SBGM, exercise, and BMI, associations that have been observed elsewhere [35–37]. While the present study showed higher HbA_{1c} values in patients aged over 54 years as well as those that attained at least secondary education, the results were not statistically significant. However, adherence to antidiabetic treatment and FPG were statistically significantly associated with higher HbA_{1c} values.

These findings are not surprising given that as a developing nation Zambia lacks the resources and capacity to manage this disease which could be associated with adherence [38].

While developed nations have processes, strategies, and infrastructures imbedded in their health care programs, including electronic continuous monitoring technology, that allow medical management of both early and late stage

TABLE 2: Glycaemic control status by characteristics/self-management behaviours of the participants at the University Teaching Hospital.

Characteristic/self-management behavior	Glycaemic control status: Good (n = 75, $HbA_{1c} \leq 48$ mmol/mol) No (%)	Glycaemic control status: Poor (n = 119, $HbA_{1c} \geq 49$ mmol/mol) No (%)	P value*
Age[a]			
15–34 years	4 (19.0)	17 (81.0)	
35–54 years	29 (38.2)	47 (61.8)	0.117
55 years and above	42 (43.3)	55 (56.7)	
Sex[a]			
Male	29 (38.2)	47 (61.8)	
Female	46 (39.0)	72 (61.0)	0.908
Education level[a]			
Never/primary	27 (36.5)	47 (63.5)	
Secondary	33 (37.5)	55 (62.5)	0.575
College/university	15 (46.9)	17 (53.1)	
Adherence[a] (N = 192)			
No	44 (30.8)	99 (69.2)	
Yes	31 (60.8)	20 (39.2)	**0.000**
SBGM[a]			
No	63 (37.5)	105 (62.5)	
Yes	12 (46.2)	14 (53.8)	0.399
SBGM means[b]			
Owning glucometer	3 (60.0)	2 (40.0)	
Public health facility	6 (46.2)	7 (53.8)	0.686
Private health facility	3 (37.5)	5 (62.5)	
Not applicable	63 (37.5)	105 (62.5)	
Exercise[a]			
No	47 (41.2)	67 (58.8)	
Yes	28 (35.0)	52 (65.0)	0.381
BMI (kg/m^2)[b] (N = 186)			
Underweight (≤18.4)	1 (16.7)	5 (83.3)	
Normal (18.5–24.9)	17 (30.4)	39 (69.6)	
Overweight (25–29.9)	31 (44.3)	39 (55.7)	0.306
Obese (≥30)	22 (40.7)	32 (59.3)	
FPG (mmol/L; mean, SD)[c]	8.47 (3.88)	10.26 (5.17)	**0.011**

[a]Pearson's Chi-Squared test, [b]Fisher's exact test, and [c]Student's t-test. *Significant P value at $P < 0.05$, SBGM: self-blood glucose monitoring, BMI: body mass index, FPG: fasting plasma glucose, and SD: standard deviation.

TABLE 3: Multivariate binary logistic regression model-determining predictors of glycaemic control status.

Predictor variable	Glycaemic control status: Good (n = 75, $HbA_{1c} \leq 48$ mmol/mol) No (%)	Glycaemic control status: Poor (n = 119, $HbA_{1c} \geq 49$ mmol/mol) No (%)	AOR (95% CI)	P value*
Adherence				
No	44 (30.8)	99 (69.2)	0.32 (0.16–0.63)	**0.001**
Yes	31 (60.8)	20 (39.2)	Ref (1.00)	
Current FPG (mmol/L; mean, SD)	8.47 (3.88)	10.26 (5.17)	0.93 (0.86–1.00)	**0.046**

HbA_{1c}: glycated haemoglobin, FPG: fasting plasma glucose, SD: standard deviation, Ref: reference category, mmol/L: millimoles per litre, and mmol/mol: millimoles per mole. *Significant P value at $P < 0.05$. AOR: adjusted odds ratio; CI: confidence interval.

disease, developing nations have inadequate capability to manage and reverse the increasing morbidity and mortality [39]. This association with adherence to antidiabetic treatment and FPG observed in this study is a common problem among individuals with diabetes [40–43]. It is therefore necessary to determine the effective behavioural interventions that can improve adherence in the Zambian diabetic patients. Consequently, this study has persuaded us to consider a focus for a changed interventional approach targeting selected factors including patient centered approaches such as understanding patient insight of the disease, and collaborative and clear communication between health care professionals and patients could impact positively on glycaemic control in these patients.

Firstly, we are aware that this was a cross-sectional study and therefore it is difficult to establish a "causal" relation between HbA_{1c} and the self-management behaviours.

Secondly, we also acknowledge that this was a small and highly selected sample from a frame of hospital attendees at a referral tertiary hospital. This limitation was augmented by the fact that the cost of purchasing laboratory materials and supplies for the study provided additional sample size limitations.

Thirdly and in addition, we also observe that there could be additional biological individual variations which could potentially bias our measurements.

Fourthly and lastly though not the least, we also report that there was incomplete data on medical records of the diabetic outpatients at the clinic, making it difficult to follow the morbidity and mortality patterns and thus reducing further the possible sample which would have improved the study power and understanding of possible determinants.

Notwithstanding the possible presence of such selection and measurement biases, we do not think these could have been important in explaining the findings as their effects are assumed to have been non-differentially distributed given the random selection of subjects that was used.

In Zambia the mortality of patients with type 2 DM is likely to continue to increase as the Zambian economy improves a factor associated with increase in western life style including diet and sedentary way of life [44]. A needs' assessment for the Noncommunicable Disease program carried out by the MoH identified deficiencies in diabetic control as having inadequacies in terms of drugs and laboratory reagents, diagnostic facilities, expertise, and community awareness for DM [18]. It may thus be not surprising to find presence of individual factors associated with poor glycaemic control status where we further argue that these are also associated with not only system supply factors but also social factors, predominantly operating at an individual level. Consequently, there is need to define DM disease burden and epidemiology with focus on determinants and thus determine potential strategies that could address these inadequacies and improve the disease outcome.

The majority of diabetic outpatients in this study had poor glycaemic control status and this could be due to a variety of factors including lack of resources and ability to buy diabetic chips and strips that allow for more frequent checks of FPG levels and/or ability to have adequate resources to store, for example, the insulin in a refrigerator which is frequently not available to many Zambians [45]. The reasons for this were not the focus of this paper and so we may only speculate regarding possible reasons for these differential glycaemic control status associations. We, however, disagree with what other evidence suggest that this can also probably be because of poor diet and exercise habits and other multiple barriers [46]. However, good glycaemic control was reported in Japan and Germany also and it has been argued that perhaps this is because of higher literacy levels in these countries resulting in improved knowledge translation about DM [47, 48].

It was interesting to note that there was a statistically significant association between adherence to antidiabetic treatment and glycaemic control status of the diabetic outpatients in this study.

This is important given that the effectiveness of drug treatment depends primarily on the efficacy of the prescribed treatment and adherence of the patient to the treatment [49]. These findings have been supported by studies elsewhere which have shown that adherence to antidiabetic treatment among diabetic patients is poor and the possible reasons have been outlined. One of the reasons is simply failure to understand and consequently failure to comply with the prescribed clinical regimen, thereby resulting in very poor outcomes [40].

In the present study, this was illustrated clearly where we observed that the diabetic outpatients who did not adhere to DM treatment had 68% decrease in the likelihood of achieving good glycaemic control status compared to those who adhered. In similar manner, in the study by Ahmad et al. [35] in Malaysia, 53.0% of the patients were nonadherent to DM treatment and the main factor which was associated with that nonadherence was age. In another study by Curkendall et al. [50] in the US, it revealed that only 45% of the patients were adherent to DM treatment. The adherence was high in the males, older patients, or patients residing in specific geographical area. The factors related to poor adherence were comorbidity, overall health level, number of drugs, and complexity of the drug regimen [51].

There is thus a critical need to understand adherence related factors so as to design prevention and control strategies that will be operable but accounting for contextual differentials even across low income countries in general. If adherence is improved this could positively improve lives of these clients. In fact, some studies have shown that an increase in adherence by as little as 10% can decrease the levels of HbA_{1c} significantly [35, 51]. Such increase is possible if behavioural linked factors such as education attainment, which has already been shown to improve glycaemic control status, are targeted [51, 52], However, tackling nonadherence is not a simple matter, as it is multifactorial and might include cost adjustments, health belief transformations, dosing frequency repackaging, and assessment of the presence of potential confounders associated with personality disorders and patient-provider relationship [40].

There is need to explore the effective behavioural interventions that can improve adherence to antidiabetic treatment among the diabetic patients in Zambia. Changing interventional approaches targeting selected factors including patient centered approaches such as understanding patient insight of the disease and collaborative and clear communication between health care professionals and patients could impact positively on glycaemic control in diabetic patients. Thus, the role of diabetic patients in the management of their diabetes remains paramount.

If this matter is critically managed, it is possible that the outcome of treatment would be much more satisfactory among diabetic outpatients and this could possibly delay the development of the complications of DM and improve the quality and length of lives for the affected individuals. There is thus need to institute prevention and control mechanism that are cost-effective, acceptable, and appropriate. Thus, combined screening with FPG and HbA_{1c} used in this study may identify patients at very high risk for diabetes when FPG and HbA_{1c} are considered together.

5. Conclusion

We conclude that, among diabetic patients, poor glycaemic control remains a challenge and this may to a greater extent be associated with "adherence to antidiabetic treatment" related factors. This may suggest limitations in past prevention and control efforts for DM at individual level as well as at care level where monitoring dynamics are limited as these patients are largely outpatients except when they are admitted to hospital for one reason or another. However, finding that FPG predicted the glycaemic control opens potential opportunities to routinely examine and identify most at risk groups, which in turn and further opens possibilities to study the associated dynamics linked to care and support. This could in turn therefore inform interventional policies and control strategies and thus improve the overall care and support of such patients. In addition, this may also be important to identify prediabetic states.

Furthermore, and given that the self-management behaviours of diabetic patients play an important role in the management of DM, there is thus need to target improvement of the efficacy of individual strategies in all prevention and control strategies for these patients.

We further argue that if this is done properly, it may consequently reduce diabetic complications and thus improve the lives of these people. The health care providers also are critical stakeholders and need to foster and place greater emphasis on counselling and improving adherence, notwithstanding the context specific differences.

Conflict of Interests

The authors declare that there is no conflict of interests regarding the publication of this paper.

Authors' Contribution

Emmanuel Mwila Musenge conceived the study. Emmanuel Mwila Musenge, Alexey Manankov, Boyd Mudenda, and Charles Michelo designed the study. Emmanuel Mwila Musenge conducted and analysed the data and wrote the paper. Alexey Manankov, Boyd Mudenda, and Charles Michelo supervised the whole study process, including the writing of the paper. All the authors read and approved the final paper. All the authors contributed equally and as stated in the paper.

Acknowledgments

The authors appreciate the University of Zambia through the Staff Development Office through the Medical Education Partnership Initiative (MEPI), for partially sponsoring the study. The authors also acknowledge faculty in Departments of Physiological Sciences and Public Health, staff at the MoH through the Managing Director, UTH for permission to conduct the study in their facilities, and Southern Africa Consortium for Research Excellence (SACORE) and Research Support Centre for guidance on data analysis. Special thanks also go to all the staff in the Department of Internal Medicine, Diabetic Clinic, and Clinical Chemistry Laboratories of the UTH for the guidance and support. Lastly, the research assistants and the participants are acknowledged for the cooperation during the study.

References

[1] World Health Organization, *Diabetes Fact Sheet No312*, World Health Organization, 2013.

[2] S. A. Tabish, "Is diabetes becoming the biggest epidemic of the twenty-first century?" *International Journal of Health Sciences*, vol. 1, no. 2, pp. 5–5, 2007.

[3] D. Cheng, "Prevalence, predisposition and prevention of type II diabetes," *Nutrition & Metabolism*, vol. 2, article 29, 2005.

[4] R. Sicree, J. Shaw, and P. Zimmert, "Heart and Diabetes Institute, the global burden: diabetes and impaired glucose," in *International Diabetes Federation: Diabetes Atlas*, vol. 4, International Diabetes Federation, 2010.

[5] International Diabetes Federation, *International Diabetes Federation Diabetes Atlas*, vol. 6, International Diabetes Federation, 2013.

[6] M. E. Cox and D. Edelman, "Tests for screening and diagnosis of type 2 diabetes," *Clinical Diabetes*, vol. 27, no. 4, pp. 132–138, 2009.

[7] A. Hartz, S. Kent, P. James, Y. Xu, M. Kelly, and J. Daly, "Factors that influence improvement for patients with poorly controlled type 2 diabetes," *Diabetes Research and Clinical Practice*, vol. 74, no. 3, pp. 227–232, 2006.

[8] M. L. Larsen, M. Hørder, and E. F. Mogensen, "Effect of long-term monitoring of glycosylated hemoglobin levels in insulin-dependent diabetes mellitus," *The New England Journal of Medicine*, vol. 323, no. 15, pp. 1021–1025, 1990.

[9] L. Roszyk, B. Faye, V. Sapin, F. Somda, and I. Tauveron, "Glycated haemoglobin (HbA1c): today and tomorrow," *Annales d'Endocrinologie*, vol. 68, no. 5, pp. 357–365, 2007.

[10] K. Mahmood and A. H. Aamir, "Glycemic control status in patients with type-2 diabetes," *Journal of the College of Physicians and Surgeons Pakistan*, vol. 15, no. 6, pp. 323–325, 2005.

[11] E. D. Moreira Jr., R. C. S. Neves, Z. O. Nunes et al., "Glycemic control and its correlates in patients with diabetes in Venezuela:

results from a nationwide survey," *Diabetes Research and Clinical Practice*, vol. 87, no. 3, pp. 407–414, 2010.

[12] E. Sobngwi, M. Ndour-Mbaye, K. A. Boateng et al., "Type 2 diabetes control and complications in specialised diabetes care centres of six sub-Saharan African countries: the Diabcare Africa study," *Diabetes Research and Clinical Practice*, vol. 95, no. 1, pp. 30–36, 2012.

[13] R. T. Erasmus, E. Blanco Blanco, A. B. Okesina, Z. Gqweta, and T. Matsha, "Assessment of glycaemic control in stable type 2 black South African diabetics attending a peri-urban clinic," *Postgraduate Medical Journal*, vol. 75, no. 888, pp. 603–606, 1999.

[14] G. M. Rwegerera, "Adherence to anti-diabetic drugs among patients with Type 2 diabetes mellitus at Muhimbili National Hospital, Dar es Salaam, Tanzania—a cross-sectional study," *Pan African Medical Journal*, vol. 17, article 252, 2014.

[15] A. B. V. Mendes, J. A. S. Fittipaldi, R. C. S. Neves, A. R. Chacra, and E. D. Moreira Jr., "Prevalence and correlates of inadequate glycaemic control: results from a nationwide survey in 6,671 adults with diabetes in Brazil," *Acta Diabetologica*, vol. 47, no. 2, pp. 137–145, 2010.

[16] N. S. Ahmad, F. Islahudin, and T. Paraidathathu, "Factors associated with good glycemic control among patients with type 2 diabetes mellitus," *Journal of Diabetes Investigation*, vol. 5, no. 5, pp. 563–569, 2014.

[17] Z. Ghazanfari, S. Niknami, F. Ghofranipour, B. Larijani, H. Agha-Alinejad, and A. Montazeri, "Determinants of glycemic control in female diabetic patients: a study from Iran. In Roszyk, L. et al. Glycated haemoglobin (HbA1c): today and tomorrow," *Annales d'Endocrinologie*, vol. 68, pp. 357–365, 2010.

[18] Ministry of Health, *National Health Strategic Plan 2011–2015: Towards Attainment of Health Related Millennium Development Goals*, Ministry of Health, 2010.

[19] University Teaching Hospital, *University Teaching Hospital Action Plan 2009/2010: Health Management Information System*, University Teaching Hospital, Lusaka, Zambia, 2010.

[20] J. Michel, C. Matlakala, R. English, R. Lessells, and M.-L. Newell, "Collective patient behaviours derailing ART roll-out in KwaZulu-Natal: perspectives of health care providers," *AIDS Research and Therapy*, vol. 10, article 20, 2013.

[21] E. A. Nyenwe, T. W. Jerkins, G. E. Umpierrez, and A. E. Kitabchi, "Management of type 2 diabetes: evolving strategies for the treatment of patients with type 2 diabetes," *Metabolism*, vol. 60, no. 1, pp. 1–23, 2011.

[22] R. V. Krejcie and D. W. Morgan, "Determining sample size for research activities," *Educational and Psychological Measurement*, vol. 30, pp. 607–610, 1970.

[23] World Health Organization, *World Health Organization STEPwise Approach to Chronic Disease Risk Factor Surveillance (STEPS) Instrument*, Version 3, World Health Organization, 2007.

[24] G. Eknoyan, "Adolphe quetelet (1796-1874)—the average man and indices of obesity," *Nephrology Dialysis Transplantation*, vol. 23, no. 1, pp. 47–51, 2008.

[25] World Health Organization, "BMI classification," Global Database on BMI, World Health Organization, 2006.

[26] D. B. Sacks, "Carbohydrates," in *TIETZ Textbook of Clinical Chemistry and Molecular Diagnostics*, C. A. Burtis, E. R. Ashood, and D. E. Burns, Eds., p. 884, Saunders Elsevier, St. Louis, Mo, USA, 2006.

[27] K. Arvind, K. M. Rajiv, and S. R. Sudhanshu, "Studies on impact of industrial pollution on biochemical and histological changes in a catfish, mystus vittatus (Bloch)," in *Industrial Pollution and Management*, A. Kumar, Ed., vol. 9, APH Publishing, 2004.

[28] International Diabetes Federation, *International Diabetes Federation Atlas*, International Diabetes Federation, 4th edition, 2009.

[29] World Health Organization, *Preventing Chronic Diseases: A Vital Investment*, World Health Organization, Geneva, Switzerland, 2010.

[30] R. E. Glasgow, K. D. McCaul, and L. C. Schafer, "Self-care behaviors and glycemic control in type I diabetes," *Journal of Chronic Diseases*, vol. 40, no. 5, pp. 399–412, 1987.

[31] S. M. S. Kurtz, "Adherence to diabetes regimens: empirical status and clinical applications," *The Diabetes Educator*, vol. 16, no. 1, pp. 50–56, 1990.

[32] R. L. Kravitz, R. D. Hays, C. D. Sherbourne et al., "Recall of recommendations and adherence to advice among patients with chronic medical conditions," *Archives of Internal Medicine*, vol. 153, no. 16, pp. 1869–1878, 1993.

[33] R. M. Anderson, J. T. Fitzgerald, and M. S. Oh, "The relationship between diabetes-related attitudes and patients' self-reported adherence," *The Diabetes Educator*, vol. 19, no. 4, pp. 287–292, 1993.

[34] S. Allemann, C. Houriet, P. Diem, and C. Stettler, "Self-monitoring of blood glucose in non-insulin treated patients with type 2 diabetes: a systematic review and meta-analysis," *Current Medical Research and Opinion*, vol. 25, no. 12, pp. 2903–2914, 2009.

[35] N. S. Ahmad, A. Ramli, and T. Paraidathathu, "Medication adehrence in atients with type 2 diabetes mellitus treated at primary health clinics in Malaysia," *Dovepress*, vol. 7, pp. 525–530, 2013.

[36] J. H. M. Quah, Y. P. Liu, N. Luo, C. H. How, and E. G. Tay, "Younger adult type 2 diabetic patients have poorer glycaemic control: a cross-sectional study in a primary care setting in Singapore," *BMC Endocrine Disorders*, vol. 13, article 18, 2013.

[37] Y. Bi, D. Zhu, J. Cheng et al., "The status of glycemic control: a cross-sectional study of outpatients with type 2 diabetes mellitus across primary, secondary, and tertiary hospitals in the jiangsu province of China," *Clinical Therapeutics*, vol. 32, no. 5, pp. 973–983, 2010.

[38] A. Mario and A. Sridevi, "Diabetes in sub-saharan Africa: Kenya, Mali, Mozambique, Nigeria, South Africa and Zambia," *International Journal of Diabetes in Developing Countries*, vol. 28, no. 4, pp. 101–108, 2008.

[39] K. Makrilakis and N. Katsilambros, "Prediction and prevention of type 2 diabetes," *HORMONES*, vol. 2, no. 1, pp. 22–34, 2003.

[40] S. B. Leichter, "Making outpatient care of diabetes more efficient: analyzing noncompliance," *Clinical Diabetes*, vol. 23, no. 4, pp. 187–190, 2005.

[41] J. N. Kalyango, E. Owino, and A. P. Nambuya, "Non-adherence to diabetic treatment at Mulgo Hospital in Uganda: prevalence and associated factors," *African Health Sciences*, vol. 8, no. 2, pp. 67–73, 2008 (Portuguese).

[42] K. Inoue, M. Matsumoto, and Y. Kobayashi, "The combination of fasting plasma glucose and glycosylated hemoglobin predicts type 2 diabetes in Japanese workers," *Diabetes Research and Clinical Practice*, vol. 77, no. 3, pp. 451–458, 2007.

[43] G. Bozkaya, E. Ozgu, and B. Karaca, "The association between estimated average glucose levels and fasting plasma glucose levels," *Clinics*, vol. 65, no. 11, pp. 1077–1080, 2010.

[44] R. BeLue, T. A. Okoror, J. Iwelunmor et al., "An overview of cardiovascular risk factor burden in sub-Saharan African countries: a socio-cultural perspective," *Globalization and Health*, vol. 5, article 10, 2009.

[45] D. Beran, J. S. Yudkin, and M. de Courten, "Access to care for patients with insulin-requiring diabetes in developing countries: case studies of Mozambique and Zambia," *Diabetes Care*, vol. 28, no. 9, pp. 2136–2140, 2005.

[46] R. L. Rothman, S. Mulvaney, T. A. Elasy et al., "Self-management behaviors, racial disparities, and glycemic control among adolescents with type 2 diabetes," *Pediatrics*, vol. 121, no. 4, pp. e912–e919, 2008.

[47] V. Reisig, P. Reitmeir, A. Döing, W. Rathmann, and A. Mielck, "Social inequalities and outcomes in type 2 diabetes in the German region of Augsburg. A cross-sectional survey," *International Journal of Public Health*, vol. 52, no. 3, pp. 158–165, 2007.

[48] K. Arai, K. Hirao, I. Matsuba et al., "The status of glycemic control by general practitioners and specialists for diabetes in Japan: a cross-sectional survey of 15,652 patients with diabetes mellitus," *Diabetes Research and Clinical Practice*, vol. 83, no. 3, pp. 397–401, 2009.

[49] H. Knobel, A. Carmona, S. Grau, J. Pedro-Botet, and A. Diez, "Adherence and effectiveness of highly active antiretroviral therapy," *Archives of Internal Medicine*, vol. 158, no. 17, pp. 1949–1953, 1998.

[50] S. M. Curkendall, N. Thomas, K. F. Bell, P. L. Juneau, and A. J. Weiss, "Predictors of medication adherence in patients with type 2 diabetes mellitus," *Current Medical Research and Opinion*, vol. 29, no. 10, pp. 1275–1286, 2013.

[51] V. W. Y. Lee and P. Y. Leung, "Glycemic control and medication compliance in diabetic patients in a pharmacist-managed clinic in Hong Kong," *American Journal of Health-System Pharmacy*, vol. 60, no. 24, pp. 2593–2596, 2003.

[52] Y. Bezie, M. Molina, N. Hernandez, R. Batista, S. Niang, and D. Huet, "Therapeutic compliance: a prospective analysis of various factors involved in the adherence rate in type 2 diabetes," *Diabetes & Metabolism*, vol. 32, no. 6, pp. 611–616, 2006.

22

Noninsulin Antidiabetic Drugs for Patients with Type 2 Diabetes Mellitus: Are We Respecting Their Contraindications?

Irene Ruiz-Tamayo,[1,2] Josep Franch-Nadal,[2,3,4] Manel Mata-Cases,[2,4,5] Dídac Mauricio,[2,4,6] Xavier Cos,[2,7] Antonio Rodriguez-Poncelas,[2,8] Joan Barrot,[2,9] Gabriel Coll-de-Tuero,[2,8] and Xavier Mundet-Tudurí[2,10,11]

[1] *Primary Health Care Center La Torrassa, Consorci Sanitari Integral, Ronda Torrassa 151-153, 08903 L'Hospitalet de Llobregat, Spain*
[2] *DAP-Cat Group, Unitat de Suport a la Recerca Barcelona Ciutat, Institut Universitari d'Investigació en Atenció Primària Jordi Gol (IDIAP Jordi Gol), Sardenya 375, 08006 Barcelona, Spain*
[3] *Primary Health Care Center Raval Sud, Gerència d'Àmbit d'Atenció Primària Barcelona Ciutat, Institut Català de la Salut, Avinguda Drassanes 17-21, 08001 Barcelona, Spain*
[4] *CIBER of Diabetes and Associated Metabolic Diseases (CIBERDEM), Instituto de Salud Carlos III (ISCIII), Monforte de Lemos 3-5, 28029 Madrid, Spain*
[5] *Primary Health Care Center La Mina, Gerència d'Àmbit d'Atenció Primària Barcelona Ciutat, Institut Català de la Salut, Mar S/N, 08930 Sant Adrià de Besòs, Spain*
[6] *Department of Endocrinology & Nutrition, Health Sciences Research Institute and Hospital Universitari Germans Trias i Pujol, Carretera Canyet S/N, 08916 Badalona, Spain*
[7] *Primary Health Care Center Sant Martí de Provençals, Gerència d'Àmbit d'Atenció Primària Barcelona Ciutat, Institut Català de la Salut, Fluvià 211, 08020 Barcelona, Spain*
[8] *Primary Health Care Center Anglès, Gerència d'Àmbit d'Atenció Primària Girona, Institut Català de la Salut, Carretera de Girona S/N, 17160 Anglès, Spain*
[9] *Primary Health Care Center Salt, Gerència d'Àmbit d'Atenció Primària Girona, Institut Català de la Salut, Manel de Falla 35, 17190 Salt, Spain*
[10] *Primary Health Care Center El Carmel, Gerència d'Àmbit d'Atenció Primària Barcelona Ciutat, Institut Català de la Salut, Murtra 130, 08032 Barcelona, Spain*
[11] *Autonomous University of Barcelona, Campus de Bellaterra, 08193 Bellaterra, Spain*

Correspondence should be addressed to Josep Franch-Nadal; josep.franch@gmail.com

Academic Editor: Simona Bo

Aim. To assess prescribing practices of noninsulin antidiabetic drugs (NIADs) in T2DM with several major contraindications according to prescribing information or clinical guidelines: renal failure, heart failure, liver dysfunction, or history of bladder cancer. *Methods.* Cross-sectional, descriptive, multicenter study. Electronic medical records were retrieved from all T2DM subjects who attended primary care centers pertaining to the Catalan Health Institute in Catalonia in 2013 and were pharmacologically treated with any NIAD alone or in combination. *Results.* Records were retrieved from a total of 255,499 pharmacologically treated patients. 78% of patients with some degree of renal impairment (glomerular filtration rate (GFR) < 60 mL/min) were treated with metformin and 31.2% with sulfonylureas. Even in the event of severe renal failure (GFR < 30 mL/min), 35.3% and 22.5% of patients were on metformin or sulfonylureas, respectively. Moreover, metformin was prescribed to more than 60% of patients with moderate or severe heart failure. *Conclusion.* Some NIADs, and in particular metformin, were frequently used in patients at high risk of complications when they were contraindicated. There is a need to increase awareness of potential inappropriate prescribing and to monitor the quality of prescribing patterns in order to help physicians and policymakers to yield better clinical outcomes in T2DM.

1. Introduction

Lifestyle modification, primarily through diet, and exercise advise are the preferred therapeutic approaches in the initial treatment of type 2 diabetes mellitus (T2DM). However, the disease tends to progress and most patients will be required to start on oral medication to maintain individualized glycemic targets. Noninsulin antidiabetic drugs (NIADs) are typically the first option for initial pharmacotherapy and include different classes of drugs with diverse modes of action, therapeutic potency, and adverse reactions [1].

Some NIADs have contraindications or must be used with caution in patients with T2DM and particular comorbid conditions. Major at-risk conditions that require tailored management of hyperglycemia include heart failure, chronic kidney disease, liver dysfunction, or history of bladder cancer. Moderate to severe renal impairment, for instance, is present in 20–40% of T2DM patients [2–4], which requires careful evaluation of risks and benefits when prescribing antihyperglycemic drugs with renal clearance. In addition, the prevalence of chronic heart failure in T2DM is 10–23%, and they have 2-fold greater risk of heart failure than their nondiabetic counterparts [5]. Suboptimal glycemic control is a predictor for its development [6]; furthermore, some glucose-lowering agents may be associated with an increased risk of heart failure [7]. Finally, T2DM patients also have an increased prevalence of the entire spectrum of liver disease, from abnormal liver enzyme levels to acute liver failure, and the use of particular antihyperglycemic agents must be avoided or they must be used with caution due to altered drug metabolism and/or hepatotoxicity [8].

Besides prescribing information enclosed in the package insert or the summary of product characteristics (SmPC), which list the labels and contraindications of each particular drug, local health authorities, international expert consensus documents, and clinical guidelines regularly publish recommendations on the use of antidiabetic drugs and indicate in which comorbid conditions they are formally contraindicated [9–12].

The appropriate use of NIADs in accordance with prescribing information or recommendations is of great importance to preserve or increase quality of life, particularly in patients with comorbid disease conditions [13]. However, a poor adherence to local and/or international guidelines on T2DM management has been reported in both primary and secondary care settings, and inappropriate or potentially inappropriate prescription of NIADs to patients with a contraindication or precautionary condition has also been documented [14–19].

The aim of this study was to investigate prescribing patterns of NIADs in a primary care setting in Catalonia, Spain, in patients with some at-risk comorbid conditions and assessed whether treatment choices agreed with the current drug's prescribing information, recommendations of expert consensus documents, or clinical guidelines when they are formally contraindicated or recommended to be used with caution.

2. Methods

2.1. Design. This was a cross-sectional, descriptive, multicenter study including all type 2 diabetes subjects between 31 and 90 years of age who attended any of the 274 primary care centers pertaining to the Catalan Health Institute (ICS) in Catalonia, Spain, in 2013. Electronic medical records were retrieved from the SIDIAP database (System for the Development of Research in Primary Care) as previously reported [4, 20]. Subjects were included in the study if they had a T2DM diagnosis (ICD-10 codes E11, E11.0–E11.9, E14, or E14.0–E14.9) in the electronic clinical record and were prescribed pharmacological treatment with any NIAD in monotherapy or in combination. Those patients exclusively treated with lifestyle modification or insulin as monotherapy were excluded.

2.2. Studied Variables. The study included data on age; gender; duration of T2DM; standardized glycated hemoglobin (HbA1c) values, using the most recent value of the preceding 15 months; and risk factors and diabetic complications, including body mass index (BMI) (most recent value in the last 24 months), microvascular complications (diabetic retinopathy, nephropathy or neuropathy), and macrovascular complications (coronary artery disease, recent myocardial infarction of a duration less than 1 year, stroke, peripheral artery disease, and heart failure). Pharmacological treatments were extracted from prescription- and pharmacy-invoicing data provided by the CatSalut general database and included the use of any NIADs as monotherapy or in combination with other glucose-lowering drugs (e.g., insulin) licensed at that time in Spain, namely, metformin, sulfonylureas, meglitinides, alpha-glucosidase inhibitors (AGIs), pioglitazone, dipeptidyl peptidase-4 inhibitors (DPP-4i), and glucagon-like peptide-1 receptor agonists (GLP-1ra).

The following major conditions were considered a potential contraindication for some drugs based on the summary of product characteristics (SmPC), international expert consensus documents, or clinical guidelines: (i) renal failure, defined as a glomerular filtration rate (GFR) $< 60\,\mathrm{mL/min/1.73\,m^2}$, and severe renal failure (GFR $< 30\,\mathrm{mL/min/1.73\,m^2}$), estimated with the Chronic Kidney Disease Epidemiology Collaboration (CKD-EPI) equation [21]; (ii) liver dysfunction, defined as hepatic enzymes over 3 times the upper limit of normal levels (either glutamyl oxaloacetic transaminase (GOT) or glutamyl pyruvic transaminase (GPT) > 120 IU/L or gamma-glutamyl transferase (GGT) > 150 IU/L); (iii) heart failure (globally and New York Heart Association (NYHA) class III or IV) functional stage [22]; and (iv) history of bladder cancer.

This study was approved by the Ethics Committee of the Primary Health Care University Research Institute (IDIAP) Jordi Gol.

2.3. Statistical Analysis. Descriptive analyses were summarized by mean and standard deviation for continuous variables and absolute frequency and percentages for categorical variables. All statistical calculations were performed using

TABLE 1: Demographic and clinical characteristics of T2DM patients included in the study.

Characteristic	$N = 255{,}499$
Age, mean (SD), years	68.0 (11.0)
Gender, n (%)	
Female	114,181 (44.7%)
Male	141,318 (55.3%)
T2DM duration, mean (SD), years	8.0 (5.6)
HbA1c, mean (SD), %*	7.3 (1.4)
BMI, mean (SD), kg/m^2	30.3 (5.2)
Renal failure (GFR < 60 mL/min), n (%)†	40,666 (20.1%)
Severe renal failure (GFR < 30 mL/min), n (%)†	2,014 (1.0%)
Complications, n (%)	
Patients with registered severe hypoglycemia episodes	463 (0.2%)
Diabetic retinopathy	19,857 (7.8%)
ACR > 300 mg/g	6,661 (2.6%)
Diabetic neuropathy	7,509 (2.9%)
Ischemic heart disease	31,145 (12.2%)
Stroke	15,158 (5.9%)
Peripheral artery disease	12,295 (4.8%)
Heart failure	13,276 (5.2%)
Any macrovascular complication	51,007 (20.0%)
Glucose-lowering treatment, alone or in combination, n (%)	
Metformin	225,753 (88.4%)
Sulfonylureas	79,472 (31.1%)
Meglitinides	16,941 (6.6%)
AGIs	1,877 (0.7%)
Pioglitazone	3,290 (1.3%)
DPP4i	39,682 (15.5%)
GLP-1ra	2,374 (0.9%)
Insulin with a NIAD	46,150 (18.1%)

*Out of 199,523 patients with available HbA1c records.
†Out of 195,674 patients with available GFR records.
ACR: albumin/creatinin ratio; AGI: alpha-glucosidase inhibitors; BMI: body mass index; DPP4i: dipeptidyl peptidase-4 (DPP-4) inhibitors; GLP-1ra: glucagon-like peptide-1 (GLP-1) receptor agonists; GFR: glomerular filtration rate; HbA1c: glycated hemoglobin; NIAD: noninsulin antidiabetic drug; SD: standard deviation; T2DM: type 2 diabetes mellitus.

StataCorp 2009 (Stata Statistical Software: Release 11. College Station, TX: StataCorp, LP).

3. Results

Clinical and demographic characteristics of the patients included in the study are shown in Table 1. Records were retrieved from a total of 255,499 patients with T2DM who during 2013 were prescribed antidiabetic pharmacological treatment based on a NIAD alone or in combination. The mean age of the patients was 68.0 years (standard deviation (SD) = 11.0), with a mean duration of T2DM of 8.0 years (SD = 5.6). The most common NIADs prescribed in pharmacologically treated cases were metformin (in 88.4% of patients), sulfonylureas (31.1%), and DPP4i (15.5%).

The clinical and demographic characteristics of the treated patients stratified by the pharmacological class of the glucose-lowering agent prescribed (alone or in combination) are shown in Table 2. In general, patients on metformin had a shorter T2DM duration, lower glycemic levels, a lower prevalence of renal failure, and fewer diabetic complications than patients treated with other NAIDs. Conversely, patients on insulin in combination with a NAID were at the other side of the spectrum and had the longest duration of the disease, highest HbA1c levels, and the highest rate of all diabetic complications.

The clinical characteristics of patients with contraindications and improper use of a NIAD are shown in Supplementary Table 1, in Supplementary Material available online at http://dx.doi.org/10.1155/2016/7502489. Patients with a contraindication were older and had a longer T2DM duration than those without a contraindication, but they did show lower HbA1c values and hence a better glycemic control.

3.1. Prescribing Patterns of NIADs in Patients with Contraindicated Comorbid Conditions. The number of T2DM patients with major contraindications and NIADs prescribed alone or in combination is shown in Table 3.

TABLE 2: Demographic and clinical characteristics of T2DM patients stratified by the pharmacological class of the glucose-lowering agents prescribed (alone or in combination).

Characteristic	Metformin (n = 225,753)	Sulfonylureas (n = 79,742)	Meglitinides (n = 16,941)	AGIs (n = 1,877)	Pioglitazone (n = 3,290)	DPP4i (n = 39,682)	GLP-1ra (n = 2,374)	Insulin with NIAD (n = 46,150)
Age, mean (SD), years	67.7 (11.4)	69.2 (11.2)	71.6 (10.9)	74.4 (9.9)	67.1 (10.6)	67.6 (10.9)	59.5 (9.5)	68.6 (11.0)
Gender, n (%)								
Female	99,082 (43.9)	34,648 (43.6)	7,867 (46.4)	850 (45.3)	1,561 (47.4)	17,199 (43.3)	1,281 (54.0)	22,679 (49.1)
Male	126,671 (56.1)	44,824 (56.4)	9,074 (53.6)	1,027 (54.7)	1,729 (52.6)	22,483 (56.7)	1,093 (46.0)	23,471 (50.9)
T2DM duration, mean (SD), years	7.9 (5.6)	9.3 (5.3)	9.9 (5.8)	10.7 (5.6)	10.6 (5.6)	9 (5.4)	8.7 (5.0)	11.4 (6.5)
HbA1c, mean (SD), %*	7.3 (1.3)	7.6 (1.4)	7.7 (1.4)	7.2 (1.3)	7.7 (1.4)	7.7 (1.4)	7.9 (1.6)	8.3 (1.6)
BMI, mean (SD), kg/m^2	30.3 (5.1)	30.0 (5.1)	29.9 (5.1)	28.7 (5.0)	32.2 (5.7)	30.4 (5.2)	37.0 (6.0)	31.0 (5.5)
ACR, mean (SD), mg/g	39.8 (143.7)	42.3 (149.7)	71.6 (223.7)	34.2 (88.3)	50.1 (191.8)	50.1 (176.7)	45.5 (137.2)	71.2 (213.3)
Complications, n (%)								
Diabetic retinopathy	17,533 (7.8)	6,594 (8.3)	2,059 (12.2)	190 (10.1)	407 (12.4)	3,766 (9.5)	308 (13.0)	9,980 (21.6)
Diabetic nephropathy†/ACR > 300 mg/g	5,455 (2.4)	2,171 (2.7)	856 (5.1)	58 (3.1)	131 (4.0)	1,312 (3.3)	105 (4.4)	2,465 (5.3)
Diabetic neuropathy	6,545 (2.9)	2,313 (2.9)	755 (4.5)	62 (3.3)	150 (4.6)	1,399 (3.5)	137 (5.8)	3,683 (8.0)
Ischemic heart disease	26,433 (11.7)	9,818 (12.4)	2,842 (16.8)	263 (14.0)	274 (8.3)	5,177 (13.0)	291 (12.3)	8,094 (17.5)
Stroke	12,777 (5.7)	4,541 (5.7)	1,363 (8.0)	123 (6.6)	148 (4.5)	2,062 (5.2)	80 (3.4)	3,904 (8.5)
Peripheral artery disease	10,470 (4.6)	3,956 (5.0)	1,272 (7.5)	86 (4.6)	155 (4.7)	2,045 (5.2)	80 (3.4)	3,954 (8.6)
Heart failure	9,711 (4.3)	4,266 (5.4)	1,698 (10.0)	120 (6.4)	82 (2.5)	2,063 (5.2)	113 (4.8)	3,780 (8.2)
Any macrovascular complication	43,440 (19.2)	16,018 (20.2)	331 (2.0)	413 (22.0)	509 (15.5)	8,105 (20.4)	388 (16.3)	13,284 (28.8)

*Out of 199,523 patients with available HbA1c records.

†Out of 195,674 patients with available GFR records.

ACR: albumin/creatinine ratio; AGI: alpha-glucosidase inhibitors; BMI: body mass index; DPP4i: dipeptidyl peptidase-4 (DPP-4) inhibitors; GLP-1ra: glucagon-like peptide-1 (GLP-1) receptor agonists; GFR: glomerular filtration rate; HbA1c: glycated haemoglobin; NIAD: noninsulin antidiabetic drug; SD: standard deviation; T2DM: type 2 diabetes mellitus.

TABLE 3: Number of T2DM patients (%) with relevant contraindications and glucose-lowering agents prescribed (alone or in combination). Percentages indicate the proportion of patients treated with each NAID with respect to the total number of patients with the condition.

Condition	Total patients with the condition	Metformin ($n = 225{,}753$)	Sulfonylureas ($n = 79{,}742$)	Meglitinides ($n = 16{,}941$)	AGIs ($n = 1{,}877$)	Pioglitazone ($n = 3{,}290$)	DPP4i ($n = 39{,}682$)	GLP-1ra ($n = 2{,}374$)
Renal failure* (GFR < 60 mL/min), *n* (%)	40,666 (20.1)	31,727 (78.0)	12,695 (31.2)	5,019 (12.3)	381 (0.9)	514 (1.3)	6,559 (16.1)	198 (0.5)
Severe renal failure* (GFR < 30 mL/min), *n* (%)	2,014 (1.0)	711 (35.3)	545 (22.5)	769 (38.1)	21 (1.0)	31 (1.5)	468 (23.2)	9 (0.4)
Heart failure, *n* (%)	13,276 (5.2)	9,711 (73.1)	4,266 (32.1)	1,698 (12.8)	120 (0.9)	82 (0.6)	2,063 (15.5)	113 (0.8)
Heart failure (NYHA functional stage)†, *n* (%)								
Class I	938	761 (81.1)	285 (30.4)	88 (9.4)	6 (0.6)	5 (0.5)	161 (17.2)	6 (0.6)
Class II	2,300	1,720 (74.8)	705 (30.7)	283 (12.3)	21 (0.9)	14 (0.6)	353 (15.3)	30 (1.3)
Class III	1,118	758 (67.8)	321 (28.7)	197 (17.6)	9 (0.8)	5 (0.4)	163 (14.6)	11 (1.0)
Class IV	104	63 (60.6)	28 (26.9)	18 (17.3)	2 (1.9)	1 (1.0)	16 (15.4)	1 (1.0)
Liver dysfunction, *n* (%)	1,447 (0.6)	1,140 (78.8)	402 (27.8)	114 (7.9)	12 (0.8)	7 (0.5)	221 (15.3)	14 (1.0)
Bladder cancer, *n* (%)	3,073 (1.2)	2,573 (83.7)	953 (31.0)	277 (9.0)	23 (0.7)	33 (1.1)	484 (15.8)	11 (0.4)

*Out of 195,674 patients with available GFR records.

†Out of 4,458 patients with available New York Heart Association (NYHA) functional classification records.

AGI: alpha-glucosidase inhibitors; DPP4i: dipeptidyl peptidase-4 (DPP-4) inhibitors; GLP-1ra: glucagon-like peptide-1 (GLP-1) receptor agonists; GFR: glomerular filtration rate.

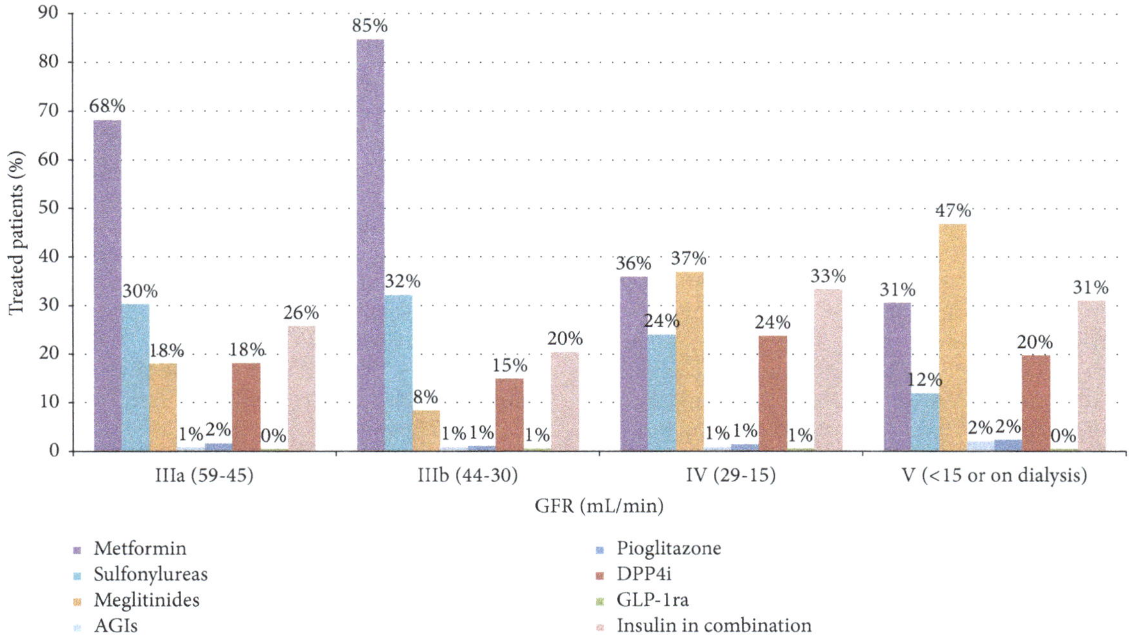

FIGURE 1: NIADs prescribed (alone or in combination) stratified by disease stage in patients with some degree of renal failure (GFR < 60 mL/min) (percentages are calculated for the total number of patients in each stage). AGI: alpha-glucosidase inhibitors; GLP-1ra: glucagon-like peptide-1 (GLP-1) receptor agonists; GFR: glomerular filtration rate; DPP4i: dipeptidyl peptidase-4 (DPP-4) inhibitors; NIAD: noninsulin antidiabetic drugs.

3.1.1. Renal Failure. A total of 40,666 patients (20.1%) had some degree of renal failure (GFR < 60 mL/min). In 78% of these cases patients were treated with metformin, and 31.2% were treated with sulfonylureas, both of them theoretically contraindicated, while other agents were prescribed in less than 16% of cases. We observed that, even in cases of severe renal failure (GFR < 30 mL/min; $n = 2{,}014$; 1% of all treated patients), when they are formally contraindicated, a significant proportion of these patients were still on metformin or sulfonylureas (35.3% and 22.5%, resp.). Based on the degree of renal impairment (Figure 1), 36% of cases in stage IV and 31% in stage V were taking metformin, and 24% and 12% of cases in stages IV and V were taking sulfonylureas, respectively. However, in both stages IV and V the most frequently prescribed agents were meglitinides (37% and 47%, resp.). Moreover, we also observed that 1% of patients with severe renal failure were taking AGIs, and 0.4% were taking GLP-1ra.

3.1.2. Heart Failure. A total of 13,276 patients (5.2%) had some degree of heart failure (Table 3). Again, metformin was the most frequently prescribed NIAD, and even in cases of moderate (class III) and severe (class IV) functional stages (a total of 1,222 patients), where metformin is formally contraindicated, it was prescribed in more than 60% of cases (67.8% in class III and 60.6% in class IV). Conversely, only 6 out of the 1,222 patients were on pioglitazone, which is also contraindicated in these 2 functional stages. In the less severe functional stages (classes I and II) only pioglitazone is contraindicated but was still prescribed in 5 out of the 938 patients in class I (0.5%) and in 14 out of the 2,300 patients in class II (0.6%) functional stage.

3.1.3. Liver Dysfunction. A total of 1,447 patients had elevated liver enzymes (liver dysfunction; Table 3). In these cases, the vast majority of patients were on metformin or sulfonylureas (78.8% and 27.8%, resp.), which are not necessarily contraindicated except in cases of advanced liver failure. However, a small proportion of patients (0.5%) were prescribed pioglitazone, which, based on the SmPC, is contraindicated in patients with baseline GPT levels >2.5 times the upper limit of normal.

3.1.4. Bladder Cancer. A history of bladder cancer was recorded for 3,073 patients (Table 3). Although the vast majority of these patients where on metformin or sulfonylureas, 33 of them (1.1%) were treated with pioglitazone, which is currently a formal contraindication in this condition.

4. Discussion

In the present study we identified a relatively high proportion of patients with T2DM and a comorbid disease with NIADs that are contraindicated or not recommended in cases of renal failure, heart failure, liver dysfunction, or history of bladder cancer.

Patients with a contraindication inappropriately taking a particular NIAD were older and had longer diabetes duration but had better glycemic control than patients without the same contraindication. This suggests that in spite of these patients being at risk of severe adverse events (e.g., hypoglycemia or lactic acidosis), treatment discontinuation could lead to a worsening of glycemic control, thus requiring a careful evaluation of the most appropriate NIADs to use in terms of efficacy and safety.

From our results, metformin, which is widely used as the initial pharmacological therapy for glycemic control in T2DM, was the NIAD that accounted for the vast majority of potentially inappropriate prescribing in patients with a comorbid disease: it was used in 35.3% of patients with severe renal failure (GFR < 30 mL/min) and in more than 60% of patients with moderate or severe heart failure. Because metformin has been associated with a risk of lactic acidosis, labeling contraindications include these conditions [10, 12, 23], but studies that have evaluated its prescribing pattern outside clinical recommendations reveal that it is actually used in a high proportion of cases in which major contraindications exist and in percentages similar to the figures that we observed [14–17]. A cross-sectional study conducted in Germany found that 73% of outpatients who were prescribed metformin had at least 1 contraindication, risk factors, or intercurrent illnesses necessitating its discontinuation [14]. A retrospective population-based study conducted in Scotland found that in 24.5% of patients who received metformin it was prescribed in spite of the presence of contraindications, and only 17.5% and 25% stopped metformin after admission with acute myocardial infarction and development of renal impairment, respectively [15]. A retrospective chart review of outpatients in the US found that about 25% of patients with 1 or more absolute contraindications (congestive heart failure or renal insufficiency) were prescribed metformin [17]. Finally, a retrospective study in Italy found that 60% of patients with 1 absolute contraindication or precautionary condition were on metformin at hospital admission, and in 41% of cases with 1 absolute contraindication it was not appropriately discontinued [16].

In the particular case of the use of metformin in patients with kidney disease, it has been consistently shown that prescribing restrictions, which recommend avoiding its use in patients with mild or moderate chronic kidney disease, are not actually followed in real-world practice [24]. Moreover, the incidence of lactic acidosis among patients on metformin is very low in stable mild-to-moderate renal dysfunction and not much different from the rates observed with other medications or the baseline incidence observed in T2DM [13, 24–26]. This has triggered some clinical guidelines to relax the cut-off, with current recommendations to stop metformin only when eGFR falls to <30 mL/min, but to reduce the dosing or use it with caution when eGFR values are between 45 and 30 mL/min [10, 12, 27, 28]. However, if we consider an eGFR <30 mL/min as the absolute contraindication, we still observed that 35.3% of patients in this stage were prescribed metformin in our setting, which is strikingly high.

The same trend has been observed with the use of metformin in patients with heart failure, with recent systematic reviews and meta-analyses showing that it is a safe option compared to other NIADs regarding the risk of heart failure or lactic acidosis [7, 29, 30]. Indeed, based on clinical evidence and these results, regulatory bodies in the US (Food and Drug Administration) in 2006 and in Canada (Health Canada) in 2010 removed the absolute contraindication of metformin in heart failure from the prescribing information and replaced it with a black box warning for its use in this population [31]. However, prescribing information has not been reviewed or modified in Europe, although the recent guideline of the European Society of Cardiology recognizes that they are widely and safely used in patients with heart failure and only recommends not to use it in case of severe renal failure or hepatic impairment [32]. Therefore, it seems reasonable to use metformin when the patient is stable and to avoid it in case of further impairment or hospitalization, as recommended by the recent American Diabetes Association guideline [10]. In our study, the rates of prescription of metformin in patients with III and IV heart failure functional stages were 67.8% and 60.6%, respectively. Moreover, we found that pioglitazone, which is also contraindicated in moderate or severe heart disease, was still prescribed to these patients (0.4% and 1% of patients with classes III and IV, resp.). In addition, the rates of inappropriate prescription of pioglitazone to patients for whom it is contraindicated in our study were <1.1% across different comorbidities (e.g., bladder cancer or liver dysfunction), which is much lower than the rate previously reported in a study conducted in Taiwan, which found that thiazolidinediones were inappropriately prescribed in about 10% of patients [33]. The reasons for this discrepancy are unclear, but the authors postulated that this high rate was due to the quick penetration of this drug class in the local market, while our low percentage could in turn be linked to a comparatively low penetrance in the Spanish market.

To our knowledge there are no studies assessing the rates of inappropriate prescription of sulfonylureas in formal contraindications, but many members of this class are associated with an increased risk of hypoglycemic episodes in patients with renal impairment or chronic liver disease [13]. We found figures that may be considered relatively high, as they were prescribed to 22.5% of patients with GFR <30 mL/min. In addition, sulfonylureas were prescribed in 27.8% of patients with liver dysfunction and metformin in 78.8% of such cases. However, they are only formally contraindicated in cases of advanced liver failure. Since we defined liver dysfunction as an elevation of liver enzymes >3 times the upper normal limits and this can be observed across different liver conditions, these do not actually correspond to real inappropriate prescriptions except in the case of pioglitazone (used in 0.5% of patients with liver dysfunction), which is specifically contraindicated when liver enzymes are elevated.

The present study has advantages and limitations that must be acknowledged. The main advantage is that we used a primary care database with high quality records that reflects real-life clinical practices in a large population of T2DM treated patients. However, and inherent to most retrospective studies, some of the studied variables were not always properly recorded in the medical records; for instance, there were 22% of patients without data on HbA1c values, 33% without data on GFR, or 66% for whom the NYHA functional class was not registered. Moreover, we cannot rule out a poor registration of comorbidities or at-risk conditions that could have underestimated the results. In addition, the retrospective design precludes determining whether clinicians were actually aware that they were prescribing against the label or clinical guidelines recommendations or the drugs were given in spite of the contraindication based on weighted individual risk-benefits. For instance, it is probable that the high rates of inappropriate or potentially inappropriate prescription of metformin is partly due to the fact that the risk-benefit in patients with nonabsolute contraindications favors its use in terms of the associated reduction of the risk of diabetes related complications, in particular macrovascular diseases. Finally, we could not estimate in what proportion of cases the particular drug was discontinued after the contraindicated condition developed and the at-risk condition was thus prevented, and we could not quantify either the incidence of adverse reactions after an inappropriate prescription (e.g., lactic acidosis, severe hypoglycemia episodes, or heart failure) or whether the drug was discontinued in case of a drug-related adverse event.

In summary, our results show that some NIADs, and in particular metformin, are frequently used in patients at high risk of complications when they are contraindicated or not recommended by the accompanying prescribing information or clinical guidelines. Prescribing of antidiabetic drugs to unsuitable patients has clinical consequences associated with an increased risk of adverse reactions and suboptimal glycemic control, and it is also associated with an economic impact relative to patients treated according to guidelines [34–37]. However, current guidelines or expert consensus does not always give clear recommendations on the use of specific NIADs in T2DM patients with a comorbid disease, probably as a result of a lack of clinical trials enrolling high-risk subjects, which may in turn result in a lack of practical advice for physicians, facilitating potentially inappropriate prescribing [13].

5. Conclusions

There is a need to increase awareness of potential inappropriate prescribing and to monitor the quality of prescribing patterns in order to help physicians and policymakers to yield better clinical outcomes in T2DM. This could be accomplished through the implementation of security reminders in the electronic clinical records so that physicians are aware of an existing complication that would require dose adjustment, discontinuing, or not even starting on a particular drug. Moreover, specific educational programs aimed at reducing the failure to recognize contraindications in patients with comorbid conditions and improving knowledge on currently available pharmaceutical products would be of great benefit to improve the management of the disease.

Disclaimer

The funding sources had no role in the design and conduct of the study; collection, management, analysis, and interpretation of the data; or preparation, review, or approval of the paper.

Conflict of Interests

The authors declare that they have no conflict of interests associated with the contents of this paper.

Acknowledgments

This study was funded by the Catalan Diabetes Association, the Catalan Health Department, and financial support provided by Boehringer-Ingelheim. CIBER of Diabetes and Associated Metabolic Diseases (CIBERDEM) is an initiative from Instituto de Salud Carlos III. The authors acknowledge Mònica Gratacòs and Amanda Prowse for providing support in the paper preparation and editing.

References

[1] M. J. Fowler, "Diabetes treatment, part 2: oral agents for glycemic management," *Clinical Diabetes*, vol. 25, no. 4, pp. 131–134, 2007.

[2] C. E. Koro, B. H. Lee, and S. J. Bowlin, "Antidiabetic medication use and prevalence of chronic kidney disease among patients with type 2 diabetes mellitus in the United States," *Clinical Therapeutics*, vol. 31, no. 11, pp. 2608–2617, 2009.

[3] A. Rodriguez-Poncelas, G. C.-D. Tuero, O. Turrò-Garriga, J. B.-D. La Puente, J. Franch-Nadal, and X. Mundet-Tuduri, "Impact of chronic kidney disease on the prevalence of cardiovascular disease in patients with type 2 diabetes in Spain: PERCEDIME2 study," *BMC Nephrology*, vol. 15, article 150, 2014.

[4] I. Vinagre, M. Mata-Cases, E. Hermosilla et al., "Control of glycemia and cardiovascular risk factors in patients with type 2 diabetes in primary care in Catalonia (Spain)," *Diabetes Care*, vol. 35, no. 4, pp. 774–779, 2012.

[5] L. Zhou, W. Deng, L. Zhou et al., "Prevalence, incidence and risk factors of chronic heart failure in the type 2 diabetic population: systematic review," *Current Diabetes Reviews*, vol. 5, no. 3, pp. 171–184, 2009.

[6] G. A. Nichols, C. M. Gullion, C. E. Koro, S. A. Ephross, and J. B. Brown, "The incidence of congestive heart failure in type 2 diabetes: an update," *Diabetes Care*, vol. 27, no. 8, pp. 1879–1884, 2004.

[7] C. Varas-Lorenzo, A. V. Margulis, M. Pladevall et al., "The risk of heart failure associated with the use of noninsulin blood glucose-lowering drugs: systematic review and meta-analysis of published observational studies," *BMC Cardiovascular Disorders*, vol. 14, article 129, 2014.

[8] K. G. Tolman, V. Fonseca, A. Dalpiaz, and M. H. Tan, "Spectrum of liver disease in type 2 diabetes and management of patients with diabetes and liver disease," *Diabetes Care*, vol. 30, no. 3, pp. 734–743, 2007.

[9] American Diabetes Association, "Standards of medical care in diabetes—2014," *Diabetes Care*, vol. 37, supplement 1, pp. S14–S80, 2014.

[10] S. E. Inzucchi, R. M. Bergenstal, J. B. Buse et al., "Management of hyperglycemia in type 2 diabetes, 2015: a patient-centered approach: update to a position statement of the american diabetes association and the european association for the study of diabetes," *Diabetes Care*, vol. 38, no. 1, pp. 140–149, 2015.

[11] P. Pozzilli, R. D. Leslie, J. Chan et al., "The A1C and ABCD of glycaemia management in type 2 diabetes: a physician's personalized approach," *Diabetes/Metabolism Research and Reviews*, vol. 26, no. 4, pp. 239–244, 2010.

[12] M. Mata, F. X. Cos, R. Morros et al., *Abordatge de la Diabetis Mellitus Tipus 2. Guies de Pràctica Clínica I Material Docent*, Institut Català de la Salut, Barcelona, Spain, 2nd edition, 2013.

[13] D. Tschöpe, M. Hanefeld, J. J. Meier et al., "The role of co-morbidity in the selection of antidiabetic pharmacotherapy in type-2 diabetes," *Cardiovascular Diabetology*, vol. 12, article 62, 2013.

[14] A. Holstein, D. Nahrwold, S. Hinze, and E.-H. Egberts, "Contra-indications to metformin therapy are largely disregarded," *Diabetic Medicine*, vol. 16, no. 8, pp. 692–696, 1999.

[15] A. M. Emslie-Smith, D. I. R. Boyle, J. M. M. Evans, F. Sullivan, and A. D. Morris, "Contraindications to metformin therapy in patients with type 2 diabetes—a population-based study of adherence to prescribing guidelines," *Diabetic Medicine*, vol. 18, no. 6, pp. 483–488, 2001.

[16] A. T. Calabrese, K. C. Coley, S. V. Dapos, D. Swanson, and R. H. Rao, "Evaluation of prescribing practices: risk of lactic acidosis with metformin therapy," *Archives of Internal Medicine*, vol. 162, no. 4, pp. 434–437, 2002.

[17] C. Horlen, R. Malone, B. Bryant et al., "Frequency of inappropriate metformin prescriptions," *The Journal of the American Medical Association*, vol. 287, no. 19, pp. 2504–2505, 2002.

[18] F. A. Masoudi, Y. Wang, S. E. Inzucchi et al., "Metformin and thiazolidinedione use in Medicare patients with heart failure," *Journal of the American Medical Association*, vol. 290, no. 1, pp. 81–85, 2003.

[19] R. Oliveira, J. Diaz Carvalho, R. Rodrigues et al., "Inappropriate prescribing of oral antidiabetics in chronic kidney disease," in *Proceedings of the 19th WONCA Europe Conference*, Lisbon, Portugal, 2014.

[20] B. Bolíbar, F. Fina Avilés, R. Morros et al., "SIDIAP database: electronic clinical records in primary care as a source of information for epidemiologic research," *Medicina Clinica*, vol. 138, no. 14, pp. 617–621, 2012.

[21] A. S. Levey, L. A. Stevens, C. H. Schmid et al., "A new equation to estimate glomerular filtration rate," *Annals of Internal Medicine*, vol. 150, no. 9, pp. 604–612, 2009.

[22] M. Dolgin, *Nomenclature and Criteria for Diagnosis of Diseases of the Heart and Great Vessels*, The Criteria Committee of the New York Heart Association, Little Brown & Co, Boston, Mass, USA, 9th edition, 1994.

[23] S. E. Inzucchi, R. M. Bergenstal, J. B. Buse et al., "Management of hyperglycemia in type 2 diabetes: a patient-centered approach: position statement of the American Diabetes Association (ADA) and the European Association for the Study of Diabetes (EASD)," *Diabetes Care*, vol. 35, no. 6, pp. 1364–1379, 2012.

[24] S. E. Inzucchi, K. J. Lipska, H. Mayo, C. J. Bailey, and D. K. McGuire, "Metformin in patientswith type 2 diabetes and kidney disease a systematic review," *The Journal of the American Medical Association*, vol. 312, no. 24, pp. 2668–2675, 2014.

[25] J. McCormack, K. Johns, and H. Tildesley, "Metformin's contraindications should be contraindicated," *Canadian Medical Association Journal*, vol. 173, no. 5, pp. 502–504, 2005.

[26] W. R. Lu, J. Defilippi, and A. Braun, "Unleash metformin: reconsideration of the contraindication in patients with renal impairment," *Annals of Pharmacotherapy*, vol. 47, no. 11, pp. 1488–1497, 2013.

[27] NICE (National Institute for Health and Clinical Excellence), Clinical guideline CG87, Type 2 diabetes: the management of type 2 diabetes, 2014, http://guidance.nice.org.uk/CG87/NiceGuidance/pdf/English.

[28] Societat Catalana de Nefrologia (SCN), *Consens Català sobre Atenció a la Malaltia Renal Crònica*, 2012, http://www.redgdps.org/index.php?idregistro=777.

[29] D. T. Eurich, F. A. McAlister, D. F. Blackburn et al., "Benefits and harms of antidiabetic agents in patients with diabetes and heart failure: systematic review," *British Medical Journal*, vol. 335, no. 7618, pp. 497–501, 2007.

[30] S. R. Salpeter, E. Greyber, G. A. Pasternak, and E. E. Salpeter, "Risk of fatal and nonfatal lactic acidosis with metformin use in type 2 diabetes mellitus," *Cochrane Database of Systematic Reviews*, vol. 4, Article ID CD002967, 2010.

[31] D. T. Eurich, D. L. Weir, S. R. Majumdar et al., "Comparative safety and effectiveness of metformin in patients with diabetes mellitus and heart failure: systematic review of observational studies involving 34,000 patients," *Circulation: Heart Failure*, vol. 6, no. 3, pp. 395–402, 2013.

[32] J. J. V. McMurray, S. Adamopoulos, S. D. Anker et al., "ESC Guidelines for the diagnosis and treatment of acute and chronic heart failure 2012: the Task Force for the Diagnosis and Treatment of Acute and Chronic Heart Failure 2012 of the European Society of Cardiology. Developed in collaboration with the Heart Failure Association (HFA) of the ESC," *European Heart Journal*, vol. 33, no. 14, pp. 1787–1847, 2012.

[33] Y.-W. Wen, Y.-W. Tsai, W.-F. Huang, F.-Y. Hsiao, and P.-S. Chen, "The potentially inappropriate prescription of new drug: thiazolidinediones for patients with type II diabetes in Taiwan," *Pharmacoepidemiology and Drug Safety*, vol. 20, no. 1, pp. 20–29, 2011.

[34] S. S. Saleh, J. Carter, C. A. Plauschinat, and S. E. Szebenyi, "Potentially inappropriate prescribing of antidiabetic drugs and impact on outcomes in patients with type 2 diabetes," in *American Diabetes Association (ADA) 67th Scientific Sessions*, p. A156, Chicago, Ill, USA, 2007.

[35] S. Y. Chen, Y. C. Lee, V. Alas, M. Greene, and D. Brixner, "Outcomes associated with concordance of oral antidiabetic drug treatments to prescribing information in patients with type 2 diabetes mellitus and chronic kidney disease," *Journal of Medical Economics*, vol. 16, no. 5, pp. 586–595, 2013.

[36] S.-Y. Chen, Y.-C. Lee, V. Alas, M. Greene, and D. Brixner, "Outcomes associated with nonconcordance to national kidney foundation guideline recommendations for oral antidiabetic drug treatments in patients with concomitant type 2 diabetes and chronic kidney disease," *Endocrine Practice*, vol. 20, no. 3, pp. 221–231, 2014.

[37] S. Y. Chen, K. Siu, B. Kovacs et al., "Clinical and economic outcomes associated with National Kidney Foundation guideline-concordant oral antidiabetic drug treatment among type 2 diabetes patients with chronic kidney disease," *Current Medical Research and Opinion*, vol. 28, no. 4, pp. 493–501, 2012.

23

Resting Heart Rate Does Not Predict Cardiovascular and Renal Outcomes in Type 2 Diabetic Patients

Vendula Bartáková,[1] Linda Klimešová,[1] Katarína Kianičková,[1] Veronika Dvořáková,[1] Denisa Malúšková,[2] Jitka Řehořová,[3] Jan Svojanovský,[4] Jindřich Olšovský,[4] Jana Bělobrádková,[3] and Kateřina Kaňková[1]

[1]*Department of Pathophysiology, Medical Faculty, Masaryk University Brno, Kamenice 5, 62500 Brno, Czech Republic*
[2]*Institute of Biostatistics and Analyses, Masaryk University Brno, Kamenice 126/3, 62500 Brno, Czech Republic*
[3]*Department of Internal Medicine-Gastroenterology, University Hospital Brno, Jihlavská 20, 62500 Brno, Czech Republic*
[4]*2nd Department of Internal Medicine, St. Anne's University Hospital, Pekařská 53, 65691 Brno, Czech Republic*

Correspondence should be addressed to Vendula Bartáková; vbartak@med.muni.cz

Academic Editor: Dirk Westermann

Elevated resting heart rate (RHR) has been associated with increased risk of mortality and cardiovascular events. Limited data are available so far in type 2 diabetic (T2DM) subjects with no study focusing on progressive renal decline specifically. Aims of our study were to verify RHR as a simple and reliable predictor of adverse disease outcomes in T2DM patients. A total of 421 T2DM patients with variable baseline stage of diabetic kidney disease (DKD) were prospectively followed. A history of the cardiovascular disease was present in 81 (19.2%) patients at baseline, and DKD (glomerular filtration rate < 60 mL/min or proteinuria) was present in 328 (77.9%) at baseline. Progressive renal decline was defined as a continuous rate of glomerular filtration rate loss ≥ 3.3% per year. Resting heart rate was not significantly higher in subjects with cardiovascular disease or DKD at baseline compared to those without. Using time-to-event analyses, significant differences in the cumulative incidence of the studied outcomes, that is, progression of DKD (and specifically progressive renal decline), major advanced cardiovascular event, and all-cause mortality, between RHR </≥65 (arbitrary cut-off) and 75 (median) bpm were not found. We did not ascertain predictive value of the RHR for the renal or cardiovascular outcomes in T2DM subjects in Czech Republic.

1. Introduction

Elevated resting heart rate (RHR) has been associated with increased risk of all-cause mortality and cardiovascular (CV) events in healthy subjects as well as those with preexisting CV disease (CVD) including hypertension, acute myocardial infarction, and heart failure or left ventricular dysfunction by numerous epidemiologic studies and recently reviewed ones by Palatini and Julius [1] and Fox et al. [2]. In a recent study of Woodward et al., individual data from 112,680 subjects in 12 cohort studies were collected and an association between RHR above 65 beats/min (bpm) and the risk of both CV and all-cause mortality has been found independent of preexisting CVD [3]. Plausible pathophysiological mechanisms were reviewed by Lang et al. [4] and include, briefly, both indirect mechanisms related to autonomic dysregulation and those directly related to an increased heart rate per se (such as increased ischaemic burden and local haemodynamic forces adversely impacting on the endothelium and arterial wall).

Several studies focused on RHR in type 2 diabetic (T2DM) subjects. Stettler et al. found an association between RHR and all-cause mortality and CVD in a cohort of 302 T2DM patients [5]. Linnemann and Janka have identified an elevated RHR as a high risk for CV death in a cohort of 475 T2DM patients [6]. Hillis et al. found a relationship between baseline higher RHR and all-cause mortality, CV death, and major CV events (nonfatal myocardial infarction or nonfatal stroke) in a cohort of 11,140 T2DM patients; the increased risk associated with a higher baseline RHR was most obvious in patients with previous macrovascular complications [7]. Hillis et al. also extended the study on the same cohort of T2DM patients on the effect of RHR and microvascular complications (nephropathy and retinopathy) and reported an increased incidence and a greater progression of [8].

There are, however, fewer data on the relationship of RHR and renal events in diabetic subjects. Miot et al. studied a cohort of 1088 T2DM patients for the association of RHR with the incidence of composite CV and renal endpoint (CV death, nonfatal myocardial infarction and/or stroke, hospitalization for heart failure, and renal replacement therapy) and also for the renal endpoint alone. While in patients without CVD no relationship was found, in the subgroup with CVD history at baseline significant association between RHR and the incidence of CV and/or renal events was ascertained [9]. However, "hard" renal end-point, an end-stage renal disease (ESRD), is impractical in majority of observational cohorts and interventional studies due to relatively short follow-up. Furthermore, diabetic kidney disease (DKD) appears to be phenotypically heterogeneous (see further) and thus pathways and mediators (e.g., RHR) leading to ESRD might differ.

As documented by recent studies in both types of diabetes, progressive renal decline (defined as continuous rate of glomerular filtration rate (GFR) loss $\geq$ 3.3% per year) might coexist with a "classical" form of DKD with increased urinary albumin excretion preceding GFR decline [10–12]. No study, so far, focused on predictive power of RHR for DKD progression considering both phenotypes (albuminuric versus nonalbuminuric DKD) in T2DM patients.

Therefore, the aims of the present study were (1) to evaluate whether RHR is associated with DKD stage or CVD at baseline, (2) to eventually replicate in our cohort of T2DM patients previous sporadic positive findings on RHR as a predictor of CVD and DKD endpoints and death in T2DM patients, and finally (3) to specifically address RHR predictive potential for progressive renal decline in our cohort.

2. Materials and Methods

2.1. Subjects. A total of 421 T2DM patients (unrelated Caucasian subjects from South Moravia region, Czech Republic), 51.5% of men, with median age 67 [IQR 61–75], median DM duration 14 years [IQR 8–21], and range of DKD stages at baseline, were enrolled into the study between 2002 and 2010. Prospective data were collected until 2013.

Severity of DKD was defined according to the urinary albumin excretion (UAE) and stage of chronic kidney disease (CKD) by GFR assessed by creatinine clearance based on 24 h urine collection. Both parameters, UAE and GFR, were repeatedly measured at least once in 6 months or more often; staging for DKD and CKD was based on two consecutive values. At baseline, the study sample consisted of normoalbuminuric subjects (UAE < 30 mg/24 h, 8.8%), microalbuminuric subjects (UAE 30–300 mg/24 h, 30.4%), macroalbuminuric subjects (UAE > 300 mg/24 h, 51.5%), and subjects with end-stage renal disease (ESRD, 9.3%). Respective staging for CKD in the same sample was CKD I (GFR $\geq$ 90 mL/min per 1.73 m^2, 17.3%), CKD II (60–89 mL/min per 1.73 m^2, 18.3%), CKD III (30–59 mL/min per 1.73 m^2, 36.9%), CKD IV (15–29 mL/min per 1.73 m^2, 16.3%), and subjects with CKD V at baseline (GFR < 15 mL/min per 1.73 m^2 or maintenance haemodialysis, 11.2%). Progressive renal decline was defined as a negative change of GFR equal to or steeper than 3.3% per year and the patient is referred to as a "decliner" and the rest as "nondecliners." Cut-off of GFR loss $\geq$ 3.3% per year has been used in previous reports [10, 11] and corresponds to the 2.5th percentile of the distribution of annual renal function loss in a general population [13]. A history of DKD at baseline (DKD-b^+) was defined as GFR < 60 mL/min/1.73 m^2 or macroalbuminuria. A history of CVD at baseline (CVD-b^+) was defined as a history of coronary artery disease, nonfatal myocardial infarction or stroke, lower limb amputation, or revascularization. RHR at baseline was determined either by 1 minute radial artery palpation or from ECG records. For detailed description of the whole group and CVD-b^+ and CVD-b^- or DKD-b^+ and DKD-b^- subgroups see Table 1.

Informed consent was obtained from each patient prior to being included in the study. The study was performed according to the recommendations of the Declaration of Helsinki and approved by the Ethical Committee of Medical Faculty, Masaryk University Brno.

2.2. Follow-Up. Subjects were prospectively followed for a median of 43 [22–77] months in diabetes and nephrology units of the two university hospitals in Brno and following end-points were considered as (1) progression of DKD defined as a decline of GFR < 60 mL/min per 1.73 m^2 during the follow-up period for those with GFR $\geq$ 60 mL/min per 1.73 m^2 at baseline or achieving ESRD, development of overt macroalbuminuria in normo- and microalbuminuric subjects at baseline, or progression of CKD by at least stage for those with CKD III and IV at baseline, (2) major adverse cardiovascular event (MACE), that is, fatal or nonfatal myocardial infarction or stroke, lower limb amputation, or revascularization, and (3) all-cause mortality (ACM). Only non-ESRD/non-CKD V at inception patients with complete follow-up information were included in the time-to-event analysis; that is, a total of 376 subjects were considered with the 48 month follow-up median [28–79].

2.3. Statistical Analysis. Data are expressed as median [interquartile range, IQR] or as percentages. Differences in continuous variables between the groups were analysed using Mann-Whitney test. Kaplan-Meier curves with log-rank testing were applied for time-to-event analysis to analyse the effect of RHR categories (< and $\geq$ actual median RHR and arbitrary cut-off 65 bpm) on studied outcomes. Standard competing risk methodology focusing on cumulative incidence was adopted for the nonparametric estimation and modelling of associations of the potential risk factors and the progression of DKD, MACE, and death. Gray test [14] was used to assess the differences in cumulative incidence of the competing risks with respect to the risk factors, and Fine and Gray model [15] was used to evaluate the predictive potential of the considered parameters. For all standard analysis,

TABLE 1: Clinical and biochemical characteristics of subjects divided according to history of CVD, baseline data.

Variables	All	CVD-b$^+$	CVD-b$^-$	P
n (%)	421	81 (19.2)	340 (80.0)	
Sex: men/women, n (%)	217 (52)/204 (48)	52 (64)/29 (36)	165 (49)/175 (51)	0.01
Age (years)	67 [61–75]	70 [63–76]	67 [60–74]	0.009
Diabetes duration (years)	14 [8–21]	16 [12–23]	13 [7–20]	1×10^{-4}
FPG (mmol/L)	8.5 [6.8–10.9]	9.3 [7.8–11.8]	8.1 [6.6–10.8]	0.02
HbA1c (%), IFCC calibration	6.4 [5.4–8.1]	6.6 [5.9–8.0]	6.4 [5.2–8.1]	NS
Creatinine (μmol/L)	142 [114–214]	188 [139–311]	135 [101–191]	$<1 \times 10^{-6}$
Urea (mmol/L)	11.0 [7.3–17.3]	16.0 [10.1–21.6]	9.9 [6.9–16.2]	$<1 \times 10^{-5}$
Albuminuria (mg/24 hours)	500 [140–2080]	1540 [350–3670]	400 [130–1740]	7×10^{-4}
Systolic blood pressure (mmHg)	144 [130–160]	145 [125–150]	142 [130–160]	NS
Diastolic blood pressure (mmHg)	80 [75–90]	80 [70–95]	80 [75–90]	NS
Total cholesterol (mmol/L)	4.9 [4.2–5.8]	4.5 [3.9–5.3]	4.9 [4.3–5.8]	0.02
Beta blockers users (%)	46.3	50.6	45.3	NS
RAAS inhibitors users (%)	62	53.1	64.1	NS
Other antihypertensive therapy (%)	69.1	71.6	68.5	NS
History of renal disease, n (%)	**328 (77.9)**	**73 (90)**	**255 (75)**	**NS**
Decliners (GFR loss ≥ 3.3% per year), n (%)	**191 (45.4)**	**36 (44)**	**155 (45.6)**	**NS**
RHR (bpm)	75 [70–80]	75 [70–84]	75 [70–80]	NS

Data are expressed as median [interquartile range] or percentages. Differences evaluated by nonparametric Mann-Whitney or chi-square test, respectively. FPG, fasting plasma glucose; HbA1c, glycated haemoglobin; GFR, glomerular filtration rate; RAAS, renin-angiotensin-aldosterone system; RHR, resting heart rate.

Statistica for Windows (Statsoft Inc., Tulsa, OK, USA) was used. $P \leq 0.05$ was considered statistically significant.

3. Results

3.1. Analysis of Baseline Data. A history of the CVD was present in 81 (19.2%) patients at baseline; DKD (GFR < 60 mL/min or proteinuria) was present in 328 (77.9%) at baseline. For characteristics of subjects, see Tables 1 and 2.

In a CVD-b$^+$ subgroup of patients (groups divided according to having or not having CVD at baseline), they were more frequently men, significantly older, and with a longer diabetes duration, higher fasting plasma glucose (FPG) levels, higher urea and creatinine plasma levels, and higher degree of albuminuria, while they did not differ in RHR, systolic (SBP) and diastolic (DBP) blood pressure, and HbA1c levels compared to CVD-b$^-$ subgroup. Finally there was no significant difference in the presence of a renal history at baseline and a proportion of decliners between subgroups.

When the patients were divided according to having or not having DKD at baseline, DKD-b$^+$ subjects had (similarly to CVD-b$^+$) higher age, longer diabetes duration, higher urea and creatinine plasma levels and higher degree of albuminuria, additionally higher DBP and higher frequency of CVD at baseline, and finally higher proportion of decliners. There was no difference in sex, FPG, HbA1c levels, SBP, and again RHR.

Comparisons of possible differences in RHR in the presence or absence of the treatment with beta-blockers, renin-angiotensin-aldosterone system blockers (i.e., sartans or angiotensin 1 receptor, 2 blockers), or other antihypertensive therapy (i.e., diuretics, Ca-blockers, and central antihypertensive drugs) revealed no statistically significant differences in the whole group or any of the CVD-b$^{+/-}$ or DKD-b$^{+/-}$ subgroups (all $P > 0.05$, Mann-Whitney test). For frequencies of each drug group prescription within the whole group or subgroups, see Tables 1 and 2 (all $P > 0.05$, chi-square test).

Finally, we assessed correlations of RHR with other clinical data (age, diabetes duration, SBP, DBP, FPG, HbA1c, creatinine, urea, and total cholesterol) and found significant correlations with FPG ($r = 0.12$, $P = 0.02$, Spearman) and SBP ($r = 0.16$, $P = 0.028$, Spearman).

3.2. Follow-Up Analysis

(A) Kaplan-Meier Analysis of Separate End-Points. During the follow-up period, cumulative incidences of DKD progression, MACE, and all-cause mortality were 48.3%, 23.1%, and 38.9%, respectively, in the whole group; for incidences in CVD-b$^{+/-}$ or DKD-b$^{+/-}$ subgroups separately, see Table 3. Of a total of 376 subjects analysed in the follow-up study, 62 had both CVD and DKD at baseline. Of those, 35 (56%) died and 27 (44%) survived ($P > 0.05$, chi-square test). Median RHR was 75 bpm in the whole group. Furthermore, 191 (45.4%) of patients were found as GFR decliners. No statistically significant difference in RHR was ascertained between decliners and nondecliners ($P > 0.05$, Mann-Whitney test).

Irrespective of non-significant differences in RHR between subjects with CVD or DKD at baseline (b$^+$) compared to those without (b$^-$), analyses were still performed for (i) the whole group and (ii) CVD-b$^{+/-}$ and (iii) DKD-b$^{+/-}$

TABLE 2: Clinical and biochemical characteristics of subjects divided according to history of DKD, baseline data.

Variables	All	DKD-b$^+$	DKD-b$^-$	P
n (%)	421	328 (77.9)	93 (22.1)	
Sex: men/women, n (%)	217 (52)/204 (48)	175(53)/153 (47)	42 (45)/51 (55)	NS
Age (years)	67 [61–75]	68 [62–75]	63 [56–71]	3×10^{-4}
Diabetes duration (years)	14 [8–21]	15 [9–22]	10 [6–15]	4×10^{-5}
FPG (mmol/L)	8.5 [6.8–10.9]	8.8 [6.9–11.2]	8.0 [6.8–9.7]	NS
HbAlc (%), IFCC calibration	6.4 [5.4–8.1]	6.5 [5.5–8.1]	6.2 [5.3–8.0]	NS
Creatinine (μmol/L)	142 [114–214]	164 [125–258]	91 [81–107]	$<1 \times 10^{-6}$
Urea (mmol/L)	11.0 [7.3–17.3]	13.3 [8.7–19.6]	6.1 [5.3–7.6]	$<1 \times 10^{-6}$
Albuminuria (mg/24 hours)	500 [140–2080]	840 [260–2350]	110 [90–150]	$<1 \times 10^{-6}$
Systolic blood pressure (mmHg)	144 [130–160]	144 [130–160]	140 [130–160]	NS
Diastolic blood pressure (mmHg)	80 [75–90]	80 [74–90]	90 [80–98]	0.001
Total cholesterol (mmol/L)	4.9 [4.2–5.8]	4.9 [4.2–5.7]	4.9 [4.3–5.9]	NS
Beta blockers at treatment (%)	46.3	48.5	33.3	NS
RAAS inhibitors at treatment (%)	62	60.7	58.1	NS
Other antihypertensive therapy (%)	69.1	71	52.7	NS
History of CV disease, n (%)	**328 (77.9)**	**73 (22)**	**8 (9)**	**0.01**
Decliners (GFR loss ≥ 3.3% per year), n (%)	**191 (45.4)**	**164 (50)**	**27 (29)**	$\mathbf{3 \times 10^{-4}}$
RHR (bpm)	75 [70–80]	74 [70–80]	74 [70–80]	NS

Data are expressed as median [interquartile range] or percentages. Differences evaluated by nonparametric Mann-Whitney or chi-square test, respectively. CV, cardiovascular; FPG, fasting plasma glucose; HbAlc, glycated haemoglobin; GFR, glomerular filtration rate; RAAS, renin-angiotensin-aldosterone system; RHR, resting heart rate.

TABLE 3: Cumulative incidence of DKD progression, MACE and all-cause mortality in the whole group and subgroups.

	DKD progressor	P	MACE	P	ALL-cause mortality	P
Whole group (n = 376)	48.3%	—	23.1%	—	38.9%	—
CKD-b$^+$ (n = 66)	51.5%	NS	22.3%	NS	53.0%	NS
CKD-b$^-$ (n = 310)	47.1%		27.3%		36.1%	
DKD-b$^+$ (n = 283)	53.4%	0.047	26.8%	0.023	48.4%	$<1 \times 10^{-4}$
DKD-b$^-$ (n = 93)	26.9%		11.7%		6.5%	

subgroups. Using time-to-event analyses, any significant differences in the cumulative incidence of the three studied outcomes were found between RHR </≥75 bpm (i.e., our median) and 65 bpm (i.e., arbitrary cut-off used in majority of meta-analyses [3]) neither in the whole group nor in the CVD-b$^{+/-}$ or DKD-b$^{+/-}$ subgroups ($P > 0.05$, log-rank test).

In spite of the fact that RHR did not significantly differ between beta-blocker users and nonusers in the whole group or any of the subgroups defined based on CVD or DKD status at baseline, we still analysed the effect of RHR (cut-off </≥65 or 75 bpm) in beta-blocker naive subjects separately (n = 145). No significant differences were assessed using this subpopulation analysis (all $P > 0.05$, log-rank test).

(B) Competing Risk Analysis. Since estimates based on the naive Kaplan-Meier curves do not consider the presence of competing risks, they apparently tend to overestimate the probability of occurrence of the individual events in time. We compared groups with initial RHR </≥ median (75 bpm) or </≥ arbitrary cut-off (65 bpm), respectively. P values in univariate analysis of competing risk model did not indicate a significant effect of the RHR on the cumulative incidence of the two competing risks (i.e., DKD progression and MACE, $P > 0.05$, Gray test). Similarly, no significance was found for all-cause death ($P > 0.05$, Gray test). Table 4 shows the results of a Fine and Gray model. Again, no significant difference between groups was found.

4. Discussion and Conclusions

In the present study we evaluated a predictive potential of baseline RHR for progression of DKD (and more specifically for rapid GFR decline), MACE, and all-cause death in T2DM patients. In the cross-sectional part of our study, we compared clinical and biochemical data between groups of diabetic subjects with or without initial DKD or CVD. Subjects in both DKD-b$^+$ and CVD-b$^+$ subgroups had significantly higher age, longer diabetes duration, worse renal parameters (higher levels of urea and creatinine and higher degree of albuminuria), higher FPG, and male predominance in a CVD-b$^+$ subgroup, while DKD-b$^+$ subgroup had higher DBP and a higher proportion of decliners.

Although previous studies found an association between RHR and prevalence of baseline CVD [7–9] or DKD [8, 9] in

TABLE 4: (a) Fine and Gray model: the effect of patient and disease characteristics on the progression of DKD (univariate analysis). (b) Fine and Gray model: the effect of patient and disease characteristics on the *MACE* (univariate analysis).

(a)

Risk factor	Risk category	Basal category	Fine and Gray model HR	95% CI	*P* value
RHR	≥65 bpm	<65 bpm	1.11	0.77–1.60	0.580
RHR	≥75 bpm	<75 bpm	0.97	0.73–1.29	0.820

(b)

Risk factor	Risk category	Basal category	Fine and Gray model HR	95% CI	*P* value
RHR	≥65 bpm	<65 bpm	0.79	0.51–1.23	0.300
RHR	≥75 bpm	<75 bpm	0.87	0.60–1.27	0.470

T2DM patients, we were not able to ascertain similar significant differences in RHR in any of those categories studied. The major focus of the study was the prospective evaluation of the predictive potential of RHR for the MACE and progression of DKD. Moreover, we believe, this is a first study dealing with RHR in relation to the progressive renal decline. The concept of progressive renal decline was proposed by Krolewski in T1DM patients as an alternative pathway to albuminuric DKD [16]. Pugliese et al. in the RIACE study on T2DM patients [12] found a reduced estimated GFR (eGFR) without albuminuria independently associated with a significant CVD burden, higher than albuminuria alone, whereas the combination of reduced eGFR and albuminuria marked a further increased risk of CVD events in an additive manner. We found a higher proportion of decliners in DKD-b$^+$ subgroup of patients, which could be explained by generally nonlinear pattern of renal disease progression; however, no such difference was found between CVD-b$^+$ and CVD-b$^-$ subgroups in spite of the fact that CVD-b$^+$ group had worse renal parameters at baseline similarly to DKD-b$^+$. This might signify a specific pathogenic mechanism unrelated to CVD and this topic warrants further study.

Since beta-blockers or RAAS blockers have an obvious influence on RHR, we adjusted our analyses for the therapy modality. There was no therapy-related effect on any of the outcomes studied and on any of subgroups.

Our finding of positive correlation of RHR with FPG and SBP corresponds with results of previous studies; for example, in a large study of a French population with almost 100,000 participants, heart rate was positively associated with blood pressure, triglycerides, glycaemia, and physical inactivity and negatively with body height [17].

In the prospective part of the study, we were unable to identify any significant relationship of an initial RHR with DKD progression, major adverse cardiovascular event, and all-cause mortality in our cohort. Since more than one end-point may occur in the same patient, a competing risk methodology for multiple risk scenario was used. Yet again, RHR was not identified as a significant risk factor for DKD progression or MACE in the univariate competing risk model. Those findings are contrary to results of previous sporadic studies. A prospective study by Hillis et al. found in a cohort of 11,140 T2DM patients with a history of CVD participating in ADVANCE study [18] an association between higher baseline RHR and a greater risk of developing microvascular endpoint (defined as a composite of new or worsening nephropathy) during 4.4-year follow-up. After adjustment for age, sex, and randomized treatment (perindopril-indapamide), a 10 bpm increase in baseline RHR was associated with an 18% increase in the observed hazard [8]. Another recent study of 1088 T2DM patients by Miot et al. [9] focused on both CV and renal parameters (briefly, 31% of patients had a history of CVD at baseline (CVD-b$^+$) and median of follow-up was 4.2 years; mean RHR was 67.7 bpm in CVD-b$^+$ subgroup and 72.4 bpm in CVD-b$^-$ subgroup) but not considering the drug therapy in the analyses ascertained RHR associated with the incidence of CV and renal morbidity/mortality ($P = 0.0002$) and also with renal risk alone adjusted for all-cause death as a competing event in the CVD-b$^+$ subgroup only ($P < 0.0001$). In the CVD-b$^-$ subgroup, no relation was found between RHR and the incidence of CV and/or renal events. We have not been able to replicate any predictive effect of the RHR for the renal or CV outcomes in T2DM population of Czech Republic. Given similar settings of our study, one of the possible explanations might certainly be a smaller sample size, slightly shorter follow-up, different definition of endpoints, or different cut-offs for RHR. Regarding the latter, of plethora of possibilities, we have chosen stratification according to two RHR cut-offs, a median RHR and an arbitrary cut-off 65 bpm in line with results of a meta-analysis by Woodward et al. [3].

There are several pathogenic mechanisms proposed by which an elevated heart rate might mediate development and progression of DKD and CVD. It has been suggested that a higher heart rate might promote microalbuminuria because of increased exposure of the glomerulus to arterial pressure waves [19]. An increased heart rate has also variety of direct detrimental cardiovascular consequences including endothelial dysfunction and atherogenic activity that are important factors in the progression of DKD too [20]. A higher heart rate also is associated with factors such as obesity, higher blood pressure, atherogenic dyslipidaemia, and reduced physical activity [21], all of which are associated with an increased risk of microvascular complications and are targets for intervention to improve outcome in patients with diabetes mellitus [22]. Finally, a faster resting heart rate is a characteristic feature of autonomic neuropathy, which is in turn associated with an increased prevalence of other complications, such as DKD or retinopathy [23]. Therefore, it is conceivable that mechanisms listed could have synergistic effects and represent potentially very important pathogenic mechanism; on the contrary, the effect might operate in stage-dependent fashion given our negative finding of increased RHR as a general predictor of DKD progression in T2DM.

We are of course aware of several limitations of our study potentially impacting on its negative outcome. First of all, current sample size is relatively small compared to previous studies. This together with the rather high representation of subjects with baseline DKD or CVD might weaken the potential predictive power of RHR in the situation of more advanced stages of cardiovascularly relevant comorbidities. Therefore, although our results indicate several trends—for example, patients with a history of CVD or DKD at baseline had more frequently beta-blockers in therapy and CVD-b^+ patients have a tendency to a higher RHR—the results were not found statistically significant in our cohort.

In conclusion, recent study analysing the potential of RHR for the prediction of progression of DKD (and specifically progressive renal decline), major cardiovascular event, and all-cause death in a cohort of Caucasian T2DM subjects did not reveal significant effect (not even in the subgroup of heart rate affecting therapy-naïve subjects). Additional studies are therefore warranted to decipher event. Additional studies are therefore warranted to decipher if RHR could be an applicable risk marker for DKD.

Conflict of Interests

The authors declare that there is no conflict of interests regarding the publication of this paper.

Authors' Contribution

Vendula Bartáková designed the study, analysed the data, and drafted the paper. Denisa Malúšková performed the statistical analysis. Veronika Dvořáková analysed the data. Jana Bělobrádková, Jitka Řehořová, Jindřich Olšovský, Linda Klimešová, Katarína Kianičková, and Jan Svojanovský contributed in recruiting participants and collecting demographic and anthropometric data. Kateřina Kaňková supervised the study and revised the paper. All authors read and approved the final paper.

Acknowledgment

This paper was supported by Grant NT/13198 from The Ministry of Health of Czech Republic.

References

[1] P. Palatini and S. Julius, "Elevated heart rate: a major risk factor for cardiovascular disease," *Clinical and Experimental Hypertension*, vol. 26, no. 7-8, pp. 637–644, 2004.

[2] K. Fox, J. S. Borer, A. J. Camm et al., "Resting heart rate in cardiovascular disease," *Journal of the American College of Cardiology*, vol. 50, no. 9, pp. 823–830, 2007.

[3] M. Woodward, R. Webster, Y. Murakami et al., "The association between resting heart rate, cardiovascular disease and mortality: evidence from 112,680 men and women in 12 cohorts," *European Journal of Preventive Cardiology*, vol. 21, no. 6, pp. 719–726, 2014.

[4] C. C. Lang, S. Gupta, P. Kalra et al., "Elevated heart rate and cardiovascular outcomes in patients with coronary artery disease: clinical evidence and pathophysiological mechanisms," *Atherosclerosis*, vol. 212, no. 1, pp. 1–8, 2010.

[5] C. Stettler, A. Bearth, S. Allemann et al., "QTc interval and resting heart rate as long-term predictors of mortality in type 1 and type 2 diabetes mellitus: a 23-year follow-up," *Diabetologia*, vol. 50, no. 1, pp. 186–194, 2007.

[6] B. Linnemann and H. U. Janka, "Prolonged QTc interval and elevated heart rate identify the type 2 diabetic patient at high risk for cardiovascular death. The Bremen diabetes study," *Experimental and Clinical Endocrinology and Diabetes*, vol. 111, no. 4, pp. 215–222, 2003.

[7] G. S. Hillis, M. Woodward, A. Rodgers et al., "Resting heart rate and the risk of death and cardiovascular complications in patients with type 2 diabetes mellitus," *Diabetologia*, vol. 55, no. 5, pp. 1283–1290, 2012.

[8] G. S. Hillis, J. Hata, M. Woodward et al., "Resting heart rate and the risk of microvascular complications in patients with type 2 diabetes mellitus," *Journal of the American Heart Association*, vol. 1, no. 5, Article ID e002832, 2012.

[9] A. Miot, S. Ragot, W. Hammi et al., "Prognostic value of resting heart rate on cardiovascular and renal outcomes in type 2 diabetic patients: a competing risk analysis in a prospective cohort," *Diabetes Care*, vol. 35, no. 10, pp. 2069–2075, 2012.

[10] A. S. Krolewski, M. A. Niewczas, J. Skupien et al., "Early progressive renal decline precedes the onset of microalbuminuria and its progression to macroalbuminuria," *Diabetes Care*, vol. 37, no. 1, pp. 226–234, 2014.

[11] A. S. Krolewski, T. Gohda, and M. A. Niewczas, "Progressive renal decline as the major feature of diabetic nephropathy in type 1 diabetes," *Clinical and Experimental Nephrology*, vol. 18, no. 4, pp. 571–583, 2014.

[12] G. Pugliese, A. Solini, E. Bonora et al., "Chronic kidney disease in type 2 diabetes: lessons from the Renal Insufficiency And Cardiovascular Events (RIACE) Italian Multicentre Study," *Nutrition, Metabolism and Cardiovascular Diseases*, vol. 24, no. 8, pp. 815–822, 2014.

[13] R. D. Lindeman, J. Tobin, and N. W. Shock, "Longitudinal studies on the rate of decline in renal function with age," *Journal of the American Geriatrics Society*, vol. 33, no. 4, pp. 278–285, 1985.

[14] R. J. Gray, "A class of K-sample tests for comparing the cumulative incidence of a competing risk," *The Annals of Statistics*, vol. 16, no. 3, pp. 1141–1154, 1988.

[15] J. P. Fine and R. J. Gray, "A proportional hazards model for the subdistribution of a competing risk," *Journal of the American Statistical Association*, vol. 94, no. 446, pp. 496–509, 1999.

[16] A. S. Krolewski, "Progressive renal decline: the new paradigm of diabetic nephropathy in type 1 diabetes," *Diabetes Care*, vol. 38, no. 6, pp. 954–962, 2015.

[17] J.-F. Morcet, M. Safar, F. Thomas, L. Guize, and A. Benetos, "Associations between heart rate and other risk factors in a large French population," *Journal of Hypertension*, vol. 17, no. 12, pp. 1671–1676, 1999.

[18] ADVANCE Management Committee, "Study rationale and design of ADVANCE: action in diabetes and vascular disease—preterax and diamicron MR controlled evaluation," *Diabetologia*, vol. 44, no. 9, pp. 1118–1120, 2001.

[19] M. Böhm, J. C. Reil, N. Danchin, M. Thoenes, P. Bramlage, and M. Volpe, "Association of heart rate with microalbuminuria in cardiovascular risk patients: data from I-SEARCH," *Journal of Hypertension*, vol. 26, no. 1, pp. 18–25, 2008.

[20] T. Nakagawa, K. Tanabe, B. P. Croker et al., "Endothelial dysfunction as a potential contributor in diabetic nephropathy," *Nature Reviews Nephrology*, vol. 7, no. 1, pp. 36–44, 2011.

[21] P. Palatini, "Elevated heart rate in cardiovascular diseases: a target for treatment?" *Progress in Cardiovascular Diseases*, vol. 52, no. 1, pp. 46–60, 2009.

[22] American Diabetes Association, "Standards of medical care in diabetes—2008," *Diabetes Care*, vol. 31, supplement 1, pp. S12–S54, 2008.

[23] A. I. Vinik, R. E. Maser, B. D. Mitchell, and R. Freeman, "Diabetic autonomic neuropathy," *Diabetes Care*, vol. 26, no. 5, pp. 1553–1579, 2003.

Prevalence of Urinary Tract Infection and Antimicrobial Susceptibility among Diabetic Patients with Controlled and Uncontrolled Glycemia in Kuwait

May Sewify,[1] Shinu Nair,[1] Samia Warsame,[2] Mohamed Murad,[1] Asma Alhubail,[1] Kazem Behbehani,[1,2] Faisal Al-Refaei,[1] and Ali Tiss[2]

[1]*Clinical Services Department, Dasman Diabetes Institute, P.O. Box 1180, 15462 Kuwait, Kuwait*
[2]*Biochemistry & Molecular Biology Unit, Dasman Diabetes Institute, P.O. Box 1180, 15462 Kuwait, Kuwait*

Correspondence should be addressed to Ali Tiss; ali.tiss@dasmaninstitute.org

Academic Editor: Giovanni Annuzzi

Diabetic patients have higher risk of urinary tract infection (UTI). In the present study, we investigated the impact of glycemic control in diabetic patients on UTI prevalence, type of strains, and their antimicrobial drugs susceptibility. This study was conducted on urine samples from 722 adult diabetic patients from which 252 (35%) samples were positive for uropathogens. Most UTI cases occurred in the uncontrolled glycemic group (197 patients) versus 55 patients with controlled glycemia. Higher glycemic levels were measured in uncontrolled glycemia group (HbA1c = 8.3 ± 1.5 and 5.4 ± 0.4, resp., $P < 0.0001$). Females showed much higher prevalence of UTI than males in both glycemic groups (88.5% and 11.5%, resp., $P < 0.0001$). In the uncontrolled glycemia group 90.9% of the UTI cases happened at ages above 40 years and a clear correlation was obtained between patient age ranges and number of UTI cases ($r = 0.94$; $P = 0.017$), whereas in the group with controlled glycemia no trend was observed. *Escherichia coli* was the predominant uropathogen followed by *Klebsiella pneumoniae* and they were together involved in 76.2% of UTI cases. Those species were similarly present in both diabetic groups and displayed comparable antibiotic resistance pattern. These results highlight the importance of controlling glycemia in diabetic patients to reduce the UTI regardless of age and gender.

1. Introduction

Urinary tract infections (UTIs) are one of the most common microbial diseases encountered in medical practice affecting people of all ages [1]. Worldwide, UTIs' prevalence was estimated to be around 150 million persons per year [2].

Diabetic patients have a higher incidence of UTI than their nondiabetic counterparts [3, 4] with a higher severity UTI which can be a cause of complications, ranging from dysuria (pain or burning sensation during urination) to organ damage and sometimes even death due to complicated UTI (pyelonephritis) [5]. In 2012, the direct medical costs associated with managing UTIs in the 22 million diabetic patients in USA were estimated to be more than $2.3 billion [6]. Moreover, diabetic patients encounter further urinary urgency and incontinence during night, a condition often manifested by painful urination and retention of urine in the bladder [7]. Furthermore, those patients frequently suffer from bacterial cystitis with higher prevalence in diabetic women including higher prevalence of both asymptomatic bacteriuria and symptomatic UTI added to recurrent complications as compared to healthy women [8, 9]. In women, premenopausal and postmenopausal periods aside with sexual activity are considered increased risk factors for developing UTI [3, 8, 10]. Finally, diabetic women have up to four times more UTI risk when they are in oral treatment or insulin injection [10].

Potential explanation of the increased UTI in diabetic patients might be the nerve damage caused by high blood glucose levels, affecting the ability of the bladder to sense the presence of urine and thus allowing urine to stay for a long time in the bladder and increasing infection probability [8, 11]. Another explanation is that high glucose levels in urine improve the growth of the bacteria in the urine [12].

Additionally, the reduced blood circulation due to prolonged diabetes mellitus may result in abnormalities of the host defense system as reflected, for example, by the decrease in certain cytokines such as IL-6 and other proinflammatory cytokines in the urine of diabetic patients [13] which may increase the risk of developing infection.

Despite the fact that *E. coli* is the most frequent bacterium in UTI, other aggressive pathogens are highly prevalent in diabetic UTIs such as fungal infections, *Klebsiella*, Gram-negative rods, *enterococci*, group B *streptococci*, *Pseudomonas*, and *Proteus mirabilis* [14, 15].

Therefore, improved control of glycemia in diabetics may help in controlling the UTIs. Accurate screening for UTI in diabetic patients is also critical to enable the appropriate treatment, avoiding related complications. Nevertheless, only scarce data are available with respect to prevalence, recurrence, and microbiological features of UTI in diabetic patients with good glycemic control as compared to those with poor glycemic control.

In this study we aimed to assess the prevalence of UTI in diabetic patients referred to our specialized center, Dasman Diabetes Institute, as well as the type of microbiologically confirmed UTI and pattern of the antimicrobial drugs susceptibility in relation to diabetes mellitus in patients with good and patients with poor glycemic control.

2. Material and Methods

2.1. Study Population. The present study was carried out between April 2011 and March 2014 at Dasman Diabetes Institute (DDI), a specialized outpatient center to help diabetic patients in controlling blood glucose levels and treating their diabetes complications. The study included 252 patients with positive UTI (see Table 1 for details) out of a total number of 722 analyzed samples. Information on patient age, gender, and history of urinary frequency was obtained from the DDI Laboratory Information System (LIS). The access and use of the anonymized data analysis from the LIS for the purpose of publication were approved by the Ethical Review Board of DDI and carried out in line with the ethical guideline of Declaration of Helsinki.

2.2. Urine Collection and Processing. Clean voided midstream urine samples were collected in sterile special urine collection cups with the assistance of trained laboratory staff at DDI. Before sample collection, each patient was provided with a brochure and instructions explaining how to collect a correct midstream urine sample to avoid contamination. All urine samples were inoculated using a calibrated inoculation needle with 10 μL of urine and each sample was inoculated on three types of media: blood agar, MacConkey agar plates, and CLED agar (Oxoid, Basingstoke, UK). All plates were incubated at 37°C for 24–48 hours for visible growth.

2.3. Identification of Isolated Microorganisms. Urine samples showing a colony count more than 10^4 cfu/mL were considered to be positive for UTI. UTI isolates were identified following standard biochemical tests. Results were not considered for more than two clinical isolates obtained from the same patient and the sample was considered to be contaminated. No-growth plates were considered as sterile.

TABLE 1: Characteristics of the study subjects with controlled and uncontrolled glycemia.

	Controlled glycemic group	Uncontrolled glycemic group
Number of patients	55 (21.8%)	197 (78.2%)
Mean age (years ± SD)	48 ± 16	63 ± 16
Type of diabetes		
Type 1	5 (9%)	15 (7.6%)
Type 2	50 (91%)	182 (92.4%)
Duration of diabetes (years)	17.26 ± 8.5	19.84 ± 8.67
HbA1c	5.4 ± 0.5	8.3 ± 1.5
Therapy		
Insulin (number)	29 (52.7%)	117 (59.4)
Metformin	27 (49.1%)	86 (43.7%)
Glimepiride	3 (5.5%)	7 (3.6%)
Sitagliptin	4 (7.3%)	12 (6.1%)

For positive urine cultures, identifications were done using automated system Microscan (Walkaway 40 SI, Siemens Healthcare Diagnostics, Sacramento, CA). Panels used for Gram-negative bacteria (NC34 and NC53) and for Gram-positive bacteria (PC21) were obtained from Siemens Healthcare Diagnostics (Sacramento, CA). For confirmation, further biochemical tests were done for both Gram-positive and Gram-negative isolates (API E20, API strep, and API staph) supplied by bioMérieux, (Durham, NC, USA).

QC strains (*Escherichia coli* ATCC 25922, *Klebsiella pneumoniae* ATCC 13883, and *Candida albicans* ATCC 10231) were supplied by American Type Culture Collection (ATCC) (Manassas, VA).

2.4. Susceptibility Testing. Susceptibilities of the common isolated bacteria (*E. coli*, *Enterococcus faecalis*, *Klebsiella pneumoniae*, *Serratia marcescens*, *Pseudomonas aeruginosa*, *Staphylococcus saprophyticus*, *Staphylococcus aureus*, and *Proteus mirabilis*) to selected antimicrobial agents causing UTI were examined. Antimicrobial sensitivity testing of all isolates was performed on diagnostic sensitivity test plates according to the Kirby-Bauer method [16] following the definition of the Committee of Clinical Laboratory International Standards (CLIS, 2014). Bacterial inoculums were prepared by suspending the freshly grown bacteria in 5 mL sterile saline. A sterile cotton swab was used to streak the surface of Mueller Hinton agar plates. Filter paper disks containing a designated concentration of the antimicrobial drugs obtained from Becton and Dickinson Company (Franklin Lakes, NJ) were used.

2.5. Statistical Analysis. Data were analyzed using the statistical software SPSS for Windows, version 17.0 (SPSS, Chicago, IL, USA). Nonparametric Mann-Whitney test was used to determine significance of difference in means between the UTI groups. Correlations between variables were calculated with Spearman's rank correlation test. $P < 0.05$ was considered to be statistically significant.

3. Results

3.1. Study Population. This study was conducted on urine samples from 722 diabetic patients received at DDI during the period between April 2011 and March 2014. Among the 722 analyzed samples, 323 (45%) were showing sterile urine samples, while 147 (20%) showed mixed growth of bacteria possibly due to improper collection of the sample. The remaining 252 (35%) samples were positive for uropathogens with colony count higher than 10^4 CFU/mL of urine and were included in the current study analysis. The studied population was classified according to the glycemic status; patients with controlled glycemia (HbA1c < 6.5) and patients with uncontrolled glycemia (HbA1c ≥ 6.5) and their main characteristics are summarized in Table 1. The number of subjects with UTI was clearly higher in the uncontrolled glycemic group ($n = 197$, 78.2%) in comparison to the controlled glycemic group ($n = 55$, 21.8%). The mean age was significantly lower for the diabetic patients with controlled glycemia (48±16 years) when compared to that (63±16 years) for the diabetic patients with uncontrolled glycemia ($P < 0.01$). As expected, significantly different levels of glycemia were measured between both groups (HbA1c = 5.4 ± 0.4 and HbA1c = 8.3 ± 1.5, resp., $P < 0.0001$). Nevertheless, no clear difference was observed in the distribution of the type of diabetes, its duration, or the used treatment between the two groups (Table 1).

3.2. UTI and Etiology of Isolates. As summarized in Table 2, females showed much higher prevalence of UTI than males as 223 (88.5%) of UTIs of the total study population were in females versus only 29 (11.5%) in males ($P < 0.0001$). Interestingly, this gender distribution pattern was very similar in both patient groups with controlled and uncontrolled glycemia.

It is worth noting that, in contrast with the controlled glycemia group, in the patients with uncontrolled glycemia there is a clear increase of UTI cases with age as 90.1% of UTI cases were observed in women with an age above 40 years (Table 2). This same trend was also observed for both males and females, despite the low number of males with UTI in our study, in particular in the controlled glycemic group. Further analysis using Spearman's correlation ranking of the distribution of UTI according to the age ranges has shown a clear increase with age of UTI cases in the uncontrolled glycemia group ($r = 0.94$; $P = 0.017$) as compared to the controlled glycemia group where there was no trend of UTI cases according to age (Figure 1).

The prevalence and the distribution of Gram-negative and Gram-positive bacteria and yeast isolated from the clinical samples are shown in Table 3 for both controlled and uncontrolled glycemia groups. These isolates from both females and males represented clinically significant pathogens. As shown in Table 3, *E. coli* was the predominant pathogen isolated from urine samples in both females and males, as well as from both patient groups including 6 ESBL positive cases, all from uncontrolled glycemia patients. Indeed, *E. coli* was isolated from 57% of UTI cases in females and 37% of UTI cases in males. In our patients, *E. coli* was similarly present in both controlled and uncontrolled glycemia groups (53.3% and 58.1%, resp.) as shown in Table 3.

The strain *K. pneumoniae* (21.8% of all cases) showed only 1 ESBL positive case also isolated from uncontrolled glycemia patients. *Enterobacter* species represented 10.5% of the isolated pathogens, whereas Gram-positive *S. agalactiae* (group B *streptococci*) were found in about 5.5% of the UTI cases and only about 1% of cases were assigned to yeast *Candida* species. Together, *E. coli* and *K. pneumoniae* strains are the most prevalent uropathogens and represent 76.2%

TABLE 2: Age and sex distribution of patients with positive UTI included in this study.

Glycemic status	Patients age groups	Gender		Total
		Male	Female	
Controlled	Average	54 ± 13	47 ± 17	48 ± 16
	20–30	2	6	8
	31–40	0	16	16
	41–50	0	7	7
	51–60	5	8	13
	61–70	0	5	5
	>70	1	5	6
	Total	**8**	**47**	**55**
Uncontrolled	Average	65 ± 12	63 ± 16	63 ± 16
	20–30	1	10	11
	31–40	0	7	7
	41–50	0	21	21
	51–60	7	25	32
	61–70	4	44	48
	>70	9	69	78
	Total	**21**	**176**	**197**

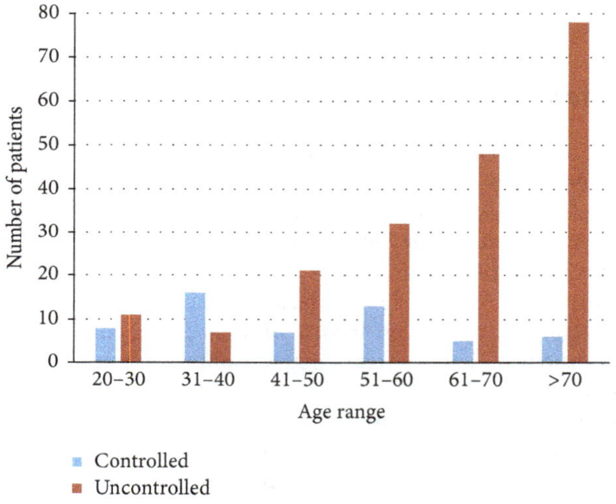

FIGURE 1: Distribution of UTI cases according to age ranges and glycemic status of our diabetic patients.

Table 3: Microbial uropathogens isolated from urine of our diabetic study population.

UTI pathogens	Uncontrolled glycemia		Controlled glycemia	
	Males	Females	Males	Females
Gram-negative microorganisms				
E. coli	6	99	5	27
K. pneumoniae	4	41	2	8
K. oxytoca	0	0	0	3
Raoultella ornithinolytica	0	5	0	0
P. aeruginosa	1	2	0	2
P. mirabilis	2	0	0	0
Citrobacter koseri	2	1	0	0
Citrobacter bummannii	0	1	0	0
Citrobacter freundii	0	1	0	0
Morganella morganii	0	1	0	0
Kluyvera species	0	1	0	0
Miscellaneous GNB	2	4	0	2
Gram-positive microorganisms				
Staphylococcus epidermidis	0	3	0	2
Staphylococcus warneri	0	2	0	0
Staphylococcus sciuri	2	2	0	0
Streptococcus agalactiae	2	9	1	2
Enterococcus faecalis	0	2	0	0
Miscellaneous GPB	0	1	0	0
Yeast				
Candida glabrata	0	1	0	0
Candida albicans	0	0	0	1
Total	21	176	8	47

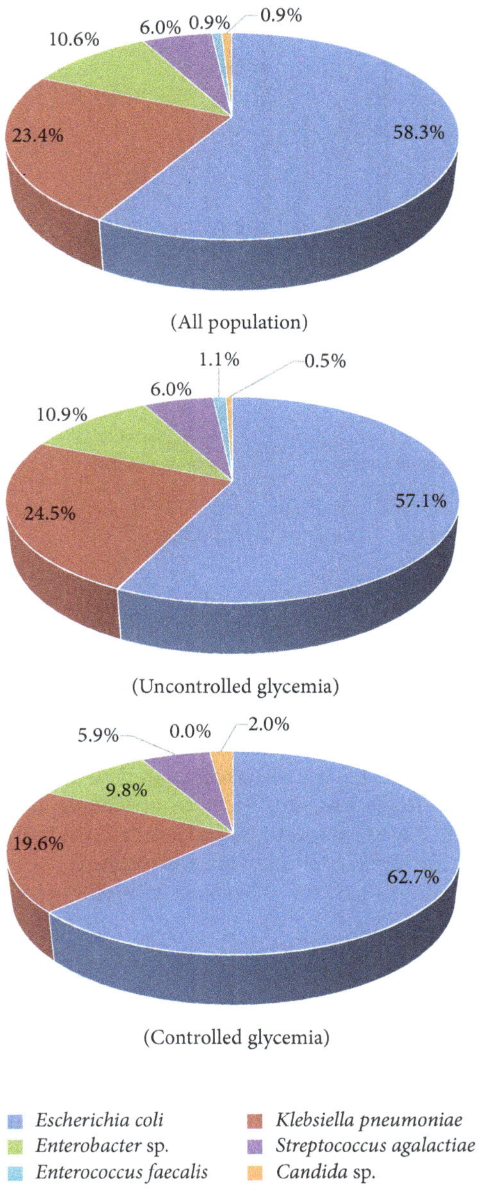

Figure 2: Distribution of most UTI prevalent pathogens in our study population groups.

of UTI cases (Table 3). In more detailed analysis and when taking into account only the 6 major strains identified in our study, the same trends in species distribution were obtained as shown in Figure 2.

3.3. Antimicrobial Susceptibility Pattern. The resistance pattern of UTI isolates from diabetic patients at DDI was analyzed and the results of antibiotic resistance of the most prevalent Gram-negative and Gram-positive pathogens are shown in Figure 3. Due to the limited number of diabetic patients with controlled glycemia, we did not analyze separately the resistance pattern of UTI isolates in this group. Gram-negative pathogens showed a comparable susceptibility pattern to most of the antibiotics, whereas the Gram-positive *Staphylococcus agalactiae* displayed completely different patterns (Figure 3). Indeed, the most prevalent pathogen, *E. coli*, displayed relatively high antimicrobial resistance rates against most of the tested antibiotics, that is, cephalothin (58%), trimethoprim-sulfamethoxazole (48%), ciprofloxacin and ampicillin/sulbactam (34%), cefotaxime (28%), ceftazidime (26%), amoxicillin/clavulanate (20%), nitrofurantoin (4%), and amikacin (2%). Likewise, *Klebsiella pneumoniae* showed similar patterns of resistance to trimethoprim-sulfamethoxazole (47%), ampicillin/sulbactam (42%), cephalothin (42%), ciprofloxacin (34%), cefotaxime (25%), amoxicillin/clavulanate (24%), ceftazidime (22%), nitrofurantoin (11%), and amikacin (2%), respectively. *Enterobacter* species resistance pattern was as follows:

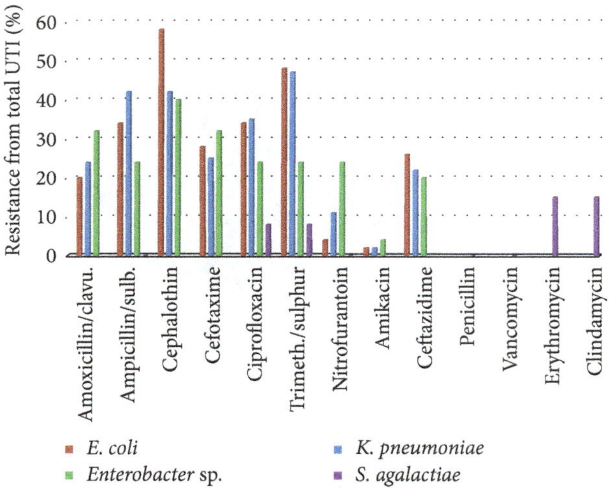

FIGURE 3: Resistance pattern for most UTI prevalent Gram-negative and Gram-positive pathogens in all population study.

cephalothin (40%), amoxicillin/clavulanate (32%), cefotaxime (32%), ciprofloxacin (24%), ampicillin/sulbactam (24%), and ceftazidime (20%), and only 4% of strains were resistant to amikacin. These species were however more resistant to nitrofurantoin (24%) and less resistant to trimethoprim-sulfamethoxazole (24%) when compared to *E. coli* and *K. pneumoniae*. Regarding *Streptococcus agalactiae*, from the 13 isolates only 2 were found to be resistant to clindamycin and erythromycin (15%). Among those 2 isolates, one was also resistant to ciprofloxacin (8%) and trimethoprim/sulphur (8%).

4. Discussion

Diabetic patients have higher risk of UTI particularly in women. In the present study, we investigated the possible impact of the glycemic control on the UTI prevalence, type of strains, and their antimicrobial drugs susceptibility in diabetic patients. Our main findings are the following: (1) there is much higher prevalence of UTI in diabetic patients with uncontrolled glycemia, (2) the glycemic control does affect the distribution of UTI according to age, but it does not affect its distribution according to gender, and (3) the etiology of the isolated strains and their antibiotic resistance pattern do not differ between patients with controlled and uncontrolled glycemia.

Analysis of our results showed that, among the 722 diabetic patients received at DDI, 35% were positive for uropathogens. This prevalence is apparently higher than the 20–30% commonly reported in diabetic patients [4, 15, 17–19]. This might be due to the fact that most of our subjects were diabetic for long periods (>10 years). Indeed, in diabetic patients, specific risk factors for UTI are usually the duration of diabetes and the presence of long-term complications, such as neuropathy, rather than current glucose control [8, 20]. It is worth mentioning that in our study there was no preselection of enrolled subjects according to gender, age, or glycemic status. Furthermore, most of the UTI cases in our study (78.2%) were found in the diabetic patients with uncontrolled glycemia in agreement with previous reports stating this trend when comparing diabetic patients (supposed to have uncontrolled glycemia) and nondiabetic subjects with normal glycemia.

Moreover, our results also showed that the majority of UTIs occurred in women (88.5%), in agreement with previous studies [19] and thereby confirming that adult women have a higher rate of UTI prevalence than men also in the diabetic population. Interestingly, this gender distribution pattern was very similar in both diabetic groups with controlled and uncontrolled glycemia suggesting that there is no impact of glycemic control on the distribution of UTI according to gender (Table 2). Similar conclusions were reported in previous studies where no significant differences were observed in the prevalence of bacteriuria both in males and in females when comparing diabetic and nondiabetic adult subjects [7, 15]. In contrast, and still comparing non-diabetic with diabetic women subjects, Geerlings et al. have reported that bacteriuria was more widespread in diabetic women with uncontrolled glycemia, [9]. As most of the previous studies on UTI in diabetic patients were carried out in women, there is limited evidence describing aspects of UTIs in diabetic men [21], and, to the best of our knowledge, the present data is the first to compare the effect of glycemic control on UTIs in males.

Despite the fact that a precise cause-effect relationship has not yet been established, multiple factors are suggested to be involved in the high occurrence of UTIs in diabetes patients. These include but are not limited to glucosuria [8], increased bacterial adherence to uroepithelial cells due to hyperglycemia [22], and neurogenic bladder [23]. In this context, Canagliflozin and Dapagliflozin, new antihyperglycemia molecules inhibiting renal glucose reabsorption and thus increasing glucosuria, were recently tested in clinical trials and were found to be associated with only a slight increase of UTI in T2D [12, 24]. This suggests that the contribution of glucosuria is limited in UTI and it does not explain its increased prevalence in diabetic patients. Nevertheless, there was a higher correlation between glucosuria and genital infection in Dapagliflozin-treated patients probably due to a greater effect of glucosuria in promoting the growth of fungal pathogens associated with genital infection as compared to bacterial pathogens typically associated with UTI [25]. In a new report, James and Hijaz have reviewed recent publications on lower urinary tract symptoms (LUTS) and UTI in diabetic women and have concluded that aging and obesity are significantly associated with worsened LUTS [26]. Glucosuria was also found to be associated with UTI and diabetic patients appeared to be at a higher risk for colonization with the virulent, extended-spectrum β-lactamase-producing *E. coli* and *Klebsiella* species in UTI [26]. In our studied population, obesity might be considered as a cofounder in the correlation between glycemic control and UTI as obesity rates are about 50% in Kuwait [27]. Unfortunately, we do not dispose of this parameter in our subjects to further investigate this potential hypothesis.

Age is a well-known risk factor for bacteriuria in non-diabetic females. Advanced age has been widely accepted as a risk factor for patients with type 2 diabetes mellitus. In our study at DDI, we confirmed that diabetes is associated with a higher risk of acute symptomatic UTI in postmenopausal women than younger women. Indeed, in our results, there was a clear correlation between age and UTI in the group with uncontrolled glycemia and most of the UTI cases occurred at older age (Figure 1). In contrast, in the controlled glycemia group, an almost equal distribution of the UTI cases was observed throughout all age ranges (Table 2) regardless of the gender, despite the limited number of patients in this group. This significant difference in the age of the two groups as well as the correlation with UTI might be explained by the fact that most of the patients with controlled glycemia are younger and thus more adhering to their treatment and healthy lifestyle as compared to old patients. The fact that 9% of patients with controlled glycemia have type 1 diabetes is not enough to explain this difference in trends with age despite knowing that type 2 diabetes prevalence and its complications are increased with age. It is worth noting that most of patients included in our study had diabetes for long periods (at least 10 years).

In the present study, *E. coli* was the predominant pathogen isolated from urine samples followed by *Klebsiella* in both females and males. Those species were similarly present in both groups with controlled and uncontrolled glycemia and hence were together involved in 76.2% of UTI cases. Comparable results were previously reported and confirm the predominance of those species in diabetic patients and in nondiabetic subjects [7, 15, 19, 28]. Those UTI etiological agents are also in line with previous data from the Kuwaiti general population previously reported [19, 29]. Furthermore, all the 6 ESBL *E. coli* identified in our study were isolated in diabetics with uncontrolled glycemia, in agreement with previous studies reporting higher prevalence of ESBL-producing *E. coli* and *Klebsiella* species in diabetic patients as compared to nondiabetics [15, 30]. Together, these observations may suggest a direct link between glycemic control and UTI with ESBL-producing strains. It is noteworthy that *Streptococcus agalactiae* represented around 6% of the UTI in our study in both diabetic patients with controlled glycemia and those with uncontrolled glycemia. Interestingly, and despite comparable prevalence already reported in general population analysis from Kuwait [19, 29], those numbers seem to be higher than what was reported in other populations where *S. agalactiae* was totally absent [15]. Al Benwan et al. have suggested that high prevalence of obesity and diabetes might explain this "Kuwaiti" specificity as diabetic patients are known to be predisposed to infection with this strain [19].

Our study also aimed to determine the resistance pattern for first-line antibiotics which are used at DDI outpatient clinics and which may help clinicians in the appropriate use of antimicrobial agents in diabetic patients. In our study we noted that Gram-negative strains including *E. coli* and *K. pneumoniae* were highly resistant (>45%) to trimethoprim-sulfamethoxazole, in agreement with previous reported studies from hospitals in Kuwait [19, 29]. Indeed, high resistance to this first-line antibiotic is of big concern to clinicians in Kuwait and other alternatives should be developed. Nevertheless, in our study, other antibiotics are displaying high sensitivity to all Gram-negative UTI isolates and these include amikacin (>96%), nitrofurantoin (75–96%), and amoxicillin/clavulanate (70–80%). Unfortunately, amikacin is potentially nephrotoxic and presents a risk of nephrotoxicity in patients with impaired renal function as well as in cases of diabetic patients [31]. Hence, the best acting antibiotics in our study were found to be nitrofurantoin, followed by amoxicillin/clavulanate and ciprofloxacin and then trimethoprim-sulfamethoxazole.

5. Conclusion

The significance of the study lies in the determination of common pathogens in diabetic patients with UTI in controlled and uncontrolled glycemia for the first time and the resistance pattern of antibiotics so that the clinicians get useful information regarding the use of antibiotics in diabetic patients. Further validation is hence anticipated in a larger diabetic population study. The study also gives evidence of differences in the etiological agents in Kuwait as compared to other regions which highlight the need of proper use of antibiotics in diabetic patients, particularly. The current study, however, has some limitations including the small number of diabetic patients with controlled glycemia analyzed and the lack of historical information on the non-UTI diabetic patients to allow detailed comparison between diabetic patients with and without UTI in relation to glycemic control. However, despite these limitations, we provided ample evidence that the control of glycemia in diabetics might help in reducing the occurrence of UTI in these vulnerable patients, specifically in aged subjects. We have also shown clear difference in the correlation between the UTI and age which seems to be directly affected by glycemic control. These findings add further evidence to the importance of tighter glycemic control in reducing the occurrence of UTI and most probably improving the clinical outcomes.

Conflict of Interests

The authors declare that there is no conflict of interests regarding the publication of this paper.

Acknowledgment

The authors would like to thank the staff at the Clinical Laboratory, Dasman Diabetes Institute, for their assistance throughout this study.

References

[1] C. M. Kunin, "Chemoprophylaxis and suppressive therapy in the management of urinary tract infections," *Journal of Antimicrobial Chemotherapy*, vol. 33, supplement A, pp. 51–62, 1994.

[2] K. Gupta, D. F. Sahm, D. Mayfield, and W. E. Stamm, "Antimicrobial resistance among uropathogens that cause community-acquired urinary tract infections in women: a nationwide analysis," *Clinical Infectious Diseases*, vol. 33, no. 1, pp. 89–94, 2001.

[3] V. de Lastours and B. Foxman, "Urinary tract infection in diabetes: epidemiologic considerations," *Current Infectious Disease Reports*, vol. 16, no. 1, article 389, 2014.

[4] J. E. Patterson and V. T. Andriole, "Bacterial urinary tract infections in diabetes," *Infectious Disease Clinics of North America*, vol. 11, no. 3, pp. 735–750, 1997.

[5] M. Saleem and B. Daniel, "Prevalence of urinary tract infection among patients with diabetes in Bangalore city," *International Journal of Emerging Sciences*, vol. 1, no. 2, pp. 133–142, 2011.

[6] A. Ward, P. Alvarez, L. Vo, and S. Martin, "Direct medical costs of complications of diabetes in the United States: estimates for event-year and annual state costs (USD 2012)," *Journal of Medical Economics*, vol. 17, no. 3, pp. 176–183, 2014.

[7] M. Bonadio, S. Costarelli, G. Morelli, and T. Tartaglia, "The influence of diabetes mellitus on the spectrum of uropathogens and the antimicrobial resistance in elderly adult patients with urinary tract infection," *BMC Infectious Diseases*, vol. 6, article 54, 2006.

[8] S. E. Geerlings, R. P. Stolk, M. J. L. Camps, P. M. Netten, T. J. Collet, and A. I. M. Hoepelman, "Risk factors for symptomatic urinary tract infection in women with diabetes," *Diabetes Care*, vol. 23, no. 12, pp. 1737–1741, 2000.

[9] S. E. Geerlings, R. P. Stolk, M. J. L. Camps et al., "Asymptomatic bacteriuria may be considered a complication in women with diabetes," *Diabetes Care*, vol. 23, no. 6, pp. 744–749, 2000.

[10] E. J. Boyko, S. D. Fihn, D. Scholes, C.-L. Chen, E. H. Normand, and P. Yarbro, "Diabetes and the risk of acute urinary tract infection among postmenopausal women," *Diabetes Care*, vol. 25, no. 10, pp. 1778–1783, 2002.

[11] S. Szucs, I. Cserhati, G. Csapo, and V. Balazs, "The relation between diabetes mellitus and infections of the unirary tract. A clinical, qualitative and quantitative bacteriological study based upon 300 diabetics and 200 controls," *The American Journal of the Medical Sciences*, vol. 240, pp. 186–191, 1960.

[12] K. M. Johnsson, A. Ptaszynska, B. Schmitz, J. Sugg, S. J. Parikh, and J. F. List, "Urinary tract infections in patients with diabetes treated with dapagliflozin," *Journal of Diabetes and its Complications*, vol. 27, no. 5, pp. 473–478, 2013.

[13] S. E. Geerlings, E. C. Brouwer, K. P. M. van Kessel, W. Gaastra, and A. M. Hoepelman, "Cytokine secretion is impaired in women with diabetes mellitus," in *Genes and Proteins Underlying Microbial Urinary Tract Virulence*, vol. 485 of *Advances in Experimental Medicine and Biology*, pp. 255–262, Springer, 2000.

[14] A. Ronald, "The etiology of urinary tract infection: traditional and emerging pathogens," *American Journal of Medicine*, vol. 113, supplement 1, pp. 14S–19S, 2002.

[15] M. Aswani Srinivas, U. K. Chandrashekar, K. N. Shivashankara, and B. C. Pruthvi, "Clinical profile of urinary tract infections in diabetics and non-diabetics," *Australasian Medical Journal*, vol. 7, no. 1, pp. 29–34, 2014.

[16] A. W. Bauer, W. M. Kirby, J. C. Sherris, and M. Turck, "Antibiotic susceptibility testing by a standardized single disk method," *American Journal of Clinical Pathology*, vol. 45, no. 4, pp. 493–496, 1966.

[17] L. M. A. J. Muller, K. J. Gorter, E. Hak et al., "Increased risk of common infections in patients with type 1 and type 2 diabetes mellitus," *Clinical Infectious Diseases*, vol. 41, no. 3, pp. 281–288, 2005.

[18] T. Benfield, J. S. Jensen, and B. G. Nordestgaard, "Influence of diabetes and hyperglycaemia on infectious disease hospitalisation and outcome," *Diabetologia*, vol. 50, no. 3, pp. 549–554, 2007.

[19] K. Al Benwan, N. Al Sweih, and V. O. Rotimi, "Etiology and antibiotic susceptibility patterns of community- and hospital-acquired urinary tract infections in a general hospital in Kuwait," *Medical Principles and Practice*, vol. 19, no. 6, pp. 440–446, 2010.

[20] K. J. Gorter, E. Hak, N. P. A. Zuithoff, A. I. M. Hoepelman, and G. E. H. M. Rutten, "Risk of recurrent acute lower urinary tract infections and prescription pattern of antibiotics in women with and without diabetes in primary care," *Family Practice*, vol. 27, no. 4, pp. 379–385, 2010.

[21] L. E. Nicolle, "Urinary tract infections in special populations. diabetes, renal transplant, HIV infection, and spinal cord injury," *Infectious Disease Clinics of North America*, vol. 28, no. 1, pp. 91–104, 2014.

[22] S. E. Geerlings, "Urinary tract infections in patients with diabetes mellitus: epidemiology, pathogenesis and treatment," *International Journal of Antimicrobial Agents*, vol. 31, supplement 1, pp. 54–57, 2008.

[23] D. Sauerwein, "Urinary tract infection in patients with neurogenic bladder dysfunction," *International Journal of Antimicrobial Agents*, vol. 19, no. 6, pp. 592–597, 2002.

[24] L. E. Nicolle, G. Capuano, A. Fung, and K. Usiskin, "Urinary tract infection in randomized phase III studies of canagliflozin, a sodium glucose co-transporter 2 inhibitor," *Postgraduate Medicine*, vol. 126, no. 1, pp. 7–17, 2014.

[25] K. M. Johnsson, A. Ptaszynska, B. Schmitz, J. Sugg, S. J. Parikh, and J. F. List, "Vulvovaginitis and balanitis in patients with diabetes treated with dapagliflozin," *Journal of Diabetes and Its Complications*, vol. 27, no. 5, pp. 479–484, 2013.

[26] R. James and A. Hijaz, "Lower urinary tract symptoms in women with diabetes mellitus: a current review," *Current Urology Reports*, vol. 15, no. 10, article 440, 2014.

[27] I. Al Rashdan and Y. Al Nesef, "Prevalence of overweight, obesity, and metabolic syndrome among adult Kuwaitis: results from community-based national survey," *Angiology*, vol. 61, no. 1, pp. 42–48, 2010.

[28] R. Simkhada, "Urinary tract infection and antibiotic sensitivity pattern among diabetics," *Nepal Medical College Journal*, vol. 15, no. 1, pp. 1–4, 2013.

[29] N. Al Sweih, W. Jamal, and V. O. Rotimi, "Spectrum and antibiotic resistance of uropathogens isolated from hospital and community patients with urinary tract infections in two large hospitals in Kuwait," *Medical Principles and Practice*, vol. 14, no. 6, pp. 401–407, 2005.

[30] S. H. MacVane, L. O. Tuttle, and D. P. Nicolau, "Impact of extended-spectrum β-lactamase-producing organisms on clinical and economic outcomes in patients with urinary tract infection," *Journal of Hospital Medicine*, vol. 9, no. 4, pp. 232–238, 2014.

[31] J. S. Sandhu, A. Sehgal, O. Gupta, and A. Singh, "Aminoglycoside nephrotoxicity revisited," *Journal, Indian Academy of Clinical Medicine*, vol. 8, no. 4, pp. 331–333, 2007.

High Intensity Aerobic Exercise Training Improves Deficits of Cardiovascular Autonomic Function in a Rat Model of Type 1 Diabetes Mellitus with Moderate Hyperglycemia

Kenneth N. Grisé,[1] T. Dylan Olver,[2] Matthew W. McDonald,[1] Adwitia Dey,[1] Mao Jiang,[1] James C. Lacefield,[3] J. Kevin Shoemaker,[2,4,5] Earl G. Noble,[1,5] and C. W. James Melling[1]

[1] *Exercise Biochemistry Laboratory, School of Kinesiology, Faculty of Health Sciences, Western University, London, ON, Canada N6A 3K7*
[2] *Neurovascular Research Laboratory, School of Kinesiology, Faculty of Health Sciences, Western University, London, ON, Canada N6A 3K7*
[3] *Department of Electrical and Computer Engineering, Department of Medical Biophysics and Robarts Research Institute, Western University, London, ON, Canada N6A 3K7*
[4] *Department of Physiology and Pharmacology, Western University, London, ON, Canada N6A 3K7*
[5] *Lawson Health Research Institute, London, ON, Canada N6C 2R5*

Correspondence should be addressed to C. W. James Melling; jmelling@uwo.ca

Academic Editor: Mark A. Yorek

Indices of cardiovascular autonomic neuropathy (CAN) in experimental models of Type 1 diabetes mellitus (T1DM) are often contrary to clinical data. Here, we investigated whether a relatable insulin-treated model of T1DM would induce deficits in cardiovascular (CV) autonomic function more reflective of clinical results and if exercise training could prevent those deficits. Sixty-four rats were divided into four groups: sedentary control (C), sedentary T1DM (D), control exercise (CX), or T1DM exercise (DX). Diabetes was induced via multiple low-dose injections of streptozotocin and blood glucose was maintained at moderate hyperglycemia (9–17 mM) through insulin supplementation. Exercise training consisted of daily treadmill running for 10 weeks. Compared to C, D had blunted baroreflex sensitivity, increased vascular sympathetic tone, increased serum neuropeptide Y (NPY), and decreased intrinsic heart rate. In contrast, DX differed from D in all measures of CAN (except NPY), including heart rate variability. These findings demonstrate that this T1DM model elicits deficits and exercise-mediated improvements to CV autonomic function which are reflective of clinical T1DM.

1. Introduction

A common and serious complication of Type 1 diabetes mellitus (T1DM) is diabetic autonomic neuropathy [1, 2]. Cardiovascular autonomic neuropathy (CAN) is a subset of diabetic autonomic neuropathy characterized by impaired autonomic control of the cardiovascular (CV) system [3]. CAN is also consistently associated with increased mortality. For instance, CAN has been reported to increase the mortality of diabetic patients by a factor of 3.45 [4]. Clinically, the most common methods for assessing CAN are heart rate variability (HRV) analysis and baroreflex sensitivity (BRS) [3, 5, 6]. In T1DM, aspects of the baroreflex arc can be impaired [7], such that both baroreceptor activity and excitability are blunted [8, 9] and the aortic depressor nerves undergo axonal atrophy [8]. As well, autonomic efferents, primarily of the parasympathetic nervous system (PSNS), have decreased activity, reduced responsiveness, and decreased neurochemical activity in the heart [10, 11]. Impairment of central nervous system regions has also been reported as the limiting factor of BRS [12, 13]. Reduced heart rate variability (HRV) is often the earliest symptom of CAN [14]. Whether measured by time domain analysis or by frequency domain analysis and whether in clinical or experimental T1DM, HRV is consistently reported to be reduced in T1DM [5, 14–17].

Exercise has been demonstrated to be an effective means of improving deficits in HRV and BRS in both clinical and experimental T1DM [18–21]. Such improvements have been attributed to improved insulin sensitivity, increased endogenous antioxidant and anti-inflammatory mediators, and improved autonomic control of the CV system [22–24]. Despite similar reductions in HRV and BRS, there are marked differences in early-stage changes to other CV parameters between clinical and experimental T1DM [25]. Specifically, in clinical T1DM, increases in heart rate (HR) and blood pressure (BP) are commonly reported in early autonomic neuropathy [1, 3, 14, 24, 26–28]. In contrast, experimental STZ-induced T1DM is regularly associated with decreased BP and HR, beginning shortly after diabetes induction [15, 16, 29–31]. Due to these opposing initial changes in BP and HR, exercise training is often observed to produce contrasting outcomes on CV parameters in experimental and clinical T1DM, namely, increased BP and HR in experimental T1DM and decreased BP and HR in clinical T1DM [19, 25, 32–34]. As a result, both the increase and decrease of these CV factors are concurrently cited as exercise-mediated improvements to CAN with little consideration of the fact that the changes are opposed between these two contexts of T1DM [25]. This is important because if animal models do not accurately reproduce T1DM pathology, then the outcomes of experimental studies may not translate to the treatment of human CAN, as the mechanisms underlying the pathology and exercise modifications may differ.

Another important difference between experimental and clinical T1DM is the common omission of insulin treatment in experimental diabetes leading to severe hyperglycemia ranging from roughly 17 to 25 mM blood glucose concentrations ([BG]) [15, 16, 29, 30]. As the severity and duration of hyperglycemia have been shown to influence the degree of diabetic neuropathy, acute and steep elevations of [BG] in STZ-induced T1DM may not only cause early onset neuropathy to the PSNS but also cause acute neuropathy of the sympathetic nervous system (SNS) and directly affect the sinoatrial (SA) node. These changes may mediate the observed reduction in BP and HR that arise acutely in experimental T1DM and in late-stage clinical T1DM [2, 35–38]. Indeed, intensive insulin therapy has been shown to restore BP and HR to non-T1DM levels in STZ-induced T1DM rats [25, 39].

Yet, despite the use of insulin therapy in clinical T1DM, it is often the case that chronic, moderate hyperglycemia is maintained as a result of difficulties in regulating [BG] in response to dynamic influences on glycemic control, such as food intake and exercise [40, 41]. This is often resultant of a tendency to err on the side of moderate hyperglycemia in order to circumvent the acute discomfort and danger associated with hypoglycemic episodes, which occur more frequently with diabetic neuropathy due to the impairment of the glucagon response [40, 42, 43]. To address this, our laboratory established a model of T1DM using a multiple low-dose STZ-treatment and insulin therapy to replicate the moderate hyperglycemia observed in clinical T1DM [44]. In our previous studies that employed this model, we observed impairments in glucose tolerance, vascular responsiveness, cardiac function, and bone health, which were improved with high intensity aerobic exercise training [44–47].

The purpose of the current study was to investigate whether our model of multiple low-dose STZ-induced T1DM with insulin therapy would induce deficits in cardiovascular autonomic function more representative of clinical T1DM, and if high intensity aerobic training could prevent those deficits. We hypothesised that (1) our model of STZ-induced T1DM would elicit indices of CAN, including a blunted BRS (bradycardia and tachycardia response), lowered HRV and intrinsic heart rate, increased vascular sympathetic tone, and increased mean arterial pressure, and (2) high intensity aerobic exercise training would prevent or ameliorate the indications of CAN.

2. Materials and Methods

2.1. Ethics Approval. The protocols used in this investigation were approved by the University of Western Ontario Council on Animal Care and conformed to the guidelines of the Canadian Council on Animal Care.

2.2. Animals. Eight-week-old male Sprague-Dawley rats were obtained from Charles River Laboratories Canada (Saint-Constant, Quebec). The rats were housed in pairs and maintained on a 12-hour dark/light cycle at a constant temperature (20±1°C) and relative humidity (50%). Rats were allowed access to standard rat chow and water *ad libitum*.

2.3. Experimental Groups. Sixty-four rats were randomly assigned to one of four groups as follows: (1) sedentary control (C, $n = 16$); (2) exercised control (CX, $n = 16$); (3) sedentary T1DM (D, $n = 16$); (4) exercised T1DM (DX, $n = 16$). All functional and blood endpoint measures were acquired 24 hours after the final exercise bout.

2.4. T1DM Induction and Insulin Dose. Upon arrival rats were acclimatized to the laboratory setting for five days. Subsequently, T1DM was induced over five consecutive days by multiple intraperitoneal (IP) injections of 20 mg/kg streptozotocin (STZ, Sigma-Aldrich) dissolved in a citrate buffer (0.1 M, pH 4.5). Diabetes was confirmed by blood glucose measurements greater than or equal to 18 mM on two consecutive days. If necessary, subsequent 20 mg/kg STZ injections were administered until diabetes was confirmed. Following the confirmation of diabetes, insulin pellets (1 pellet; 2 U insulin/day; Linplant, Linshin Canada, Inc., Toronto, Ontario, Canada) were implanted subcutaneously in the abdominal region. Insulin pellet doses were then monitored for 1 week and adjusted (±0.5 pellets) in order to obtain daily nonfasting blood glucose concentrations in the moderate hyperglycemic range of 9–17 mM. Insulin dose was determined by multiplying the total quantity of pellet implanted (0.5 pellet increments) by the amount of insulin released per pellet (2 units of insulin/day/pellet) divided by the body weight (Kg) of the rat.

2.5. Body Weight and Blood Glucose Concentration. Body weights and nonfasting blood glucose concentrations were obtained weekly. Blood was obtained from the saphenous vein by venous puncture with a 30-gauge needle and measured via Freestyle Lite Blood Glucose Monitoring System (Abbott Diabetes Care Inc., Mississauga, Ontario, Canada).

2.6. Intravenous Glucose Tolerance Test. Intravenous glucose tolerance tests (IVGTT) were performed on all animals prior to T1DM induction (pre-T1DM) and at the end of week 10 of the exercise training period. Rats were fasted for approximately 8 to 12 hours prior to the assay and did not perform exercise on the day of their IVGTT. A sterile-filtered dextrose solution (50% dextrose, 50% ddH_2O) was injected (1 g/kg) into the lateral tail vein of the conscious rat. Following dextrose infusion, blood glucose was measured at 5 minutes, at 10 minutes, and then at 10-minute intervals thereafter until blood glucose levels plateaued.

2.7. Exercise Protocol. Prior to the initiation of the exercise training program, rats were familiarized with the exercise equipment on two consecutive days. The familiarization consisted of two 15-minute sessions of running at progressive treadmill speeds up to 30 meters per minute (m/min). The treadmill was a custom-built apparatus fabricated by the physical plant at University of Western Ontario and has been used in many previous studies [44–47]. The exercise training program consisted of 1 hour of motor-driven treadmill running per day at 27 m/min with a 6-degree incline, 5 days per week, for 10 weeks. The exercise intensity was determined based on earlier research that investigated oxygen uptake in rats at various treadmill speeds. The chosen intensity was found to represent approximately 75–85% VO_{2max} [48, 49].

2.8. Preparative Surgery and Instrumentation. To achieve a surgical plane of anesthesia, rats were placed in an induction chamber circulating 4% isoflurane (96% O_2). Once motor reflexes were undetectable, rats were transferred to a nosecone delivering 3% isoflurane (97% O_2) and placed on a hot water pad (37°C). Rats were cannulated with saline-infused polyethylene (PE90) catheters in the right jugular vein and carotid artery and each catheter was attached to a three-way stopcock. The jugular vein catheter was used for drug infusions and the carotid artery catheter was connected in series with a pressure transducer (PX272, Edwards Life Sciences, Irvine, California, USA) for arterial blood pressure measurements.

At the end of the preparative surgery, rats were injected IP with a 25 mg/Kg "cocktail" of urethane (16 mg/mL) and α-chloralose (100 mg/mL), an anesthetic cocktail that has been shown to have the least inhibition of baseline CV control and autonomic function [50]. A total of 10 mL of urethane/α-chloralose was made, 5 mL of which was diluted to 50% with ddH_2O and was used as needed to maintain anesthesia throughout data collection. Isoflurane anesthesia was gradually removed, whereby urethane/α-chloralose was the primary anesthesia used during data collection.

2.9. Basal Heart Rate, Systolic Blood Pressure, and Mean Arterial Pressure. Heart rate (HR), systolic blood pressure (SBP), and mean arterial pressure (MAP) were determined from the blood pressure pulse waveform and were collected while the rats were under urethane/α-chloralose anesthesia in the supine position. The pressure transducer was calibrated using a standard analog manometer. Data were obtained using a PowerLab data acquisition system, digitized, and recorded at 1000 Hz using the bundled LabChart 7 Pro software (ADInstruments, Colorado Springs, CO, USA).

2.10. Heart Rate Variability. Prior to drug infusions, 5 minutes of spontaneous electrocardiogram data was sampled at 1000 Hz and analyzed with LabChart HRV analysis software (ADInstruments). Time domain analysis of the standard deviation between normal peak pulses of the pressure pulse waveform (SDNN) was quantified as a measure of the total variability of the HR. Frequency domain analysis of the high frequency (HF) band of the Fast Fourier Transform (FFT) of the data was assessed as an index of parasympathetically mediated HRV.

2.11. Baroreflex Sensitivity. Baroreflex sensitivity (BRS) was assessed using the modified Oxford technique [51, 52]. The BRS was quantified using the slope of the linear regression line representing the linear portion of the sigmoidal heart rate-systolic blood pressure relationship (ΔHR {BPM}/ ΔSBP $\{mmHg\}^{-1}$) after rapid bolus injections (~5 s) of phenylephrine (PE, 12 μg/Kg, 10 μg/mL) and sodium nitroprusside (SNP, 60 μg/Kg, 110 μg/mL) dissolved in ddH_2O. The rationale for this method is detailed by Studinger et al. (2007) [54]. For each drug, the catheter was first filled with a 0.2 mL volume to ensure accuracy of the drug dose. After a stable baseline was obtained, a bolus injection of SNP was rapidly infused and the reflex SNS mediated tachycardia response was measured. The analysis began at the onset of SBP decrease after SNP infusion and ended when SBP reached its nadir. This was followed by a saline flush to washout any remaining SNP in the catheter. After a stable baseline was reestablished, this same procedure was then followed using PE to measure PSNS mediated reflex bradycardia, except that analysis began at the onset of SBP increase and ended when SBP reached its zenith. Responses to PE and SNP were plotted separately and only regression lines (slopes) with correlation coefficients (r) ≥ 0.70 and $p < 0.05$ were accepted [53, 54].

2.12. Vascular Sympathetic Tone. To measure the sympathetic contribution to baseline vascular resistance, MAP was assessed before and after a bolus injection of the α-adrenergic receptor blocker, prazosin (85 μg/Kg, 500 μg/mL). Following this protocol, animals were euthanized via exsanguination while still under urethane/α-chloralose anesthesia.

2.13. Neuropeptide Y ELISA. To ensure physiological testing did not confound serum neuropeptide Y concentration

[NPY] measurement, a subset of animals from each group did not undergo surgery for heart rate variability, baroreflex sensitivity, mean arterial pressure, or vascular sympathetic tone measurements. Rather, at the end of the 10-week exercise training period these animals were anesthetized via intraperitoneal injection of sodium pentobarbital (65 mg/kg) and blood serum samples for [NPY] measurement were collected upon euthanasia. Serum [NPY] was measured using an NPY ELISA kit (USCN Life Sciences Inc.) according to the manufacturer's instructions.

2.14. Intrinsic Heart Rate. A Langendorff preparation was used to measure intrinsic heart rate. Following the euthanasia of animals for blood [NPY] measurement, hearts were extracted and immediately arrested by placing them in ice cold Krebs-Henseleit buffer (KHB). Hearts were cannulated for unpaced retrograde aortic constant flow perfusion (15 mL/min) of coronary arteries with KHB (containing 120 mM NaCl, 4.63 M KCl, 1.17 mM KH_2PO_4, 1.25 mM $CaCl_2$, 1.2 mM $MgCl_2$, 20 mM $NaHCO_3$, and 8 mM glucose gassed with 95% O_2 and 5% CO_2) that was maintained at 37°C [55]. Hearts were equilibrated for 30 min to determine baseline intrinsic heart rate.

2.15. Data Analysis and Statistics. Body weight and blood glucose concentrations were compared using a two-way repeated measures ANOVA, while endpoint measures were compared by two-way ANOVA, with the exception of endpoint insulin dose, which was compared using a one-tailed t-test. When significance was found, pairwise comparisons were made using the Fisher LSD post hoc test. Data are represented as mean ± standard error, with a significance level set at $p < 0.05$.

3. Results

3.1. Animal Characteristics. All groups increased in body weight over the course of the study ($p < 0.05$, Figure 1(a)). At the end of the study, the body weights of the T1DM groups (D and DX) were lower than non-T1DM groups (C and CX), and exercised groups (CX and DX) weighed less than their nonexercised counterparts (C and D; $p < 0.05$). Following the confirmation of diabetes, weekly [BG] was mostly maintained in the targeted range of 9–17 mM; however, the [BG] did move outside of this range periodically. The [BG] in the T1DM groups were elevated in comparison to the non-T1DM groups ($p < 0.05$; Figure 1(b)). Within the non-T1DM and T1DM groups, there was no difference in [BG] between nonexercised and exercised groups (C versus CX and D versus DX; $p > 0.05$).

3.2. Intravenous Glucose Tolerance Test and Insulin Dosages. The glucose clearance rate (K_G) of the diabetic groups (D and DX) decreased from pre-T1DM to week 10 of training ($p < 0.05$), whereas K_G of the CX group increased ($p < 0.05$; Figure 2(a)). Both diabetic groups had significantly lower K_G values than both the control groups (C and CX) at week 10 ($p < 0.05$; Figure 2(a)). However, there was not a significant interaction between diabetes and exercise on K_G. The amount of insulin supplementation that the DX group received was significantly less than the amount the D group received at week 10 ($p < 0.05$; Figure 2(b)).

3.3. Mean Arterial Pressure, Heart Rate, and Intrinsic Heart Rate. For resting HR and MAP, there was not a significant difference between groups at week 10 (Figures 3(a) and 3(b), resp.). However, for the intrinsic heart rate (IHR), there was main effect of both exercise and T1DM, where T1DM decreased the IHR, while exercise increased IHR ($p < 0.05$, Figure 3(c)). Further, within the T1DM groups (D and DX), exercise increased IHR, while within the nonexercised groups (C and D) T1DM decreased IHR ($p < 0.05$).

3.4. Heart Rate Variability. Total HRV at week 10, as measured by the standard deviation of the normal pulse wave peaks (SDNN), was not significantly different between groups (Figure 4(a)). However, there was a main effect of exercise on the HF contribution to HRV, where exercise increased HF HRV ($p < 0.05$, Figure 4(b)). Particularly, within the T1DM groups (D and DX), exercise increased HF HRV ($p < 0.05$).

3.5. Baroreflex Sensitivity. In response to SNP infusion, there was not a significant difference between groups in the tachycardia BRS response (Figure 5(a)). However, a significant interaction between T1DM and exercise was observed for BRS during the bradycardia response to phenylephrine ($p < 0.05$, Figure 5(b)). More specifically, within the T1DM groups (D and DX) exercise prevented the reduction in BRS that was observed in the D group ($p < 0.05$).

3.6. Vascular Sympathetic Tone and Serum NPY. An interaction between T1DM and exercise was observed for the prazosin-induced change in MAP ($p < 0.05$, Figure 6(a)). Within the nonexercised groups (C and D), T1DM resulted in an increased change in MAP ($p < 0.05$). Within the T1DM groups (D and DX) exercise prevented the increased change in MAP observed in the D group ($p < 0.05$). There was also a main effect of T1DM on [NPY] ($p < 0.05$, Figure 6(b)). Within the nonexercised groups (C and D) and exercised groups (CX and DX), serum [NPY] was increased by T1DM ($p < 0.05$).

4. Discussion

This study demonstrated that a multiple low-dose STZ model with moderate hyperglycemia, maintained using insulin therapy, produced deficits in cardiovascular autonomic function without inducing the resting bradycardia or hypotension typical of other STZ models. This study also showed that high intensity aerobic exercise training can prevent deficits of cardiovascular autonomic function caused by T1DM. Furthermore, because [BG] was held within a moderate hyperglycemic range, the observed exercise-mediated improvements to indications of CAN were independent of changes in [BG] and, instead, may primarily have been the result of

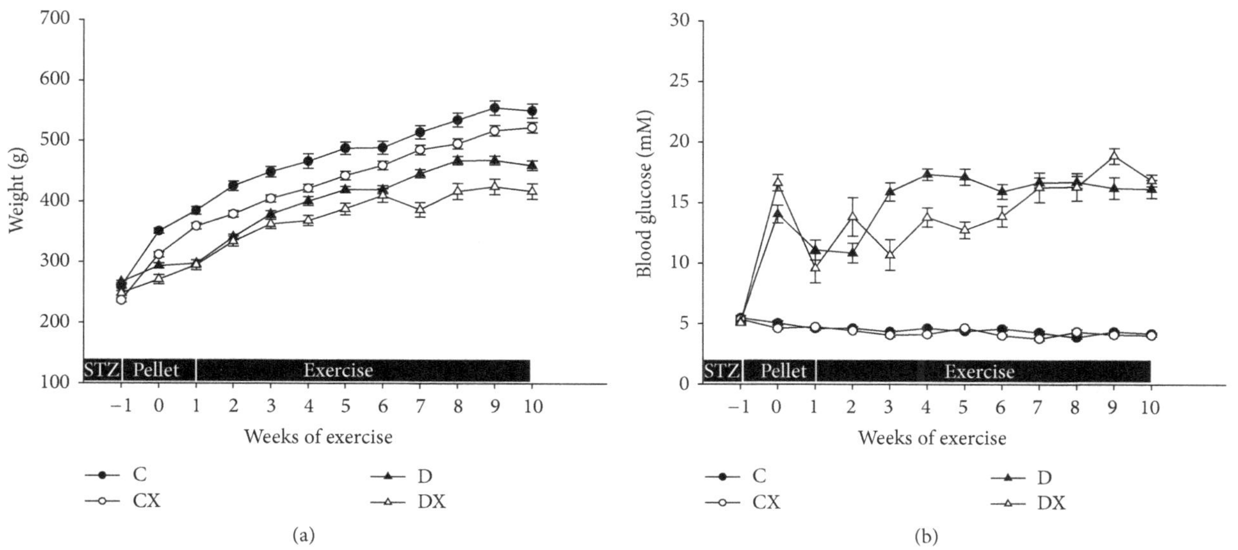

FIGURE 1: (a) Weekly body weights: C, sedentary control ($n = 16$); CX, control exercise ($n = 16$); D, sedentary T1DM ($n = 15$); DX, T1DM exercise ($n = 12$). (b) Weekly blood glucose concentrations: C ($n = 16$); CX ($n = 15$); D ($n = 15$); DX ($n = 13$). STZ, pellet, and exercise indicate the periods of STZ injection, insulin pellet implantation, and aerobic exercise, respectively. Significantly different groups ($p < 0.05$). Data are mean ± SE. There was significant difference in body weight between T1DM and non-T1DM groups, while a significant difference was evident between exercised and nonexercised groups. The blood glucose concentrations in the T1DM groups were significantly different than non-T1DM groups.

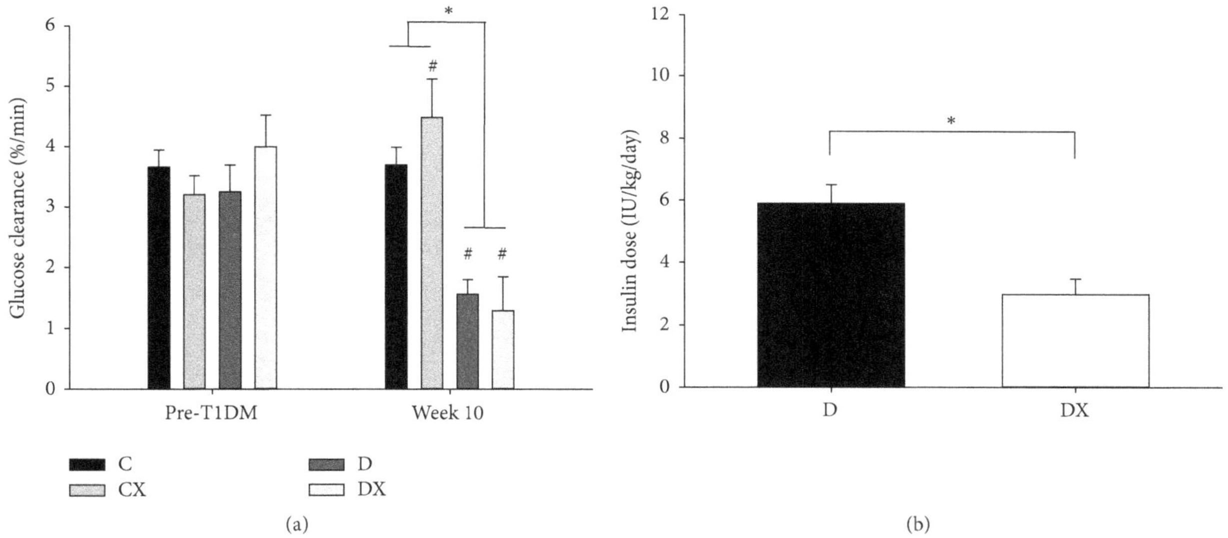

FIGURE 2: (a) IVGTT glucose clearance rate (K_G) values prior to T1DM induction (pre-T1DM) and week 10 of exercise training: C, sedentary control ($n = 16$); CX, control exercise ($n = 15$); D, sedentary T1DM ($n = 15$); DX, T1DM exercise ($n = 15$). (b) Insulin dosages at week 10: D ($n = 16$); DX ($n = 16$). *Significantly different groups ($p < 0.05$). #Significantly different from week 1. Data are mean ± SE.

improvements to other aspects of glucoregulation and/or the preservation of autonomic nervous system function.

Although we found time domain analysis of total HRV, as measured by the SDNN, did not demonstrate differences between groups, frequency domain analysis exposed a reduction in the HF power in the D group compared with the DX group. Since the HF power corresponds to the level of vagally mediated parasympathetic HRV, these results demonstrate not only the detrimental effects of T1DM on autonomic cardiac control but also the benefits of exercise training toward ameliorating those effects. These findings are similar to those of other experiments of both experimental [16, 21] and clinical diabetes [18, 56, 57]. For example, Mostarda et al. (2009) reported that STZ-induced T1DM reduced the HF component of HRV, which was improved by exercise [21]. Also, they found that the vagal tonus of the control exercised

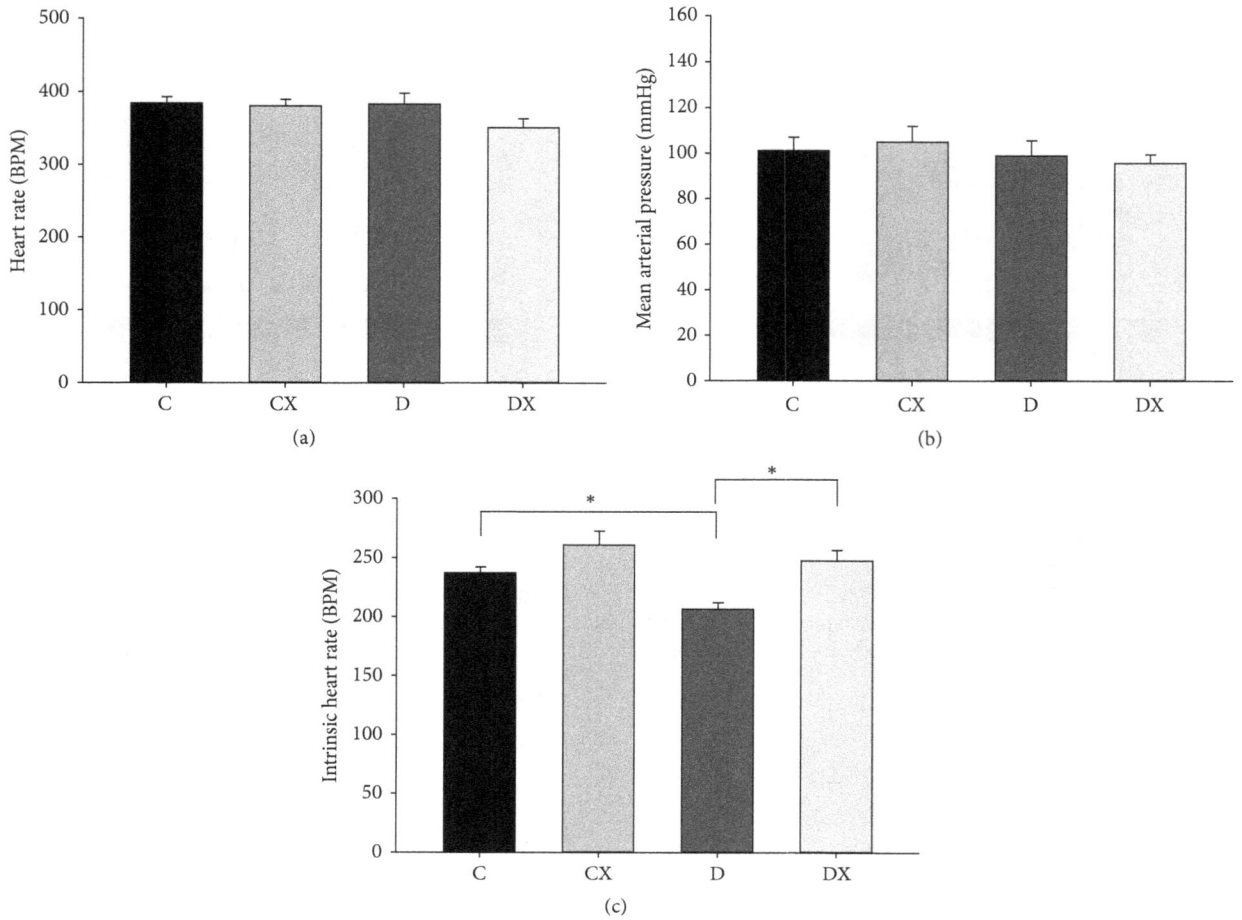

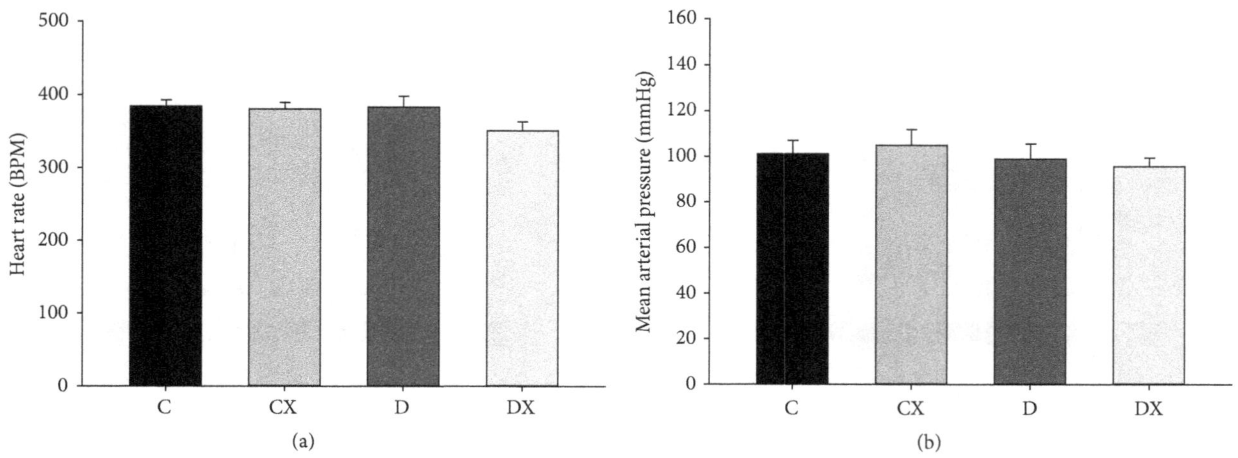

Figure 3: (a) Heart rate (beats per minute) and (b) mean arterial pressure at week 10. C, sedentary control ($n = 7$); CX, control exercise ($n = 7$); D, sedentary T1DM ($n = 8$); DX, T1DM exercise ($n = 10$). (c) Intrinsic heart rate (IHR) at week 10. C ($n = 10$); CX ($n = 11$); D ($n = 12$); DX ($n = 9$). *Significantly different groups ($p < 0.05$). Data are mean ± SE.

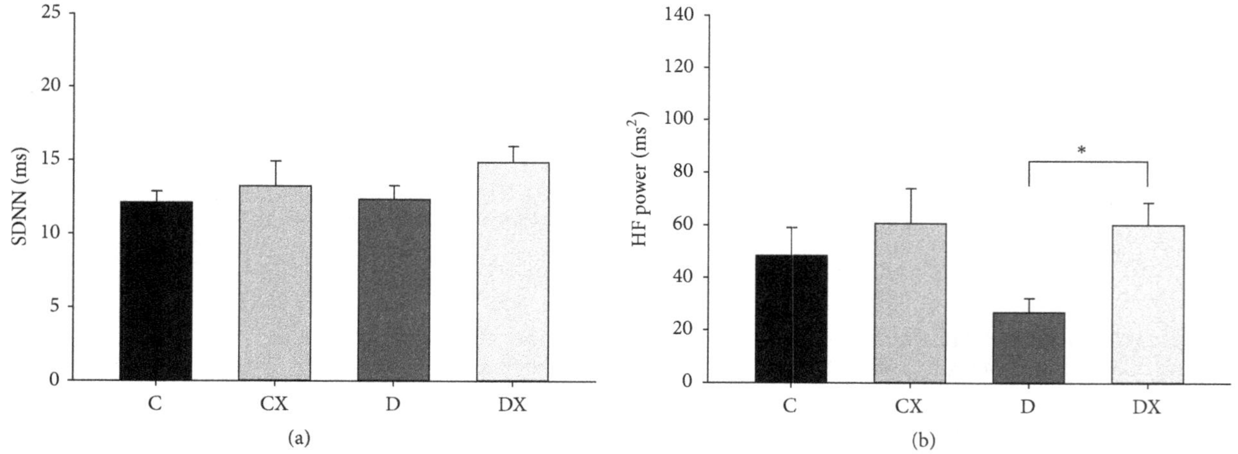

Figure 4: (a) Total HRV (SDNN) at week 10: C, sedentary control ($n = 5$); CX, control exercise ($n = 7$); D, sedentary T1DM ($n = 8$); DX, T1DM exercise ($n = 8$). (b) High Frequency (HF, parasympathetic) HRV component at week 10: C ($n = 6$); CX ($n = 7$); D ($n = 8$); DX ($n = 8$). *Significantly different groups ($p < 0.05$). Data are mean ± SE.

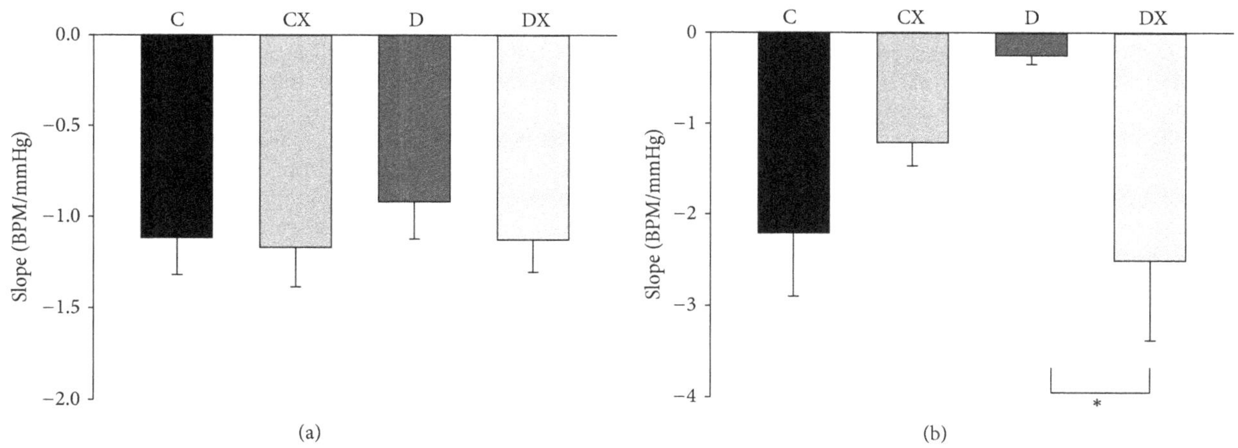

FIGURE 5: (a) Tachycardia baroreflex response sensitivity to sodium nitroprusside at week 10: C, sedentary control ($n = 7$); CX, control exercise ($n = 6$); D, sedentary T1DM ($n = 6$); DX, T1DM exercise ($n = 10$). (b) Bradycardia baroreflex response to phenylephrine at week 10: C ($n = 7$); CX ($n = 5$); D ($n = 7$); DX ($n = 10$). *Significantly different groups ($p < 0.05$). Data are mean ± SE.

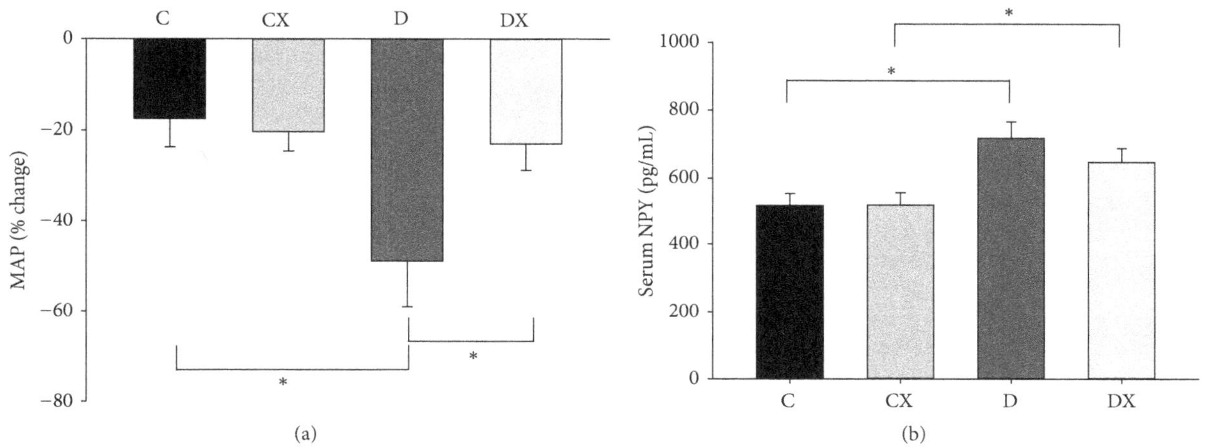

FIGURE 6: (a) Vascular sympathetic tone (VST) at week 10. This was determined by measuring the percent change in MAP after prazosin treatment at week 10: C, sedentary control ($n = 8$); CX, control exercise ($n = 7$); D, sedentary T1DM ($n = 5$); DX, T1DM exercise ($n = 7$). (b) Serum NPY at week 10: C ($n = 6$); CX ($n = 6$); D ($n = 6$); DX ($n = 6$). *Significantly different groups ($p < 0.05$). Data are mean ± SE.

rats did not differ from sedentary controls [21]. Likewise, Chen et al. (2008) reported that children with T1DM who performed a high level of physical activity did not differ from controls in HRV; however, children with T1DM who had low level of physical activity had significantly reduced HRV compared to both active children with T1DM and non-T1DM children [18]. Thus, the current study provides support that exercise can be an effective means to improve HRV in T1DM.

Both tachycardia and bradycardia responses were studied in the context of BRS analysis in order to explore the control features related to unloading or loading of the baroreceptors, respectively. Some discrepancy exists between different experimental models of T1DM and their impact on BRS measures. Investigations using the hyperglycemic Non-Obese Diabetic (NOD) T1DM mouse model have shown elevations in BRS measures rather than attenuated responses [58]. In contrast, tachycardic-SNP and bradycardic-PE responses have been shown to be lower in STZ-induced T1DM hyperglycemic rats in comparison to non-T1DM controls [21] but were improved with exercise training [59]. In the current study, the slope of the hypotensive tachycardia response was not significantly different between any of the groups suggesting that responses to baroreceptor unloading are not affected by T1DM or exercise. However, T1DM reduced the bradycardia response to baroreceptor loading, which was nullified by concurrent exercise training. These findings are in line with previous reports demonstrating a bradycardia change in PE-BRS without an accompanying change in SNP-BRS [60], which was improved following aerobic exercise [61]. Discrepancies in BRS responses in T1DM models seem to be closely associated with both the duration and the severity of diabetes. A recent study examining the time-course of BRS changes in response to STZ-induced hyperglycemia reported that alteration of the SNP-BRS was not evident until 12 weeks of diabetes, while a change in PE-BRS was evident as early as 4 weeks after induction [62]. Interestingly, the animals in the aforementioned study were moderately hyperglycemic (16–18 mM), suggesting that the severity of the hyperglycemia may play a role in the progression of this neuropathy. This relationship has also been demonstrated in humans. Vinik and Ziegler (2007) reported that poor glycemic control [63] and duration of diabetes [64] play a central role in progression of cardiovascular autonomic neuropathy. Yet, it is not clear what role insulin therapy may play in the neuropathy. Insulin supplementation to STZ-induced T1DM rats can modify the changes in BRS sensitivity evident at 48 weeks of T1DM [65]. Indeed, in clinical T1DM patients, intensive therapy is well documented to slow the progression and delay the appearance of abnormal autonomic function [66].

However, the current study provides evidence that the ability of exercise to ameliorate cardiovascular autonomic dysfunction may be independent of its ability to reduce [BG], which challenges the direct relationship between [BG] and CAN suggested by previous studies [67–69]. The IVGTT performed at the conclusion of the 10-week exercise period demonstrated an increased glucose clearance rate (K_G) and therefore glucose tolerance, in the CX group compared to the preexercise training period. However, in both the sedentary and exercise diabetic groups there was an equal decline in K_G to nearly the same rate. This decrease was significantly different from pre-T1DM values and the week 10 values of the C and CX groups. While this would normally indicate that both of the diabetic groups developed equally impaired glucose tolerance, it was also the case that the DX group required approximately half of the dosage of exogenous insulin compared to the D group to maintain their [BG] in the 9–17 mM range. With double the insulin dose, it is likely that the total serum insulin over a given time during IVGTT would have been greater in the D than DX group, and with their K_G being equal, that would indicate that there was a greater insulin sensitivity in the diabetic exercise group [70, 71]. Together, these IVGTT results demonstrate that exercise training improved glucose tolerance and insulin sensitivity [67]. Furthermore, since the [BG] of the diabetic groups in this study was held in a constant range, any abovementioned exercise-induced improvements to CV autonomic function would not have been mediated through a reduction in systemic [BG] but may have been the result of improvements in insulin sensitivity and glucose utilization [72, 73]. This should be borne in mind when considering the effects of diabetes and exercise on indices of CV autonomic function, such as HRV and BRS.

An alternative mechanism by which exercise can influence BRS was reported by Bernardi et al. (2011), who elucidated the importance of tissue oxygenation in T1DM [74]. They demonstrated that a reduced parasympathetic BRS in patients with T1DM was improved by both oxygen supplementation and deep breathing to the same degree, which indicated the increased respiration and oxygen delivery resultant of exercise could have been mediating increases in BRS. This led the authors to suggest that hypoxia in T1DM functionally restrains parasympathetic activity. However, reduced BRS could also be attributed to defects in the baroreceptors, baroreceptor afferent nerves, CNS structures, or efferent fibres of the baroreflex circuit [7, 8, 61]. In the present study, the finding that the tachycardia response of the baroreflex was unimpaired by T1DM, while the bradycardia response was, suggests that the afferent arm and central regulators of the baroreflex were not dysfunctional and that the observed decrement of baroreflex bradycardia may have been caused partly by alterations in efferent parasympathetic outflow [8, 29]. The smaller HF HRV in the D group is consistent with this interpretation.

Another interesting outcome of the current study was the alteration of sympathetic vasomotor control in the D group, which was also modified by concurrent exercise training. In this study, prazosin treatment resulted in a drop in MAP that was approximately twofold greater in the D group compared to the C and DX groups, which is indicative of a much greater sympathetic contribution to the maintenance of baseline vascular resistance [75, 76]. Similarly, Martinez-Nieves and Dunbar (1999) reported that male T1DM rats had a greater decrease in MAP after a bolus injection of prazosin compared to their control cohorts [77]. However, they postulated that an elevated prazosin response could be the result of increased α_1-adrenergic receptor sensitivity [77]. Yet, in this study, the finding that treatment with PE, an α_1-adrenergic receptor agonist, did not result in a greater peak SBP, nor a greater percent increase in SBP from baseline in the T1DM group (data not shown), argues against a receptor-based sensitivity mechanism and, rather, suggests that efferent sympathetic outflow may have been elevated in the D group. However, we cannot determine the mechanism that resulted in prazosin showing a preferential decrease in MAP in the D group versus DX or C based on the data in this study. Yet, in line with the current results, such elevations in resting sympathetic activity would make activation of the BRS response to SNP-induced hypotension more difficult.

The conclusion above regarding sympathetic hyperactivity in the D group is supported by measurements of neuropeptide Y [NPY] obtained in this study. [NPY] is coreleased with norepinephrine from perivascular and cardiac sympathetic nerve terminals during sympathetic activation [78, 79]. In clinical T1DM, a diabetes-related decrease in [NPY] is attributed to impaired sympathetic function, whereas increased [NPY] is attributed to sympathetic overactivity [79–81]. In the current study, serum [NPY] was greater in both of the T1DM groups in comparison to their control groups. This finding is consistent with elevated sympathetic outflow in clinical T1DM [81]. Interestingly, no major impact of exercise was observed on serum [NPY]. Thus, despite the ability of exercise to preserve reflex cardiac function in T1DM, hyperglycemia itself appears to have impacted basal vascular adrenergic activity in both T1DM groups. This observation is consistent with the sympathoexcitatory effect of hyperglycemia [82]. As both T1DM groups were maintained at equally elevated [BG], there may have been a correspondingly similar stimulation of peripheral sympathetic activation and NPY release [79, 82, 83].

Despite improvements by exercise training to deficits of cardiovascular autonomic function, no observable statistical differences in either MAP or HR were evident between any of the groups. Indeed, it has been shown that alterations in autonomic function occur before or without alterations in MAP and HR and are uncorrelated to changes in sympathetic tone [84]. The observed changes in basal sympathetic activity may assist in the maintenance of blood pressure, ventricular function, and cardiac output during the early stage of diabetes, which is supported by our findings that inhibition of sympathetic activity results in a greater decrease in MAP in diabetic rats than normal rats [85]. In that respect, we previously reported that although T1DM animals demonstrated significant alterations in myocardial dimensions and structure, measurements of cardiac performance (ejection fraction, fractional shortening, and cardiac output measurements) were unchanged [44].

To evaluate the heart rate of these animals without neural influence, we measured the beat rate of denervated hearts using the isolated Langendorff technique. We found that the IHR of the D group was lower than both C and DX groups, which would support the notion that decreased IHR masked the effects of sympathetic overactivity in the current study. Further, it supports evidence that STZ-induced diabetes may have a direct effect on heart rate by modifying the heart itself [86, 87]. Interestingly, in some studies, insulin therapy was only able to partially reverse bradycardia and it was shown that STZ-treatment itself could lengthen the action potential duration in the SA node, slowing the HR [88]. However, if hyperglycemia or STZ directly affected cardiac muscle or the SA node and caused a decreased IHR in the D group, it is also the case that exercise training rescued or prevented the deficit, as the IHR of the DX group was not different from the CX group. Thus, previous experimental T1DM studies that reported that STZ-induced bradycardia and hypotension were caused by CAN, and that exercise-induced normalization of HR and BP was evidence of improvements in autonomic function, may really have been observing changes in intrinsic cardiac function which were independent of autonomic control. Such changes could instead have been due to depressed sarcoplasmic reticulum function or impaired calcium handling [87, 89, 90]. Therefore, the direct effects of STZ on the heart and IHR require further examination and should be taken into consideration in future studies that investigate the autonomic regulation of CV function in STZ-induced T1DM models.

An important consideration regarding the design of the current study was the use of anesthetized rats. In order to accurately reflect cardiovascular parameters in such a state, we selected an anaesthetic regime that provides the lowest level of influence on baseline and reflexive CV control attainable in rodent models [50]. A light plane anesthesia 0.5–1.2 g/kg has been shown to maintain the integrity of the cardiovascular system, where higher doses of urethane (above 1.5 g/kg) can produce hypotension and bradycardia, as well as high rates of mortality [91, 92]. In the current study we used a minimal dose of 25 mg/kg, which was reported in previous studies by our laboratory to have little influence on neurovascular blood flow measures [93–95]. That being said, it cannot be determined to what extent, if at all, the autonomic nervous system was augmented by the urethane-chloralose treatment in comparison to conscious animals. Further work examining a comparison of our anesthesia regime with freely moving conscious animals (using telemetry devices) will better address this matter.

5. Conclusions

In this study, T1DM induced indications of parasympathetic withdrawal, sympathetic overactivity, and, despite a decreased IHR, no change in resting MAP or HR. However, concurrent exercise training with T1DM maintained the sensitivity of the parasympathetically mediated baroreflex bradycardia, prevented an increase in vascular sympathetic tone, maintained a higher bodyweight, and prevented a decrease in IHR. The ability of exercise training to preserve parasympathetic function in this model of T1DM indicates that the exercise-mediated improvements to parasympathetic function are independent of alterations in [BG]. However, the finding that [NPY] remained elevated suggests that hyperglycemia has a direct impact on adrenergic activity. Taken together, our T1DM model of progressive STZ induction and insulin treatment induced autonomic impairments similar to those observed in clinical T1DM and demonstrates the novelty of this model for investigating the effectiveness of high intensity aerobic exercise training as a means to prevent the progression of CAN in T1DM. Thus, although not examined in this study, the mechanisms that underlie the physiological changes caused by T1DM and exercise can be the focus of future investigations using this model.

Abbreviations

BG: Blood glucose
BP: Blood pressure
BRS: Baroreflex sensitivity
C: Sedentary control
CAN: Cardiovascular autonomic neuropathy
CX: Exercised control
CV: Cardiovascular
D: Sedentary T1DM
DX: Exercised T1DM
HF: High frequency
HR: Heart rate
HRV: Heart rate variability
IHR: Intrinsic heart rate
MAP: Mean arterial pressure
NPY: Neuropeptide Y
PE: Phenylephrine
SBP: Systolic blood pressure
SNP: Sodium nitroprusside
SNS: Sympathetic nervous system
STZ: Streptozotocin
T1DM: Type 1 diabetes mellitus.

Conflict of Interests

The authors declare that there is no conflict of interests regarding the publication of this paper.

Authors' Contribution

Kenneth N. Grisé contributed to the study design, data collection, data analysis, and writing. T. Dylan Olver, Matthew W. McDonald, Adwitia Dey, and Mao Jiang contributed to the study design and data collection. James C. Lacefield and Earl G. Noble facilitated the data collection. J. Kevin Shoemaker provided data analysis and writing. C. W. James Melling contributed to the study design, data analysis, and writing.

Acknowledgments

This study was supported by the Canadian Institute of Health Research Grant (nos. CCT-83029 and 217532) and the Natural Sciences and Engineering Council Discovery Grant (RGPGP-2015-00059).

References

[1] A. I. Vinik, R. E. Maser, B. D. Mitchell, and R. Freeman, "Diabetic autonomic neuropathy," *Diabetes Care*, vol. 26, no. 5, pp. 1553–1579, 2003.

[2] S. V. P. Fazan, C. C. A. De Vasconcelos, M. M. Valencia, R. Nessler, and K. C. Moore, "Diabetic peripheral neuropathies: a morphometric overview," *International Journal of Morphology*, vol. 28, no. 1, pp. 51–64, 2010.

[3] M. Kuehl and M. J. Stevens, "Cardiovascular autonomic neuropathies as complications of diabetes mellitus," *Nature Reviews Endocrinology*, vol. 8, no. 7, pp. 405–416, 2012.

[4] R. E. Maser, B. D. Mitchell, A. I. Vinik, and R. Freeman, "The association between cardiovascular autonomic neuropathy and mortality in individuals with diabetes," *Diabetes Care*, vol. 26, no. 6, pp. 1895–1901, 2003.

[5] M. Lishner, S. Akselrod, V. M. Avi, O. Oz, M. Divon, and M. Ravid, "Spectral analysis of heart rate fluctuations. A non-invasive, sensitive method for the early diagnosis of autonomic neuropathy in diabetes mellitus," *Journal of the Autonomic Nervous System*, vol. 19, no. 2, pp. 119–125, 1987.

[6] A. Boysen, M. A. G. Lewin, W. Hecker, H. E. Leichter, and F. Uhlemann, "Autonomic function testing in children and adolescents with diabetes mellitus," *Pediatric Diabetes*, vol. 8, no. 5, pp. 261–264, 2007.

[7] Y. Li, "Cardiovascular autonomic dysfunction in diabetes as a complication: cellular and molecular mechanisms," in *Type 1 Diabetes Complications*, D. Wagner, Ed., 2011.

[8] H. C. Salgado, R. Fazan Júnior, V. P. Fazan, V. J. Da Silva, and A. A. Barreira, "Arterial baroreceptors and experimental diabetes," *Annals of the New York Academy of Sciences*, vol. 940, no. 55, pp. 20–27, 2001.

[9] Y.-L. Li, T. P. Tran, R. Muelleman, and H. D. Schultz, "Blunted excitability of aortic baroreceptor neurons in diabetic rats: involvement of hyperpolarization-activated channel," *Cardiovascular Research*, vol. 79, no. 4, pp. 715–721, 2008.

[10] C. Y. Maeda, T. G. Fernandes, H. B. Timm, and M. C. Irigoyen, "Autonomic dysfunction in short-term experimental diabetes," *Hypertension*, vol. 26, no. 6, part 2, pp. 1100–1104, 1995.

[11] D. D. Lund, A. R. Subieta, B. J. Pardini, and K. S. K. Chang, "Alterations in cardiac parasympathetic indices in STZ-induced diabetic rats," *Diabetes*, vol. 41, no. 2, pp. 160–166, 1992.

[12] H. Gu, P. N. Epstein, L. Li, R. D. Wurster, and Z. J. Cheng, "Functional changes in baroreceptor afferent, central and efferent components of the baroreflex circuitry in type 1 diabetic mice (OVE26)," *Neuroscience*, vol. 152, no. 3, pp. 741–752, 2008.

[13] H.-Y. Chen, J.-S. Wu, J.-J. Chen, and J.-T. Cheng, "Impaired regulation function in cardiovascular neurons of nucleus tractus solitarii in streptozotocin-induced diabetic rats," *Neuroscience Letters*, vol. 431, no. 2, pp. 161–166, 2008.

[14] M. Schönauer, A. Thomas, S. Morbach, J. Niebauer, U. Schönauer, and H. Thiele, "Cardiac autonomic diabetic neuropathy," *Diabetes & Vascular Disease Research*, vol. 5, no. 4, pp. 336–344, 2008.

[15] F. C. Howarth, M. Jacobson, O. Naseer, and E. Adeghate, "Short-term effects of streptozotocin-induced diabetes on the electrocardiogram, physical activity and body temperature in rats," *Experimental Physiology*, vol. 90, no. 2, pp. 237–245, 2005.

[16] B. D. Schaan, P. Dall'Ago, C. Y. Maeda et al., "Relationship between cardiovascular dysfunction and hyperglycemia in streptozotocin-induced diabetes in rats," *Brazilian Journal of Medical and Biological Research*, vol. 37, no. 12, pp. 1895–1902, 2004.

[17] B. Yang and K. H. Chon, "Assessment of diabetic cardiac autonomic neuropathy in type I diabetic mice," in *Proceedings of the Annual International Conference of the IEEE Engineering in Medicine and Biology Society (EMBC '11)*, pp. 6560–6563, Boston, Mass, USA, August 2011.

[18] S.-R. Chen, Y.-J. Lee, H.-W. Chiu, and C. Jeng, "Impact of physical activity on heart rate variability in children with type 1 diabetes," *Child's Nervous System*, vol. 24, no. 6, pp. 741–747, 2008.

[19] B. K. Pedersen and B. Saltin, "Evidence for prescribing exercise as therapy in chronic disease," *Scandinavian Journal of Medicine and Science in Sports*, vol. 16, supplement 1, pp. 3–63, 2006.

[20] H. Komine, J. Sugawara, K. Hayashi, M. Yoshizawa, and T. Yokoi, "Regular endurance exercise in young men increases arterial baroreflex sensitivity through neural alteration of baroreflex arc," *Journal of Applied Physiology*, vol. 106, no. 5, pp. 1499–1505, 2009.

[21] C. Mostarda, A. Rogow, I. C. M. Silva et al., "Benefits of exercise training in diabetic rats persist after three weeks of detraining," *Autonomic Neuroscience: Basic and Clinical*, vol. 145, no. 1-2, pp. 11–16, 2009.

[22] S. Golbidi, M. Badran, and I. Laher, "Antioxidant and anti-inflammatory effects of exercise in diabetic patients," *Experimental Diabetes Research*, vol. 2012, Article ID 941868, 16 pages, 2012.

[23] E. J. Henriksen and V. Saengsirisuwan, "Exercise training and antioxidants: relief from oxidative stress and insulin resistance," *Exercise and Sport Sciences Reviews*, vol. 31, no. 2, pp. 79–84, 2003.

[24] A. I. Vinik, R. E. Maser, and D. Ziegler, "Autonomic imbalance: prophet of doom or scope for hope?" *Diabetic Medicine*, vol. 28, no. 6, pp. 643–651, 2011.

[25] K. K. Hicks, E. Seifen, J. R. Stimers, and R. H. Kennedy, "Effects of streptozotocin-induced diabetes on heart rate, blood pressure and cardiac autonomic nervous control," *Journal of the Autonomic Nervous System*, vol. 69, no. 1, pp. 21–30, 1998.

[26] A. R. Lafferty, G. A. Werther, and C. F. Clarke, "Ambulatory blood pressure, microalbuminuria, and autonomic neuropathy in adolescents with type 1 diabetes," *Diabetes Care*, vol. 23, no. 4, pp. 533–538, 2000.

[27] J. J. Chillarón, M. P. Sales, J. A. Flores-Le-Roux et al., "Insulin resistance and hypertension in patients with type 1 diabetes," *Journal of Diabetes and its Complications*, vol. 25, no. 4, pp. 232–236, 2011.

[28] F. Collado-Mesa, H. M. Colhoun, L. K. Stevens et al., "Prevalence and management of hypertension in type 1 diabetes mellitus in Europe: the EURODIAB IDDM complications study," *Diabetic Medicine*, vol. 16, no. 1, pp. 41–48, 1999.

[29] P. Dall'Ago, V. O. K. Silva, K. L. D. De Angelis, M. C. Irigoyen, R. Fazan Jr., and H. C. Salgado, "Reflex control of arterial pressure and heart rate in short-term streptozotocin diabetic rats," *Brazilian Journal of Medical and Biological Research*, vol. 35, no. 7, pp. 843–849, 2002.

[30] R. Fazan Jr., G. Ballejo, M. C. O. Salgado, M. F. D. Moraes, and H. C. Salgado, "Heart rate variability and baroreceptor function in chronic diabetic rats," *Hypertension*, vol. 30, no. 3, part 2, pp. 632–635, 1997.

[31] K. C. Tomlinson, S. M. Gardiner, R. A. Hebden, and T. Bennett, "Functional consequences of streptozotocin-induced diabetes mellitus, with particular reference to the cardiovascular system," *Pharmacological Reviews*, vol. 44, no. 1, pp. 103–150, 1992.

[32] D. Lucini and M. Pagani, "Exercise: should it matter to internal medicine?" *European Journal of Internal Medicine*, vol. 22, no. 4, pp. 363–370, 2011.

[33] A. D. Harthmann, K. De Angelis, L. P. Costa et al., "Exercise training improves arterial baro- and chemoreflex in control and diabetic rats," *Autonomic Neuroscience*, vol. 133, no. 2, pp. 115–120, 2007.

[34] K. L. D. De Angelis, A. R. Oliveira, P. Dall'Ago et al., "Effects of exercise training on autonomic and myocardial dysfunction in streptozotocin-diabetic rats," *Brazilian Journal of Medical and Biological Research*, vol. 33, no. 6, pp. 635–641, 2000.

[35] Y. Harati, "Diabetic neuropathies: unanswered questions," *Neurologic Clinics*, vol. 25, no. 1, pp. 303–317, 2007.

[36] T. J. Orchard, C. E. Lloyd, R. E. Maser, and L. H. Kuller, "Why does diabetic autonomic neuropathy predict IDDM mortality? An analysis from the Pittsburgh Epidemiology of Diabetes Complications study," *Diabetes Research and Clinical Practice*, vol. 34, supplement 1, pp. S165–S171, 1996.

[37] K. L. De Angelis, B. D. Schaan, C. Y. Maeda, P. Dall'Ago, R. B. Wichi, and M. C. Irigoyen, "Cardiovascular control in experimental diabetes," *Brazilian Journal of Medical and Biological Research*, vol. 35, no. 9, pp. 1091–1100, 2002.

[38] G. Monckton and E. Pehowich, "Autonomic neuropathy in the streptozotocin diabetic rat," *Canadian Journal of Neurological Sciences*, vol. 7, no. 2, pp. 135–142, 1980.

[39] F. C. Howarth, M. Jacobson, M. Shafiullah, and E. Adeghate, "Long-term effects of streptozotocin-induced diabetes on the electrocardiogram, physical activity and body temperature in rats," *Experimental Physiology*, vol. 90, no. 6, pp. 827–835, 2005.

[40] W. H. Polonsky, C. L. Davis, A. M. Jacobson, and B. J. Anderson, "Hyperglycaemia, hypoglycaemia, and blood glucose control in diabetes: symptom perceptions and treatment strategies," *Diabetic Medicine*, vol. 9, no. 2, pp. 120–125, 1992.

[41] J. J. Valletta, A. J. Chipperfield, G. F. Clough, and C. D. Byrne, "Metabolic regulation during constant moderate physical exertion in extreme conditions in type 1 diabetes," *Diabetic Medicine*, vol. 29, no. 6, pp. 822–826, 2012.

[42] G. J. Taborsky and T. O. Mundinger, "Minireview: the role of the autonomic nervous system in mediating the glucagon response to hypoglycemia," *Endocrinology*, vol. 153, no. 3, pp. 1055–1062, 2012.

[43] D. J. Cox, L. A. Gonder-Frederick, J. A. Shepard, L. K. Campbell, and K. A. Vajda, "Driving safety: concerns and experiences of parents of adolescent drivers with type 1 diabetes," *Pediatric Diabetes*, vol. 13, no. 6, pp. 506–509, 2012.

[44] C. W. J. Melling, K. N. Grisé, C. P. Hasilo et al., "A model of poorly controlled type 1 diabetes mellitus and its treatment with aerobic exercise training," *Diabetes & Metabolism*, vol. 39, no. 3, pp. 226–235, 2013.

[45] K. E. Hall, M. W. McDonald, K. N. Grisé, O. Campos, E. G. Noble, and C. W. J. Melling, "he role of resistance and aerobic exercise training on insulin sensitivity measures in STZ-induced Type 1 diabetic rodents," *Metabolism*, vol. 62, no. 10, pp. 1485–1494, 2013.

[46] J. M. Murias, K. N. Grise, M. Jiang, H. Kowalchuk, C. W. J. Melling, and E. G. Noble, "Acute endurance exercise induces changes in vasorelaxation responses that are vessel-specific," *The American Journal of Physiology: Regulatory, Integrative and Comparative Physiology*, vol. 304, no. 7, pp. R574–R580, 2013.

[47] J. M. Murias, A. Dey, O. A. Campos et al., "High-intensity endurance training results in faster vessel-specific rate of vasorelaxation in type 1 diabetic rats," *PLoS One*, vol. 8, no. 3, Article ID e59678, 2013.

[48] T. G. Bedford, C. M. Tipton, N. C. Wilson, R. A. Oppliger, and C. V. Gisolfi, "Maximum oxygen consumption of rats and its changes with various experimental procedures," *Journal of Applied Physiology*, vol. 47, no. 6, pp. 1278–1283, 1979.

[49] B. Rodrigues, D. M. Figueroa, C. T. Mostarda, M. V. Heeren, M.-C. Irigoyen, and K. De Angelis, "Maximal exercise test is a useful method for physical capacity and oxygen consumption determination in streptozotocin-diabetic rats," *Cardiovascular Diabetology*, vol. 6, article 38, 2007.

[50] C. W. Usselman, L. Mattar, J. Twynstra, I. Welch, and J. K. Shoemaker, "Rodent cardiovascular responses to baroreceptor unloading: effect of plane of anaesthesia," *Applied Physiology, Nutrition and Metabolism*, vol. 36, no. 3, pp. 376–381, 2011.

[51] B. Gribbin, T. G. Pickering, P. Sleight, and R. Peto, "Effect of age and high blood pressure on barorefiex sensitivity in man," *Circulation Research*, vol. 29, no. 4, pp. 424–431, 1971.

[52] B. E. Hunt, L. Fahy, W. B. Farquhar, and A. Taylor J, "Quantification of mechanical and neural components of vagal baroreflex in humans," *Hypertension*, vol. 37, no. 6, pp. 1362–1368, 2001.

[53] L. Rudas, A. A. Crossman, C. A. Morillo, J. R. Halliwill, U. O. Kari, and T. A. Kuusela, "Human sympathetic and vagal baroreflex responses to sequential nitroprusside and phenylephrine," *The American Journal of Physiology—Heart and Circulatory Physiology*, vol. 76, no. 5, part 2, pp. H1691–H1698, 1999.

[54] P. Studinger, R. Goldstein, and J. A. Taylor, "Mechanical and neural contributions to hysteresis in the cardiac vagal limb of the arterial baroreflex," *The Journal of Physiology*, vol. 583, part 3, pp. 1041–1048, 2007.

[55] Z. Paroo, J. V. Haist, M. Karmazyn, and E. G. Noble, "Exercise improves postischemic cardiac function in males but not females: consequences of a novel sex-specific heat shock protein 70 response," *Circulation Research*, vol. 90, no. 8, pp. 911–917, 2002.

[56] G. Zoppini, V. Cacciatori, M. L. Gemma et al., "Effect of moderate aerobic exercise on sympatho-vagal balance in Type 2 diabetic patients," *Diabetic Medicine*, vol. 24, no. 4, pp. 370–376, 2007.

[57] S.-R. Chen, Y.-J. Lee, H.-W. Chiu, and C. Jeng, "Impact of glycemic control, disease duration, and exercise on heart rate

variability in children with type 1 diabetes mellitus," *Journal of the Formosan Medical Association*, vol. 106, no. 11, pp. 935–942, 2007.

[58] V. Gross, J. Tank, H.-J. Partke et al., "Cardiovascular autonomic regulation in Non-Obese Diabetic (NOD) mice," *Autonomic Neuroscience: Basic and Clinical*, vol. 138, no. 1-2, pp. 108–113, 2008.

[59] K. A. D. S. Silva, R. D. S. Luiz, R. R. Rampaso et al., "Previous exercise training has a beneficial effect on renal and cardiovascular function in a model of diabetes," *PLoS ONE*, vol. 7, no. 11, Article ID e48826, pp. 1–10, 2012.

[60] T. M. Murça, T. C. S. Almeida, M. K. Raizada, and A. J. Ferreira, "Chronic activation of endogenous angiotensin-converting enzyme 2 protects diabetic rats from cardiovascular autonomic dysfunction," *Experimental Physiology*, vol. 97, no. 6, pp. 699–709, 2012.

[61] L. Jorge, D. Y. da Pureza, D. da Silva Dias, F. F. Conti, M.-C. Irigoyen, and K. De Angelis, "Dynamic aerobic exercise induces baroreflex improvement in diabetic rats," *Experimental Diabetes Research*, vol. 2012, Article ID 108680, 5 pages, 2012.

[62] L.-Z. Hong, Y.-C. Chan, M.-F. Wang et al., "Modulation of baroreflex function by rosiglitazone in prediabetic hyperglycemic rats," *Physiological Research*, vol. 61, no. 5, pp. 443–452, 2012.

[63] A. I. Vinik and D. Ziegler, "Diabetic cardiovascular autonomic neuropathy," *Circulation*, vol. 115, no. 3, pp. 387–397, 2007.

[64] D. Ziegler, "Diabetic cardiovascular autonomic neuropathy: prognosis, diagnosis and treatment," *Diabetes/Metabolism Reviews*, vol. 10, no. 4, pp. 339–383, 1994.

[65] K. S. Chang and D. D. Lund, "Alterations in the baroreceptor reflex control of heart rate in streptozotocin diabetic rats," *Journal of Molecular and Cellular Cardiology*, vol. 18, no. 6, pp. 617–624, 1986.

[66] R. Pop-Busui, P. A. Low, B. H. Waberski et al., "Effects of prior intensive insulin therapy on cardiac autonomic nervous system function in type 1 diabetes mellitus: the diabetes control and complications trial/epidemiology of diabetes interventions and complications study (DCCT/EDIC)," *Circulation*, vol. 119, no. 22, pp. 2886–2893, 2009.

[67] G. Tancrede, S. Rousseau-Migneron, and A. Nadeau, "Beneficial effects of physical training in rats with a mild streptozotocin-induced diabetes mellitus," *Diabetes*, vol. 31, no. 5, part 1, pp. 406–409, 1982.

[68] J. A. Wegner, D. D. Lund, J. M. Overton, J. G. Edwards, R. P. Oda, and C. M. Tipton, "Select cardiovascular and metabolic responses of diabetic rats to moderate exercise training.," *Medicine & Science in Sports & Exercise*, vol. 19, no. 5, pp. 497–503, 1987.

[69] S. Chipkinn, S. Klugh, and L. Chasan-Taber, "Exercise and diabetes," *Cardiology Clinics*, vol. 19, no. 3, pp. 489–505, 2001.

[70] A. Tura, S. Sbrignadello, E. Succurro, L. Groop, G. Sesti, and G. Pacini, "An empirical index of insulin sensitivity from short IVGTT: validation against the minimal model and glucose clamp indices in patients with different clinical characteristics," *Diabetologia*, vol. 53, no. 1, pp. 144–152, 2010.

[71] R. G. Hahn, S. Ljunggren, F. Larsen, and T. Nyström, "A simple intravenous glucose tolerance test for assessment of insulin sensitivity," *Theoretical Biology and Medical Modelling*, vol. 8, no. 1, article 12, 2011.

[72] J. Paulson, J. Dennis, R. Mathews, and J. Bow, "Metabolic effects of treadmill exercise training on the diabetic heart," *Journal of Applied Physiology*, vol. 73, no. 1, pp. 265–271, 1992.

[73] T. L. Broderick, P. Poirier, and M. Gillis, "Exercise training restores abnormal myocardial glucose utilization and cardiac function in diabetes," *Diabetes/Metabolism Research and Reviews*, vol. 21, no. 1, pp. 44–50, 2005.

[74] L. Bernardi, M. Rosengård-Bärlund, A. Sandelin, V. P. Mäkinen, C. Forsblom, and P.-H. Groop, "Short-term oxygen administration restores blunted baroreflex sensitivity in patients with type 1 diabetes," *Diabetologia*, vol. 54, no. 8, pp. 2164–2173, 2011.

[75] I. Rodríguez-Gómez, Y. Baca, J. M. Moreno et al., "Role of sympathetic tone in BSO-induced hypertension in mice," *American Journal of Hypertension*, vol. 23, no. 8, pp. 882–888, 2010.

[76] D. S. DeLorey, J. B. Buckwalter, S. W. Mittelstadt, M. M. Anton, H. A. Kluess, and P. S. Clifford, "Is tonic sympathetic vasoconstriction increased in the skeletal muscle vasculature of aged canines?" *The American Journal of Physiology—Regulatory Integrative and Comparative Physiology*, vol. 299, no. 5, pp. R1342–R1349, 2010.

[77] B. Martinez-Nieves and J. Dunbar, "Vascular dilatatory responses to sodium nitroprusside (SNP) and alpha-adrenergic antagonism in female and male normal and diabetic rats," *Proceedings of the Society for Experimental Biology and Medicine*, vol. 222, no. 2, Article ID 44433, pp. 90–98, 1999.

[78] J. M. Lundberg, A. Franco-Cereceda, J. S. Lacroix, and J. Pernow, "Neuropeptide Y and sympathetic neurotransmission," *Annals of the New York Academy of Sciences*, vol. 611, pp. 166–174, 1990.

[79] C. Wahlestedt, R. Hakanson, C. A. Vaz, and Z. Zukowska-Grojec, "Norepinephrine and neuropeptide Y: vasoconstrictor cooperation in vivo and in vitro," *The American Journal of Physiology—Regulatory Integrative and Comparative Physiology*, vol. 258, no. 3, pp. R736–R742, 1990.

[80] A. Ejaz, F. W. LoGerfo, and L. Pradhan, "Diabetic neuropathy and heart failure: role of neuropeptides," *Expert Reviews in Molecular Medicine*, vol. 13, article e26, 2011.

[81] P. C. Perin, S. Maule, and R. Quadri, "Sympathetic nervous system, diabetes, and hypertension," *Clinical and Experimental Hypertension*, vol. 23, no. 1-2, pp. 45–55, 2001.

[82] S. Villafaña, F. Huang, and E. Hong, "Role of the sympathetic and renin angiotensin systems in the glucose-induced increase of blood pressure in rats," *European Journal of Pharmacology*, vol. 506, no. 2, pp. 143–150, 2004.

[83] D. Giugliano, R. Marfella, L. Coppola et al., "Vascular effects of acute hyperglycemia in humans are reversed by L-arginine. Evidence for reduced availability of nitric oxide during hyperglycemia," *Circulation*, vol. 95, no. 7, pp. 1783–1790, 1997.

[84] M. Pagani, G. Malfatto, S. Pierini et al., "Spectral analysis of heart rate variability in the assessment of autonomic diabetic neuropathy," *Journal of the Autonomic Nervous System*, vol. 23, no. 2, pp. 143–153, 1988.

[85] L. Zhang, X.-Q. Xiong, Z.-D. Fan, X.-B. Gan, X.-Y. Gao, and G.-Q. Zhu, "Involvement of enhanced cardiac sympathetic afferent reflex in sympathetic activation in early stage of diabetes," *Journal of Applied Physiology*, vol. 113, no. 1, pp. 47–55, 2012.

[86] M. A. Malone, D. D. Schocken, S. K. Hanna, X. Liang, and J. I. Malone, "Diabetes-induced bradycardia is an intrinsic metabolic defect reversed by carnitine," *Metabolism*, vol. 56, no. 8, pp. 1118–1123, 2007.

[87] S. Penpargkul, F. Fein, E. Sonnenblick, and J. Scheur, "Sarcoplasmic from diabetic reticular rats function," *Journal of Molecular and Cellular Cardiology*, vol. 13, no. 3, pp. 303–309, 1981.

[88] F. C. Howarth, R. Al-Sharhan, A. Al-Hammadi, and M. A. Qureshi, "Effects of streptozotocin-induced diabetes on action

potentials in the sinoatrial node compared with other regions of the rat heart," *Molecular and Cellular Biochemistry*, vol. 300, no. 1-2, pp. 39–46, 2007.

[89] P. K. Ganguly, G. N. Pierce, K. S. Dhalla, and N. S. Dhalla, "Defective sarcoplasmic reticular calcium transport in diabetic cardiomyopathy," *The American Journal of Physiology*, vol. 244, no. 6, pp. E528–E535, 1983.

[90] L. Ligeti, O. Szenczi, C. M. Prestia et al., "Altered calcium handling is an early sign of streptozotocin-induced diabetic cardiomyopathy," *International Journal of Molecular Medicine*, vol. 17, no. 6, pp. 1035–1043, 2006.

[91] W. B. Severs, L. C. Keil, P. A. Klase, and K. C. Deen, "Urethane anesthesia in rats. Altered ability to regulate hydration," *Pharmacology*, vol. 22, no. 4, pp. 209–226, 1981.

[92] K. J. Field, W. J. White, and C. M. Lang, "Anaesthetic effects of chloral hydrate, pentobarbitone and urethane in adult male rats," *Laboratory Animals*, vol. 27, no. 3, pp. 258–269, 1993.

[93] T. D. Olver, M. W. McDonald, K. N. Grisé, A. Dey, M. D. Allen, P. J. Medeiros et al., "Exercise training enhances insulin-stimulated nerve arterial vasodilation in rats with insulin-treated experimental diabetes," *The American Journal of Physiology: Regulatory, Integrative and Comparative Physiology*, vol. 306, no. 12, pp. R941–R950, 2014.

[94] T. D. Olver, L. Mattar, K. N. Grise et al., "Glucose-stimulated insulin secretion causes an insulin-dependent nitric oxide-mediated vasodilation in the blood supply of the rat sciatic nerve," *The American Journal of Physiology: Regulatory, Integrative and Comparative Physiology*, vol. 305, no. 2, pp. R157–R163, 2013.

[95] T. D. Olver, K. N. Grisé, M. W. McDonald, A. Dey, M. D. Allen, C. L. Rice et al., "The relationship between blood pressure and sciatic nerve blood flow velocity in rats with insulin-treated experimental diabetes," *Diabetes and Vascular Disease Research*, vol. 11, no. 4, pp. 281–289, 2014.

Characteristics of Type 2 Diabetes with Ketosis in Baoshan, Yunnan of China

Shichun Du,[1] Xia Yang,[2] Degang Shi,[2] and Qing Su[1]

[1] *Department of Endocrinology, Xinhua Hospital Affiliated to Shanghai Jiaotong University School of Medicine, Shanghai 200092, China*
[2] *Department of Endocrinology, Baoshan People's Hospital, Yunnan 678000, China*

Correspondence should be addressed to Qing Su; suqingxinhua@163.com

Academic Editor: Raffaele Marfella

Objectives. The study provided data to demonstrate the characteristics of type 2 diabetes (T2D) with ketosis in rural parts of south-west border of China in order to help health professionals with optimizing diabetic care. *Methods.* All hospitalized adult diabetic patients consecutively between January 2011 and July 2015 in Baoshan People's Hospital, Yunnan province of China, were evaluated. T2D with ketosis, ordinary T2D (without ketosis), and type 1 diabetes (T1D) patients were analyzed according to the clinical and biochemical parameters and chronic complications in these subjects. *Results.* The prevalence of T2D with ketosis was 12% in the whole study subjects. Overweight and obese patients were predominant (49.1%) in T2D patients with ketosis. The mean HbA1c (13.3 ± 3.1%, $P = 0.01$), fasting plasma glucose (16.9 ± 6 mmol/L, $P < 0.0001$), and plasma triglyceride (4.0 ± 4.0 mmol/L, $P < 0.0001$) in T2D patients with ketosis were significantly higher than ordinary T2D patients without ketosis. Infections were the most common inducements in T2D patients with ketosis. Chronic complications including peripheral neuropathy (34.9%), retinopathy (12.7%), diabetic foot (18.1%), and persistent microalbuminuria (11.7%) were common in T2D patients with ketosis. *Conclusions.* This study indicated the poor glycemic control in diabetic patients in rural areas of south-west part of China. More efforts were urgently required to popularize public health education and improve medical quality in diabetic treatment in these regions.

1. Introduction

The outbreak of type 2 diabetes (T2D) is one of the largest public health problems around China [1–3]. Up till now, the prevalence of diabetes in adults of China has been 11.6% [2], while the current situations of diabetic control in rural areas are not clear. It is commonly acknowledged that diabetes is developing faster in urban areas than rural ones [2, 3]. However, the rural areas are becoming the disaster zone of diabetes due to the rapid changes in lifestyle with the development of economy and lack of adequate health education [4]. Many T2D patients are diagnosed with extreme hyperglycemia combined with ketosis on admission in south-west border of China.

T2D associated with ketosis presents most commonly in uncontrolled hyperglycemia with or without precipitating factors [5]. In rural areas, it is commonly seen due to lack of prior diagnosis or lack of proper medical treatment after diabetes diagnosis [5]. T2D patients with ketosis differ in so many respects from the typical type 1 diabetes (T1D) patients and are not completely the same with ordinary T2D patients without ketosis [6]. In this study, we examined the clinical characteristics of diabetic inpatients in order to find the same difference in clinical, biochemical, and chronic complications in T2D patients with ketosis compared to ordinary T1D and T2D patients. Furthermore, we aimed to provide health professional regional data for improvement of medical care quality in diabetic patients.

2. Methods

We retrospectively collected data from 3129 diabetic inpatients (1563 males and 1566 females) aged 12 years or older in the endocrinology department of Baoshan People's Hospital

TABLE 1: Anthropometric and biochemical characteristics of participants.

	T2DK	T1D	T2D	$P1$	$P2$
Subjects (%total)	371 (12%)	104 (3%)	2654 (85%)	—	—
Age (yr)	49 ± 13	26 ± 14	47 ± 14	<0.0001	0.85
Gender (male %)	66	44	48	<0.0001	<0.0001
Family history (%)	35	11	37	0.03	0.89
Height (cm)	162 ± 9	150 ± 11	158 ± 8	0.04	0.23
Weight (kg)	64.6 ± 14	45.3 ± 9.7	57.4 ± 11	<0.0001	0.21
Body mass index (kg/m^2)	25 ± 4	19 ± 3	23 ± 3	<0.0001	0.76
Overweight or obese (%)	49.1	11.7	43.5	<0.0001	0.62
Systolic pressure (mmHg)	120 ± 21	123 ± 28	120 ± 27	0.41	0.87
Diastolic pressure (mmHg)	79 ± 12	77 ± 18	80 ± 14	0.83	0.92
Fasting glucose (mmol/L)	16.9 ± 6	20.1 ± 6	10.3 ± 4	0.0003	<0.0001
Postprandial 2-hour glucose (mmol/L)	24.1 ± 7	30.2 ± 7	18.4 ± 6	0.0002	0.0001
Fasting C-peptide (nmol/L)	0.65 ± 0.2	0.47 ± 0.1	0.98 ± 0.9	0.11	0.08
Postprandial 2-hour C-peptide (nmol/L)	2.04 ± 0.8	0.69 ± 0.1	2.18 ± 1.0	0.001	0.75
Hemoglobin A1c (%)	13.3 ± 3.1	14.1 ± 4.7	10.2 ± 2.1	0.43	0.01
Fructosamine (mmo/L)	3.82 ± 0.8	3.79 ± 0.9	3.14 ± 0.7	0.91	0.08
Ketoacidosis (%)	12.1	65.4	—	<0.0001	—
Total cholesterol (mmo/L)	5.3 ± 1.7	5.7 ± 1.7	4.9 ± 1.6	0.48	0.11
Triglyceride (mmo/L)	4.0 ± 4.0	4.3 ± 3.0	2.8 ± 2.7	0.47	<0.0001
Serum creatinine (μmol/L)	85.6 ± 34.1	77.1 ± 38.5	80.2 ± 38	0.73	0.83

T2DK, type 2 diabetes with ketosis; T1D, type 1 diabetes; T2D, type 2 diabetes; $P1$, T2DK versus T1D; $P2$, T2DK versus T2D.

of Yunnan province from January 2011 to July 2015. Those with surgery, serious trauma, pregnancy, and secondary or pancreatic exocrine diseases were excluded. Patients with unconsciousness were also excluded. There were 3 groups in our study: T2D with ketosis (T2DK), T1D, and T2D without ketosis groups. Diabetes was diagnosed according to diagnostic criteria of American Diabetes Association [7]. Overweight and obesity were defined by body mass index (BMI) ≥24 (standard criteria for China set forth by the Chinese Obesity Working Group) [8, 9]. Patients were classified to T1D if they had repeated C-peptide deficiency and positive diabetes associated autoantibodies or are dependent on insulin treatment at follow-up. Patients were assigned to the T2D group if they were overweight, managed with oral hypoglycemic agents, or noncompliant with drug treatment after diabetes diagnosis. T2DK group was diagnosed according to T2D clinical and metabolic features (BMI and age at presentation, etc.) in combination with preserved β cell function and positive urine ketone body results. Subjects with new diagnosed diabetes or not more than 6 months after onset were recognized as new-onset. All the enrolled patients had no history of secondary diabetes. Urinary ketone body was detected using sodium nitroprusside method (Arkray Factory Inc.). Ketosis positive was diagnosed with urinary acetoacetate increased over 15 mg/dL. Plasma glucose was measured by hexokinase method. C-peptide was measured by chemiluminescent immunometric method (Roche Cobas e601). Hemoglobin A1c (HbA1c) was detected by Bio-Rad D10 automatic HbA1c analyzers. Lipids were measured by using Siemens ADVIA1800. Data were collected on clinical presentations (age, gender, family history of diabetes, height, weight, etc.) and biological parameters including plasma glucose, total cholesterol, triglycerides, HbA1c, C-peptide, and serum creatinine. All of the blood samples were performed once at the time on admission in a fasting state except for the 2 h plasma glucose and C-peptide. The chronic diabetic complications were evaluated during the hospitalization.

All data were analyzed using JMP 9.0 (SAS Institute, Cary, NC). The ANOVA test, Kruskal-Wallis test, and Mann-Whitney test were used for statistical analysis according to continuous or categorical variables. The data were expressed as means ± SD. Two-tailed P values <0.05 were considered significant.

3. Results

Among total 3129 patients, 371 (12%), 104 (3%), and 2654 (85%) patients were categorized as T2DK, T1D, or ordinary T2D (without ketosis) groups. 3084 (>98%) patients enrolled were of Han nationality and 45 patients of other origins. Table 1 showed the demographic and laboratory data of all the enrolled subjects. The age of patients in T2DK groups (49 ± 13 yrs) was significantly older than T1D patients (26 ± 14 yrs, $P < 0.0001$), and similar to T2D patients (47 ± 14 yrs, $P = 0.85$). Male proportion was higher in T2DK (66%) group compared to T1D (44%) and T2D (48%) group. The family history was positive in about 35% T2DK patients, which was similar ($P = 0.89$) to T2D, but predominantly higher ($P = 0.03$) than T1D. BMI at admission was higher in T2DK group (25 ± 4 kg/m^2) compared with that in T1D (19 ± 3 kg/m^2, $P < 0.0001$), while similar to that in ordinary T2D (23 ± 3 kg/m^2, $P = 0.76$). Significantly more patients with overweight or

Table 2: Comparison of new-onset and old diagnosed diabetes.

	T2DK	T1D	T2D	*P*1	*P*2
Duration					
New-onset (months)	1.73 ± 2.5	0.67 ± 0.5	2.1 ± 3.2	<0.0001	0.75
Old diagnosed (years)	6.3 ± 5.3	4.4 ± 6.2	10.1 ± 9.0	0.73	0.02
Triggers of diabetic ketosis (%)					
New-onset	13.8	5.0	—	0.01	—
Old diagnosed	38.7	20.0	—	0.02	—
Weight reduction (kg)					
New-onset	7.3 ± 4.4	2.1 ± 2.3	4.5 ± 5.3	0.02	0.04
Old diagnosed	9.2 ± 6.3	15.2 ± 7.2	10.4 ± 6.1	0.0014	0.79

T2DK, type 2 diabetes with ketosis; T1D, type 1 diabetes; T2D, type 2 diabetes; *P*1, T2DK versus T1D; *P*2, T2DK versus T2D.

obese patients were in the group of T2DK (49.1%) and T2D (43.5%). There were no differences in systolic blood pressure and diastolic blood pressure among the three groups at the time of admission.

Patients of T2DK showed remarkably elevated plasma fasting glucose (16.9 ± 6 versus 10.3 ± 4 mmol/L, $P < 0.0001$ T2Dk versus T2D) and HbA1c (13.3 ± 3.1 versus 10.2 ± 2.1%, $P = 0.01$ T2Dk versus T2D) level compared to T2D upon admission. Fasting C-peptide (0.65 ± 0.2 nmol/L) in T2DK was similar to that in T1D (0.47 ± 0.1 nmol/L, $P = 0.11$), and slightly lower than that in T2D (0.98 ± 0.9 nmol/L, $P = 0.08$). However, the postprandial 2-hour C-peptide was significantly higher in T2DK (2.04 ± 0.8 nmol/L) than that in T1D (0.69 ± 0.1 nmol/L, $P = 0.001$), and similar to that in T2D (2.18 ± 1.0 nmol/L, $P = 0.75$). The patients of T2D with ketosis group had significantly higher plasma triglyceride (4.0 ± 4.0 mmol/L) than patients of ordinary T2D without ketosis group (2.8 ± 2.7 mmol/L, $P < 0.0001$), and similar to T1D group (4.3 ± 3.0 mmol/L, $P = 0.47$). Meanwhile, the total plasma cholesterol was similar in T2DK compared with T1D and T2D (5.3 ± 1.7, 5.7 ± 1.7, and 4.9 ± 1.6 mmol/L, resp., in T2DK, T1D, and T2D, $P = 0.48$ T2DK versus T1D; $P = 0.11$ T2DK versus T2D).

Diabetic patients experienced reduction of body weight on admission. For those new-onset T2DK, weight reduction was 7.3 ± 4.4 kg, significantly higher than T1D (2.1 ± 2.3 kg, $P = 0.02$) and T2D (4.5 ± 5.3 kg, $P = 0.04$) groups. For those old diagnosed diabetic subjects in T2DK, weight reduction was 9.2 ± 6.3 kg, less than T1D (15.2 ± 7.2 kg, $P = 0.0014$), and similar to T2D (10.4 ± 6.1 kg, $P = 0.79$) groups (Table 2). Moreover, among patients with existing diabetes in the T2DK group, most patients (83%) had seldom or never received regular drug treatment for diabetes, and nearly no one (<1%) had adequate glycemic control (data not shown).

Unlike most of the T1D patients who were cases of spontaneous ketosis, in the group of T2DK, most patients were admitted with obvious inducements. The provoked ketosis was 13.8% in new-onset and 38.7% in the previously diagnosed T2D (Table 2). The predominant factors were infections. Among them, respiratory, urinary, and digestive system infections were frequent inducements in T2DK (Figure 1).

The patients with T2DK had more atherosclerosis (19% versus 7%, resp., in T2DK and T1D, $P < 0.0001$) and fatty liver disease (21% versus 11%, resp., in T2DK and T1D, $P < 0.0001$) compared with those with T1D. Retinopathy was less in T2DK compared to T1D (12.7% versus 25%, $P = 0.02$ T2DK versus T1D). There were more cases of persistent microalbuminuria on admission in the T2DK (11.7%) compared with T2D (8.1%, $P = 0.01$). No significant differences were found in peripheral neuropathy among T2DK (34.9%), T1D (41.3%), and T2D (31.8%). The histogram of the diabetic chronic complications was demonstrated (Figure 2).

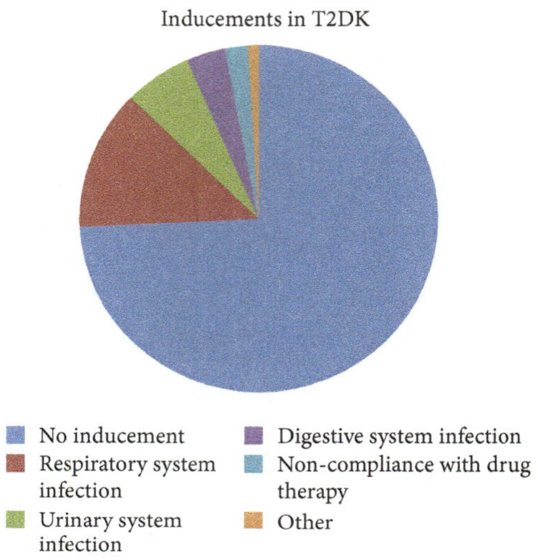

Figure 1: Inducements in type 2 diabetes with ketosis.

4. Discussion

In this study, we showed characteristics of T2D with ketosis comparing with those ordinary T2D and T1D in a tertiary hospital in Baoshan, Yunnan province of China. The T2D patients with ketosis had prominent characteristics of overweight and positive family history of diabetes. Prior to their admission, the blood glucose of most type 2 diabetes with ketosis patients in our study was poorly controlled, as reflected by elevated HbA1c levels. HbA1c could be used to determine the average blood glucose levels over 2 to 3 months. High HbA1c levels indicated the previously undiagnosed or poorly controlled diabetes.

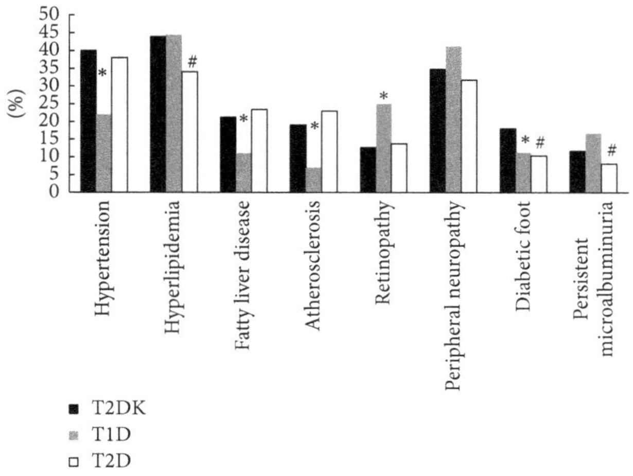

FIGURE 2: Chronic complications of diabetes. T2DK, type 2 diabetes with ketosis; T1D, type 1 diabetes; T2D, type 2 diabetes. $^*P < 0.05$, T2DK versus T1D; $^\#P < 0.05$, T2DK versus T2D.

Patients with type 2 diabetes were susceptible to ketosis or ketoacidosis under long-term uncontrolled hyperglycemia especially with inducement conditions such as infections, surgery, or trauma. Most type 2 diabetic patients irregularly or never got treatment after their first diabetic diagnosis in poor regions. Infections were common inducements in T2D with ketosis in these study subjects. In rural areas, patients with hyperglycemia were delayed for diagnosis and treatment because of the backward of economy, education, and medicine.

Type 2 diabetes with ketosis was characterized by marked hyperglycaemia, ketosis (or even ketoacidosis), and severe insulin deficiency [10, 11]. Accumulating evidence has shown that not only severe glucotoxicity but also lipotoxicity might contribute to the β cell dysfunction [12–16]. Our study indicated that patients in T2DK group had significantly higher plasma triglyceride than those in ordinary T2D group, which was consistent with previous study [17]. It was concluded from our study that male and overweight patients were prone to ketosis and these data confirmed the results of previous studies [14, 18]. Mechanisms underlying the reason why males were susceptible to ketosis in type 2 diabetes population were not clear up to now. A large population study [19] reported that adherence of diabetes medications was significantly associated with sex (male versus female, odds ratio 1.14, $P < 0.0001$), which might be an important reason why male predominated in T2DK group. At the same time, it has been suggested that some factors including body fat distribution, hormonal factors, and differences in the lifestyle such as alcohol abuse and smoking habits might contribute to the gender difference [14, 18, 20]. In our study, 35% male T2D ketosis patients had the habits of smoking or drinking, while the figure in female is 0.8% (data not shown).

Chronic diabetic complications were commonly seen in these study subjects, which were true with some previous studies [21, 22]. We found that T2D with ketosis patients had a similar risk of chronic diabetic complications with ordinary T2D in some aspects. However, T2D patients with ketosis were prone to suffer from diabetic foot and persistent microalbuminuria compared to ordinary T2D patients. The possible reason might be the long-term worse glucose control in the T2DK than in T2D group in our study groups. Further prolonged and large scale population studies were needed to gain definite conclusions.

There were some limitations in this report. First, the study subjects were not available for plasma ketosis test, which was more sensitive and specific than urine test. Second, this was a single-center study with limitations of study number and region; thus, the multicenter studies should be performed to further clarify the characteristics of diabetes in the south-west rural parts of China.

In summary, T2D with ketosis group occupied a large proportion on admission in total study patients. These subjects were in need of tighter glucose control due to the severe chaos of glucose and lipids metabolism and more chronic complications. The results indicated that diabetes has become a public health problem even in rural areas of China. More efforts such as intensive health education and medical resources targeted at the prevention and treatment of diabetes are urgently needed in the rural population in Yunnan province, China.

Conflict of Interests

The authors state that they have no conflict of interests.

Acknowledgments

The study was supported by the research Grant of Shanghai Municipal Commission of Health and Family Planning, no. 20144Y0140, and the research Grant of cooperation between medicine and engineering techniques of Shanghai Jiaotong University, no. YG2015QN43.

References

[1] D. Hu, P. Fu, J. Xie et al., "Increasing prevalence and low awareness, treatment and control of diabetes mellitus among Chinese adults: the InterASIA study," *Diabetes Research and Clinical Practice*, vol. 81, no. 2, pp. 250–257, 2008.

[2] Y. Xu, L. Wang, J. He, Y. Bi, M. Li et al., "Prevalence and control of diabetes in Chinese adults," *The Journal of the American Medical Association*, vol. 310, no. 9, pp. 948–959, 2013.

[3] J. C. N. Chan, V. Malik, W. Jia et al., "Diabetes in Asia: epidemiology, risk factors, and pathophysiology," *The Journal of the American Medical Association*, vol. 301, no. 20, pp. 2129–2140, 2009.

[4] D. S. Prasad, Z. Kabir, A. K. Dash, and B. C. Das, "Prevalence and risk factors for diabetes and impaired glucose tolerance in Asian Indians: a community survey from urban Eastern India," *Diabetes & Metabolic Syndrome*, vol. 6, no. 2, pp. 96–101, 2012.

[5] B. Liu, C. Yu, Q. Li, and L. Li, "Ketosis-onset diabetes and ketosis-prone diabetes: same or not?" *International Journal of Endocrinology*, vol. 2013, Article ID 821403, 6 pages, 2013.

[6] H. Lu, F. Hu, Y. Zeng et al., "Ketosis onset type 2 diabetes had better islet β-cell function and more serious insulin resistance," *Journal of Diabetes Research*, vol. 2014, Article ID 510643, 6 pages, 2014.

[7] American Diabetes Association, "Diagnosis and classification of diabetes mellitus," *Diabetes Care*, vol. 27, supplement 1, pp. S5–S10, 2004.

[8] C. Chen and F. C. Lu, "The guidelines for prevention and control of overweight and obesity in Chinese adults," *Biomedical and Environmental Sciences*, vol. 17, supplement 1, pp. 1–36, 2004.

[9] B. F. Zhou and Coorperative Meta-Analysis Group of China Obesity Task Force, "Predictive values of body mass index and waist circumference to risk factors of related diseases in Chinese adult population," *Zhonghua Liu Xing Bing Xue Za Zhi*, vol. 23, no. 1, pp. 5–10, 2002.

[10] G. E. Umpierrez, D. Smiley, and A. E. Kitabchi, "Narrative review: ketosis-prone type 2 diabetes mellitus," *Annals of Internal Medicine*, vol. 144, no. 5, pp. 350–357, 2006.

[11] E. Sobngwi, S. P. Choukem, F. Agbalika et al., "Ketosis-prone type 2 diabetes mellitus and human herpesvirus 8 infection in sub-Saharan Africans," *The Journal of the American Medical Association*, vol. 299, no. 23, pp. 2770–2776, 2008.

[12] S. Tangvarasittichai, "Oxidative stress, insulin resistance, dyslipidemia and type 2 diabetes mellitus," *World Journal of Diabetes*, vol. 6, no. 3, p. 456, 2015.

[13] G. E. Umpierrez, D. Smiley, A. Gosmanov, and D. Thomason, "Ketosis-prone type 2 diabetes: effect of hyperglycemia on β-cell function and skeletal muscle insulin signaling," *Endocrine Practice*, vol. 13, no. 3, pp. 283–290, 2007.

[14] X. Wang and H. Tan, "Male predominance in ketosis-prone diabetes mellitus," *Biomedical Reports*, vol. 3, pp. 439–442, 2015.

[15] D. Smiley, P. Chandra, and G. E. Umpierrez, "Update on diagnosis, pathogenesis and management of ketosis-prone Type 2 diabetes mellitus," *Diabetes Management*, vol. 1, no. 6, pp. 589–600, 2011.

[16] V. Poitout, I. Briaud, C. Kelpe, and D. Hagman, "Glucolipotoxicity of the pancreatic beta cell," *Annales d'Endocrinologie*, vol. 65, no. 1, pp. 37–41, 2004.

[17] H. Tan, Y. Zhou, and Y. Yu, "Characteristics of diabetic ketoacidosis in Chinese adults and adolescents—a teaching hospital-based analysis," *Diabetes Research and Clinical Practice*, vol. 97, no. 2, pp. 306–312, 2012.

[18] G. Goodstein, A. Milanesi, and J. E. Weinreb, "Ketosis-prone type 2 diabetes in a veteran population," *Diabetes Care*, vol. 37, no. 4, pp. e74–e75, 2014.

[19] M. S. Kirkman, M. T. Rowan-Martin, R. Levin et al., "Determinants of adherence to diabetes medications: findings from a large pharmacy claims database," *Diabetes Care*, vol. 38, no. 4, pp. 604–609, 2015.

[20] E. A. Nyenwe, R. S. Loganathan, S. Blum et al., "Active use of cocaine: an independent risk factor for recurrent diabetic ketoacidosis in a city hospital," *Endocrine Practice*, vol. 13, no. 1, pp. 22–29, 2007.

[21] L. Salvotelli, V. Stoico, F. Perrone et al., "Prevalence of neuropathy in type 2 diabetic patients and its association with other diabetes complications: the Verona Diabetic Foot Screening Program," *Journal of Diabetes and Its Complications*, vol. 29, no. 8, pp. 1066–1070, 2015.

[22] S. M. S. Islam, D. S. Alam, M. Wahiduzzaman et al., "Clinical characteristics and complications of patients with type 2 diabetes attending an urban hospital in Bangladesh," *Diabetes and Metabolic Syndrome*, vol. 9, no. 1, pp. 7–13, 2015.

27

Decrease in (Major) Amputations in Diabetics: A Secondary Data Analysis by AOK Rheinland/Hamburg

Melanie May,[1] Sebastian Hahn,[2] Claudia Tonn,[1] Gerald Engels,[3,4] and Dirk Hochlenert[5]

[1] *AOK Rheinland/Hamburg, Die Gesundheitskasse, Unternehmensbereich Ambulante Versorgung, Geschäftsbereich Selektivverträge, Kasernenstrasse 61, 40213 Düsseldorf, Germany*
[2] *AOK Rheinland/Hamburg, Die Gesundheitskasse, Unternehmensbereich M-RSA/Finanzen/Controlling, Geschäftsbereich Controlling, Kasernenstrasse 61, 40213 Düsseldorf, Germany*
[3] *Chirurgische Praxis am Bayenthalgürtel, Bayenthalgürtel 45, 50968 Köln, Germany*
[4] *Ltd. Arzt Abteilung, Wundchirurgie St. Vinzenz Hospital Köln, Merheimer Strasse 221, 50733 Köln, Germany*
[5] *Centrum für Diabetologie, Endoskopie und Wundheilung, Merheimer Strasse 217, 50733 Köln, Germany*

Correspondence should be addressed to Melanie May; melanie.may@rh.aok.de

Academic Editor: Alberto Piaggesi

Aim. In two German regions with 11.1 million inhabitants, 6 networks for specialized treatment of DFS were implemented until 2008. Data provided for accounting purposes was analysed in order to determine changes in the rate of diabetics requiring amputations in the years before and after the implementation. *Method.* Data covering 2.9 million people insured by the largest insurance company between 2007 and 2013 was analysed by the use of log-linear Poisson regression adjusted for age, gender and region. *Results.* The rate of diabetics needing major amputations fell significantly by 9.5% per year ($p < 0.0001$) from 217 to 126 of 100,000 patients per year. The rate of diabetics needing amputations of any kind fell from 504 to 419 of 100,000 patients per year ($p = 0.0038$). *Discussion.* The networks integrate health care providers in an organised system of shared care. They educate members of the medical community and the general public. At the same time, a more general disease management program for people with diabetes was implemented, which may also have contributed to this decrease. At the end of the observation period, the rate of diabetics requiring amputations was still high. For this reason, further expansion of organised specialized care is urgently needed.

1. Introduction

Diabetic foot syndrome (DFS) is a lifelong consequence of diabetes mellitus which occurs in active and inactive phases. It may place the mobility of those affected under threat and consequently their independence, quality of life, and ability to work. In some cases, it may be fatal. In particular, after amputations above the ankle, mobility is impaired, as half of those affected are no longer able to walk independently [1, 2]. An important aim in the care of people with active DFS is therefore to avoid these so-called major amputations. According to the data currently available, 5–10% of people with active DFS are affected by this in standard care, while the figure in specialised care is 2–3.5% [3–5].

A substantial proportion of the spending on diabetes care in Germany is attributable to the DFS [6, 7]. Major amputations in particular, with their follow-up costs, entail significant levels of spending [8]. The development of care for people with DFS receives high priority all over the world [9].

Delivery of care to the patient is unavoidably of an interdisciplinary and interprofessional nature. It requires coordinated cooperation between all of the parties involved, which in the regions of Rhineland (9.4 million inhabitants) and Hamburg (1.7 million) joint forces into six separate regional networks since 2002. These networks integrate hospital departments, doctors and nurses working in the outpatient field, and orthopaedic shoemakers and podiatrists as healthcare service providers working in independent facilities. Coordinated treatment paths, regular quality circles, visiting physician programmes, and open benchmarking are some of the methods used in shared patient care.

Within the German health care system, baseline medical care is covered by contracts between insurance companies and organised physicians. They are called "collective contracts" because all adequately specialized physicians are free to participate. These contracts are highly regulated by federal and regional law. Disease management programs are among these collective contracts. Additionally, insurance companies can conclude contracts with groups of health care providers to offer extra services to their customers. For these contracts called "selective contracts," insurance companies are allowed to select the participating providers. AOK Rhineland/Hamburg (AOK RH) is a prime insurance company in these regions and aims to improve the care given to people with diabetes. To achieve this, in addition to a disease management program (DMP Diabetes), AOK RH together with other insurance companies supported the development of networks for the treatment of people with a diabetic foot syndrome since 2005 through selective contracts (DFS SC). After a trial period from 2005 to 2008, these contracts were concluded with network participants throughout the entire area covered by the AOK RH. From the very beginning of the contract, the aim was to produce an effect on the region as a whole. Therefore, the networks began at an early stage to make offers of further education to other facilities within the contract region. To this same aim, second-opinion procedures prior to major amputations were made available and awareness campaigns were conducted.

Publications on the incidence of amputations in Germany have so far been limited to the analysis of hospital stays with amputation events without reference to individuals. It has been argued that a change of strategy from partial amputations performed consecutively towards a unique procedure could result in reduced amputation figures in spite of an increase in the number of individuals affected and therefore a distortion of the perception of the result. The present work identifies not only the hospital stays with amputations performed, but also the number of people affected.

2. Materials and Methods

We analysed accounting data for the years 2007 to 2013 of the AOK RH in accordance with Sections 295, 300, and 301 of Social Security Code Book Five. This data contains information on the diagnoses according to the International Classification of Disease (ICD-10 GM), drug prescriptions according to the Anatomical Therapeutic Chemical- (ATC-) code, and surgical procedures according to the German Procedure Classification (OPS). The diagnosis of diabetes was considered to have been confirmed if indicated by more than one statement independently. These were similar to other investigations from the German healthcare system [10–12]:

(i) A 3-digit diagnosis (ICD E10* to E14*) in at least 3 of 4 consecutive quarters at the level "certain" according to the ICD 10 GM.

(ii) At least two prescriptions of antidiabetic agents (ATC A10) within 12 months.

(iii) A prescription of antidiabetic agents and a diabetes diagnosis or a glucose or HbA1c measurement within 12 months.

Major amputations were considered to be those performed at the level of the ankle or above (OPS 5-864, 5-869.0), whereas minor amputations were amputations below the ankle (OPS 5-865), which is also analogous to earlier investigations [13, 14].

Absolute frequencies were normalised to 100,000 diabetics. Adjusted amputation frequencies were presented by means of regression analysis.

The figures were compiled separately for each of the 27 regions in Rhineland and Hamburg and presented together. The breakdown corresponds to the administrative structures of AOK RH and takes into account regional specificities.

2.1. Statistics: Poisson Regression. For each of the 27 regions in Rhineland and Hamburg, the number of diabetics and their gender and age distribution, as well as the amputations themselves were determined for each year during the period investigated. This took into account possible changes in demographic developments resulting from changes in age and gender distribution or the number of insured individuals.

Using a log-linear Poisson regression [15], the annual frequency of amputations within each region was modelled with adjustments according to age and gender. We additionally applied two different offset variables: in Model 1, the offset was the absolute number of diabetics in the year under consideration within each region; in Model 2, it was the number of diabetics in the year 2007 held constant over all years. The second modelling procedure was added in order to eliminate the possible effect of any change in coding behaviour over the years.

The Poisson regression was performed using SAS version 9.2 of PROC GENMOD.

3. Results

3.1. General. Among approximately 2.9 million individuals insured by AOK RH in 2007, the diabetes prevalence was 8.2%. This figure rose in 2013 to 9.9%, with levels being 10.9% in Hamburg and 9.8% in Rhineland, respectively (Figure 1). The proportion of women was 37.2% overall and the average patient age was 69.3 (±13.8). The total number of hospital stays with amputations carried out on 6,958 diabetics in the period from 2007 to 2013 was 11,436 (3,607 with major and 7,829 with minor amputations).

3.2. Structured Care. In 2013, over 10,000 people with diabetes and DFS received structured care in networks in accordance to contracts provided by the AOK RH. In addition to the increasing numbers of participants in structured care, the proportion of diabetics cared for in the Disease Management Program (DMP) also rose to around 65% and therefore amounted to over 180,000 individuals in 2013 in absolute terms (Figure 2). Of all policyholders with diabetes who underwent amputations, 777 (11.2%) were cared for

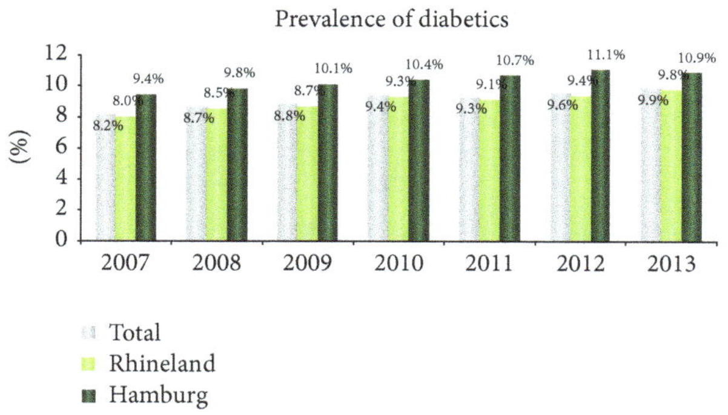

FIGURE 1: Prevalence of diabetics covered by AOK RH, 2007–2013.

in networks (SC), with 22.4% of these undergoing major amputations (Table 1).

TABLE 1: Overview of selective contract (SC) participants and amputation frequency.

People with diabetes and amputation from 2007 to 2013	6,958
SC participants with amputation (major or minor)	777
SC participants with major amputation	174
SC participants with minor amputation	613
Proportion of SC participants undergoing major amputations compared to the total number of amputations	22.4%

3.3. Amputations. It was shown that over the course of seven years up to 2013, there was a significant reduction of 41.7% in the number of patients undergoing a major amputation ($p < 0.0001$). The proportion of people with minor amputations fell by 2.1% ($p = 0.6624$) (Table 2, Figures 3(a) and 3(b)). The proportion of those who required any form of amputation fell by 17.0% ($p < 0.0001$) (results normalised in each case to 100,000 diabetics). In total, 1,537 (22.1%) diabetics underwent multiple amputations over the years and can therefore be assigned to more than one year.

The results of the Poisson regression did not provide any indications of over- or underdispersion (deviance/df = 1.35 (Model 1) and 1.10 (Model 2)).

When adjusted for age and gender distribution for each region, a significant reduction in the number of individuals undergoing major amputations of 9.5% ($p < 0.0001$) is found across all of the years. If it is assumed that the number of diabetics remains constant (Model 2), an annual decline of 8.50% ($p = 0.0002$) is recorded. The number of people affected by amputations, regardless of whether these were major or minor, fell annually by 3.7% ($p = 0.0038$).

4. Discussion

The incidence of major amputations varies worldwide between 56 and 6,000 for every 100,000 people with diabetes [16]. This variability is caused not only by differences in health care, but also by uncertainties regarding the diagnosis of the diabetic disease and whether all of the amputation events performed are recorded [17]. The incidence also varies within countries. For example, at 151 Primary Care Trusts (PCTs) in England between 2007 and 2010, the figures varied from 64 to 525 per 100,000 [18]. In Ipswich (UK), the introduction of specialised care which completely replaced the previous form of care observed a reduction in major amputations in the years 1995 to 2005 from 364 to 67 per 100,000 people with diabetes [19]. In the study presented here, the number of those affected fell from 217 to 126 per 100,000 diabetics. The number of hospital stays with an event decreased from 263 to 146 per 100,000 diabetics. This need for improvement which still exists in the international comparison might be attributable to specific aspects of the German healthcare system. Generally speaking, all hospitals with their own surgical departments can charge fees for major amputations. The complete replacement of the existing form delivering care by an alternative form is not possible here.

The specialised care is provided as an additional offer to the standard care. Indeed, only a minority of the amputations examined here were performed on patients who received care in the networks of the selective contract. The fact that the care would only be partially taken over by the networks was already foreseeable when the intervention was planned; therefore, the introduction was accompanied by a number of measures such as advanced training courses, offers of second opinions, and awareness campaigns in order to achieve a broad effect.

Two previous population-based studies of the care for people with DFS in Leverkusen, a city within the area studied here, showed a decrease in the number of amputations over the entire period under investigation (1990–2005) [20] which had not yet been seen in the years 1990–1998 [21]. In this survey, the reduction was attributed to a change in the type of care, which also formed part of the development of the regional networks.

Previous evaluations of amputation incidence from accounting data [22–24] were case and not individual related. Therefore, it was not possible to state how many people with diabetes underwent amputations and the extent to which the development in the absolute surgical figures affected the number of patients involved. This is illustrated by the study presented here, which covers the insured from two major regions and uses the figures of the largest health insurance company in these regions.

Furthermore, the analysis of the number of patients affected shows for the first time that in Germany there has been a significant decrease in the number of people with diabetes who require amputations. The number of people affected by minor amputations is falling only by a lesser extent, which is partly attributable to the fact that minor amputations are being carried out instead of major amputations.

The limitations of the study relate in particular to the selection of the patients affected due to their membership of AOK RH and the development in the incidence of the diabetes diagnoses documented. However, the selection bias remained constant over the observed period; since there were no mergers of AOK RH with other health insurance

TABLE 2: Absolute number of hospital stays with amputation events and diabetics, proportion of diabetics with amputation compared to total number of diabetics.

Year	Number of the insured	Number of insured diabetics	Number of hospital stays with amputations			Number of diabetics with amputation			Number of diabetics with amputation/100,000 diabetics		
			Major	Minor	Amputation (major + minor)	Major	Minor	Amputation*	Major	Minor	Amputation*
2007	2,908,300	237,164	619	975	1,594	514	761	1,196	217	321	504
2008	2,857,963	247,690	511	1,083	1,594	431	844	1,190	174	341	480
2009	2,850,008	251,623	559	1,120	1,679	456	869	1,253	181	345	498
2010	2,863,114	269,432	566	1,130	1,696	456	861	1,243	169	320	461
2011	2,881,479	267,708	515	1,120	1,635	429	884	1,245	160	330	465
2012	2,867,117	274,092	421	1,198	1,619	365	897	1,201	133	327	438
2013	2,817,703	278,647	416	1,163	1,579	352	875	1,167	126	314	419

*Patients were counted only once in the corresponding year irrespective of the type of amputation (major and/or minor).

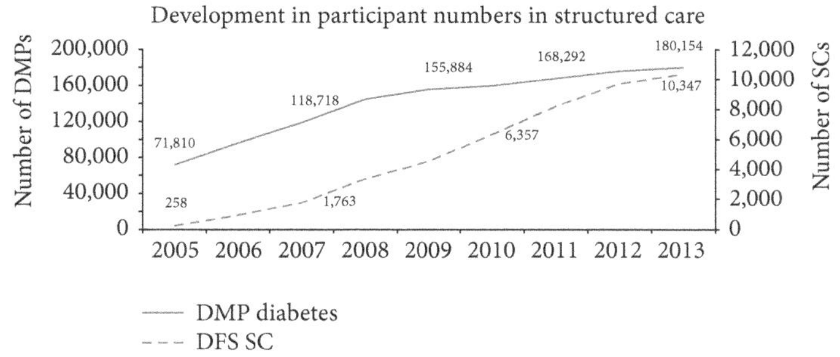

FIGURE 2: Development in participant numbers in the DMP and DFS selective contract (SC).

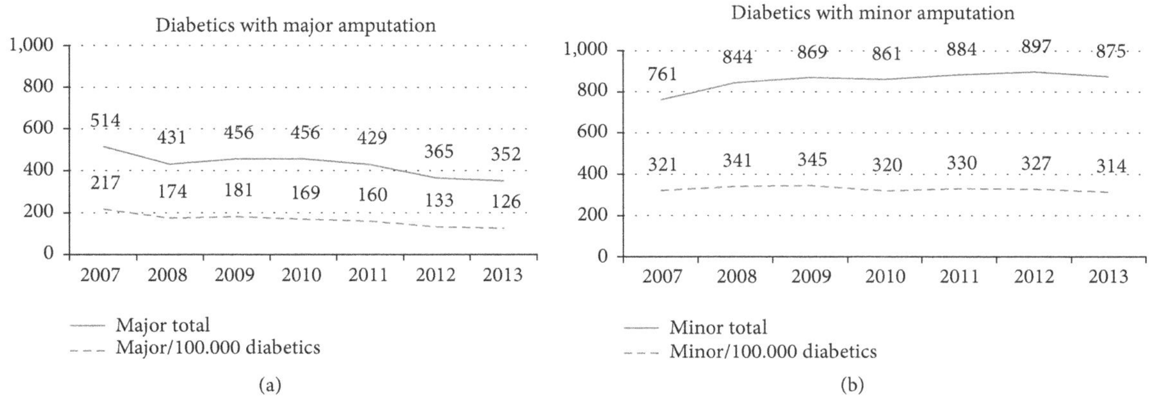

FIGURE 3: Number of diabetics with major or minor amputation, 2007–2013.

companies, no other trends became apparent among the insured and the number of insured individuals remained more or less the same. The increase in the number of diagnosed diabetes cases might have been attributable in part to a change in coding behaviour. For this reason, a second modelling procedure was carried out which assumed that the prevalence of diabetes remained unchanged. In this evaluation, there was also a very clear and significant reduction in the incidence of insured individuals undergoing amputations in particular major amputations.

5. Summary Assessment

The figures presented, which are based on routine data, confirm a very significant improvement in the care of people with DFS. The number of people affected who underwent major amputations with their serious consequences fell dramatically during the seven years after the introduction of organised specialised care. Both the structured treatment program DMP Diabetes and the specialized "DFS" contract are used by a large proportion of affected people in Rhineland and in Hamburg. However, the majority of those who underwent an amputation event did not use specialized care offered by the contract. The increasing number of patients in this contract alongside with the efforts to induce advances in the nonspecialized standard care might explain that improvement and should be investigated in further studies. For this reason, the expansion of the care of people with diabetic foot syndrome in structured foot networks is indispensable in the future.

Conflict of Interests

The authors declare that there is no conflict of interests regarding the publication of this paper.

References

[1] M. R. Nehler, J. R. Coll, W. R. Hiatt et al., "Functional outcome in a contemporary series of major lower extremity amputations," *Journal of Vascular Surgery*, vol. 38, no. 1, pp. 7–14, 2003.

[2] T. Schoppen, A. Boonstra, J. W. Groothoff, J. De Vries, L. N. Göeken, and W. H. Eisma, "Physical, mental, and social predictors of functional outcome in unilateral lower-limb amputees," *Archives of Physical Medicine and Rehabilitation*, vol. 84, no. 6, pp. 803–811, 2003.

[3] D. Hochlenert and G. Engels, "Low major amputation rate and low recurrence in networks for treatment of the DFS," in *Abstract Book, X. Diabetic Foot Study Group Meeting Seminaris See Hotel, Berlin-Potsdam, Germany, 28–30 September*, 2012.

[4] D. Hochlenert, G. Engels, and L. Altenhofen, "Integrated health care delivery for patients with diabetic foot syndrome in Cologne," *Deutsches Arzteblatt*, vol. 103, no. 24, pp. A1680–A1683, 2006.

[5] R. Lobmann, O. Achwerdov, S. Brunk-Loch et al., "The diabetic foot in Germany 2005–2012: analysis of quality in specialized diabetic foot care centers," *Wound Medicine*, vol. 4, pp. 27–29, 2014.

[6] I. Köster, E. Huppertz, H. Hauner, and I. Schubert, "Direct costs of diabetes mellitus in Germany—CoDiM 2000–2007," *Experimental and Clinical Endocrinology & Diabetes*, vol. 119, no. 6, pp. 377–385, 2011.

[7] H. Hauner, "The costs of diabetes mellitus and its complications in Germany," *Deutsche Medizinische Wochenschrift*, vol. 131, supplement 8, pp. S240–S242, 2006.

[8] J. Apelqvist, G. Ragnarson-Tennvall, J. Larsson, and U. Persson, "Long-term costs for foot ulcers in diabetic patients in a multidisciplinary setting," *Foot and Ankle International*, vol. 16, no. 7, pp. 388–394, 1995.

[9] W. Jeffcoate and K. Bakker, "World Diabetes Day: footing the bill," *The Lancet*, vol. 365, no. 9470, p. 1527, 2005.

[10] A. Icks, B. Haastert, C. Trautner, G. Giani, G. Glaeske, and F. Hoffmann, "Incidence of lower-limb amputations in the diabetic compared to the non-diabetic population. Findings from nationwide insurance data, Germany, 2005–2007," *Experimental and Clinical Endocrinology & Diabetes*, vol. 117, no. 9, pp. 500–504, 2009.

[11] I. Köster, H. Hauner, and L. von Ferber, "Heterogeneity of costs of diabetic patients: the Cost of Diabetes Mellitus Study," *Deutsche Medizinische Wochenschrift*, vol. 131, no. 15, pp. 804–810, 2006.

[12] H. Hauner, I. Koster, and L. von Ferber, "Prevalence of diabetes mellitus in Germany 1998–2001. Secondary data analysis of a health insurance sample of the AOK in Hesse/KV in Hesse," *Deutsche Medizinische Wochenschrift*, vol. 128, no. 50, pp. 2632–2637, 2003.

[13] G. Heller, C. Gunster, and H. Schellschmidt, "How frequent are diabetes-related amputations of the lower limbs in Germany? An analysis on the basis of routine data," *Deutsche Medizinische Wochenschrift*, vol. 129, no. 9, pp. 429–433, 2004.

[14] G. Heller, C. Gunster, and E. Swart, "The frequency of lower limb amputations in Germany," *Deutsche Medizinische Wochenschrift*, vol. 130, no. 28-29, pp. 1689–1690, 2005.

[15] A. C. Cameron and P. K. Trivedi, *Regression Analysis of Count Data*, Cambridge University Press, New York, NY, USA, 1998.

[16] P. W. Moxey, P. Gogalniceanu, R. J. Hinchliffe et al., "Lower extremity amputations—a review of global variability in incidence," *Diabetic Medicine*, vol. 28, no. 10, pp. 1144–1153, 2011.

[17] G. Rayman, S. T. M. Krishnan, N. R. Baker, A. M. Wareham, and A. Rayman, "Are we underestimating diabetes-related lower-extremity amputation rates? Results and benefits of the first prospective study," *Diabetes Care*, vol. 27, no. 8, pp. 1892–1896, 2004.

[18] N. Holman, R. J. Young, and W. J. Jeffcoate, "Variation in the recorded incidence of amputation of the lower limb in England," *Diabetologia*, vol. 55, no. 7, pp. 1919–1925, 2012.

[19] S. Krishnan, F. Nash, N. Baker, D. Fowler, and G. Rayman, "Reduction in diabetic amputations over 11 years in a defined U.K. population: benefits of multidisciplinary team work and continuous prospective audit," *Diabetes Care*, vol. 31, no. 1, pp. 99–101, 2008.

[20] C. Trautner, B. Haastert, P. Mauckner, L. M. Gätcke, and G. Giani, "Reduced incidence of lower-limb amputations in the diabetic population of a German city, 1990–2005: results of the Leverkusen Amputation Reduction Study (LARS)," *Diabetes Care*, vol. 30, no. 10, pp. 2633–2637, 2007.

[21] C. Trautner, B. Haastert, M. Spraul, G. Giani, and M. Berger, "Unchanged incidence of lower-limb amputations in a German City, 1990–1998," *Diabetes Care*, vol. 24, no. 5, pp. 855–859, 2001.

[22] G. Heller, *Häufigkeit von Amputationen—aktuelle Zahlen*, Vortrag an der 41, Jahrestagung der Deutschen Diabetesgesellschaft, Leipzig, Germany, 2005.

[23] G. Heller, C. Günster, and H. Schellschmidt, "Wie häufig sind Diabetes-bedingte Amputationen unterer Extremitäten in Deutschland," *Deutsche Medizinische Wochenschrift*, vol. 129, pp. 429–433, 2004.

[24] F. Santosa, T. Moysidis, S. Kanya, Z. Babadagi-Hardt, B. Luther, and K. Kröger, "Decrease in major amputations in Germany," *International Wound Journal*, vol. 12, no. 3, pp. 276–279, 2013.

28

Comparison of the Effects of Continuous Subcutaneous Insulin Infusion and Add-On Therapy with Sitagliptin in Patients with Newly Diagnosed Type 2 Diabetes Mellitus

Heng Wan,[1] Defu Zhao,[1] Jie Shen,[1] Lu Lu,[2] Tong Zhang,[1] and Zhi Chen[1]

[1] *Department of Endocrinology and Metabolism, The Third Affiliated Hospital of Southern Medical University, Guangzhou 510630, China*
[2] *School of Traditional Chinese Medicine, Southern Medical University, Guangzhou 510515, China*

Correspondence should be addressed to Jie Shen; shenjiedr@163.com

Academic Editor: Mitsuhiko Noda

To identify a new regimen to optimize treatment for patients with newly diagnosed type 2 diabetes (T2DM) by short-term continuous subcutaneous insulin infusion (CSII) alone. *Methods.* 60 patients with newly diagnosed T2DM were randomized into two groups ($n = 30$ each) and treated for 2 weeks with CSII alone (CSII group) or with CSII plus sitagliptin (CSII + Sig group). The glycemic variability of the patients was measured using a continuous glucose monitoring system (CGMS) for the last 72 hours. A standard meal test was performed before and after the interventions, and the levels of glycated albumin, fasting glucose, fasting C-peptide, postprandial 2 h blood glucose, and postprandial 2 h C-peptide were examined. *Results.* Compared with the CSII group, the indicators of glycemic variability, such as the mean amplitude of glycemic excursion (MAGE) and the standard deviation of blood glucose (SDBG), were decreased significantly in the CSII + Sig group. The changes before and after treatment in the C-peptide reactivity index (ΔCPI) and the secretory unit of islet in transplantation index (ΔSUIT) indicated a significant improvement in the CSII + Sig group. *Conclusions.* Add-on therapy with sitagliptin may be an optimized treatment for patients with newly diagnosed T2DM compared with short-term CSII alone.

1. Introduction

Type 2 diabetes mellitus (T2DM) is a chronic disease that is characterized by progressive β-cell dysfunction that leads to insulin deficiency. At the time of diagnosis, β-cell function may be reduced by as much as 50% compared with healthy control subjects and will progressively deteriorate over time, irrespective of lifestyle and pharmacological interventions, as revealed in the UK Prospective Diabetes Study [1]. Recent studies have suggested that short-term intensive insulin therapy, with continuous subcutaneous insulin infusion (CSII) potentially being the best current therapeutic option [2, 3], can rapidly relieve newly diagnosed T2DM patients of high glucose toxicity, ameliorate the state of insulin resistance, and restore islet β-cell function [4, 5]. However, glycemic variability and hypoglycemia are risks associated with this type of therapy [6, 7].

Studies suggest that glycemic variability, an HbA1c-independent risk factor, is another important factor leading to chronic complications of diabetes [8–10]. Some studies have even suggested that glycemic variability has more deleterious effects than sustained hyperglycemia in the development of diabetic complications [11, 12]. Therefore, glycemic variability should be one of the criteria for evaluating glycemic control.

A continuous glucose monitoring system (CGMS) can provide information concerning glucose concentrations throughout the day by monitoring levels every 5 min, thus helping to detect trends in glycemic variability, hyperglycemia, and hypoglycemia that are more difficult to detect using conventional self-monitoring of blood glucose [13].

Our previous study [14] showed that the area under the curve of glucagon-like peptide-l (GLP-1) in patients with T2DM was significantly lower than that in patients with normal glucose tolerance or impaired glucose tolerance. However, the dipeptidyl peptidase-4 (DPP-4) inhibitor sitagliptin can increase active GLP-1 concentrations and thereby enhance insulin secretion by β-cells and inhibit glucagon release from α-cells in a glucose-dependent manner [15]. Therefore, our present study uses CGMS to evaluate the impact of glycemic variability when adding sitagliptin to the CSII therapy of newly diagnosed T2DM patients.

In addition, previous studies have suggested that sitagliptin can restore α-cell function, ameliorate insulin resistance (HOMA-IR), and improve pancreatic β-cell function (HOMA-β) in patients [16]. In our study, sitagliptin is added to short-term CSII to control the glucose of newly diagnosed T2DM patients to determine whether there is an improvement in pancreatic β-cell function.

The aim of this randomized controlled trial is to compare the effects of CSII alone with those of CSII combined with sitagliptin in newly diagnosed T2DM patients in an attempt to optimize a therapeutic regimen for such patients.

2. Methods

2.1. Subjects. Sixty inpatients newly diagnosed with T2DM according to the 1999 World Health Organization diagnostic criteria were recruited in The Third Affiliated Hospital, Southern Medical University, Guangzhou, China, from September 2014 to May 2015. The following inclusion criteria were used: (1) age between 30 and 70 years, fasting plasma glucose (FPG) between 8 and 16.7 mmol/L, glycosylated hemoglobin (HbA1C) ≥8.0%, and a body mass index (BMI) between 18 and 28 kg/m^2; (2) negative for glutamic acid decarboxylase autoantibody (GAD-Ab), anti-islet cell autoantibody (ICA-Ab), and anti-insulin autoantibody (IAA-Ab); and (3) no previous treatment with an antidiabetic or antihyperlipidemic medication. The following exclusion criteria were used: (1) type 1 diabetes, gestational diabetes, or diabetes with an identifiable secondary cause; (2) significant renal impairment (estimated creatinine clearance <50 mL/min) or elevated alanine or aspartate aminotransferase (ALT or AST, resp.); (3) occurrence of any severe diabetic complications or severe infection in the previous 3 months; and (4) scheduled surgery or serious trauma. Other patients whom the investigator judged to be inappropriate for the study were also excluded.

2.2. Study Design and Treatment. The eligible patients were randomized (1:1) using a random number table into treatment groups receiving either CSII alone (A: CSII group) or CSII combined with 100 mg sitagliptin once daily (B: CSII + Sig group) for 2 weeks. All patients were treated with insulin aspart (Novo Nordisk, Bagsvaerd, Denmark) using insulin pumps (MiniMed 712E, Medtronic, Northridge, CA, USA). The initial daily insulin dosage was calculated as follows: total insulin dose daily = 0.5 unit × body weight (kg). The basal rate (units/h) was calculated as 50% of the total insulin dose, and the other 50% was administered as a preprandial bolus before each of the three daily meals. The initial basal dose was divided into six doses that were administered during the following six periods of the day: 00:00 to 03:00 h, 03:00 to 07:00 h, 07:00 to 12:00 h, 12:00 to 17:00 h, 17:00 to 22:00 h, and 22:00 to 24:00 h. Capillary blood glucose was monitored eight times per day (before and 2 h after each meal, at bedtime, and at 03:00 h). The basal and bolus doses of insulin infusion were adjusted daily by one doctor by 2 to 10 units according to the capillary blood glucose level to achieve euglycemia (fasting blood glucose <7.0 mmol/L and postprandial blood glucose <10.0 mmol/L). The CSII was suspended after 2 weeks of treatment, and glucose levels were monitored by CGMS (Medtronic MiniMed, Northridge, CA, USA) during the last three days (72 h) of treatment.

A standard meal tolerance test using a meal consisting of 2037 kcal, 54.8 g of carbohydrate, 25.8 g of fat, and 9.4 g of protein was administered before and after the suspension of CSII treatment. Blood was collected at 0 and 120 min after the meal start. No antihyperlipidemic agents were used during the intervention.

All of the subjects underwent an education program on diabetes self-management, including diet and exercise counseling. A diabetic diet consisting of 50% carbohydrate (200 g), 35% fat, and 15% protein was provided for all subjects during intervention. The distribution of caloric intake was 20% for breakfast, 40% for lunch, and 40% for dinner. Regular physical exercise, such as walking, jogging, or stair climbing, for 30 min after meals was recommended.

This work was approved by the Medical Research and Ethics Committee of the Third Affiliated Hospital of Southern Medical University (Guangzhou, People's Republic of China) and registered at chictr.org (Chinese Clinical Trial Registry) with trial registration identifier number ChiCTR-TRC-14005224. An informed consent was obtained from all participants in this study.

2.3. Measurements. Anthropometric and laboratory data, including height, weight, age, BMI, FPG, 2 h postprandial plasma glucose (PPG), glycated hemoglobin (HbA1c), glycated albumin (GA), fasting C-peptide (FC-P), 2 h postprandial C-peptide (PC-P), triglycerides (Tg), total cholesterol (TC), high-density lipoprotein-cholesterol (HDL-C), and low-density lipoprotein-cholesterol (LDL-C), were measured before and after CSII treatment with the exception of HbA1c, which was not measured after treatment. The secretory unit of islet in transplantation (SUIT) index and C-peptide reactivity index (CPI) were used to estimate β-cell function. The following formulas were used: SUIT index $= 250 \times$ FC-P (ng/mL)/(FPG (mg/dL) $- 3.43$); CPI = FC-P (ng/mL)/FPG (mg/dL) $\times 100$.

The mean amplitude of glycemic excursions (MAGE), standard deviation of blood glucose levels (SDBG), largest amplitude of glycemic excursions (LAGE), mean blood glucose level (MBG), proportion (%) of time in hyperglycemia (>10 mmol/L) (PT10.0), proportion (%) of time in hypoglycemia (<3.9 mmol/L) (PT3.9), 1 h fasting MBG, and 3 h postprandial MBG were obtained by CGMS.

The difference in insulin dosage (Δinsulin) and the change in body mass index (ΔBMI) before and after treatment

TABLE 1: Baseline comparisons between the CSII and CSII + Sig groups before treatment.

Characteristic	Group		P value
	CSII	CSII + Sig	
Patients	30	30	—
Gender (F/M)	15/15	16/14	—
Age (years)	45.18 ± 7.10	46.40 ± 5.14	0.49
Weight (kg)	63.14 ± 6.45	65.99 ± 9.90	0.19
BMI (kg/m^2)	23.56 ± 1.48	23.76 ± 3.01	0.74
HbAlc (%)	10.06 ± 1.82	10.47 ± 1.33	0.32
GA (%)	33.42 ± 4.68	34.11 ± 3.86	0.53
FPG (mmol/L)	10.39 ± 0.96	10.23 ± 0.92	0.50
PPG (mmol/L)	17.97 ± 1.48	18.52 ± 1.45	0.15
FC-P (ng/mL)	1.65 ± 0.59	1.48 ± 0.71	0.32
PC-P (ng/mL)	3.99 ± 2.14	4.20 ± 1.70	0.67
CPI	0.89 ± 0.33	0.82 ± 0.42	0.49
SUIT	2.26 ± 0.84	2.09 ± 1.07	0.49
TC (mmol/L)	5.17 ± 0.72	5.25 ± 0.65	0.69
HDL-C (mmol/L)	1.35 ± 0.29	1.40 ± 0.27	0.50
LDL-C (mmol/L)	2.78 ± 0.64	2.90 ± 0.77	0.51
Tg (mmol/L)	1.94 ± 0.62	2.06 ± 0.96	0.57

Note: data are presented as the means ± SD. CSII group: CSII monotherapy group; CSII + Sig group: CSII therapy in combination with sitagliptin group; GA: glycated albumin; FPG: fasting plasma glucose; PPG: postprandial plasma glucose; FC-P: fasting C-peptide; PC-P: 2-h postprandial C-peptide; CPI: C-peptide reactivity index; SUIT: secretory unit of islet in transplantation index; TC: total cholesterol; Tg: triglycerides; HDL-C: high-density lipoprotein-cholesterol; LDL-C: low-density lipoprotein-cholesterol.

were calculated, and the number of hours in which the target blood glucose was reached was recorded.

2.4. Statistical Methods. All statistical analyses were performed using SPSS 13.0 software (SPSS, Inc., Chicago, IL, USA). The variables were then examined independently and subjected to normality and homogeneity of variance tests. The data for normally distributed variables are reported as the means ± SD, and the data nonnormally distributed variables are reported as medians and interquartile ranges. Count data are expressed as rates. The independent-samples t-test was used to test for differences between two groups. The paired t-test was used to test for differences before and after the intervention. Fisher's exact test was used to analyze enumeration data. A two-sided value of $P < 0.05$ was considered statistically significant.

3. Results

3.1. Baseline Characteristics and General Treatment Efficacy. Sixty patients with newly diagnosed T2DM were recruited for the study and randomized into two groups. No patients dropped out, and no serious adverse effects were observed during the intervention. The baseline features and clinical characteristics of the patients (age, gender, weight, and BMI) were similar between the two groups ($P > 0.05$, Table 1). There were also no significant differences between the groups in glucose levels (HbA1c, GA, FPG, and PPG), lipid profile (TC, HDL-C, LDL-C, and Tg), or indices of β-cell secretion (CPI, SUIT) at the beginning of the study ($P > 0.05$, Table 1).

TABLE 2: Glycemic variability between the CSII and CSII + Sig groups after the suspension of continuous subcutaneous insulin infusion.

Characteristic	Group		P value
	CSII	CSII + Sig	
MAGE (mmol/L)	3.98 ± 0.55	2.84 ± 0.92	<0.01
SDBG (mmol/L)	2.01 ± 0.37	1.42 ± 0.37	<0.01
LAGE (mmol/L)	6.81 ± 1.29	5.55 ± 1.27	<0.01
MBG (mmol/L)	7.95 ± 0.57	6.64 ± 0.37	<0.01
PT10.0 (%)	6.25 ± 1.48	1.50 ± 1.83	<0.01
PT3.9 (%)	2.42 ± 3.60	0.29 ± 0.73	0.04
1 h MBG			
Before breakfast (mmol/L)	6.42 ± 0.45	6.04 ± 0.68	0.01
Before lunch (mmol/L)	6.68 ± 1.03	6.16 ± 0.66	0.02
Before supper (mmol/L)	6.71 ± 0.89	6.17 ± 0.56	0.01
3 h MBG			
After breakfast (mmol/L)	9.78 ± 1.60	7.51 ± 0.64	<0.01
After lunch (mmol/L)	8.78 ± 1.49	7.59 ± 0.56	<0.01
After supper (mmol/L)	9.29 ± 1.78	7.50 ± 0.61	<0.01

Note: MAGE: mean amplitude of glycemic excursions; SDBG: standard deviation of blood glucose; LAGE: largest amplitude of glycemic excursions; MBG: mean blood glucose; PT3.9: proportion (%) of time in hypoglycemia (<3.9 mmol/L); PT10.0: proportion (%) of time in hyperglycemia (>10 mmol/L). Independent-samples t-tests were employed.

3.2. Comparison of Glycemic Excursions. The values of the indices of glycemic excursions derived from the CGMS during the last three days of treatment are shown in Table 2. The LAGE, MAGE, and SDBG of the patients in the CSII + Sig group were all significantly lower than those of the CSII group after the intervention ($P < 0.01$). Similarly, the preprandial 1 h MBG level, the postprandial 3 h MBG level, and the MBG level during the last 72 h of treatment were significantly lower in the CSII + Sig group than in the CSII group ($P < 0.05$). During treatment, the incidence of patients who experienced hypoglycemia (PG < 3.9 mmol/L), as indicated by self-monitoring of blood glucose (SMBG), in the CSII + Sig group was 16.7% (5/30), which was lower than that observed in the CSII group (23.3%; 7/30). However, this difference was not significant ($P > 0.05$). Furthermore, CGMS showed that the PT3.9 of the CSII + Sig group was significantly lower than that of the CSII group ($P = 0.04$). In addition, the PT10.0 of the CSII + Sig group was significantly lower than that of the CSII group ($P < 0.01$).

3.3. Changes in GA. After 2 weeks of treatment, the GA reduction from baseline in the CSII + Sig group was 8.02% (final mean GA, 26.09%), and the reduction in the CSII group was 4.82% (final mean GA, 28.60%); both of these changes were significant ($P < 0.01$). The reduction in the GA (ΔGA) in the CSII + Sig group was significantly greater than the reduction in the CSII group ($P < 0.01$, Table 3).

TABLE 3: Comparison of the changes in in insulin dosage and clinical features from before to after treatment between the CSII and CSII + Sig groups.

Characteristic	Group		P value
	CSII	CSII + Sig	
Δdosage of insulin (U)	4.14 ± 8.59	−2.02 ± 7.50	<0.01
Δbasal insulin dose (U)	1.27 ± 4.59	0.38 ± 4.24	0.44
Δbolus insulin dose (U)	2.87 ± 5.81	−2.40 ± 3.65	<0.01
Δbasal/bolus ratio	0.05 ± 0.89	0.22 ± 0.20	0.31
Δweight (kg)	−0.04 ± 1.38	−0.54 ± 1.18	0.14
ΔBMI (kg/m^2)	−0.02 ± 0.51	−0.19 ± 0.41	0.15
Time to achieve euglycemia (h)	127.92 ± 27.60	92.88 ± 18.72	<0.01
ΔGA (%)	−4.82 ± 2.75	−8.02 ± 2.90	<0.01
ΔFPG (mmol/L)	−3.85 ± 1.39	−4.39 ± 1.23	0.12
ΔPPG (mmol/L)	−4.20 ± 2.32	−6.45 ± 3.13	<0.01
ΔFC-P (ng/mL)	0.09 ± 0.37	0.21 ± 0.54	0.29
ΔPC-P (ng/mL)	1.46 ± 1.26	1.76 ± 1.57	0.41
ΔCPI	0.63 ± 0.32	0.84 ± 0.42	0.03
ΔSUIT	1.64 ± 0.86	2.20 ± 1.10	0.03
ΔTC (mmol/L)	−0.35 ± 0.40	−0.39 ± 0.65	0.74
ΔHDL-C (mmol/L)	−0.04 ± 0.19	−0.05 ± 0.16	0.82
ΔLDL-C (mmol/L)	−0.12 ± 0.29	−0.22 ± 0.51	0.40
ΔTg (mmol/L)	−0.13 ± 0.20	−0.29 ± 0.50	0.10

Note: Δ: change from before treatment to after. Data are presented as the means ± SD. Paired t-tests were employed.

3.4. Effects on Glucose Level and β-Cell Function. All of the patients in the two groups achieved euglycemia within the two weeks of intervention. However, in both the CSII + Sig and CSII groups, significant reductions from baseline in FPG (5.84 ± 1.05 and 6.55 ± 0.93, resp.) and PPG (12.07 ± 2.79 and 13.77 ± 1.92, resp.) were observed after treatment ($P <$ 0.01 and $P <$ 0.01, resp.). In addition, the values of SUIT (4.29 ± 1.47 and 3.90 ± 1.39, resp.), CPI (1.66 ± 0.56 and 1.51 ± 0.53, resp.), and PC-P (5.97 ± 2.55 and 5.45 ± 2.40, resp.) were significantly elevated from baseline in both the CSII + Sig and CSII groups ($P < 0.01$, $P < 0.01$, and $P < 0.01$, resp.). The FC-P (1.69±0.51) of the CSII + Sig group increased significantly ($P = 0.04$) after treatment, whereas the FC-P (1.73 ± 0.49) of the CSII group was comparable to baseline ($P > 0.05$).

The changes in β-cell function between the two groups were also compared. The increases in SUIT and CPI (ΔSUIT and ΔCPI) from baseline to after treatment were greater in the CSII + Sig group than in the CSII group ($P = 0.03$ and $P = 0.03$, resp., Table 3). The decrease in PPG (ΔPPG) was greater in the CSII + Sig group than in the CSII group ($P <$ 0.01, Table 3), whereas the decrease in FPG (ΔFPG) and the increases in C-P and PC-P (ΔC-P and ΔPC-P) did not differ between the groups (all $P > 0.05$, Table 3).

3.5. Influence of the Lipid Profile. The lipid profile improved to some extent in both groups. Significant suppression of the fasting TC, LDL-c, and Tg levels was observed in both the CSII ($P < 0.01$, $P = 0.03$, and $P < 0.01$, resp., Figure 1) and CSII + Sig ($P < 0.01$, $P = 0.03$, and $P < 0.01$, resp., Figure 1) groups compared with baseline, whereas the change in HDL-c from baseline to after treatment was not significant in either group (both $P > 0.05$, Figure 1). However, the reductions in the fasting lipid profile (ΔTC, ΔLDL-c, ΔHDL-c, and ΔTg) were comparable between the two groups (all $P > 0.05$, Table 3).

3.6. Evaluation of Time to Achieve Euglycemia, Dosage of Insulin, and Weight. As shown in Table 3, there was a significantly shorter time to achieve euglycemia and a significant decline in the daily insulin dosage (Δdosage of insulin) in the CSII + Sig group compared with the CSII group ($P < 0.01$ and $P < 0.01$, resp., Table 3). The decline in the bolus insulin dose (Δbolus insulin dose) was significantly greater in the CSII + Sig group than in the CSII group ($P < 0.01$, Table 3), but the changes in the basal insulin dose (Δbasal insulin dose) and the basal/bolus ratio (Δbasal/bolus ratio) were comparable between the groups ($P > 0.05$ and $P > 0.05$, resp., Table 3). No differences were found in the changes in body weight and BMI (Δweight and ΔBMI) between the two groups (both $P > 0.05$, Table 3).

4. Discussion

This study assessed the clinical efficacy of sitagliptin in patients with newly diagnosed T2DM receiving CSII treatment, including the reduction in glucose excursion and differences in glucose amelioration, β-cell function, and lipid metabolism.

Based on the overview of the available evidence provided by Nalysnyk et al., it appears that glucose variability, characterized by extreme glucose excursions, could be a predictor of diabetic complications, independent of HbA1c levels, in patients with T2DM [17]. Glucose variability also has been shown to be associated with the activation of oxidative stress and the innate immune system, which increases the risk of diabetic complications [18]. Previous studies have suggested that add-on sitagliptin therapy is significantly well tolerated and improves HbA1c, fasting blood glucose, and postprandial blood glucose compared with placebo in T2DM [19–23]. One study suggested that sitagliptin added to CSII treatment decreases glucose variability, such as MAGE [23]. However, in that study, glucose variation was calculated by measuring capillary blood glucose rather than through CGMS; this is a limitation because intermittent glucose monitoring only allows the variation to be estimated. Here, we assessed glucose variability by CGMS and found that the addition of sitagliptin to CSII therapy produced significant reductions in MAGE, LAGE, and SDBG, indicating that add-on sitagliptin therapy can improve glucose variability in patients with newly diagnosed T2DM who receive CSII treatment. This improvement may be attributed to dipeptidyl peptidase-4 inhibitors, which are reported to inhibit the degradation of the endogenous incretin hormones glucagon-like peptide-1

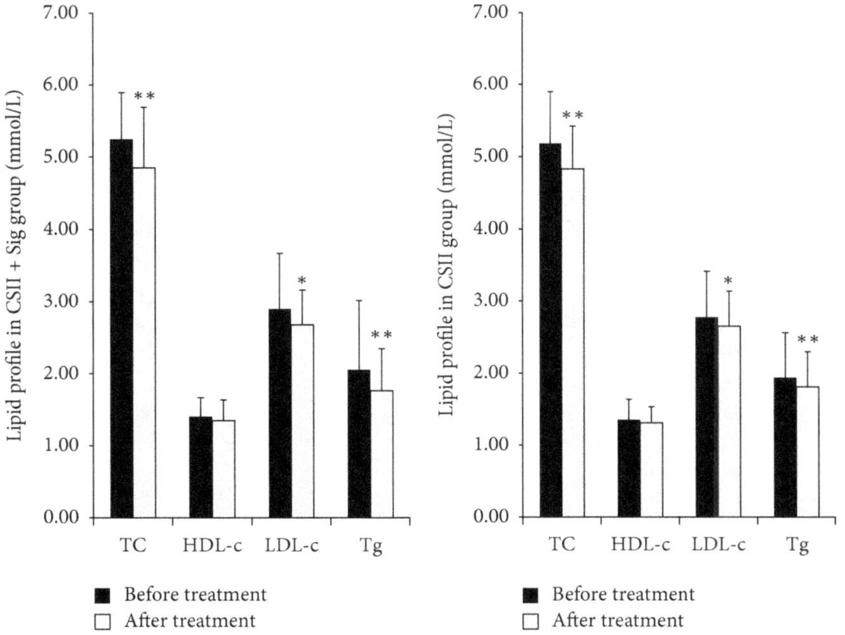

FIGURE 1: Changes in lipid profile before and after treatment for both groups. Note: $^{*}P < 0.05$ and $^{**}P < 0.01$; paired t-tests (after versus before treatment) were conducted. TC: total cholesterol; HDL-c: high-density lipoprotein-cholesterol; LDL-c: low-density lipoprotein-cholesterol; Tg: triglycerides.

and gastric inhibitory polypeptide, which in turn glucose-dependently promote insulin secretion and inhibit glucagon secretion, thus helping to correct hyperglycemic states [24]. In this regard, our results also suggest that the risk of hypoglycemia may be reduced by add-on sitagliptin therapy as the PT3.9 was decreased in the CSII + Sig group.

Although an improvement in glycemic control using the combination of a DPP-4 inhibitor and insulin was demonstrated in previous studies [19–21], the intervention time in those studies was longer than 3 months. In patients with T2DM receiving CSII with add-on sitagliptin for 2 weeks, HbA1c was also significantly decreased compared with that in patients receiving CSII alone in a study by Yuan et al. [22] However, HbA1c is an indicator of glycemic control over a 3-month period. In our study, GA was used to monitor the glycemic control state, as it is an indicator of glycation, over a 2-3 week period in diabetic patients. Our finding that GA had a greater improvement in the CSII + Sig group than in the CSII group is consistent with previous studies. Because it is influenced by the improvement of postprandial blood glucose, GA is a better indicator of glucose excursion than HbA1c [25]. Our study showed that the 1 h MBG before meals, 3 h MBG after meals, and glucose excursion were ameliorated when sitagliptin was added to the CSII treatment. The greater improvement in glycemic control in patients receiving CSII with sitagliptin may help to restore islet β-cell function more effectively.

As glucotoxicity is corrected rapidly, β-cell function can be improved in newly diagnosed T2DM patients treated with short-term intensive insulin therapy [5]. Treatment with sitagliptin has also been shown to improve measures of β-cell function [16, 26]. Moreover, in previous clinical studies using concomitant therapy of insulin and sitagliptin, the effect of add-on sitagliptin on improving β-cell function was investigated in long-term interventions of at least 12 weeks [19–21]. In a study by Yuan et al. [22], the levels of insulin and C-peptide were strikingly increased and HOMA-β (the homeostasis model assessment of β-cell function) was improved in the CSII plus sitagliptin group compared with the CSII group. In our study, SUIT and CPI were used to assess β-cell responsiveness. Similar to the results of Yuan et al.'s study [22], the indicators of β-cell function, SUIT and CPI, were increased. These improvements were most likely due to the improvement of glycemic control in the CSII + Sig group compared with the CSII group. Therefore, the benefits of sitagliptin on β-cell function cannot be ignored.

As noted in the position statements of the American Diabetes Association and the European Association for the Study of Diabetes (ADA/EASD), the problems of weight and economics should be considered in the management of hyperglycemia in T2DM. Sitagliptin has been shown to be effective and well tolerated in various treatment regimens with a neutral effect on body weight, possibly because sitagliptin treatment augments GLP-1 levels [27]. Additionally, previous studies have indicated that add-on therapy of sitagliptin to various insulin regimens (not including CSII) could decrease daily insulin doses and improve glycemic control without severe hypoglycemia or weight gain [19–21]. With insulin therapy, further improvement is needed for a glycemic control that will not increase hypoglycemia and weight gain to limit the insulin dose when high doses are needed. In our study, there were great improvements in the state of glucose with an insulin dose decrease and without weight gain (sitagliptin in combination with CSII therapy group versus CSII monotherapy group). It is worth noting that significantly fewer days were required to achieve euglycemia when sitagliptin was added to CSII in the present study, which suggests that the combined therapy may shorten hospital stays and reduce hospitalization expenses for T2DM patients. Therefore, add-on therapy with sitagliptin added to CSII can be cost effective by decreasing the insulin dose and shortening the time to achieve euglycemia.

An unfavorable effect on lipids was thought to be one of the potentially modifiable risk factors for coronary artery disease in patients with T2DM according to the UK Prospective Diabetes Study (UKPDS) [28]. As indicated in this and previous studies, lipotoxicity can be eliminated by short-term CSII-based intensive treatment. In our study, the lipid profiles of both groups after 2 weeks of intensive treatment were significantly improved compared with those before treatment as both treatments lowered TC, LDL-c, and Tg levels. However, the favorable effect on lipids was comparable between CSII alone and CSII combined with sitagliptin. Possible explanations for this finding include the following: (1) the length of our study was only 2 weeks; (2) a previous study showed that postprandial plasma levels of TG-rich lipoproteins were reduced after treatment with sitagliptin for 6 weeks [29], whereas only fasting plasma lipids were measured in our study; and (3) there were an insufficient number of samples in our study.

In summary, our randomized trial in which sitagliptin was added to a CSII-based short-term intensive treatment in patients with newly diagnosed T2DM was very effective in improving glycemic excursions, glucose levels, GA, and β-cell function; additionally, a reduced incidence of hypoglycemia, a shorter time to achieve euglycemia, a significant reduction in the insulin dosage, and no weight gain were observed compared with CSII alone. CSII plus sitagliptin appears to be a beneficial regimen, particularly for individuals with newly diagnosed T2DM, and it should be tested in a larger, long-term clinical trial.

Consent

An informed consent was obtained from all participants in this study.

Conflict of Interests

The authors declare that no competing financial interests that may pose a conflict of interests exist.

Authors' Contribution

Heng Wan and Defu Zhao are equal contributors to this work.

Acknowledgments

This study was supported by the Science and Technology Commission of Guangdong Province, China (2011B010500027, 2011B060500011, and 2009B11400036), and the Natural Science Foundation of Guangdong Province, China (S2013010016045).

References

[1] U.K. Prospective Diabetes Study Group, "U.K. Prospective diabetes study 16. Overview of 6 years' therapy of type II diabetes: a progressive disease," *Diabetes*, vol. 44, no. 11, pp. 1249–1258, 1995.

[2] W.-S. Lv, L. Li, J.-P. Wen et al., "Comparison of a multiple daily insulin injection regimen (glargine or detemir once daily plus prandial insulin aspart) and continuous subcutaneous insulin infusion (aspart) in short-term intensive insulin therapy for poorly controlled type 2 diabetes patients," *International Journal of Endocrinology*, vol. 2013, Article ID 614242, 6 pages, 2013.

[3] H. Yang, X. Heng, C. Liang et al., "Comparison of continuous subcutaneous insulin infusion and multiple daily insulin injections in Chinese patients with type 2 diabetes mellitus," *Journal of International Medical Research*, vol. 42, no. 4, pp. 1002–1010, 2014.

[4] C. K. Kramer, B. Zinman, and R. Retnakaran, "Short-term intensive insulin therapy in type 2 diabetes mellitus: a systematic review and meta-analysis," *The Lancet Diabetes and Endocrinology*, vol. 1, no. 1, pp. 28–34, 2013.

[5] J. Weng, Y. Li, W. Xu et al., "Effect of intensive insulin therapy on beta-cell function and glycaemic control in patients with newly diagnosed type 2 diabetes: a multicentre randomised parallel-group trial," *The Lancet*, vol. 371, no. 9626, pp. 1753–1760, 2008.

[6] S. M. Pastores, "ACP Journal Club. Review: intensive insulin therapy does not reduce mortality but increases severe hypoglycemia in hospitalized patients," *Annals of Internal Medicine*, vol. 155, no. 2, pp. Cl–C12, 2011.

[7] E. Nyenwe, "Intensive insulin therapy in hospitalised patients increases the risk of hypoglycaemia and has no effect on mortality, infection risk or length of stay," *Evidence-Based Medicine*, vol. 17, no. 1, pp. 8–9, 2012.

[8] E. L. Johnson, "Glycemic variability in type 2 diabetes mellitus: oxidative stress and macrovascular complications," *Advances in Experimental Medicine and Biology*, vol. 771, pp. 139–154, 2012.

[9] M. Brownlee, "Biochemistry and molecular cell biology of diabetic complications," *Nature*, vol. 414, no. 6865, pp. 813–820, 2001.

[10] M. Brownlee, "The pathobiology of diabetic complications: a unifying mechanism," *Diabetes*, vol. 54, no. 6, pp. 1615–1625, 2005.

[11] A. Ceriello, K. Esposito, L. Piconi et al., "Oscillating glucose is more deleterious to endothelial function and oxidative stress than mean glucose in normal and type 2 diabetic patients," *Diabetes*, vol. 57, no. 5, pp. 1349–1354, 2008.

[12] L. Piconi, L. Quagliaro, R. Assaloni et al., "Constant and intermittent high glucose enhances endothelial cell apoptosis through mitochondrial superoxide overproduction," *Diabetes/Metabolism Research and Reviews*, vol. 22, no. 3, pp. 198–203, 2006.

[13] J. Zhou, H. Li, X. Ran et al., "Reference values for continuous glucose monitoring in Chinese subjects," *Diabetes Care*, vol. 32, no. 7, pp. 1188–1193, 2009.

[14] J. Shen, Z. Chen, C. Chen, X. Zhu, and Y. Han, "Impact of incretin on early-phase insulin secretion and glucose excursion," *Endocrine*, vol. 44, no. 2, pp. 403–410, 2013.

[15] Y. Zhao, L. Yang, and Z. Zhou, "Dipeptidyl peptidase-4 inhibitors: multitarget drugs, not only antidiabetes drugs," *Journal of Diabetes*, vol. 6, no. 1, pp. 21–29, 2014.

[16] D. M. Riche, H. E. East, and K. D. Riche, "Impact of sitagliptin on markers of β-cell function: a meta-analysis," *American Journal of the Medical Sciences*, vol. 337, no. 5, pp. 321–328, 2009.

[17] L. Nalysnyk, M. Hernandez-Medina, and G. Krishnarajah, "Glycaemic variability and complications in patients with diabetes mellitus: evidence from a systematic review of the literature," *Diabetes, Obesity & Metabolism*, vol. 12, no. 4, pp. 288–298, 2010.

[18] M. R. Rizzo, M. Barbieri, R. Marfella, and G. Paolisso, "Reduction of oxidative stress and inflammation by blunting daily acute glucose fluctuations in patients with type 2 diabetes: role of dipeptidyl peptidase-IV inhibition," *Diabetes Care*, vol. 35, no. 10, pp. 2076–2082, 2012.

[19] T. Katsuno, H. Ikeda, K. Ida, J.-I. Miyagawa, and M. Namba, "Add-on therapy with the DPP-4 inhibitor sitagliptin improves glycemic control in insulin-treated Japanese patients with type 2 diabetes mellitus," *Endocrine Journal*, vol. 60, no. 6, pp. 733–742, 2013.

[20] E. S. Hong, A. R. Khang, J. W. Yoon et al., "Comparison between sitagliptin as add-on therapy to insulin and insulin dose-increase therapy in uncontrolled Korean type 2 diabetes: CSI study," *Diabetes, Obesity & Metabolism*, vol. 14, no. 9, pp. 795–802, 2012.

[21] T. Vilsbøll, J. Rosenstock, H. Yki-Järvinen et al., "Efficacy and safety of sitagliptin when added to insulin therapy in patients with type 2 diabetes," *Diabetes, Obesity & Metabolism*, vol. 12, no. 2, pp. 167–177, 2010.

[22] G. Yuan, J. Jia, C. Zhang et al., "Safety and efficacy of sitagliptin in combination with transient continuous subcutaneous insulin infusion (CSII) therapy in patients with newly diagnosed type 2 diabetes," *Endocrine Journal*, vol. 61, no. 5, pp. 513–521, 2014.

[23] G. Yuan, H. Hu, S. Wang et al., "Improvement of β-cell function ameliorated glycemic variability in patients with newly diagnosed type 2 diabetes after short-term continuous subcutaneous insulin infusion or in combination with sitagliptin treatment: a randomized control trial," *Endocrine Journal*, vol. 62, no. 9, pp. 817–834, 2015.

[24] K. J. Hare, T. Vilsbøll, M. Asmar, C. F. Deacon, F. K. Knop, and J. J. Holst, "The glucagonostatic and insulinotropic effects of glucagon-like peptide 1 contribute equally to its glucose-lowering action," *Diabetes*, vol. 59, no. 7, pp. 1765–1770, 2010.

[25] K. Yoshiuchi, M. Matsuhisa, N. Katakami et al., "Glycated albumin is a better indicator for glucose excursion than glycated hemoglobin in type 1 and type 2 diabetes," *Endocrine Journal*, vol. 55, no. 3, pp. 503–507, 2008.

[26] L. Xu, C. D. Man, B. Charbonnel et al., "Effect of sitagliptin, a dipeptidyl peptidase-4 inhibitor, on beta-cell function in patients with type 2 diabetes: a model-based approach," *Diabetes, Obesity & Metabolism*, vol. 10, no. 12, pp. 1212–1220, 2008.

[27] A. Karasik, P. Aschner, H. Katzeff, M. J. Davies, and P. P. Stein, "Sitagliptin, a DPP-4 inhibitor for the treatment of patients with type 2 diabetes: a review of recent clinical trials," *Current Medical Research and Opinion*, vol. 24, no. 2, pp. 489–496, 2008.

[28] R. C. Turner, H. Millns, H. A. W. Neil et al., "Risk factors for coronary artery disease in non-insulin dependent diabetes mellitus: united Kingdom prospective diabetes study (UKPDS: 23)," *British Medical Journal*, vol. 316, no. 7134, pp. 823–828, 1998.

[29] A. J. Tremblay, B. Lamarche, C. F. Deacon, S. J. Weisnagel, and P. Couture, "Effect of sitagliptin therapy on postprandial lipoprotein levels in patients with type 2 diabetes," *Diabetes, Obesity & Metabolism*, vol. 13, no. 4, pp. 366–373, 2011.

Permissions

All chapters in this book were first published in JDR, by Hindawi Publishing Corporation; hereby published with permission under the Creative Commons Attribution License or equivalent. Every chapter published in this book has been scrutinized by our experts. Their significance has been extensively debated. The topics covered herein carry significant findings which will fuel the growth of the discipline. They may even be implemented as practical applications or may be referred to as a beginning point for another development.

The contributors of this book come from diverse backgrounds, making this book a truly international effort. This book will bring forth new frontiers with its revolutionizing research information and detailed analysis of the nascent developments around the world.

We would like to thank all the contributing authors for lending their expertise to make the book truly unique. They have played a crucial role in the development of this book. Without their invaluable contributions this book wouldn't have been possible. They have made vital efforts to compile up to date information on the varied aspects of this subject to make this book a valuable addition to the collection of many professionals and students.

This book was conceptualized with the vision of imparting up-to-date information and advanced data in this field. To ensure the same, a matchless editorial board was set up. Every individual on the board went through rigorous rounds of assessment to prove their worth. After which they invested a large part of their time researching and compiling the most relevant data for our readers.

The editorial board has been involved in producing this book since its inception. They have spent rigorous hours researching and exploring the diverse topics which have resulted in the successful publishing of this book. They have passed on their knowledge of decades through this book. To expedite this challenging task, the publisher supported the team at every step. A small team of assistant editors was also appointed to further simplify the editing procedure and attain best results for the readers.

Apart from the editorial board, the designing team has also invested a significant amount of their time in understanding the subject and creating the most relevant covers. They scrutinized every image to scout for the most suitable representation of the subject and create an appropriate cover for the book.

The publishing team has been an ardent support to the editorial, designing and production team. Their endless efforts to recruit the best for this project, has resulted in the accomplishment of this book. They are a veteran in the field of academics and their pool of knowledge is as vast as their experience in printing. Their expertise and guidance has proved useful at every step. Their uncompromising quality standards have made this book an exceptional effort. Their encouragement from time to time has been an inspiration for everyone.

The publisher and the editorial board hope that this book will prove to be a valuable piece of knowledge for researchers, students, practitioners and scholars across the globe.

List of Contributors

Rina Su, Jie Yan and Huixia Yang
Department of Obstetrics and Gynecology, Peking University First Hospital, No. 8, Xishiku Street, Xicheng District, Beijing 100034, China

Masanori Abe, Kazuyoshi Okada, Noriaki Maruyama, Hiroyuki Takashima and Osamu Oikawa
Division of Nephrology, Hypertension and Endocrinology, Department of Internal Medicine, Nihon University School of Medicine, Tokyo 173-8610, Japan

Masayoshi Soma
Division of Nephrology, Hypertension and Endocrinology, Department of Internal Medicine, Nihon University School of Medicine, Tokyo 173-8610, Japan
Division of General Medicine, Department of Internal Medicine, Nihon University School of Medicine, Tokyo 173-8610, Japan

Milton-Omar Guzmán-Ornelas and Fernanda-Isadora Corona-Meraz
Instituto de Investigación en Reumatología y del Sistema Musculo Esquelético, Centro Universitario de Ciencias de la Salud, Universidad de Guadalajara, Sierra Mojada No. 950, Colonia Independencia, 44340 Guadalajara, JAL, Mexico
UDG-CA-701, Grupo de Investigación Inmunometabolismo en Enfermedades Emergentes (GIIEE), Centro Universitario de Ciencias de la Salud, Universidad de Guadalajara, Sierra Mojada No. 950, Colonia Independencia, 44340 Guadalajara, JAL, Mexico

Marcelo Heron Petri
Instituto de Investigación en Reumatología y del Sistema Musculo Esquelético, Centro Universitario de Ciencias de la Salud, Universidad de Guadalajara, Sierra Mojada No. 950, Colonia Independencia, 44340 Guadalajara, JAL, Mexico
Translational Cardiology, Center for Molecular Medicine, Department of Medicine, Karolinska Institutet, L8:03, 17176 Stockholm, Sweden

Mónica Vázquez-Del Mercado
Instituto de Investigación en Reumatología y del Sistema Musculo Esquelético, Centro Universitario de Ciencias de la Salud, Universidad de Guadalajara, Sierra Mojada No. 950, Colonia Independencia, 44340 Guadalajara, JAL, Mexico
Departamento de Biología Molecular y Genómica, Centro Universitario de Ciencias de la Salud, Universidad de Guadalajara, Sierra Mojada No. 950, Colonia Independencia, 44340 Guadalajara, JAL, Mexico
Servicio de Reumatología, División de Medicina Interna, Hospital Civil "Dr. Juan I. Menchaca", Universidad de Guadalajara, Salvador de Quevedo y Zubieta No. 750, 44340 Guadalajara, JAL, Mexico

Efraín Chavarría-Ávila
Instituto de Investigación en Reumatología y del Sistema Musculo Esquelético, Centro Universitario de Ciencias de la Salud, Universidad de Guadalajara, Sierra Mojada No. 950, Colonia Independencia, 44340 Guadalajara, JAL, Mexico
UDG-CA-701, Grupo de Investigación Inmunometabolismo en Enfermedades Emergentes (GIIEE), Centro Universitario de Ciencias de la Salud, Universidad de Guadalajara, Sierra Mojada No. 950, Colonia Independencia, 44340 Guadalajara, JAL, Mexicow
Departamento de Disciplinas Filosófico, Metodológico e Instrumentales, Centro Universitario de Ciencias de la Salud, Universidad de Guadalajara, Sierra Mojada No. 950, Colonia Independencia, 44340 Guadalajara, JAL, Mexico

Sandra-Luz Ruíz-Quezada
UDG-CA-701, Grupo de Investigación Inmunometabolismo en Enfermedades Emergentes (GIIEE), Centro Universitario de Ciencias de la Salud, Universidad de Guadalajara, Sierra Mojada No. 950, Colonia Independencia, 44340 Guadalajara, JAL, Mexico
Departamento de Farmacobiología, Centro Universitario de Ciencias Exactas e Ingenierías, Universidad de Guadalajara, Boulevard Marcelino García Barragán No. 1421, 44430 Guadalajara, JAL, Mexico

Perla-Monserrat Madrigal-Ruíz
Instituto de Investigación en Reumatología y del Sistema Musculo Esquelético, Centro Universitario de Ciencias de la Salud, Universidad de Guadalajara, Sierra Mojada No. 950, Colonia Independencia, 44340 Guadalajara, JAL, Mexico
UDG-CA-701, Grupo de Investigación Inmunometabolismo en Enfermedades Emergentes (GIIEE), Centro Universitario de Ciencias de la Salud, Universidad de Guadalajara, Sierra Mojada No. 950, Colonia Independencia, 44340 Guadalajara, JAL, Mexico
Departamento de Biología Molecular y Genómica, Centro Universitario de Ciencias de la Salud, Universidad de Guadalajara, Sierra Mojada No. 950, Colonia Independencia, 44340 Guadalajara, JAL, Mexico

Jorge Castro-Albarrán
UDG-CA-701, Grupo de Investigación Inmunometabolismo en Enfermedades Emergentes (GIIEE), Centro Universitario de Ciencias de la Salud, Universidad de Guadalajara, Sierra Mojada No. 950, Colonia Independencia, 44340 Guadalajara, JAL, Mexico

Flavio Sandoval-García
Instituto de Investigación en Reumatología y del Sistema Musculo Esquelético, Centro Universitario de Ciencias de la Salud, Universidad de Guadalajara, Sierra Mojada No. 950, Colonia Independencia, 44340 Guadalajara, JAL, Mexico

Rosa-Elena Navarro-Hernández
Instituto de Investigación en Reumatología y del Sistema Musculo Esquelético, Centro Universitario de Ciencias de la Salud, Universidad de Guadalajara, Sierra Mojada No. 950, Colonia Independencia, 44340 Guadalajara, JAL, Mexico
UDG-CA-701, Grupo de Investigación Inmunometabolismo en Enfermedades Emergentes (GIIEE), Centro Universitario de Ciencias de la Salud, Universidad de Guadalajara, Sierra Mojada No. 950, Colonia Independencia, 44340 Guadalajara, JAL, Mexico
Departamento de Biología Molecular y Genómica, Centro Universitario de Ciencias de la Salud, Universidad de Guadalajara, Sierra Mojada No. 950, Colonia Independencia, 44340 Guadalajara, JAL, Mexico
Departamento de Farmacobiología, Centro Universitario de Ciencias Exactas e Ingenierías, Universidad de Guadalajara, Boulevard Marcelino García Barragán No. 1421, 44430 Guadalajara, JAL, Mexico

Shirong Zheng, Lu Cai and Paul N. Epstein
Department of Pediatrics, University of Louisville, Louisville, KY 40202, USA

Susan Coventry
Department of Pathology, University of Louisville, Louisville, KY 40202, USA

David W. Powell
Department of Medicine, University of Louisville, Louisville, KY 40202, USA

Venkatakrishna R. Jala and Bodduluri Haribabu
Department of Microbiology and Immunology, University of Louisville, Louisville, KY 40202, USA

Hong Feng
Department of Endocrinology, Affiliated Hospital of Luzhou Medical College, Luzhou, Sichuan 646000, China
Department of Internal Medicine, Nan'an District People's Hospital, Chongqing 400060, China

Junling Gu
Department of Endocrinology,The Fifth People's Hospital of Chongqing, Chongqing 400062, China

Fang Gou, Wei Huang, Chenlin Gao, Guo Chen, Yang Long, Xueqin Zhou, Maojun Yang, Shuang Liu, Shishi Lü, Qiaoyan Luo and Yong Xu
Department of Endocrinology, Affiliated Hospital of Luzhou Medical College, Luzhou, Sichuan 646000, China

Matej Samoš, František Kovál, Michal Mokáň, Tomáš Bolek, Peter Galajda and Marián Mokáň
Department of Internal Medicine I, Jessenius Faculty of Medicine in Martin, Comenius University in Bratislava, 036 59 Martin, Slovakia

Marián Fedor and Peter Kubisz
National Center of Hemostasis and Thrombosis, Department of Hematology and Blood Transfusion, Jessenius Faculty of Medicine in Martin, Comenius University in Bratislava, 036 59 Martin, Slovakia

Uazman Alam, Yasar Amjad and Omar Asghar
Centre for Endocrinology and Diabetes, Institute of Human Development, University of Manchester and the Manchester Royal Infirmary, Central Manchester Hospital Foundation Trust, Manchester M13 9NT, UK

Ioannis N. Petropoulos and Anges Wan Shan Chan
Department of Medicine, Barts and the London School of Medicine and Dentistry, London E1 2AD, UK

Rayaz A. Malik
Centre for Endocrinology and Diabetes, Institute of Human Development, University of Manchester and the Manchester Royal Infirmary, Central Manchester Hospital Foundation Trust, Manchester M13 9NT, UK
Weill Cornell Medical College in Qatar, Doha, Qatar

Ekta Lachmandas, Corina N. A.M. van den Heuvel, Michelle S. M. A. Damen, Maartje C. P. Cleophas,Mihai G. Netea and Reinout van Crevel
Department of Internal Medicine and Radboudumc Center for Infectious Diseases, Radboud University Medical Center, Internal Postal Code 463, P.O. Box 9101, 6500 HB Nijmegen, Netherlands

Helena H. Chowdhury, Jelena Velebit, Nataša RadiT and Robert Zorec
Laboratory for Neuroendocrinology-Molecular Cell Physiology, Institute of Pathophysiology, Faculty of Medicine, University of Ljubljana, Zaloska 4, SI-1000 Ljubljana, Slovenia
Celica Biomedical Center, Tehnološki Park 24, SI-1000 Ljubljana, Slovenia

Vito FranIiI
Celica Biomedical Center, Tehnološki Park 24, SI-1000 Ljubljana, Slovenia

Marko Kreft
Laboratory for Neuroendocrinology-Molecular Cell Physiology, Institute of Pathophysiology, Faculty of Medicine, University of Ljubljana, Zaloska 4, SI-1000 Ljubljana, Slovenia
Celica Biomedical Center, Tehnološki Park 24, SI-1000 Ljubljana, Slovenia
Department of Biology, Biotechnical Faculty, University of Ljubljana, Večna Pot 111, SI-1000 Ljubljana, Slovenia

Xiaoyu Ma
Geriatrics Department, The First Hospital of China Medical University, Shenyang, Liaoning, China

Canlu Lu, Can Wu and Qiuyue Wang
Endocrine Department, The First Hospital of China Medical University, Shenyang, Liaoning, China

Chuan Lv
Endocrine Department, The People Hospital of Liaoning Province, Shenyang, Liaoning, China

Zhimei Lv, Mengsi Hu, Xiaoxu Ren, Jiangong Lin, Nannan Ding, QunWang and RongWang
Department of Nephrology, Provincial Hospital Affiliated to Shandong University, Jinan 250021, China

Minghua Fan
Department of Obstetrics and Gynecology, Second Hospital of Shandong University, Jinan 250033, China

Junhui Zhen
Department of Pathology, Medical School of Shandong University, Jinan 250012, China

Liqun Chen
Department of Nephrology, First Affiliated Hospital of Chongqing Medical University, Chongqing 400042, China

Yaa Obirikorang, Nyalako Dzah and Caroline Nkrumah Akosah
Department of Nursing, Faculty of Health and Allied Sciences, Garden City University College (GCUC), Kenyasi, Kumasi, Ghana

Christian Obirikorang, Emmanuel Acheampong and Emmanuella Batu Nsenbah
Department of Molecular Medicine, School of Medical Science, Kwame Nkrumah University of Science and Technology (KNUST), Kumasi, Ghana

Enoch Odame Anto
Department of Molecular Medicine, School of Medical Science, Kwame Nkrumah University of Science and Technology (KNUST), Kumasi, Ghana
Royal Ann College of Health, Department of Medical Laboratory Technology, Atwima Manhyia, Kumasi, Ghana

Nicolai J.Wewer Albrechtsen, Simon Veedfald, Astrid Plamboeck, Carolyn F. Deacon, Bolette Hartmann and Jens J. Holst
Department of Biomedical Sciences, Faculty of Health and Medical Sciences, University of Copenhagen, 2200 Copenhagen, Denmark
Novo Nordisk Foundation Center for Basic Metabolic Research, Faculty of Health and Medical Sciences, University of Copenhagen, 2200 Copenhagen, Denmark

Filip K. Knop
Department of Biomedical Sciences, Faculty of Health and Medical Sciences, University of Copenhagen, 2200 Copenhagen, Denmark
Novo Nordisk Foundation Center for Basic Metabolic Research, Faculty of Health and Medical Sciences, University of Copenhagen, 2200 Copenhagen, Denmark
Center for Diabetes Research, Gentofte Hospital, University of Copenhagen, 2900 Heller up, Denmark

Tina Vilsboll
Center for Diabetes Research, Gentofte Hospital, University of Copenhagen, 2900 Heller up, Denmark

Elideth Martínez-Ladrón de Guevara, Alejandro Martínez Martínez and Vicente Hernández-García
Institute of Biomedical Sciences, Autonomous University of Ciudad Juárez, 32310 Ciudad Juárez, CHIH, Mexico

Nury Pérez-Hernández, David Guillermo Pérez-Ishiwara and Juan Santiago Salas-Benito
National School of Medicine and Homeopathy, National Polytechnic Institute, 07320 Mexico City, DF, Mexico

Miguel Ángel Villalobos-López
Centre for Research in Applied Biotechnology, National Polytechnic Institute, 90700 Tepetitla, TLAX, Mexico

Wenping Li
Key Lab for Pharmacology of Ministry of Education, Department of Pharmacology, Zunyi Medical College, Zunyi 563003, China
Chengdu Chronic Diseases Hospital, Chengdu 610083, China

Wenwen Zhao and Xiuping Chen
State Key Laboratory of Quality Research in Chinese Medicine, Institute of Chinese Medical Sciences, University of Macau, Macau

QinWu, Yuanfu Lu and Jingshan Shi
Key Lab for Pharmacology of Ministry of Education, Department of Pharmacology, Zunyi Medical College, Zunyi 563003, China

C. Di Filippo, B. Ferraro, R. Maisto, M. C. Trotta, N. Di Carluccio, F. Rossi and M. D'Amico
Department of Experimental Medicine, Section of Pharmacology "L. Donatelli", Second University of Naples, 80138 Naples, Italy

S. Sartini and C. La Motta
Department of Pharmacy, University of Pisa, 56126 Pisa, Italy

F. Ferraraccio
Department of Clinical, Public and Preventive Medicine, Second University of Naples, 80138 Naples, Italy

Jo Satoh
NTT-EAST Tohoku Hospital, 2-29-1 Yamato-machi, Wakabayashi-ku, Sendai, Miyagi 984-8560, Japan

Nobuo Kohara
Department of Neurology, Kobe City Medical Center General Hospital, 4-6 Minatojima-Nakamachi, Chuo-ku, Kobe, Hyogo 650-0046, Japan

Kenji Sekiguchi
Division of Neurology, Kobe University Graduate School of Medicine, 7-5-2 Kusunoki-cho, Chuo-ku, Kobe, Hyogo 650-0017, Japan

Yasuyuki Yamaguchi
Sumitomo Dainippon Pharma, Co., Ltd., 6-8 Doshomachi 2-chome, Chuo-ku, Osaka 541-0045, Japan

Xiao-na Zhang, Ze-jun Ma, YingWang, Yu-zhu Li, Bei Sun, Xin Guo, Cong-qing Pan and Li-ming Chen
2011 Collaborative Innovation Center of Tianjin for Medical Epigenetics, Key Laboratory of Hormone and Development of Ministry of Health, Metabolic Disease Hospital and Tianjin Institute of Endocrinology, Tianjin Medical University, Tianjin 300070, China

Bingyan Cao, Chunxiu Gong, Di Wu, Xiaoqiao Li, Min Liu, Wenjing Li, Chang Su, Xuejun Liang and Yi Gu
Department of Pediatric Endocrinology and Genetic Metabolism, Beijing Children's Hospital, Capital Medical University, Beijing 100045, China

Chaoxia Lu and Fang Liu
Institute of Basic Medical Sciences, Peking Union Medical College, Beijing 100730, China

Xiaojing Liu and Yingxian Zhang
Department of Endocrinology and Genetic Metabolism, Zhengzhou Children's Hospital, Zhengzhou 450053, China

Zhan Qi
Department of Pediatrics, Beijing Children's Hospital, Capital Medical University, Beijing 100045, China

Mei Feng
Department of Endocrinology, Shanxi Children's Hospital, Taiyuan 030013, China

Marcin Braun, Bartlomiej Tomasik, EwaWrona, Wojciech Fendler, Agnieszka Szadkowska, Agnieszka ZmysBowska and Wojciech Mlynarski
Department of Pediatrics, Oncology, Hematology and Diabetology, MedicalUniversity of Lodz, Sporna 36/50, 91-738 Lodz, Poland

Przemyslawa Jarosz-Chobot
Department of Pediatrics, Endocrinology and Diabetology, Medical University of Silesia, Medykow 16, 40-752 Katowice, Poland

JayneWilson
Cancer Research UK Clinical Trials Unit, School of Cancer Sciences, University of Birmingham, Vincent Drive, Edgbaston, Birmingham B15 2TT, UK

Emmanuel Mwila Musenge and AlexeyManankov
Department of Physiological Sciences, School of Medicine, University of Zambia, Ridgeway Campus, P.O. Box 50110, 10101 Lusaka, Zambia

Charles Michelo and BoydMudenda
Department of Public Health, Section for Epidemiology and Biostatistics, School of Medicine, University of Zambia, Ridgeway Campus, P.O. Box 50110, 10101 Lusaka, Zambia

Irene Ruiz-Tamayo
Primary Health Care Center La Torrassa, Consorci Sanitari Integral, Ronda Torrassa 151-153, 08903 L'Hospitalet de Llobregat, Spain
DAP-Cat Group, Unitat de Suport a la Recerca Barcelona Ciutat, Institut Universitari d'Investigació en Atenció Primária Jordi Gol (IDIAP Jordi Gol), Sardenya 375, 08006 Barcelona, Spain

Josep Franch-Nadal
DAP-Cat Group, Unitat de Suport a la Recerca Barcelona Ciutat, Institut Universitari d'Investigació en Atenció Primária Jordi Gol (IDIAP Jordi Gol), Sardenya 375, 08006 Barcelona, Spain
Primary Health Care Center Raval Sud, Gerência Ámbit d'Atenció Primária Barcelona Ciutat, Institut Català de la Salut, Avinguda Drassanes 17-21, 08001 Barcelona, Spain

ManelMata-Cases
DAP-Cat Group, Unitat de Suport a la Recerca Barcelona Ciutat, Institut Universitari d'Investigació en Atenció Primária Jordi Gol (IDIAP Jordi Gol), Sardenya 375, 08006 Barcelona, Spain
CIBER of Diabetes and Associated Metabolic Diseases (CIBERDEM), Instituto de Salud Carlos III (ISCIII), Monforte de Lemos 3-5, 28029 Madrid, Spain
Primary Health Care Center La Mina, Gerência d' Àmbit d'Atenció Primària Barcelona Ciutat, Institut Català de la Salut, Mar S/N, 08930 Sant Adrià de Besós, Spain

DídacMauricio
DAP-Cat Group, Unitat de Suport a la Recerca Barcelona Ciutat, Institut Universitari d'Investigació en Atenció Primária Jordi Gol (IDIAP Jordi Gol), Sardenya 375, 08006 Barcelona, Spain
CIBER of Diabetes and Associated Metabolic Diseases (CIBERDEM), Instituto de Salud Carlos III (ISCIII), Monforte de Lemos 3-5, 28029 Madrid, Spain
Department of Endocrinology & Nutrition, Health Sciences Research Institute and Hospital Universitari Germans Trias i Pujol, Carretera Canyet S/N, 08916 Badalona, Spain

Xavier Cos
DAP-Cat Group, Unitat de Suport a la Recerca Barcelona Ciutat, Institut Universitari d'Investigació en Atenció Primária Jordi Gol (IDIAP Jordi Gol), Sardenya 375, 08006 Barcelona, Spain
Primary Health Care Center Sant Martí de Provençals, Gerência d' Àmbit d'Atenció Primària Barcelona Ciutat, Institut Català de la Salut, Fluvià 211, 08020 Barcelona, Spain

Antonio Rodriguez-Poncelas and Gabriel Coll-de-Tuero
DAP-Cat Group, Unitat de Suport a la Recerca Barcelona Ciutat, Institut Universitari d'Investigació en Atenció Primária Jordi Gol (IDIAP Jordi Gol), Sardenya 375, 08006 Barcelona, Spain
Primary Health Care Center Anglés, Gerência d' Àmbit d'Atenció Primària Girona, Institut Catalàde la Salut, Carretera de Girona S/N, 17160 Anglés, Spain

Joan Barrot
DAP-Cat Group, Unitat de Suport a la Recerca Barcelona Ciutat, Institut Universitari d'Investigació en Atenció Primária Jordi Gol (IDIAP Jordi Gol), Sardenya 375, 08006 Barcelona, Spain
Primary Health Care Center Salt, Gerência d' Àmbit d'Atenció Primària Girona, Institut Català de la Salut, Manel de Falla 35, 17190 Salt, Spain

Xavier Mundet-Tudurí
DAP-Cat Group, Unitat de Suport a la Recerca Barcelona Ciutat, Institut Universitari d'Investigació en Atenció Primária Jordi Gol (IDIAP Jordi Gol), Sardenya 375, 08006 Barcelona, Spain
Primary Health Care Center El Carmel, Gerência d'Àmbit d'Atenció Primària Barcelona Ciutat, Institut Català de la Salut, Murtra 130, 08032 Barcelona, Spain
Autonomous University of Barcelona, Campus de Bellaterra, 08193 Bellaterra, Spain

Vendula Bartáková, Linda Klimešová, Katarína KianiIková, Veronika Dvoláková and Katelina Kaňková
Department of Pathophysiology, Medical Faculty, Masaryk University Brno, Kamenice 5, 62500 Brno, Czech Republic

Denisa Malúšková
Institute of Biostatistics and Analyses, Masaryk University Brno, Kamenice 126/3, 62500 Brno, Czech Republic

Jitka keholová and Jana Bjlobrádková
Department of Internal Medicine-Gastroenterology, University Hospital Brno, Jihlavskà 20, 62500 Brno, Czech Republic

Jan Svojanovský and Jindlich Olšovský
42nd Department of Internal Medicine, St. Anne's University Hospital, Pekařsk´a 53, 65691 Brno, Czech Republic

May Sewify, Shinu Nair, MohamedMurad, Asma Alhubail and Faisal Al-Refaei
Clinical Services Department, Dasman Diabetes Institute, P.O. Box 1180, 15462 Kuwait, Kuwait

SamiaWarsame and Ali Tiss
Biochemistry & Molecular Biology Unit, Dasman Diabetes Institute, P.O. Box 1180, 15462 Kuwait, Kuwait

Kazem Behbehani
Clinical Services Department, Dasman Diabetes Institute, P.O. Box 1180, 15462 Kuwait, Kuwait
Biochemistry & Molecular Biology Unit, Dasman Diabetes Institute, P.O. Box 1180, 15462 Kuwait, Kuwait

Kenneth N. Grisé, Matthew W. McDonald, Adwitia Dey, Mao Jiang and C.W. James Melling
Exercise Biochemistry Laboratory, School of Kinesiology, Faculty of Health Sciences, Western University, London, ON, Canada N6A 3K7

T. Dylan Olver
Neurovascular Research Laboratory, School of Kinesiology, Faculty of Health Sciences, Western University, London, ON, Canada N6A 3K7

James C. Lacefield
Department of Electrical and Computer Engineering, Department of Medical Biophysics and Robarts Research Institute, Western University, London, ON, Canada N6A 3K7

J. Kevin Shoemaker
Neurovascular Research Laboratory, School of Kinesiology, Faculty of Health Sciences, Western University, London, ON, Canada N6A 3K7
4Department of Physiology and Pharmacology, Western University, London, ON, Canada N6A 3K7
5Lawson Health Research Institute, London, ON, Canada N6C 2R5

Earl G. Noble
Exercise Biochemistry Laboratory, School of Kinesiology, Faculty of Health Sciences, Western University, London, ON, Canada N6A 3K7
Lawson Health Research Institute, London, ON, Canada N6C 2R5

Shichun Du and Qing Su
Department of Endocrinology, Xinhua Hospital Affiliated to Shanghai Jiaotong University School of Medicine, Shanghai 200092, China

Xia Yang and Degang Shi
Department of Endocrinology, Baoshan People's Hospital, Yunnan 678000, China

MelanieMay and Claudia Tonn
AOK Rheinland/Hamburg, Die Gesundheitskasse, Unternehmensbereich Ambulante Versorgung, Geschäftsbereich Selektivverträge, Kasernenstrasse 61, 40213 Düsseldorf, Germany

Sebastian Hahn
AOK Rheinland/Hamburg, Die Gesundheitskasse, Unternehmensbereich M-RSA/Finanzen/Controlling, Geschäftsbereich Controlling, Kasernenstrasse 61, 40213 Düsseldorf, Germany

Gerald Engels
Chirurgische Praxis am Bayenthalgürtel, Bayenthalgürtel 45, 50968 Köln, Germany
Ltd. Arzt Abteilung, Wundchirurgie St. Vinzenz Hospital Köln, Merheimer Strasse 221, 50733 Köln, Germany

Dirk Hochlenert
Centrum für Diabetologie, Endoskopie und Wundheilung, Merheimer Strasse 217, 50733 Köln, Germany

Heng Wan, Defu Zhao, Jie Shen, Tong Zhang and Zhi Chen
Department of Endocrinology and Metabolism, The Third Affiliated Hospital of Southern Medical University, Guangzhou 510630, China

Lu Lu
School of Traditional Chinese Medicine, Southern Medical University, Guangzhou 510515, China

www.ingramcontent.com/pod-product-compliance
Lightning Source LLC
Chambersburg PA
CBHW080459200326
41458CB00012B/4028
9781632413987